MEANING-CENTERED PSYCHOTHERAPY IN THE CANCER SETTING

MEANING-CENTERED PSYCHOTHERAPY IN THE CANCER SETTING

Finding Meaning and Hope in the Face of Suffering

EDITED BY

WILLIAM BREITBART, MD

Chairman, Department of Psychiatry and Behavioral Sciences
The Jimmie C. Holland Chair in Psychiatric Oncology
Chief, Psychiatry Service
Memorial Sloan-Kettering Cancer Center
Professor of Clinical Psychiatry
Weill Medical College of Cornell University
New York, New York

OXFORD
UNIVERSITY PRESS

OXFORD
UNIVERSITY PRESS

Oxford University Press is a department of the University of Oxford. It furthers the University's objective of excellence in research, scholarship, and education by publishing worldwide. Oxford is a registered trade mark of Oxford University Press in the UK and certain other countries.

Published in the United States of America by Oxford University Press
198 Madison Avenue, New York, NY 10016, United States of America.

Library of Congress Cataloging-in-Publication Data
Names: Breitbart, William, 1951– editor.
Title: Meaning-centered psychotherapy in the cancer setting : finding meaning and hope in the face of suffering / edited by William Breitbart.
Description: Oxford ; New York : Oxford University Press, [2017] | Includes bibliographical references and index.
Identifiers: LCCN 2016045419 (print) | LCCN 2016046124 (ebook) | ISBN 9780199837229 (alk. paper) |
ISBN 9780199837236 (ebook) | ISBN 9780190462789 (ebook) | ISBN 9780199390748 (online)
Subjects: | MESH: Neoplasms—psychology | Psychotherapy—methods | Quality of Life | Hope |
Stress, Psychological—therapy | Culturally Competent Care
Classification: LCC RC271.M4 (print) | LCC RC271.M4 (ebook) | NLM QZ 200 | DDC 616.99/40651—dc23
LC record available at https://lccn.loc.gov/2016045419

9 8 7 6 5 4 3 2 1

Printed by Sheridan Books, Inc., United States of America

For my parents, Rose and Moses Breitbart, who gave me life and the courage to live.

For my wife, Rachel Breitbart, and our son, Samuel Benjamin Breitbart, who gave me love and the courage to love.

In memory of my nephew, Ross Evan Breitbart, who had the courage to live and the courage to love, and gave me the courage to face what lies beyond.

In memory of Lillian Epstein, who gave life to my beloved wife Rachel and gave me the gift of understanding the beauty of generosity.

In memory of my niece, Renata Horowitz, who taught me that life is meant to be lived fully every moment of every day.

Sweet Ross, Lillian, Renata, you are all remembered.

CONTENTS

FOREWORD

MEANING THROUGH TIME AND GENERATIONS

We have struggled in our fields of psycho-oncology and palliative care to find a therapeutic approach that helps patients with cancer address their existential concerns of an uncertain future. I recall clearly several years ago when Bill said, "I have been reading *Man's Search for Meaning* by Viktor Frankl and I think his ideas would be very helpful in talking with patients with advanced cancer." Frankl was an academic psychiatrist in Vienna until World War II, when he was forced from his work, home, and family and lived as an inmate for 3 years in Auschwitz, Dachau, and other concentration camps. His book recounts his rich insights into how he and his colleagues coped with unbelievable brutality there. He held tenaciously to his belief that the one thing they could not take away was the meaning that he gave to his own life. When he was released, he wrote about his observations from the camps and also described a new psychotherapy, called logotherapy, which incorporated his existential view—that people's basic need is for meaning in their life no matter how short or how long. Bill has devoted the past 10 years to using Frankl's concepts to develop a model applicable for cancer patients, called meaning-centered psychotherapy. At last, there is a validated therapeutic approach based on helping patients find meaning in their lives.

It has been a pleasure to watch the development and dissemination of meaning-centered psychotherapy. Bill has engaged others in the work to extend the concepts and apply them first, specifically to patients with cancer, but over time the group has found the approach valuable with caregivers, with grieving people, and with any group for whom life is precarious and existential issues are of concern.

I am said to be the "mother of psycho-oncology," and it is with great pride that I look on the many contributions that have carried the field forward. I also am pleased to be "mother" of our Department of Psychiatry and Behavioral Sciences at Memorial Sloan Kettering Cancer Center. The department has spawned some remarkable psycho-oncologists over the years since 1977. Bill and colleagues stand out because they have given us a tool with which to approach the weighty conversations we have with patients around these issues. Bill represents the second generation of psycho-oncologists from Memorial, similar to his being second generation to his parents who experienced the Holocaust. I am sure that this work has special meaning for him from his personal existential perspective as well as professional. I am honored to be part of the "family" and to write this foreword for such an important book for our field.

Jimmie Holland, MD
Wayne E. Chapman Chair in Psychiatric Oncology
Attending Psychiatrist
Department of Psychiatry and Behavioral Sciences
Memorial Sloan Kettering Cancer Center
New York, New York
April, 2016

ACKNOWLEDGMENTS

I am indebted to my family for its love and support, and I remember those precious to me, both family and patients, who have died during the period of time we conducted the work on meaning-centered psychotherapy (MCP) reflected in this text.

I am indebted to all of my colleagues at Memorial Sloan Kettering who played central roles in the development and conduct of the four randomized controlled trials of both MCP formats. Special thanks to Mindy Greenstein, Shannon Poppito, Hayley Pessin, Barry Rosenfeld, Wendy Lichtenthal, Allison Applebaum, and the many research collaborators, research assistants, interventionists, pre- and postdoctoral fellows, and research managers and coordinators.

I am immensely grateful to all of my colleagues and collaborators and friends who contributed outstanding chapters describing not only individual and group MCP for advanced cancer patients but also the growing number of MCP adaptations for various cancer populations and for novel purposes. I am especially grateful to my international colleagues for contributing their work in MCP to this text. A special note of thanks to my editors at Oxford University Press, Andrea Knobloch and Rebecca Suzan.

My thanks to the National Institutes of Health, the National Cancer Institute, the National Center for Complementary and Alternative Medicine, the American Cancer Society, the Fetzer Institute, and the Kohlberg Foundation, which provided funding for MCP clinical trials research at Memorial Sloan Kettering Cancer Center.

Finally, my gratitude is extended to the many hundreds of patients who participated in the clinical trials of MCP and their devoted families and caregivers. Although many of the patients who participated in the clinical trials of MCP at Memorial Sloan Kettering Cancer Center are no longer with us, their legacies are alive and affect the course and meaning of the lives they touched in profound ways. I carry their wisdom in my heart—a heart now more fully open to the love and suffering in the world and the search for meaning and peace.

William Breitbart, MD
Chairman, Department of Psychiatry and Behavioral Sciences
The Jimmie C. Holland Chair in Psychiatric Oncology
Chief, Psychiatry Service
Memorial Sloan Kettering Cancer Center
New York, New York
Professor of Clinical Psychiatry
Weill Medical College of Cornell University
New York, New York

CONTRIBUTORS

Allison J. Applebaum, PhD
Assistant Attending Psychologist
Department of Psychiatry and Behavioral Sciences
Memorial Sloan Kettering Cancer Center
New York, New York

William Breitbart, MD
Chairman
Department of Psychiatry and Behavioral Sciences
The Jimmie C. Holland Chair in Psychiatric Oncology
Chief
Psychiatry Service
Memorial Sloan Kettering Cancer Center
New York, New York
Professor of Clinical Psychiatry
Weill Medical College of Cornell University
New York, New York

Angela Chen
Immigrant Health and Cancer Disparities Service
Department of Psychiatry and Behavioral Sciences
Memorial Sloan Kettering Cancer Center
New York, New York

Rosario Costas-Muñiz, PhD
Assistant Attending Psychologist
Department of Psychiatry and Behavioral Sciences
Immigrant Health and Cancer Disparities Service
Memorial Sloan Kettering Cancer Center
New York, New York

Caraline Craig, MPH
Department of Psychiatry and Behavioral Sciences
Memorial Sloan Kettering Cancer Center
New York, New York

Gali Elinger, MA
Department of Psychology
Bar-Ilan University
Ramat Gan, Israel
Department of Psycho-Oncology
Institute of Oncology
Assuta Medical Center
Tel Aviv, Israel

Natalie Fenn, BA
Department of Psychiatry and Behavioral Sciences
Memorial Sloan Kettering Cancer Center
New York, New York

Lise Fillion, PhD, RN
Professor of Nursing
Laval University
CHU de Québec
Quebec City, Quebec, Canada

Jennifer S. Ford, PhD
Associate Attending
Department of Psychiatry and Behavioral Sciences
Department of Pediatrics
Memorial Sloan Kettering Cancer Center
New York, New York

Clara Fraguell, MA
Psychologist
Mutuam-EAPS Barcelona Stress and Health Research Group
Faculty of Psychology
Universitat Autònoma de Barcelona
Barcelona, Spain

Pierre Gagnon, MD, FRCPC
Professor of Pharmacy
Laval University
CHU de Québec and Maison Michel-Sarrazin
Quebec City, Quebec, Canada

Francesca Gany, MD, MS
Chief, Immigrant Health and Cancer Disparities Service
Memorial Sloan Kettering Cancer Center
New York, New York
Department of Healthcare Policy and Research
Weill Cornell Medical College
New York, New York

Olga Garduño-Ortega, BA
Immigrant Health and Cancer Disparities Service
Department of Psychiatry and Behavioral Sciences
Memorial Sloan Kettering Cancer Center
New York, New York

Francisco Gil, PhD
Director, Psycho-Oncology Department
Institut Català d'Oncologia
Clinical Psychologist
Associate Professor of Psychology
Stress and Health Research Group
Faculty of Psychology
Universitat Autònoma de Barcelona
Barcelona, Spain

Gil Goldzweig, PhD
Associate Professor
Dean, School of Behavioral Sciences
The Academic College of Tel-Aviv
Yaffo, Israel

Carlos Javier González, MA
Linguistics/Cultural Responsiveness Program Manager
Immigrant Health and Cancer Disparities Service
Department of Psychiatry and Behavioral Sciences
Memorial Sloan Kettering Cancer Center
New York, New York

Ilanit Hasson-Ohayon, PhD
Associate Professor
Bar-Ilan University
Ramat Gan, Israel

Xiaoxiao Huang, MA
Immigrant Health and Cancer Disparities Service
Department of Psychiatry and Behavioral Sciences
Memorial Sloan Kettering Cancer Center
New York, New York

Greta Jankauskaite, BA
Department of Psychiatry and Behavioral Sciences
Memorial Sloan Kettering Cancer Center
New York, New York

Julia A. Kearney, MD
Assistant Professor
Department of Psychiatry and Behavioral Sciences
Department of Pediatrics
Memorial Sloan Kettering Cancer Center
New York, New York

Anat Laronne, MA
Department of Psycho-Oncology
Institute of Oncology
Assuta Medical Center
Tel Aviv, Israel

Jennifer Leng, MD, MPH
Immigrant Health and Cancer Disparities Service
Department of Psychiatry and Behavioral Sciences
Memorial Sloan Kettering Cancer Center
New York, New York
Department of Healthcare Policy and Research
Weill Cornell Medical College
New York, New York

Wendy G. Lichtenthal, PhD
Assistant Attending Psychologist
Department of Psychiatry and Behavioral Sciences
Memorial Sloan Kettering Cancer Center
New York, New York

Joaquín T. Limonero, PhD
Health Psychologist
Lecturer (Acreditated Professor of Psychology), Stress and Health Research Group
Faculty of Psychology
Universidad Autónoma de Barcelona
Barcelona, Spain

Florence Lui
Department of Clinical Psychology
The City College of New York
New York, New York
Immigrant Health and Cancer Disparities Service
Memorial Sloan Kettering Cancer Center
New York, New York

Melissa Masterson, MA
Fordham University
Department of Psychology
Bronx, New York

Stephanie Napolitano, MA
Department of Psychiatry and Behavioral Sciences
Memorial Sloan Kettering Cancer Center
New York, New York

Hayley Pessin, PhD
Department of Psychiatry and Behavioral Sciences
Memorial Sloan Kettering Cancer Center
New York, New York

Noam Pizem, MA
Division of Oncology
Chaim Sheba Medical Center
Tel Hashomer
Ramat Gan, Israel

Kailey E. Roberts, MA
Department of Psychiatry and Behavioral Sciences
Memorial Sloan Kettering Cancer Center
New York, New York

Xiomara Rocha-Cadman, MD
Assistant Attending Psychiatrist
Department of Psychiatry and Behavioral Sciences
Memorial Sloan Kettering Cancer Center
New York, New York

Barry Rosenfeld, PhD
Professor of Psychology
Fordham University
New York, New York

Katherine Sharpe, MTS
Senior Vice President, Patient and Caregiver Support
American Cancer Society
Atlanta, Georgia

Elizabeth Slivjak, BA
Department of Psychiatry and Behavioral Sciences
Memorial Sloan Kettering Cancer Center
New York, New York

Corinne Sweeney, PhD
Department of Psychiatry and Behavioral Sciences
Memorial Sloan Kettering Cancer Center
New York, New York

Mélanie Vachon, PhD
Department of Psychology
Université du Québec à Montréal
Montréal, Quebec, Canada

Nadia van der Spek, PhD
Department of Clinical Psychology
IDC Center for Psycho-Oncology OLVG Hospital
Vrije Universiteit Amsterdam
Amsterdam, the Netherlands

Irma Verdonck-de Leeuw, PhD
Professor of Clinical Psychology
Vrije Universiteit Amsterdam
Department of Otolaryngology—Head and Neck Surgery
VU University Medical Center
Amsterdam, the Netherlands

Reut Wertheim, MA
Department of Psychology
Bar-Ilan University
Ramat Gan, Israel

Dawn Wiatrek, PhD
Strategic Director, Cancer Treatment Access
American Cancer Society
Atlanta, Georgia

INTRODUCTION

FINDING MEANING IN THE FACE OF SUFFERING: A PERSONAL JOURNEY OF MEANING

This textbook, *Meaning-Centered Psychotherapy in the Cancer Setting*, which I am proud to edit and have published by Oxford University Press, is a culmination of more than a decade and a half of work conducted by the Psychotherapy Laboratory within the Department of Psychiatry and Behavioral Sciences at Memorial Sloan Kettering Cancer Center. I am the founding Director of the Psychotherapy Laboratory, and our group of laboratory faculty members, research personnel, and collaborators has produced a body of research on issues related to what I refer to as "meta-diagnostic constructs"—existential issues leading to despair, suffering, hopelessness, and loss of spiritual well-being and meaning that often leads to desire for hastened death, poor quality of life, and poor psychosocial outcomes.[1–19] This body of work has led to a focus on the importance of "meaning" and the psychosocial and quality of life benefits of sustaining and enhancing meaning in advanced cancer patients.

The recent publication of several randomized controlled trials of meaning-centered group psychotherapy (MCGP) and individual meaning-centered psychotherapy (IMCP),[19–21] as well as the publication of two treatment manuals—*Meaning-Centered Group Psychotherapy for Patients with Advanced Cancer*[22] and *Individual Meaning-Centered Psychotherapy for Patients with Advanced Cancer*[23]—represent the culmination of many years of effort to develop an effective meaning-centered psychotherapy intervention for cancer patients—a research effort that was born out of clinical experience with thousands of advanced cancer patients who taught me and my research team the importance of sustaining meaning in order to still have the courage and will to live life, even in the face of death. These patients taught me that experiencing meaningful moments could be accompanied by the emotion of joy, which made it possible to better tolerate suffering and uncertainty. The randomized controlled trials of MCP in fact demonstrate that by enhancing meaning, patients with advanced cancer have significantly improved quality of life and spiritual well-being and significantly less anxiety, depression, hopelessness, desire for hastened death, and symptom burden distress—all mediated through enhanced meaning. We have in fact demonstrated the power of meaning in the amelioration of suffering and despair.

A famous Talmudic question asks, "What is truer than the truth?" The answer: "The story." What follows is the "story" of meaning-centered psychotherapy for cancer patients. Like many stories, it involves multiple characters as well as twists and turns in the narrative; and like all stories, it has its origins in an important legacy that has been given, and represents what these characters have created with this given legacy.

Perhaps the most important source of legacy given in the story of meaning-centered psychotherapy is the inspiration of the work of Viktor Frankl.[24,25] Meaning-centered psychotherapy was inspired, to a great degree, by the works of Frankl and his elucidation of the importance of meaning in human behavior and existence. It is the conviction that there is always the possibility for meaning, the experience of meaning, the creation or search for meaning, even in the setting of advanced cancer and the limitations of time in the face of death that is the essence of meaning-centered psychotherapy for advanced cancer patients.

Frankl's seminal work, *Man's Search for Meaning*,[24] reminds us that finding meaning in our existence is a defining characteristic of human beings. Meaning cannot be given by one human being to another; rather, each of us must go through the process of searching for the meaning in our lives. Before describing meaning-centered psychotherapy in terms of its scientific rationale, structure, and practice, I want to start with the "truth"; the story; my story, which is one of "a personal journey in search of meaning: from the camp to the cancer center."

I am a child of Holocaust survivors. This is an identity that has defined me because of the profound legacy and source of meaning it has imparted to me. It is what Life has given me, and I have made the choice to respond to this legacy of death, and loss, and perceived meaninglessness by using it as a source for compassion to ease those in despair with advanced cancer and help them reclaim a life of meaning in the face of loss, suffering, and limitations.

I am a physician. I am trained and certified in both internal medicine and general psychiatry. I am also trained and certified in the subspecialty of psychiatry called psychosomatic medicine, specifically the field of psycho-oncology. Psycho-oncology is a new field, developed primarily during the past 35 years, which focuses on the psychosocial care of cancer patients and their families.

I am a physician, and my mission is to care for cancer patients and their families. I began my training in psycho-oncology in 1984 as a clinical fellow in psycho-oncology at Memorial Sloan Kettering Cancer Center in New York City, working closely with my mentor, Dr. Jimmie Holland. I made Dr. Holland's mission, to create the field of psycho-oncology in order to provide comprehensive psychosocial care to cancer patients throughout the world, my mission as well. I have worked toward this goal, for almost 32 years, as a clinician, researcher, educator, administrator, writer, lecturer, and advocate.

I am a psychiatrist/psycho-oncologist who was searching to find a way to ameliorate the despair of patients with advanced cancer who saw no meaning, value, or purpose in living in the face of the limitations of approaching death. In my search, I found that the belief in the possibility of experiencing or creating meaning, even in the last months or days of life, sustained hope and diminished despair and suffering. This is the story of my personal journey in search of meaning, and the development of an approach to care for advanced cancer patients I came to call "meaning-centered psychotherapy."

THE LEGACY OF THE HOLOCAUST

My parents, Rose and Moses Breitbart, were Holocaust survivors. After disrupting their lives at ages 14 and 17, respectively, my parents survived the Holocaust by hiding, fighting as partisans in the forests of Poland, and finally in a displaced persons camp outside of Munich called Fahrenvald. They married there in 1949, and they spent their wedding night in a borrowed "wedding bed." Arriving on the Lower East Side of Manhattan, New York City, they had nothing of their own but the will to live and the courage to love; and with that will to live and courage to love they created a life of meaning in a meaningless world. They had the fight. They had the insight.

I was the first born of two sons. The legacy of the Holocaust remained alive and lived with us in our two-bedroom apartment on Grand Street. The Holocaust did not have its own room; it lived in every room, and on the walls, and in the drawers, in pictures, in documents in files, and in prayer books and tefilin saved from the flames of war.

"Why am I here?" My mother asked this question of herself every morning of my life and urged me to ask the same question of myself every day. "Why am I here? And so many others are not!" This in fact is the more complete question my mother asked. Both my parents lost so much—parents, siblings, cousins, aunts, uncles, schoolmates, friends.

I grew up with a legacy of loss and suffering, but in a home filled with love, compassion, and the need to find meaning and purpose and significance. I accepted the responsibility and the burden of living not only my life but also the lives of those who did not survive.

I commit a great deal of time and energy to this mission, sometimes working 80 hours a week and spending many evenings and weekends in the hospital or traveling to lecture or participate in scientific meetings. It did not come as a surprise to me when my wife of 30years recently expressed that she and my 25-year-old son occasionally "feel lonely" and miss my presence at home. I am blessed to have an understanding and loving family.

I am a psychiatrist whose mission is to care for cancer patients and their families, too often at the expense of caring for my own family. So it is no surprise that when I received a telephone call several years ago, on a Saturday morning of a weekend when I was not scheduled for hospital coverage or supervision of trainees, I immediately went into the hospital to help a patient in distress. I did not know that I was about to have a "transformative" experience.

THE CASE OF TRANSFORMATION

The call was not from a doctor or nurse at the hospital but, rather, from one of my neighbors on the Upper East Side of Manhattan. Her best friend was a patient in the hospital at Memorial Sloan Kettering Cancer Center and was in extreme emotional distress. She did not call to ask me to see her friend in the hospital but, rather, to ask me how she could best comfort her friend and how to help her in her current state of despair, grappling with a profound sense of loss of hope and meaning. After eliciting details of her friend's dilemma, I quickly volunteered to go in to see her friend myself—not only as an act of compassion but also out of a sense of responsibility in my role as Chief of the Psychiatry Service at the hospital.

This is a brief summary of the details of the case prior to my meeting the patient:

> She is the 47-year-old mother of 2 children, ages 8 and 11. She has spent the last 20 years of her life working to become the successful head of a legal firm in New York City. She is a woman of accomplishment, achievement, and will. She is a woman who is beloved and loves well. When she learned of a diagnosis of cancer, she quickly used her powerful connections to receive her cancer treatment at Memorial Sloan Kettering Cancer Center in New York, from the "best" oncologists and surgeons in the country. Initially, the most remarkable part of her cancer experience was that she was misdiagnosed. She was thought to have ovarian cancer, and, despite the shock and fear, had adapted to the news and held on to the hope of a possibly favorable outcome. But the diagnosis was wrong, and the prognosis was suddenly dramatically changed, for the worse. Intraoperatively it became clear that this was not ovarian cancer, but in fact a rare presentation of metastatic colon cancer (Meig's syndrome) that had spread to the ovaries and the lower pelvis. Now her prognosis was dire. The shift in expectations was dramatic; different treatment, different course trajectory, different time expectations in terms of survival. From potential cure or long-term survival, to preparing for death. The fear of death overwhelmed her. The profound sadness of a life cut short, of children not fully raised, of the loss of all those she loved and the life she was so fully living. She was in great despair and suffering terribly. She needed someone to give her guidance and comfort.

THE JOURNEY LEADING TO THIS PATIENT'S BEDSIDE

I was called to see her by her dearest friend, who perceived the great need to help ameliorate the fear of death in her friend but felt she had no idea how to help; what words to use to comfort, what path of guidance to provide. "How do I help my friend overcome her fear of death? How do I help her maintain a sense of meaning and hope in the face of death?" were the questions posed to me. These were familiar questions—ones I had contemplated and grappled with through my clinical and research career for more than two decades. As I made my way to the hospital, in anticipation of my encounter with this patient, I had a relatively clear sense of what I felt would be helpful in our encounter. My sense of clarity, about what constituted an effective approach to patients with advanced cancer who were in despair and turmoil in the face of death, came from thousands of clinical experiences with dying patients; a series of clinical research studies my group had conducted during the past decade on despair and desire for death near the end of life; an awakening to the importance of existential psychotherapy and our group's experience in conducting intervention trials of a novel psychotherapy I had developed that we called meaning-centered psychotherapy; and my rediscovery of existential philosophy (particularly the works of Frankl), the importance of lessons provided by my personal Holocaust legacy, and the ancient and sacred texts of my heritage. As I made my journey to this patient's bedside, I recalled the journey I had made during the past decades that led me to the sense that I was the right person for this patient to see today, and that my ideas about a psychotherapeutic approach to the problem of living life with meaning, in the face of death, could be potentially helpful to her and patients like her.

THE IMPORTANCE OF MEANING IN END-OF-LIFE CARE

My research group has conducted a series of studies examining the importance of meaning and spiritual well-being in end-of-life care.[4-10] We demonstrated a central role for spiritual well-being, and, in particular, meaning, as a buffering agent, protecting against depression, hopelessness, and desire for hastened death among terminally ill cancer patients. We also found that spiritual well-being was significantly associated with end-of-life despair (as defined by hopelessness, desire for hastened death, and suicidal ideation), even after controlling for the influence of depression. Moreover, when spiritual well-being was divided into two components, one measuring a sense of meaning and another measuring spirituality linked to religious faith, the inability to maintain a sense of meaning was much more strongly associated with end-of-life despair than was the faith component of spiritual well-being (i.e., the ability to sustain a sense of meaning was associated with lower levels of hopelessness, desire for hastened death, and suicidal ideation). These findings are significant in the face of what we have come to learn about the consequences of depression and hopelessness in cancer patients. Depression and hopelessness are associated with dramatically higher rates of suicide, suicidal ideation, and desire for hastened death and interest in physician-assisted suicide.[1-3] Our findings[3] demonstrate that hopelessness is an independent and synergistic predictor of desire for death that is as powerful an influence on desire for death as (and independent of) depression. Such data (demonstrating that loss of meaning and hopelessness, independent of depression, lead to despair at the end of life) strongly suggested to us that nonpharmacologic, psychotherapeutic interventions must be developed to help patients with loss of meaning and hopelessness at the end of life. We set out to develop such a set of interventions using Frankl's concepts of the importance of meaning in human existence.

MEANING-CENTERED PSYCHOTHERAPY FOR ADVANCED CANCER PATIENTS

The importance of spiritual well-being and the role of "meaning" in particular in moderating depression, hopelessness, and desire for death in terminally ill cancer and AIDS patients demonstrated by our research group led us to look beyond the role of antidepressant treatment for depression in this population and to focus new efforts on developing nonpharmacologic (psychotherapy) interventions that can address such issues as hopelessness, loss of meaning, and spiritual well-being in patients with advanced cancer at the end of life. In fact, two studies of pharmacologic treatment of depression in advanced cancer and AIDS patients demonstrated that if depression is effectively treated, desire for hastened death remits; however, a significant proportion of patients with desire for hastened death were not clinically depressed but had loss of meaning and hopelessness independent of depression.[11-13] Thus, clearly a nonpharmacologic approach to enhance meaning and hope was needed. This effort led to an exploration and analysis of the work of Frankl and his concepts of logotherapy or meaning-based psychotherapy.[24,25] Although Frankl's logotherapy was not designed for the treatment of cancer patients or those with life-threatening illness, his concepts of meaning and spirituality clearly, in our view, had applications in psychotherapeutic work with advanced cancer patients, many of whom seek guidance and help in dealing with issues of sustaining meaning, hope, and understanding cancer and impending death in the context of their lives. Frankl's main contributions to human psychology have been to raise awareness of the spiritual component of human experience and the central importance of meaning (or the will to meaning) as a driving force or instinct in human psychology. Frankl's basic concepts include the following:

1. Meaning of life: Life has meaning and never ceases to have meaning even up to the last moment of life; meaning may change in this context, but it never ceases to exist.
2. Will to meaning: The desire to find meaning in human existence is a primary instinct and basic motivation for human behavior.
3. Freedom of will: We have the freedom to find meaning in existence and to choose the attitude toward suffering.
4. The three main sources of meaning in life are derived from creativity (work, deeds, and dedication to causes), experience (art, nature, humor, love, relationships, and roles), and attitude—the attitude one takes toward suffering and existential problems.
5. Meaning exists in a historical context; thus, legacy (past, present, and future) is a critical element in sustaining or enhancing meaning.

The novel intervention we developed and call "meaning-centered psychotherapy" is based on the concepts described previously and the principles of Frankl's logotherapy. It is designed to help patients with advanced cancer sustain or enhance a sense of meaning, peace, and purpose in their lives even as they approach the end of life. We initially conducted a pilot randomized trial of an 8-week (1½-hour weekly sessions) meaning-centered *group* psychotherapy (MCGP) intervention, based on the concepts of meaning as elucidated by Frankl, that utilized a highly developed treatment manual incorporating a mixture of didactics, discussion, and experiential exercises that focus around particular themes related to meaning and advanced cancer. Our findings[19] suggested that MCGP is a highly effective intervention, increasing a sense of meaning, spiritual well-being, and hope while decreasing end-of-life despair. Subsequent randomized controlled trials of MCGP and a more flexible individual format of MCP (IMCP) in fact demonstrate that by enhancing meaning, patients with advanced cancer have significantly improved quality of life and spiritual well-being and significantly less anxiety, depression, hopelessness, desire for hastened death, and symptom burden distress—all mediated through enhanced meaning.[19–21]

BEYOND MEANING: INTEGRATING CONCEPTS OF WILL, MEANING, AND CARE

I had gained a great deal of therapeutic insights into the care of the cancer patient facing death through my work in developing and conducting clinical trials with a manualized, structured, meaning-centered psychotherapy intervention. However, a persistent sense remained with me that there was much more to be learned and further insights needed in order to be able to more effectively work with patients facing death. There was much more for me to learn and more transformation required in me and my approach to patients. I began to turn my attention to the works of the existential philosophers, and to several sacred texts, to take me further on this journey.

Those of us who work in palliative medicine ignore the lessons of the great books and sacred texts of our civilizations at our own peril. Wisdom lies in works as disparate as Leo Tolstoy's *The Death of Ivan Illyich*, the Book of Job, or Martin Heidegger's *Being and Time*. It is becoming a more common practice in palliative care and psycho-oncology training programs for trainees to be exposed to the humanities in an effort to learn about the care of "humans." Reading and discussing *The Death of Ivan Illyich* is now quite a popular means of teaching our younger colleagues about the process of dying and the potential for redemption and growth even in the last moments before death. The Book of Job, however, has eluded many of us in palliative care as a source of lessons that can be applied to clinical intervention in palliative medicine. I suspect there are multiple reasons: (1) The Book of Job is seen as a purely religious text with few secular applications; (2) the lessons of the Book of Job are perhaps arcane, unclear, and subject to extensive and divergent interpretations; and (3) although not the final reason, I suspect that too many of us have not really bothered to actually read the Book of Job and only know what we hear from others of the lessons that may lie within. The truth is that during the past 23 years, I have been working in the care of the dying, referred to Job hundreds if not thousands of times in the context of discussing suffering, and yet I had never really taken the time to read the text myself—completely and with an open mind.

Reading the Book of Job turns out to not be an easy task. There are many versions, of varying lengths and with differing story lines. There is also no paucity of controversy as to which is the accurate version. In addition, there is no dearth of commentary on the interpretations of the lessons of this epic poem. Great thinkers ranging from Spinoza to Carl Jung have responded to Job's story with great thought, insight, and differing conclusions as to what it reveals about the relationship between man and God. Most of the debates have focused on the questions of Theodicy (Can God and evil coexist?) and whether God is a "personal" God, involved in the affairs of human beings, punishing those who sin, rewarding those who are deserving, and responding to prayer, or whether God is a "natural" God who is unknowable, mysterious—one whose actions cannot be understood by human beings. These are primarily religious questions about the nature of God, yet they are questions that arise in the palliative care setting quite frequently. "Why did this happen to me?" "What did I do to deserve this?" These are questions we are asked frequently as palliative care clinicians. Although these are often religious questions that relate to an individual's relationship to God, they are also in essence universal existential concerns that are being expressed. Patients often turn to us a clinicians for comfort, solace, and even answers.

I recently set out to read the Book of Job. I chose to read the Book of Job translated and with an introduction by Stephen Mitchell,[26] who is a Brooklyn-born poet and translator of sacred texts whose work I was familiar with and had enjoyed reading in the past. I have particularly enjoyed his translations of the poetry of Rainer Maria Rilke and his translation of the Psalms. Mitchell does not merely provide a modern accessible translation but also gives historical context and references that enrich the experience of the reading. This was definitely the case in my reading of his translation of the Book of Job. For example, I learned that we do not really know who is the author of the Book of Job. There is little evidence as to who the author is, when and where he or she wrote it, or for what kind of audience. One of the greatest paradoxes of this greatest Jewish work of art is that the hero is a gentile, as might have been the author. Some authorities estimate that this dramatic epic poem, which treats the problem of the suffering of the innocent, and of retribution, was written between the seventh and fifth century BC. Despite the uncertainty as to the Jewish origins of the author or hero of this poem, the theme of Job is the great Jewish theme of the post-Holocaust age—the theme of the innocent victim. As a child of Holocaust survivors, I was of course drawn to some of these elements.

Indeed, there are a myriad of existential and spiritual themes that one can become immersed in when reading the Book of Job. I focused on two themes really, because of their relevance to my work as a clinician who cares for those who suffer during the dying process. First, I was struck by the relevance of Job's experience of suffering to the experience of so many of the patients we care for. When Job is afflicted with disease of his flesh and bones, the description of his experience reminded me of the experience of a patient with leukemia whom I had cared for. After undergoing a bone marrow transplant, this patient was suffering from severe graft-versus-host disease. Job felt his bone marrow swell in pain, his skin was cracked and oozing, and he cried out in despair, even begging for death to end his suffering. "This is exactly what I experienced, I was praying to die so that my suffering could end," my patient recounted as we discussed Job's experience. I was impressed by the accuracy of the description of suffering. Second, I was struck by the repeated themes of being "upright" and "whole." I recognized these themes as being useful clinical and psychotherapeutic concepts in the care of those who are suffering in the face of death.

We first encounter the terms "upright" and "whole" in the prologue of the poem, in which God says to the Accuser (Satan), "Did you notice my servant Job? There is no one on earth like him: an *upright* and *whole* man, who fears God and avoids evil." These terms are likely used here to describe Job as a man who shuns evil, a man of integrity and goodness, and a pious man who fears God. As the story of Job progresses, the concepts of being "upright" and "whole" return repeatedly, with an even richer, more powerful meaning and wisdom attached to them.

Our next encounter with the concepts of "upright" and "whole" occurs quickly after Job is told that all of his material wealth has been lost and that all of his sons and daughters have been killed. Job stands up. He tears his robe. He shaves his head. He lays down with his face in the dust, pouring earth on his head. He then says, "Naked I came from my mother's womb, and naked I will return there. The Lord gave, and the Lord has taken; may the name of the Lord be blessed." Now some may focus on Job's acceptance of God's will; I, however, was struck by Job's initial acts of (1) falling to the ground from an "upright," standing position and literally humbling himself in the dust from which he was formed (the humus of humanity); and (2) tearing his clothes, symbolically representing the disintegration or rupture of the "whole" that was his identity prior to losing all that gave his life meaning. Now Job's actions might also strike some as being similar to the Jewish act of "Teshuvah" or repentance for a sin committed against God. It is interesting to note that the term *Teshuvah* also means "to return," implying that Job's actions are intended to lead God to restore him to a state of being "upright" and "whole" through repentance. In fact, at the end of the Book of Job, God does restore all of Job's wealth, provides an even greater number of children and grandchildren, and fully restores Job's identity and his relationship to the transcendent. Job is restored to a state of being "upright" and "whole."

I became interested in how these concepts of being "upright" and "whole" might be of benefit in my clinical work with dying patients. I have conceptualized being "upright" as a manifestation of *will*. When one is "upright," one is capable of exerting his or her will in the world. Exerting one's will, or free will, in the case of a terminally ill patient may take the form of having the "courage to continue to live in the face of death"; to have the courage to still have wishes, wants, and desires in life, despite the finiteness of life; and to reassess priorities in the face of a limited prognosis and decide to focus on those priorities (e.g., spending time with family, deciding to not take palliative chemotherapy and focusing on pain and symptom control, creating a generativity document, or continuing to work as long as possible). When patients are forced to lay in bed with fatigue or uncontrolled pain (not upright, but literally on their backs) and robbed of their ability to enact their will, they clearly suffer. The concept of remaining "upright" for as long as possible in the face of the dying process is, in my opinion, a useful construct to utilize in terms of treatment planning and goals of care.

I have begun to conceptualize the concept of being "whole" as the ability of a patient facing a life-threatening illness "to remain connected to all that gives *meaning*, value, and purpose" to one's life, even during the dying process—to remain connected to loved ones and to resist the "isolation" that comes from couples "protecting" each other from their fears and concerns but, rather, to "relate" to each other by sharing these fears and concerns and to be closer and more connected at a time when such connectedness is so very vital. Being "whole" represents an effort to "preserve one's identity" for as long as possible, despite the real or threatened losses and ravages of progressive disease.

Recently, in working with an older man who was struggling with advanced myeloma, we discussed these concepts of facing the dying process "upright" and whole" in our psychotherapy. These concepts were quite attractive to him, and I sensed they resonated strongly with his wishes for how he could find a "way to live while he was dying." "upright" and "whole" as guides for how to live in the face of death seemed to be helpful concepts, but I felt something was missing. If I used the metaphor of "upright" and "whole" as two legs of a stool, the stool seemed a bit unstable, unfinished. One more basic principle, one more leg of the stool (a three-legged stool), seemed necessary to make it stable, complete, and truly useful. That is when I discovered "care."

BEING CAREFUL

Martin Heidegger was an influential, and somewhat controversial, German existential philosopher whose best known work is *Being and Time*.[27] Heidegger elaborated our further understanding of the nature (or experience) of "being," the "intentionality of being" (consciousness is "about" something), the temporality of our existence, and such important existential concepts as "responsibility" and "angst." Heidegger also describes what he refers to as a "care structure" of "being" (Dasein), and "being in the world" is essentially "care." Admittedly, Heidegger's concepts of "care" and a "care structure" are complex, but I began to understand this concept of "care" as twofold. On the one hand, "care" refers to our being engaged in the world as a willful agent, with people, causes, and ideas that we deeply care about. On the other hand, "care" refers to "self-care" or caring for one's self. Self-care is the realization that one must preserve one's self (through taking care of one's self) in order to be able to care for others and the world. In our meaning-centered group psychotherapy, we conduct an experiential exercise in one of our session on "responsibility." Members of the group are asked to respond to the stimulus question, "Who and what are you responsible to or for?" In co-facilitating these sessions, I have been consistently surprised by the responses of the terminal cancer patients in these groups. Almost universally, cancer patients respond, "First, I am responsible for myself. If I do not care for myself, I cannot be responsible for anyone or anything else." I am surprised by this response because my list of answers never included "taking care of myself." It was not selfishness, I soon learned, but rather an important lesson of life that those of us in good health often ignore but that life-threatening illnesses, such as cancer, remind us in profound ways.

As I traveled to the hospital to meet the patient in despair, I thought of these concepts of being "upright" and "whole"—but how to incorporate this third notion of "care" (including the importance of caring for one's self)? The words came to me as an epiphany. "Careful." "Full of care." "Carefully." I smiled to myself at the prospect of being able to give the following answer to a very profound question: "Doctor, how can I manage to live in the face of death?" The answer: "Very carefully." As the taxi pulled up to the main entrance of the hospital, I felt that perhaps I had finally constructed that stable, three-legged stool: "Upright, whole, and careful." Did I have an answer to the question, "How do I live in the face of death?" I was about to find out if this approach (Box I) would open a path out of despair for the patient who waited for me on the 10th floor of the hospital.

BOX I HOW TO LIVE (BE) IN THE FACE OF DEATH

- *Upright*: Realization that one is still alive and standing, not lying beneath the ground; continuing to have wants and wishes, to exert one's will, to have courage
- *Whole*: To remain connected to all that gives meaning, value, and purpose in life; to relate, not isolate
- *Careful*: To remember to care for one's self, one's loved ones, one's legacy; rippling effect

AT THE PATIENT'S BEDSIDE

The following is a brief summary of my meeting with the patient:

> As I entered the room, she smiled, despite her despair, perhaps because she anticipated that I could help ease the turmoil she was experiencing so acutely. "You look like a psychiatrist should look!" she said aloud. Her husband was off on an errand, and we decided to find a private, quiet room to talk, rather than speaking at her bedside in her room, which she shared with another patient. "I'm in turmoil!" The distress was apparent on her face as she began to weep. She described the events of the past 3 weeks. First a diagnosis of ovarian cancer. Then a process of information gathering, finding the best doctors, starting to adapt to her altered life trajectory and the tasks that lied ahead of her, hopeful that her prognosis would be favorable and that life could be resumed at some point down the line. Then the news after surgery, just 2 days ago, that this was metastatic colon cancer, with a new set of information to learn and process, and a new prognosis to make sense of. I quickly normalized for her the sense of turmoil she was experiencing. With any diagnosis of cancer, one must go through a process of "assimilation" and "accommodation." Hearing the news, digesting it, believing it is really you with this cancer, and then a process of accommodating to this new reality through cognitive coping, emotional coping, active coping, and meaning-focused coping. I explained that she had just gone through one process of assimilation and accommodation and was now forced to suddenly start the assimilation and accommodation process anew. She had successfully done this before and I predicted she would again, and in fact pointed out where she had already started the processes. Then came a torrent of emotions: fear of death, anger at the misdiagnosis, anger at the injustice of a shortened life, deep profound sadness at the anticipated loss of her life as she knew it, leaving her children, her husband; all unbearably sad. She initially spoke of her fear of death and the overwhelming anxiety it produced. Soon it became clear through my questioning that fear was not her only emotional response to death. There was the anger, sadness, guilt. We spoke of her religious beliefs and dissected her fear of death. In fact she was comforted by her religious beliefs, and had her own ideas of death being in fact a serene and not unpleasant experience. It was, in fact, not death that challenged her so, but rather the impossibility of how she could live through the period of time from now until death that really overwhelmed and frightened her. "Doctor, how can I live in the face of death?" She asked the question I had been waiting for; the question I had been struggling and working for so long to find an answer to. "Carefully, very carefully," I said. I then explained to her my experiences with patients during the past 24 years and how I had begun to evolve what I thought might be a useful answer to this question. We talked about the Book of Job, which she had read as a young person. And the lessons I had learned from Job's experience. I outlined an approach for how to live (be) in the face of death by being "upright, whole, and careful." I explained each concept. "Upright" meant the following. She was still alive, standing above ground, not dead yet. She needed to have the courage to continue to live and exert her will; to continue to have wishes, desires, hopes, wants; to live fully for as long as possible. "Whole" meant she needed to remain connected to all that gave her life meaning. To stay connected to her loved ones, her children, her husband, even perhaps to work. "Careful" meant she needed to take care of herself. The road ahead was going to be difficult, with

chemotherapy and other treatments. She needed to be kind to herself, to rest, and to give herself time. She also needed to have the courage to still care for and love the people she most treasured, resisting the impulse to withdraw because of how much it would hurt to lose them when the time came. We talked at length about these three concepts and how they related to her life. Her mask of despair began to crumble, and the person beneath began to re-emerge. Everything about her seemed calmer. "This has been helpful, thank you," she said. The plans for her care involved her returning to her home in another city in several days. I referred her to a respected colleague close to her home. We embraced and said goodbye.

Two days later, I receive a handwritten card from her best friend who had first contacted me for help and advice. It was a truly moving note:

> I don't know exactly what you said to my dear friend in the hospital, but whatever it was, it helped her in a very profound way. She is no longer in despair and feels she has a path and direction to follow now. I wish that I could have been there to hear what you discussed. It sounded as if I would have benefited from the discussion as well. All I know at this point is that I should pick up the Book of Job and read it again.

THE GOALS OF PSYCHOTHERAPY IN ADVANCED CANCER

There is an evolution taking place regarding the nature and scope of the clinical goals of psychotherapeutic or counseling interventions in the palliative care setting. Most psychotherapists and counselors would agree that until recently, there were two basic constructs that were universally accepted as the basis of the counseling intervention with a dying patient: support and non-abandonment. Supportive counseling is, at its essence, allying with a patient's defenses and coping strategies and supporting or reinforcing them. So the patient who is dying, and is using denial in the face of the proximity of death, would be supported by the therapist in this way of coping. We all find ourselves allying with hopes, even unrealistic ones, expressed by patients and families in the dying process. However, experienced clinicians also create possibilities for patients to discuss death and dying by gentle questioning. Non-abandonment or presence is a second basic principle of counseling the terminally ill. The therapist makes a commitment to escort or accompany the patient through the course of treatment and the dying process. There is power in the presence of the therapist in accompanying the patient on this too often lonely path. The goals of psychotherapy with advanced cancer patients often consist of applying the practices of "compassion" (Box II). The question many of us are have been asking in recent years is "Can we accomplish something more ambitious in psychotherapy with the terminally ill?"

The "more ambitious" goal of psychotherapy with the terminally ill is to help patients come to a sense of acceptance of a life lived and, thus, ultimately an acceptance of death (i.e., being able to face death with a sense of peace and equanimity). Many suggest such a goal of care is not achievable by all, and perhaps inappropriate for many. I suggest that tasks of life completion are achievable and essential at this phase of life. Acknowledging or facing death (i.e., the finiteness of life) is the impetus for transformation. Facing death forces us to turn around and face life—the life one has lived. When one examines the life one has lived and struggles to accept that lived life, one is faced with a number of challenges and tasks

BOX II GOALS OF PSYCHOTHERAPY IN PALLIATIVE CARE: THE PRACTICES OF COMPASSION

- *Hospitality*: Creating the setting for community and communication—recognizing we share the human condition and we are connected
- *Presence*: To give the other our full attention: "attending" physician; to be fully present for the other transcending our own concerns
- *Listening*: To hear and to respond in a way that makes the patient know he or she has been "understood"; empathy

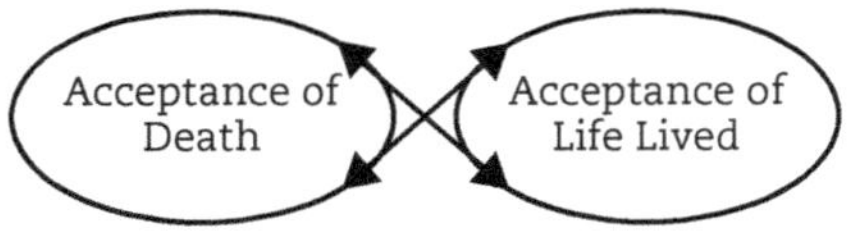

FIGURE I The end-of-life dynamic.

of dying (Box III). Facing death can enhance the process of pursuing a sense of coherence, meaning, and completion of one's life. It allows for realization that the last chapter of one's life is the last opportunity to live to one's full potential; to leave behind an authentic legacy, to connect with the beyond, and to transcend life as we know it. The goal is to preserve the idea that there is still life to be lived, still time to become, so that one can die with a sense of peace, equanimity, and acceptance of the life one lived. The paradox of the end-of-life dynamic is through acceptance of the life one has lived comes acceptance of death (Figure I).

BOX III EXISTENTIALLY INFORMED END-OF-LIFE CARE GOALS: GROWTH AND TASKS IN THE DYING PROCESS

- Sense of life completion
- Sense of coherent meaning about one's life
- Leaving legacy
- Facing death with peace and equanimity
- Acceptance of death
- Acceptance of a life lived

CONCLUSION

I am a physician whose mission is to care for cancer patients and their families, too often at the expense of caring for my own family. In the process of searching for a means of integrating concepts of will, meaning, and care into an approach to ameliorate the despair experienced by patients facing death, I had a transformative experience that led me to appreciate the importance of caring for myself and my family, while still "being in the world." The lessons of the dying are to inform the living of the value of life. Perhaps we die so that we can appreciate the importance of living.

—William Breitbart

REFERENCES

1. Breitbart W, Rosenfeld B, Passik S. Interest in physician assisted suicide among ambulatory HIV infected patients. *Am J Psychiatry.* 1996;153:238–242.
2. Breitbart W, Rosenfeld B. Physician-assisted suicide: The influence of psychosocial issues. *Cancer Control.* 1999;6:146–161.
3. Breitbart W, Rosenfeld B, Pessin H, et al. Depression, hopelessness, and desire for hastened death in terminally ill cancer patients. *J Am Med Assoc.* 2000;284:2907–2911.
4. Nelson C, Rosenfeld B, Breitbart W, et al. Spirituality, depression and religion in the terminally ill. *Psychosomatics.* 2002;43:213–220.
5. McClain C, Rosenfeld B, Breitbart W. The influence of spirituality on end-of-life despair among terminally ill cancer patients. *Lancet.* 2003;361:1603–1607.
6. Breitbart W. Spirituality and meaning in supportive care: Spirituality- and meaning-centered group psychotherapy interventions in advanced cancer. *Support Care Cancer.* 2002;10(4):272–280.
7. Breitbart W, Gibson C, Poppito SR, et al. Psychotherapeutic interventions at the end of life: A focus on meaning and spirituality. *Can J Psychiatry.* 2004;49(6):366–372.
8. McClain-Jacobson C, Rosenfeld B, Kosinski A, et al. Belief in an afterlife, spiritual well-being and end-of-life despair in patients with advanced cancer. *Gen Hosp Psychiatry.* 2004;26:484–486.
9. Breitbart W. Spirituality and meaning in supportive care: Spirituality and meaning-centered group psychotherapy intervention in advanced cancer. *Support Care Cancer.* 2002;10:272–278.
10. Breitbart W, Gibson C, Poppito S, et al. Psychotherapeutic interventions at the end of life: A focus on meaning and spirituality. *Can J Psychiatry.* 2004;49:366–372.
11. Breitbart W, Rosenfeld B, Gibson C, et al. Impact of treatment for depression on desire for hastened death in patients with advanced AIDS. *Psychosomatics.* 2010;51(2):98–105.
12. Rosenfeld B, Breitbart W, Gibson C, et al. Desire for hastened death among patients with advanced AIDS. *Psychosomatics.* 2006;47:6:504–512.
13. Rosenfeld B, Pessin H, Marziliano A, et al. Does desire for hastened death change in terminally ill cancer patients? *Social Sci Med.* 2014;111:35–40.
14. Rosenfeld B, Gibson C, Kramer M, et al. Hopelessness and terminal illness: The construct of hopelessness in patients with advanced AIDS. *Palliat Support Care.* 2004;2:43–53.

15. O'Mahony S, Goulet J, Kornblith A, et al. Desire for hastened death, cancer pain and depression: Report of a longitudinal observational study. *J Pain Symptom Manage.* 2005;5:446–457.
16. Abbey JG, Rosenfeld B, Pessin H, et al. Hopelessness at the end of life: The utility of the hopelessness scale with terminally ill cancer patients. *Br J Health Psychol.* 2006;11:173–183.
17. Rosenfeld B, Pessin H, Lewis C, et al. Assessing hopelessness in terminally ill cancer patients: Development of the Hopelessness Assessment in Illness Questionnaire (HAI). *Psychol Assess.* 2011;23(2):325–336.
18. Chochinov HM, Kristjanson LJ, Breitbart W, et al. Effect of dignity therapy on distress and end-of-life experience in terminally ill patients: A randomized controlled trial. *Lancet Oncol.* 2011;12(8):753–762.
19. Breitbart W, Rosenfeld B, Gibson C, et al. Meaning-centered group psychotherapy for patients with advanced cancer: A pilot randomized controlled trial. *Psycho-oncology.* 2010;19:21–28.
20. Breitbart W, Poppito S, Rosenfeld B, et al. A pilot randomized controlled trial of individual meaning-centered psychotherapy for patients with advanced cancer. *J Clin Oncol.* 2012;30:1304–1309.
21. Breitbart W, Rosenfeld B, Pessin H, et al. Meaning-centered group psychotherapy: An effective intervention for reducing despair in patients with advanced cancer. *J Clin Oncol.* 2015;33(7):749–54.
22. Breitbart W, Poppito S. *Meaning-Centered Group Psychotherapy for Patients with Advanced Cancer.* New York, NY: Oxford University Press; 2014.
23. Breitbart W, Poppito S. *Individual Meaning-Centered Psychotherapy for Patients with Advanced Cancer.* New York, NY: Oxford University Press; 2014.
24. Frankl VF. *Man's Search for Meaning.* 4th ed. New York, NY: Simon &Schuster; 1959.
25. Frankl VF. *The Will to Meaning.* 2nd ed. New York, NY: Penguin; 1969.
26. Mitchell S. *The Book of Job.* New York, NY: HarperCollins; 1992.
27. Heidegger M, Stambaugh J. *Being and Time: A Translation of Sein and Zeit* (SUNY Series in Contemporary Continental Philosophy). New York, NY: State University of New York Press; 1996.

1

The Existential Framework of Meaning-Centered Psychotherapy

WILLIAM BREITBART

As If I Were an Angel

It's as if I were an angel
flying through the clouds.
As if that could be.
Me.
An angel.
As if there could be
a future
I could not know.
A future without death
being the end,
but a beginning.
As if that could be.
Me.
An angel.
A lapsed Jewish angel
with wings to fly.
As if I would transcend
what I ever could have imagined.
Me.
As if that could possibly be
Me,
An angel.
Not alone.
But with other angels.
Angels like me
who never imagined love beyond limits.

WILLIAM BREITBART, MD[1]

INTRODUCTION

Through the writings of Viktor Frankl,[2–5] Irvin Yalom,[6] and many other existentialist philosophers and psychotherapists,[7–17] our group began to conceptualize and then incorporate into meaning-centered psychotherapy (MCP) an existential framework and context for MCP in the cancer setting, especially in advanced cancer patients who were facing death, in despair, struggling with hopelessness and a loss of meaning in what was now a life "limited" by time, and facing suffering and loss. The process of developing MCP, and the subsequent testing of meaning-centered group psychotherapy (MCGP) and individual meaning-centered psychotherapy (IMCP) in randomized controlled trials,[18–24] started approximately 15 years ago. Our group in the Psychotherapy Laboratory of the Department of Psychiatry and Behavioral Sciences at Memorial Sloan Kettering Cancer Center (MSKCC), which I lead, realized at a very early stage that MCP was not only an intervention for advanced cancer patients with loss of meaning, adapted from Frankl's insights into the importance of meaning in human existence and the sources of meaning available to all human beings (elaborated in a more complex manner as a logotherapy intervention for a general, healthy population—not specific to cancer), but also in fact existed within a long-standing existential philosophical and psychotherapeutic context. A clinician delivering MCP would clearly benefit from familiarity with the existential underpinnings not only of Frankl's work but also of MCP in particular.

THE ONTOLOGY OF ONCOLOGY

Ontology is the study of the nature of "being" and "existence." Existentialism is the branch of philosophy that concerns itself with the question of the nature of existence. Existential psychotherapy is a branch of psychotherapy that utilizes the insights of existential philosophy and incorporates these ideas into a psychotherapeutic approach for a variety of clinical problems. In the oncology setting, and especially in a setting of advanced cancer where patients are faced with the "existential" crisis of impending death, psychotherapeutic approaches that incorporate the contributions of existential philosophy and psychology are highly relevant, applicable, and apparently beneficial.[2–24]

As human beings (*Homo sapiens*—"sapient" meaning wise or capable of higher thought), we, as opposed to other creatures, tend to be concerned with a variety of existential, spiritual, and religious questions as to the nature of our existence, the meaning and purpose of our lives, the question of our place in the universe, and the mystery of death. Human beings often struggle with three basic questions:

1. Where did I come from?
2. Why am I here?
3. Where am I going (i.e., what lies beyond death)?

These questions are the central questions of the religious or spiritual experience. Carl Sagan[11] writes that the quintessential human *spiritual* act is the pursuit of an understanding of one's place in the vast mystery of the universe. This in fact may be, at its most basic, a *religious* act as well. The word "religion" derives from the Latin *religio*, whose roots *re* (again) and *ligare* (to bind) essentially refer to an effort to "re-connect" or "bind together." The attempt of human beings to bind or tie together these questions of where we came from, why we are here, and where we are ultimately going is in essence a *religious* task. The pursuit of transcendence or connectedness to something greater than one's self is also, at its most basic and simple form, a *religious* endeavor (no matter whether one is a theist, a deist, or an atheist).

The notion of "symmetry" is also raised by these three basic questions, particularly in the sense that "where we are going" (what lies beyond death) and "where we came from" are in fact similar if not the same places (or states of being or of nonbeing or nothing). This concept of "symmetry," first attributed to the ancient Greek philosopher Epicurus,[25] suggests that we go back from whence we came. For the individual whose religious faith system involves the concepts of an immortal soul and of life after death, these questions may be provided with comforting answers. For the individual who does not have such a belief system, the concept of symmetry can still provide some comfort and ameliorate some of the fears associated with the notion of being relegated to "oblivion" after death. Epicurus did not believe in the immortality of the soul or life after death. He believed that after death there was nothing (no thing); nothing to fear, no pain, no retribution, no judgment. Epicurus did, however, believe in symmetry and that where we go is similar to where we came from, suggesting that the experience of death is most like the experience "before birth." For many of my patients who fear death (especially nonexistence, obliteration), there may be something comforting about the fact that their experience before birth was not distressing or torturous, and that their experience after death may be quite similarly benign. I recently investigated the etymology of the word "oblivion," a word often used to describe the state we enter upon death. It has many negative connotations,

BOX 1.1 THE UNIQUE EXISTENTIAL NATURE OF HUMAN BEINGS

- Human beings are uniquely aware of our existence.
  - Awe: dread paradox, finiteness, responsibility, guilt, culture
- Meaning-making is the defining characteristic of human beings as a species.
- Connection/connectedness is essential to human survival and is the essence of the human experience.
  - To each other, past, present, future, something greater
- The capacity for transformation is unique to human beings
  - Growth, benefit finding, attitude toward suffering

among them "obliteration," "annihilation," and "nothingness"; however, I did come across a more comforting variation on the meaning of "oblivion." This meaning of the word "oblivion" related to the concept of forgetting and forgiving, as in amnesty. I have begun to try to think of "oblivion" as a place where all is forgiven and nothing is remembered—a state of peace, with no past, no future, only the present.

THE UNIQUE EXISTENTIAL NATURE OF HUMAN BEINGS

Human beings are unique among living creatures and most advanced animals in several specific ways, as described by numerous existential philosophers and thinkers.[2–17] Box 1.1 summarizes the four major ways in which human beings are unique existential animals: (1) Human beings are uniquely aware of our existence, (2) meaning-making is the defining characteristic of human beings as a species, (3) connection/connectedness is essential to human survival and is at the essence of the human experience, and (4) the capacity for transformation is unique to human beings.

Human Beings Are Uniquely Aware of Our Existence

Human beings are unique among living creatures in that we are "aware of our existence"—we can objectively contemplate ourselves. Almost 200 years ago, Kierkegaard postulated that as a result of this, we experience two emotions: "awe" and "dread." It is awesome to be alive. Yet it is dreadful to recognize that we all die and that death can come at any moment. Kierkegaard described the resulting experience of living this "aware" human life as a "struggle of being against nonbeing."

This awareness of our existence as human beings also results in an existential and biological imperative to somehow "respond" to the fact of our existence. This "ability to respond" to existence is embodied in the existential principle of *responsibility*. We thus have a responsibility to create a life (related directly to Frankl's concept of "creative" sources of meaning—all the ways in which we derive meaning from creating a life and becoming "who" we strive to be in the world). This responsibility to create a life involves creating a unique life (one only we could have lived—authentic to us) and to live this life to its fullest potential—thus creating a life of meaning, purpose, direction, growth, and transformation, becoming a valued members of a culture and world on meaning (as described by Ernest Becker). Most, if not all, of us fail at this impossible task. Falling short of this responsibility leads to what existentialists describe as *existential guilt*, the notion that I could have done more and that I missed opportunities or failed in some ways. This concept is well exemplified by what were reported to be Albert Einstein's last words on his deathbed, which were "If only I had known more mathematics."

Meaning-Making Is the Defining Characteristic of Human Beings as a Species

There are three central themes of Frankl's work that are basic concepts utilized in MCP:

1. *The will to meaning*: The need to find meaning in our existence is a basic primary motivating force shaping human behavior. Meaning-making is a defining characteristic of human beings.
2. *Life has meaning*: Frankl believed that life has meaning and never ceases to have

meaning, or the potential for meaning, from the first moments of life until the last, although what is meaningful may sometimes change over time as people's circumstances change. Perhaps more broadly, in MCP we have adapted this concept as follows: The possibility to create or experience meaning exists throughout our lives, even in the last months, weeks, days, or even hours of life. If we believe that life is "meaningless," it is not because there is no meaning in our lives (or the possibility of creating or experiencing meaning); it is because we have become disconnected from meaning or have become so demoralized that we see no possibility of creating or experiencing meaning. The imperative then is to constantly "search" for meaning. It is this search that is as important perhaps as actually arriving at a meaningful destination. Many existential philosophers believed that there is no externally given meaning to human existence and that it is solely left to human beings to create the meaning in their lives.[9,10] Others held out the possibility of some "ultimate" externally determined meaning given to human beings by a creator, and that it is our responsibility to "search" for this ultimate meaning to our lives.[2–5,16]

3. *Freedom of will*: We have the "freedom" to find meaning in our existence and to choose our attitude toward suffering. Although there are many aspects of suffering that we have no control over, Frankl suggests that perhaps the last ultimate vestige of freedom that we have as human beings is to consider and choose our attitude toward suffering, even when almost every other freedom has been taken from us. Frankl came to this realization in a concentration camp. Certainly, cancer illness and treatment are not to be compared to a concentration camp experience; however, cancer illness and treatment do in fact create significant limitations, suffering, and relinquishing of a great deal of control. The belief that despite all the limitations imposed by cancer, one does have the freedom to choose how one responds, and the attitude one takes, to the cancer experience.is central to the concept of deriving meaning through choice.

Central to both Frankl's work and MCP is the concept that there are several predictable and easily accessible sources of meaning in human life, which include "creative sources" of meaning (e.g., work), "experiential sources" of meaning (e.g., love), "attitudinal sources" of meaning (e.g., turning a tragedy into a triumph), and "historical sources" of meaning (e.g., the legacy you are given, the legacy you live, and the legacy you give). Most of us live lives of meaning without consciously being aware that we are utilizing these sources of meaning. When plunged into turmoil by a terminal cancer diagnosis, it appears to be helpful for patients to have these sources of meaning delineated, described, experienced, and brought to conscious awareness so that one can "reach" for "each" source of meaning when overcome by a sense of loss or disconnection from the experience of personal meaning.

Connection/Connectedness Is Essential to Human Survival and Is the Essence of the Human Experience

Many animal species have an innate biological sense that their survival is enhanced by traveling and living in herds. Human beings have elaborated the concept of connectedness to a much greater existential and spiritual level. We do not merely stay close to each other to better survive the possibility of external attack by predators but, rather, have come to understand that the essence of the human experience is anchored in a lived connection between fellow human beings, between us and nature, between us and time, and between us and something transcendent. The experience of connection is directly related to the concept of transcendence. Our lives as human beings derive more of a sense of meaning when we can transcend our own individual concerns and engage in life and connect to live in caring, compassionate, and enriching ways. Connectedness involves not only love and care to others but also an indebtedness to care for one's own life and to be connected to one's authentic self. It involves an attitude of self care as well as care for others. Somehow the struggle of life is more bearable when we know we are not alone and that we have not been the first of our species to confront this struggle. Connectedness also refers to connectedness to time: the past, present, and future. Frankl's "experiential" source of meaning is meaning derived primarily from all of these varying forms of connectedness: love, caring, transcendence, time, nature, beauty, and the continuum of human life. *Transcendence* is connection and also an attitude. "Attitudinal" sources of meaning relate primarily to the ability to choose to not be defined by limitations. Transcendence is the result of this attitude to rise above limitations, and it is often achieved through the knowledge that we are not alone and that connectedness is the road to transcendence. I often make the analogy of escalators at the airport. We know what the "ascending" escalators are—they are the escalators that take us up. The "descending" escalators are the escalators that take us down. So where are the "transcending" escalators? They are the moving walkways that take us to all of the various gates from which planes fly to all areas of the world, connecting us from our geographically defined and limited circumstances to destinations throughout the world.

The Capacity for Transformation Is Unique to Human Beings (Growth, Benefit Finding, and Attitude Toward Suffering)

Human beings are unique in that we have the capacity to grow in response to failures, losses, and adverse events or tragedies. We can learn from our mistakes and adopt an attitude that we will not be defined by our limitations or handicaps or circumstances. Certainly with a cancer diagnosis, we encounter multiple limitations, including confrontation with the ultimate limitation of death. It is our attitude toward suffering that allows us to transform and grow. Human beings are the only species that build cancer centers in response to the traumatic effects of cancer, and we are the only species that undergoes plastic surgery to achieve an appearance that is not limited by our genetics. Karl Jaspers[14] defined suffering as a human being's experience encounter with any limitation. Thus, "attitudinal" sources of meaning in MCP focus on choosing an attitude or a response to limitations, suffering, or an uncertain future. Courage, connectedness, and values given by one's ancestors in the form of a legacy given are important factors allowing us to choose constructive, transcendent attitudes, as in the basic will to meaning—the basic human drive to experience or create meaning in one's life.

Frankl[2–5] described what he called the "tragic triad" or the existential facts of life—the fact that in life, sooner or later, one will inevitably have to encounter death, suffering, and guilt. Guilt here refers to existential guilt—the fact that none of us ever truly live our lives to their unique and fullest potential. So there are unfinished life tasks, regrets, and shortcomings that produce this existential guilt. The task of dying is to relieve this guilt by completing life tasks; asking for forgiveness; forgiving oneself for being imperfectly human; trying to create a coherent sense of meaning of one's life; accepting who one is; and, it is hoped, accepting the life one has lived. Suffering is experienced whenever we encounter any limitation or infringement on our freedom, and death is the ultimate limitation. On the one hand, all these issues can cause distress and make life seem meaningless. On the other hand, they can also be sources for finding meaning in life. Finding a sense of purpose and meaning can help alleviate the distress that these facts of life cause. Frankl quotes the philosopher Nietzche,[26] who wrote that "He who has a why to live for can bear with almost any how." Although sooner or later everyone must confront these existential issues, receiving a cancer diagnosis may bring them into much greater focus—sooner and more intensively.

EXISTENTIAL CONCERNS CONFRONTING HUMAN BEINGS, ESPECIALLY THOSE WITH ADVANCED CANCER

Yalom[6] described four ultimate basic human existential concerns: death, freedom, meaninglessness, and isolation. Box 1.2 expands the number and types of existential concerns common in patients with advanced cancer. These existential concerns all have salience and applications during the delivery of MCP, particularly in advanced cancer patients.

Death, or the inevitability of death, is a constant dread that lies just beneath the surface in all human beings. Death anxiety breaks through when our efforts to adapt to, minimize, or deny death fail us, particularly at moments of loss, the death of those close to us, or when we are confronted with the limitations of life such as when we are diagnosed with a life-threatening illness like cancer. Death is the ultimate limitation. A nightmare has been described as a failed dream in which death anxiety breaks through. Panic attacks have similarly been described as

BOX 1.2 COMMON EXISTENTIAL ISSUES IN ADVANCED CANCER

- The inevitability of death: death anxiety, the ultimate limitation, separation
- Freedom: responsibility, existential guilt, will, groundlessness, courage, commitment, attitude
- Existential isolation: Our ultimate aloneness transcendence, connection, prayers
- Meaninglessness: search for meaning, connection, culture, values
- Hopelessness and an uncertain future
- Time: momentary living
- End of life task completion: forgiveness, the nature of Being, Who versus What
- Acceptance of death: acceptance of a life lived

examples of death anxiety breaking through. Kierkegaard used the terms "angst" or "dread" when referring to what we call "death anxiety" or what social psychologists refer to as "existential terror."[27,28] Angst is often thought to refer merely to fear or anxiety. Interestingly, "angst" derives from the German root *angust*, which is also the term for anger. This implies that anxiety and anger both comprise the duality of emotions related to death. Angst also refers to guilt or remorse, and many existentialists think of the term "angst" as related to the concept of existential guilt, the idea that one has not achieved enough in one's life—not lived a unique life to its fullest potential. This sense of existential guilt, many existentialists hypothesize, is the root of death anxiety and anger at impending death. Hence, several existentially oriented interventions at the end of life focus on concepts of completing life tasks, making amends, forgiving and asking for forgiveness, and trying to accept the life that one has lived.[19] Ernest Becker[27] hypothesized that in order to mitigate against death anxiety, human beings create "culture"—humanly constructed beliefs about reality that reduce death anxiety. All "cultures" elucidate the origins of the universe; prescribe appropriate behaviors, values, and virtues; and offer literal or symbolic paths to immortality. Humans thus manage existential terror by believing that life is meaningful and by the self-esteem obtained by meeting or exceeding cultural values. Thus, Becker and psychologists such as Sheldon Solomon who study "terror management"[27,28] highlight the importance of sustaining and enhancing a personal sense of meaning and purpose individually, and perhaps in the world as well, as critical to the mitigation of "death anxiety." In fact, Solomon and colleagues' work suggests that self-esteem and sense of meaning bolster against death anxiety when individuals are confronted with a "mortality salient" scenario.

Freedom, or the fact that we have the freedom to make our lives as we will—to be the authors of our own lives—is another source of existential distress. The concept of existential freedom suggests an absence of external structure imposed upon the course and shape of our lives (perhaps with the exception of the genetic predispositions with which we have been born, such as height, gender, intelligence, and diseases) and a frightening existential groundlessness resulting from the idea that we are primarily responsible for our lives. The concepts of responsibility, will, and existential guilt all are derived from this ultimate freedom. The need to respond to life or "responsibility" becomes central when one is aware of existential freedom. It is through exerting our will (and choosing our attitude) that we create the life that only we were meant to live, the person we want to become. Existential guilt arises when one is distracted from or impeded from exerting one's will and responsibility in living up to one's unique potential (never lives up to one's potential).

Responsibility implies that it is completely up to us to create ourselves, our lives, and the meaning in our lives. No externally given destiny or meaning leaves us "groundless," and this often is experienced as anxiety and angst. It is up to us to create our lives. In MCP, "creative sources" of meaning are especially important to human existence and are central to the existential obligation (understood as the concept of "responsibility") that all human beings experience when they become aware of their existence. Driven by both biology and existential imperative, once we realize that we exist, we must respond to the fact of our existence by "creating a life." We each are driven to create a unique life, with direction and meaning and also growth and transformation to become an effective and useful member of a larger culture or society in a world that we imbue with meaning. What drives this need or will to create a life has been the subject of much philosophical debate. Is it the will to meaning? Is it love or procreation, or mere survival? My understanding of creative sources of meaning has evolved over time. For much of the past 15 years spent in the development of MCP for advanced cancer patients in the Psychotherapy Laboratory I lead at Memorial Sloan Kettering, I had thought of creative sources of meaning as those aspects, values, efforts, and so on that go into the process of creating one's life. Frankl would often refer to "work" as the central creative source of meaning. But counseling advanced cancer patients, for whom work was no longer an available expression or source of meaning, I realized that work could not possibly be the sole element of this source of meaning. It soon became clear that "creative" sources of meaning also referred to what one really cared about in the world and the pursuit of fostering and creating that person, entity, attitude, value, and virtue into being. Enacting one's responsibility to create a life of meaning and authenticity, of growth and transformation and self-actualization, in fact really involved the process of creating "who" you become in the world as well as the "what" (or work) that allows you to express who you are.

Thus, the process of becoming a "who" in order to discover the "what" in one's life took on greater significance for me as an element of a meaning-centered psychotherapy. What comprises the "who" of a human being, and how does one create who one becomes? There are values, virtues, emotions, cognitions, and physical functions that all seemed like reasonable candidates in some combination or permutation. Ultimately, it is "attitude" that is at the core of "who" you are. The process of creating yourself, at its essence, involves the creation of the attitude you take toward life; life, love, and suffering. Creating your attitude is essentially creating your soul (from the Greek philosophical perspective: your mind and spirit). Suddenly it becomes clear why being loving, empathic, generous, and caring to others brings so much personal reward. It is because this is how we create, feed, and grow our attitude in the world and thus give birth to and nurture our very own souls.

Meaninglessness is a basic existential concern. Human beings respond to the existential concern of meaninglessness through the will, search, and creation of meaning in order to bear one's life. In the absence of an obvious, externally imposed meaning to life, we search for meaning in an uncertain and groundless world. This search for meaning generates our sense of values; when there is a "why," there is a "how." Meaning-making is the defining characteristic of human beings as a species. Frankl[2–5] proposed that the "will to meaning"—the need to find or create or experience meaning in life—is a basic motivating force of human behavior. Central to both Frankl's work[2–5] and MCP is the concept that there are several predictable and easily accessible sources of meaning in human life, including "creative sources" of meaning (engaging in life; e.g., work), "experiential sources" of meaning (connecting to life; e.g., love), "attitudinal sources" of meaning (transcending limitations; e.g., turning a tragedy into a triumph), and "historical sources" of meaning (life as a continuum; e.g., the legacy you are given, the legacy you live, and the legacy you give). Most of us live lives of meaning without consciously being aware that we are utilizing these sources of meaning. When plunged into turmoil by a terminal cancer diagnosis, it appears to be helpful for patients to have these sources of meaning delineated, described, experienced, and brought to conscious awareness so that one can "reach" for "each" (*e*xperiential, *a*ttitudinal, *c*reative, and *h*istorical (EACH)) source of meaning when overcome by a sense of loss or disconnection from the experience of personal meaning.

Defining Meaning

Meaning can be defined or conceptualized in cognitive as well as experiential forms. Having a sense that one's life has meaning involves the conviction that one is fulfilling a unique role and purpose in a life that is a gift—a life that comes with a responsibility to live to one's full potential as a human being and, in so doing, being able to achieve a sense of peace, contentment, or even transcendence through connectedness with something greater than one's self. Meaning is the experience of feeling fully alive, of being in love with "being"; the experience of "connectedness, love, care, and indebtedness" to one's life, one's self, one's loved ones, and to the past, present, and future; and connection to the authentic self (the "who" and not the" what" I am) to others, to the transcendent, to meaningful moments. Meaning is the experience of "love, beauty, joy, and life" in all its duality.

Meaning is the experience of "freedom"—being free to be our true selves. Meaning is a state, as opposed to a trait. Meaning is not an absolute; it is not permanent or long-lasting; it needs to be created and experienced anew constantly. This characteristic of meaning is not only the reason it is so common for human beings confronting the tragic facts of life to lose their sense of meaning but also what makes it possible to develop an intervention such as MCP to help create, sustain, or enhance a sense of meaning in patients experiencing profound limitations, suffering, loss, and existential guilt.

Existential isolation or our ultimate aloneness is a critically important existential concern, particularly as we contemplate our deaths. Existential isolation does not refer to intra- or interpersonal loneliness or social isolation but, rather, to the knowledge that we must face the ultimate challenges of our existence alone (e.g., birth and death). Death has been described as the ultimate limitation, but death is also the ultimate separation—separation from consciousness, ourselves, our essence. It is hoped that we will be accompanied by those who love us, but ultimately they cannot take the entire journey with us. Existential isolation is ameliorated by our drives as human beings to love and be loved, to transcend ourselves, and to connect to that which is greater than ourselves.

What We Can Learn from Carl Sagan About Existential Isolation

Carl Sagan the astrophysicist and biologist was admired greatly as both a scientist and a writer for the public. His public writings and lectures did not merely focus on the science of astronomy and astrophysics but also dealt with existential and spiritual issues from a scientific perspective.[11] In 2006, Ann Druyan, Sagan's widow, edited and posthumously published Sagan's Gifford Lectures on natural theology as a book titled *The Varieties of Scientific Experience: A Personal View of the Search for God*, in which he expressed his views on the existence of God in the natural world.[11] This edited volume of lectures is a must-read for anyone interested in the integration of science and spirituality. Sagan died at age 62 after three bone marrow transplantations for myelodysplastic syndrome. Certainly he had contemplated his mortality, his spirituality, and his place in the universe. More than most of us, he had a rather extensive knowledge of the nature of the universe, its vastness, its origins, and the laws of nature and physics that guide natural phenomena. In the editor's introduction to *The Varieties of Scientific Experience*, Druyan writes that

> as a child growing up in Brooklyn, Carl would recite the Hebrew V'Ahavta prayer from Deuteronomy at Temple Services. He knew the prayer by heart, and it may have been the inspiration for him to first ask, What is love without understanding? What allows us to live in the universe if not love?

The prayer V'Ahavta literally means "and Love." Although Carl Sagan may not be the only cosmologist and astrophysicist to both achieve scientific recognition from his peers and become a popular translator of cosmology and science for the public, he is, I believe, the only astrophysicist to have written a fiction novel and the screenplay for the adaptation of that novel into a major Hollywood motion picture. *Contact*[29] is a science fiction novel written by Carl Sagan and published in 1985. It deals with the theme of contact between humanity and a more technologically advanced, extraterrestrial life form. The novel originated as a screenplay in 1979. When development of the film stalled, Sagan decided to convert the stalled film into a novel. The film concept was subsequently revived and eventually released in 1997 as the film *Contact* starring Jodie Foster. On the surface, the film is about a young woman scientist's often challenging search for extraterrestrial life in the vast universe. She and her team of scientists use radiofrequency satellite telescopes listening for sounds of life from the far reaches of the universe. The subplot is a romance between her (a staunch empirical scientist who requires extraordinary evidence for extraordinary claims—and takes nothing on faith) and a young theologian who develops faith in God because of an inexplicable personal revelatory experience. This difference between the two leads to their breakup. Naturally, "contact" is made with earthlings by highly intelligent life forms from a far distant part of the galaxy. The story unfolds. The aliens send blueprints for the manufacture of a spacecraft to bring a human to them. Our female scientist is the astronaut selected. She travels through wormholes in the craft and meets a representative of the alien species. The alien, in the form of her deceased father, meets with her and tells her about the beauty of the universe. The female scientist/astronaut returns abruptly to earth. She has had a 48-hour experience, but she is told that there was a terrible malfunction and her space capsule in fact just fell through the centrifuge-like spacecraft, taking barely a few seconds. There is no video or audio evidence confirming anything she experienced. In Congressional hearings aimed at shaping the entire debacle into some form of hoax, the female scientist is forced to state (I am paraphrasing),

> I admit there is no single shred of evidence to prove what I experienced, but I did experience it. And it was life changing, but I cannot prove it. I suppose I am asking you to take what I am saying as a matter of faith!

The first few times I watched *Contact*, I was moved and entertained by the issues of faith versus science and the truth of science versus the truth of experience. But watching it more recently, I saw a different layer and aspect of Sagan's message, a message I had come to cherish doing the work I do with the dying—specifically, the problem of existential isolation and the concept of transcendence. Existential isolation is a primary existential concern, a fear, of mortal humans—the idea that we are born alone, die alone, and perhaps ultimately really only live alone our entire lives. Alone, isolated, disconnected. In the film *Contact*, Sagan is referring to not only contact between two life forms in the vast universe but also basic human contact with each other. Connection, connectedness, the essence of transcendence (transcending our limitations our existential isolation that disconnects us from each other). In the film, the alien tells the female scientist,

> You're an interesting species, you humans. You're capable of such beautiful dreams, and such horrible nightmares. You feel so lost, so cut off, so alone, only you're not. See, in all our searching, the only thing we've found that makes the emptiness bearable, is each other.

Hopelessness and an uncertain future are existential concerns and challenges for patients with advanced cancer. The maintenance of "hope versus despair" is a constant struggle for patient suffering and living in the face of death. We are born. We live. We die. In between birth and death is a life that is filled with joy and sadness, laughter and tears, tragedy and triumph, suffering and healing. This life can be long or short in duration. The events in our lives can be given meaning or appear to be absent of meaning. The events in our lives can be given value and judged as "good" or "bad," "just" or "unjust," or they can be interpreted as random valueless events. Our perspective on these aspects and events of human existence is often shaped by our religious beliefs—or lack of them—our experiences, and our instincts. Ultimately, however, the task of every human being is to find the means by which one can live a mortal life that is inevitably characterized by finiteness and the existential truths that have been described in this chapter. Simply stated, the challenge of life is to learn how to balance hope and despair, to learn how to live with the inevitability of death and suffering. Hope is inextricably bound to both the future and the possibility of experiencing meaning. Hope is the act of creating an uncertain future.

The Uncertain Future

So many of our patients struggle with the idea of the future—either the uncertainty of the future or the certainty of death in the future. What many find difficult is how to deal with being in that space (that time) between now and death, struggling somehow to not give into despair and meaninglessness. They are trying to find something that can still be created in the face of death; within the limitations and constraints of the finiteness of life. Recently, a patient wrote me an email asking how he could possible feel he had any future at all, given that he had metastatic pancreatic cancer. I had just read and then watched a video clip of Jacques Derrida[12,13] speaking about the future, so I wrote him the following:

> I think of the future constantly, perhaps to the detriment of living fully in the present. But your question is a basic human question that deals directly with the nature of our existence. I've recently begun to understand that there are probably two kinds of future. The predictable, basic, universal, mediocre future, and the unpredictable, uncertain, unique future. The predictable future is the future where time marches on, the sun will set and rise, we are all born and live and die, we have little role to play in creating or controlling this future. The unpredictable future is the only future in which we have agency in creating or shaping the future through our choices and our attitude. The unpredictable future is more about "what (or who) comes, unpredictably, into our lives and how we respond to it" the people the events. The "others" who come into our lives and we choose to allow this to change our lives and our future. A friend, a love, creative ideas, . . . So while one element of the future is predictable (death), *there is so much of the future that is unpredictable and that we take a part in*

> *creating*. So never stop trying to create your future because there is always hope that something or someone will unpredictably enter it.

Prayers and Lies and the Future

Another patient wrote me that he was an atheist but had an impulse to pray and was confused by it. Was it a betrayal of all he believed? Was it a lack of courage on his part? I wrote him the following email in reply:

> So the question is—Why would someone who is an agnostic or an atheist pray? I have prayed and sometimes pray even though I am at least an agnostic. Who am I praying to? And why am I praying? And what am I praying for? Do I expect my prayers to be answered? Well, one of the last times I prayed was a plea to god to take my son's diabetes from him and give it to me. Did I expect god to hear me? Or respond to my prayer? No. My prayer was a hopeless act but not a useless act. It was an act of love. It was an act of connection to my son, to nature and the universe, an act connecting me to myself, my past and my future. It was a prayer meant for me to hear, exhorting me to bring to bear my love and courage and caring to deal with this uncertainly in my family's life, and take part in creating our future. *The act of creating an uncertain future is hope. The act of creating an uncertain future is love. The act of creating an uncertain future is our debt to life.*

I received an email from a patient with far advanced disease after one of our sessions. He wrote,

> Thank you for another helpful session. I wonder if you can expand on why you said it was important to learn how to lie? What does lying entail, when is it okay, and how far can or should one go? Of course I understand the gross definition and the obvious areas where it is not okay to lie, but what I'm trying to understand is when it is okay or even beneficial to lie to one's self, and to others?

Well now the entire world (or at least the readers of this text) knows that I occasionally point out the value of the importance of knowing how to lie in order to live in the world! I had not recalled saying this to the patient, but clearly the subject of lies had come up and had an effect on this patient. What are lies? What purposes do they serve? All human beings lie. Perhaps it is even unique to us as a species. Is there an existential purpose, I wondered. I wrote the following email after watching a Derrida[13] video clip:

> Glad the session was helpful. This business about lying can be complex as you suggest, but let's make it simple: The lie is about the future. The truth is about the past. In order to live with hope one has to be creating an uncertain future. Lies give this uncertain future a direction.

Time is not only a central question of inquiry in the field of physics but also a primary existential concern related to both the nature of "being" and the nature of "death." The questions have always been: How can we live knowing that we are mortal and we die? Is life worth living, knowing that it is finite? How can we live in the face of death? How can a human being with a diagnosis of metastatic incurable cancer and a prognosis of several months manage to *not* focus on the clock and the nearness of death but, rather, live each day (or at least some days) experiencing moments of joy, meaning, and appreciation that he or she is alive today? These questions raise our awareness of the temporality of life, the nature of time, the relationship of being to time, and the concepts of infinity and finiteness. Living in the "moment" is certainly a common recommendation of clinicians, particularly those who view mindfulness meditation practice as beneficial. Jon Kabat-Zinn[30] writes that "this moment is all we really have to work with. . . . In every moment we find ourselves at the crossroads of here and now." The here and now is also often described as the "present"; however, the concept of living "in the moment" or the "present" has many limitations as a concept for me as a clinician and practically as a method of living, in my experience, for my patients. Part of the difficulty is that the "moment" or the "present" is quite brief and fleeting. It is difficult to hold onto or grasp. The "present" is gone the moment you realize that it is here, and then you are in the future and a new present. On a practical level, it seems more like there is only the past and the future, and the present is with us for too short a moment to appreciate or do anything with. This is particularly true if we experience the temporality of life or time in "chronological" terms.

Momentary Living

The fact is that in the modern era we live "lives coupled to chronological time." The ticking of seconds, minutes, hours, days, months, years—we experience life as a time-based commodity that we are always running out of. The ancient Greeks had more complex and varied concepts of time that may be particularly helpful for those who are confronting the finiteness of life in direct and almost inescapable manner due to life-threatening illness. The ancient Greeks had two words for time, "Chronos" and "Kairos." "Chronos" refers to chronological time or sequential time—the concept of time that we universally use today. "Kairos," however, refers not to chronological time but, rather, to profound moments or milestones or events in life, particularly those that are most meaningful or transformative. The ancient Greeks also saw time as not necessarily only linear but also as "cyclical." The concept of cyclical time reflects the constant experience of the past and the future in each moment of the present. As we move through life and experience moments of profound emotion or meaning, we imbue that lived experience (moment) with the contributions of the past legacy we have inherited and experiences that have shaped the present moment, while anticipating how we will enact and shape the direction of the uncertain future that we are creating.

Interestingly, the ancient Greeks saw the past as lying before us because we could see it and examine it. They believed the future was behind us because we could not yet see it. These alternative concepts of time—the past, present, and future—can be very informative and helpful. Perhaps they can help us move toward an attitude of "living life uncoupled from chronological time"—a way of "living momentarily": living life focused on the moments and events and milestones of our lives that bring the experience of meaning and the sense of being more fully alive.

"Momentary living" is thus not an exhortation to live "in the moment" but, rather, to live life uncoupled from chronological time—to live life for the moments of profound and meaningful experiences (living from moment to moment). Patients confronting their mortality and facing death in more concrete terms because of life-threatening illness could benefit from this attitudinal shift in the perception of time from a chronological one to one based on meaningful moments and experiences. A cyclical concept of time is also intriguing and somehow resonates as being innate to our human experience as well. Old-fashioned round clocks actually do tell time in a cyclical manner. The hands of the clock go round and round, and the hours keep repeating. In the digital era, we see time reflected to us as a commodity that we are quickly running out of. "I just have so much time left!" It can be activating and a call to life, a call to action. But too often it is paralyzing and causes panic. The concepts of finiteness and infinity are also quite interesting to examine. A finite period of chronological time can be measured, but infinity cannot. Infinity is not a measure of time. Life is finite in time. We live in finite lives based on chronologic time. Can we live an infinity within a finite lifetime. Infinity may in fact be a representation of cyclical time—a constant movement between the past, present, and future that is constantly at play in each of our lived moments of meaningful experiences. What may be paradoxical is that true freedom (and the experience of the infinite in life) may be most tangible and possible within the limits of a finite, mortal, human life.

End of life task completion is an existential challenge central to the relief of existential guilt and the goal of acceptance of a life lived. The task of dying, according to Frankl,[2–5] is to relieve oneself of existential guilt through whatever means possible (e.g., forgiveness, acceptance, making amends, and completing end of life tasks). Karen Steinhauser[31] explored the most important end of life tasks of concern to patients with advanced cancer (Box 1.3). Her research revealed that patient priorities near the end of life include saying goodbye to important people, resolving unfinished business with family and friends, sharing time with friends and family, and remembering personal accomplishments. Ira Byock,[32] in his book *Dying Well*, reminds us that with dying, just as with the end of any relationship, it is important for human beings to acknowledge and say five

BOX 1.3 END-OF-LIFE TASK COMPLETION: WHAT IS IMPORTANT TO DYING PATIENTS

- Say goodbye to important people
- Resolve unfinished business with family or friends
- Share time with friends and family
- Remember personal accomplishments

things: "I love you"; "Thank you for loving me"; "I forgive you"; "Please forgive me"; and "Goodbye." Steinhauser's work[31] further suggests that patients yearn to have physicians who understand them as people and see them for "who" they are as opposed to "what" they are (a stage IV pancreatic cancer patient). This in fact is central to the nature of Being and how clinicians relate to human "beings" at the end of life.

The Nature of Being: Who or What

> The question of Being, to return to philosophy—because the first question of philosophy is: What is it "to Be"? What is Being? The question of being is itself always already divided between "the who and the what." Is Being "someone or something"?
>
> Jacques Derrida[13]

There are many challenges that face clinicians who choose to work or train in palliative medicine. There is of course the challenge of mastering various medical diagnostic and treatment skills. There is a growing body of evidence-based medicine in the field of palliative care, and most training programs in palliative medicine spend an appropriately significant amount of time teaching trainees to become expert diagnosticians and clinicians. It soon becomes obvious, with clinical experience, that skills in sensitive, empathic, and effective communication with patients and families also are extraordinarily vital to master if one is to have a career in palliative medicine. Goals of care and how a clinician measures "success" or "failure" are also critical to an understanding of one's identity as a palliative care clinician. Often, a conscious dedication to minimizing avoidable suffering, rather than prolonging life at the cost of suffering, becomes the mark of provision of "good care." In this way, patient deaths are not the metric of meaningful and significant work but, rather, the manner of death and one's ability to ameliorate suffering are the measure of the quality of one's skills. These are all such complex and challenging skills and attitudes necessary to master in the process of training as a palliative care clinician, but we have not yet even mentioned the problem of how palliative care clinicians manage their own death anxiety and their grief while bearing constant witness to death day in and day out. It was these latter problems of dealing with the impact of confronting death daily, and its impact on palliative care trainees, for which the palliative medicine fellowship training program director at MSKCC asked me to try to find some way to help our trainees. We started with a series of individual meetings (or debriefings as we called them unofficially) between the palliative medicine clinical fellows and myself in my office at the cancer center. I recently completed a series of such meetings, and I find myself reflecting on these meetings with a sense that while I may have been of some help to these trainees, I left with the gift of a new understanding of the "creative" process. By that I mean the process by which we as human beings respond to our existence by creating a life and becoming "who" we aspire to become in the world.

Invariably, in addition to discussions of personal death anxiety, managing the experience of grief over patient deaths, and the notion of existential guilt related to perceptions of a good clinical outcome, our discussions touched on the question of why the trainees chose palliative medicine as a career and how that choice fit into their notion of the trajectory of the lives that they were creating. What became clear rather quickly was that most of the trainees were focused on becoming a "good palliative care clinician." They had great difficulty in even grasping the idea of the notion of becoming a person with a set of values and passions who did palliative care medicine as their work but also held creating a family or dedicating their lives to some greater cause as essential to who they were. This was too abstract for them at first. Jacques Derrida[12] would often discuss the importance of the distinction between "the who and the what" (*le Qui et le Quoi*). Do you aspire to become a "who" or a "some one" in the world, or do you aspire to become a "what" or a "something" in the world? So in reflecting on my discussions with the trainees, I noticed how many of our young and brightest, those who in fact choose the amelioration of suffering as their life's work, find it so much more comfortable to talk about becoming a "something" rather than a "someone."

It is ironic that when we speak of "end of life care goals" for our patients, we are much more focused on preserving the "who" of the patient, preserving the someone who that patient has been in life and allowing that to be what is most meaningful and significant as the patient faces death. Those of us who are responsible for the training of young palliative care clinicians would serve them well to help them understand that their "life goals" should also incorporate the "who," the someone they want to become and create, not merely the "what," the type of clinician they want to become. This requires an opportunity for trainees to reflect on who they are becoming as human beings in this world and how palliative medicine is just one important expression of who they are becoming through the process of training. Perhaps such an understanding would help our trainees become more comfortable communicating with patients on a human level, with the knowledge that we are all in the same existential boat, mortal human beings—with the main difference being that we as palliative care clinicians have knowledge, skills, and experience that we can share that may ultimately relieve suffering. After all, that is "who" we are.

Acceptance of death is the ultimate existential challenge. The goal of psychotherapy with the terminally ill is to help patients come to a sense of acceptance of a life lived and thus, ultimately, an acceptance of death (i.e., being able to face death with a sense of peace and equanimity). Many suggest such a goal of care is not achievable by all and perhaps inappropriate for many. I suggest that tasks of life completion are achievable and essential at this phase of life. Acknowledging or facing death (i.e., the finiteness of life) is the impetus for transformation. Facing death forces us to turn around and face life—the life one has lived. When one examines the life one has lived and struggles to accept that lived life, one is faced with a number of challenges and tasks of dying (Boxes 1.3 and 1.4). Facing death can enhance the process of pursuing a sense of coherence, meaning, and completion of one's life. It allows for realization that the last chapter of one's life is the last opportunity to live to one's full potential, to leave behind an authentic legacy, to connect with the beyond, and to transcend life as we know it. The goal is to preserve the idea that there is still life to be lived, still time to become, so that one can die with a sense of peace, equanimity, and acceptance of the life one lived. The paradox of the end of life dynamic is that through acceptance of the life one has lived comes acceptance of death.

BOX 1.4 EXISTENTIALLY INFORMED END-OF-LIFE GOALS

- Sense of life completion
- Sense of coherent meaning about one's life
- Leaving legacy
- Facing death with peace and equanimity
- Acceptance of a life lived
- Acceptance of death

SUMMARY

Meaning-centered psychotherapy was developed and is informed by a long-standing existential philosophical and psychotherapeutic context and framework. This chapter provided a brief overview of some of the most basic and central existential concepts and concerns of human beings—particularly those facing suffering, death, loss, and guilt—that are relevant to a theoretical understanding of MCP as well as the practice of MCP. A clinician delivering MCP would clearly benefit from familiarity with these existential underpinnings of MCP. The following chapters present specifics about the theoretical, empirical, and practical bases of delivering MCP in a variety of formats to a wide variety of patients in the oncology setting.

REFERENCES

1. Breitbart W. As if I were an angel. *Palliat Support Care*. 2013;11:447.
2. Frankl VF. *Man's Search for Meaning*. 4th ed. Boston, MA: Beacon; 1959/1992.
3. Frankl VF. *The Doctor and the Soul*. New York, NY: Random House; 1955/1986.
4. Frankl VF. *Man's Search for Ultimate Meaning*. New York, NY: Plenum; 1975/1997.
5. Frankl VF. *The Will to Meaning: Foundations and Applications of Logotherapy*. New York, NY: New American Library; 1988.
6. Yalom ID. *Existential Psychotherapy*. New York, NY: Basic Books; 1980.
7. Kierkegaard S, Hong H, Hong E. *Fear and Trembling/Repetition*. Princeton, NJ: Princeton University Press; 1983.
8. Heidegger M. *Being and Time*. Stambaugh J, trans. Albany, NY: State University of New York Press; 1996.
9. Camus A. *The Myth of Sisyphus*. New York, NY: Knopf; 1955.
10. Sartre J-P. *Being and Nothingness*. Barnes HE, trans. London: Routledge; 2003.
11. Sagan C. The God hypothesis. In: Druyan A, ed. *The Varieties of Scientific Experience: A Personal View of the Search for God*. New York, NY: Penguin; 2006:147–168.
12. Kamuf P, ed. *A Derrida Reader: Between the Blinds*. New York, NY: Columbia University Press; 1991.

13. *Derrida*; A documentary film directed by K Dick and A Ziering Kofman. Shown at the Sundance Film Festival; 2002.
14. Jaspers K. *Reason and Existenz*. Earle W, trans. New York, NY: Noonday; 1955.
15. May R. *The Courage to Create*. New York, NY: Norton; 1994.
16. Tillich P. *The Courage to Be*. New Haven, CT: Yale University Press; 1952.
17. Beals C. *Levinas and the Wisdom of Love*. Houston, TX: Baylor University Press; 2007.
18. Greenstein M, Breitbart W. Cancer and the experience of meaning: A group psychotherapy program for people with cancer. *Am J Psychother*. 2000;54(4):486–500.
19. Breitbart W. Spirituality and meaning in supportive care: Spirituality and meaning-centered group psychotherapy interventions in advanced cancer. *Support Care Cancer*. 2002;10(4):272–280.
20. Breitbart W, Rosenfeld B, Gibson C, et al. Meaning-centered group psychotherapy for patients with advanced cancer: A pilot randomized controlled trial. *Psycho-Oncology*. 2010;19:21–28.
21. Breitbart W, Poppito S, Rosenfeld B, et al. A pilot randomized controlled trial of individual meaning-centered psychotherapy for patients with advanced cancer. *J Clin Oncol*. 2012;30:1304–1309.
22. Breitbart W, Rosenfeld B, Pessin H, et al. Meaning-centered group psychotherapy: An effective intervention for reducing despair in patients with advanced cancer. *J Clin Oncol*. 2015;33(7):749–754.
23. Breitbart W, Poppito S. *Meaning Centered Group Psychotherapy for Patients with Advanced Cancer*. New York, NY: Oxford University Press; 2014.
24. Breitbart W, Poppito S. *Individual Meaning Centered Psychotherapy for Patients with Advanced Cancer*. New York, NY: Oxford University Press; 2014.
25. Epicurus. *The Epicurus Reader: Selected Writings and Testimonia*. Inwood B, Gerson, LP, ed. and trans. Indianapolis, IN: Hackett; 1994.
26. Nietzsche F. *Human, All too Human: A Book for Free Spirits*. Cambridge, UK: Cambridge University Press; 1986.
27. Becker E. *The Denial of Death*. New York, NY: Free Press; 1973.
28. Maxfield M, Pyszczysnki T, Solomon S. Finding meaning in death: Terror management among the terminally ill. In: Straker N, ed. *Facing Cancer and the Fear of Death: A Psychoanalytic Perspective on Treatment*. New York, NY: Aronson; 2012:41–60.
29. Sagan C. *Contact*. New York, NY: Simon & Schuster; 1985.
30. Kabat-Zinn J. *Wherever You Go There You Are*. New York, NY: Hyperion; 1994.
31. Steinhauser KE, Alexander SC, Byock IR, George LK, Tulsky JA. Seriously ill patients' discussions of preparation and life completion: an intervention to assist with transition at the end of life. *Palliat Support Care*. 2009 Dec;7(4):393–404. doi: 10.1017/S147895150999040X
32. Byock I. *Dying Well: The Prospect for Growth at the End of Life*. New York, NY: Riverhead/ Putnam; 1977.

2

Meaning-Centered Group Psychotherapy for Advanced Cancer Patients

WILLIAM BREITBART, ALLISON J. APPLEBAUM, AND MELISSA MASTERSON

INTRODUCTION

A famous Talmudic question asks, "What is truer than the truth?" The answer: "The story." This, dear reader, is the story of meaning-centered group psychotherapy (MCGP), at least in an abbreviated form. Like many clinical interventions in our field of psycho-oncology, meaning-centered psychotherapy (MCP) arose from a need to deal with a challenging clinical problem—a problem for which no effective intervention was, as yet, available. In fact, it was through the fortunate collision of encountering a clinical problem in the context of being inspired by the works of pioneers in existential philosophy and psychiatry that MCP was conceived, developed, tested, and ultimately demonstrated to be an effective intervention. The clinical problem was despair, hopelessness, and desire for hastened death in advanced cancer patients who were in fact not suffering from a clinical depression[1] but, rather, confronting an existential crisis of loss of meaning, value, and purpose in the face of a terminal prognosis. Although our group ultimately demonstrated that desire for hastened death in the presence of a clinical depression could be reversed with adequate antidepressant therapy,[2] no effective intervention was available for loss of meaning and hopelessness in the absence of clinical depression. Inspired primarily by the works of Viktor Frankl[3–6] and further informed by the contributions of Irvin Yalom,[7] our research group adapted Frankl's concepts of the importance of meaning in human existence (and his "logotherapy") and initially created a meaning-centered intervention in a group format (MCGP), intended primarily for advanced cancer patients. The goal of the intervention was to diminish despair, demoralization, hopelessness, and desire for hastened death by sustaining or enhancing a sense of meaning, even in the face of death. Although MCP relies heavily on Frankl's concepts of meaning and sources of meaning as resources to reconnect with meaning in the midst of suffering (see the sections in this chapter on the format and content of the MCGP intervention), MCP also incorporates important and fundamental existential concepts and concerns that do not directly focus on meaning but are clearly related to the search, connection, and creation of meaning. MCGP is an 8-week intervention composed of didactics and experiential exercises. It is designed to help advanced cancer patients understand the importance and relevance of sustaining, reconnecting with, and creating meaning in their lives through common and reliable sources of meaning that may serve as resources of meaning that help to diminish despair near the end of life.

BACKGROUND

As we continue to develop our understanding of the psychosocial needs of palliative care patients, it is becoming more apparent that our present concepts of adequate care must be expanded in their focus beyond simple pain and physical symptom control to include psychiatric, psychosocial, existential and spiritual domains of end-of-life care.[8–12] Although physical symptoms are indeed distressing to patients with advanced disease, it is clear that symptoms relating to psychological distress and existential concerns are even more prevalent than pain and other physical symptoms.[13] Acknowledging the psychological as well as spiritual domains of end-of-life care has been identified as a priority by both medical professionals and cancer patients.

Defining Spirituality as a Construct of Meaning and/or Faith

The Consensus Conference on Improving Spiritual Care as a Dimension of Palliative Care defined spirituality as "the aspect of humanity that refers to the way individuals seek and express meaning and purpose and the way they experience their connectedness to the moment, to self, to others, to nature, and to the significant or sacred."[14] Others have also defined spirituality as a construct that involves concepts of both meaning and religious faith.[15,16] Meaning, or having a sense that one's life has meaning, involves the conviction that one is fulfilling a unique role and purpose in a life that is a gift. This life comes with a responsibility to live to one's full potential as a human being; in so doing, one is able to achieve a sense of peace, contentment, or even transcendence, through connectedness with something greater than one's self.[4] Faith is differentiated from meaning as a belief in a higher transcendent power, not necessarily identified as God and not necessarily through participation in the rituals or beliefs of a specific organized religion. The faith component of spirituality is most often associated with religion and religious belief, whereas the meaning component of spirituality appears to be a more universal concept that can exist in religious or non-religiously identified individuals.

Spiritual Well-Being/Meaning and Its Impact on Psychosocial Outcomes in Advanced Cancer

There has been great interest in the role in palliative care of faith and religious beliefs on health outcomes.[17–21] Recent studies have found that religion and spirituality generally play a positive role in patients' coping with illnesses such as cancer or HIV.[17,22,23] The link between religion and health is weaker and less consistent than that between spirituality/meaning and health outcomes.[24,25] Importantly for this work, researchers theorize that religious beliefs may serve to help patients construct meaning in suffering inherent to illness, which may in turn facilitate acceptance of their situation.[19]

There is extensive evidence that demonstrates the significance of spiritual well-being for patients at the end of life. For example, in a qualitative study, Singer and colleagues found that "achieving a sense of spiritual peace" was a domain of end-of-life care that was most important from the patients' perspective.[26] Moadel and colleagues surveyed 248 cancer patients and asked them what their most important needs were.[27] Of these patients, 51% said they needed help overcoming fears, while 41% needed help finding hope, 40% needed help finding meaning in life, 43% needed help finding peace of mind, and 39% needed help finding spiritual resources. In a sample of 162 Japanese hospice inpatients, psychological distress was related to meaninglessness in 37%, hopelessness in 37%, and loss of social role and feeling irrelevant in 28%.[28] Finally, in a survey conducted by Meier and colleagues on the reasons for patient requests for assisted suicide, physicians reported that "loss of meaning in life" accounted for 47% of the requests.[29] Clearly, from patient and physician perspectives alike, issues of spirituality are essential elements of quality end-of-life care.

Several published studies highlight the importance of these concepts in end-of-life care. Brady and colleagues found that cancer patients who reported a high degree of meaning in their lives were able to report higher satisfaction with their quality of life and to tolerate severe physical symptoms better than patients who reported lower levels of meaning/peace.[30] Our research group[1,23] has demonstrated a central role for spiritual well-being (i.e., meaning) as a buffering agent, protecting against depression, hopelessness, and desire for hastened death among terminally ill cancer patients. McClain and colleagues found that spiritual well-being was significantly associated with end-of-life despair (as defined by hopelessness, desire for hastened death, and suicidal ideation), even after controlling for the influence of depression.[31] Yanez and colleagues similarly found that increases in meaning/peace in breast cancer survivors significantly predicted better mental health and lower distress, whereas increases in faith did not.[32]

This research highlights the role of meaning as a buffer against depression, hopelessness, suicidal ideation, and desire for hastened death, and it is significant in the face of what we know about the consequences of depression and hopelessness in cancer patients. Depression, hopelessness, and loss of meaning are associated with poorer survival[33] and higher rates of suicide, suicidal ideation, and desire for hastened death.[1,34–37] In addition, hopelessness and loss of meaning have been shown to be independent of depression as predictors of desire for death, and they are as influential on desire for death as depression.[1] Therefore, there is a critical need for the development of psychosocial interventions for the terminally ill that address loss of meaning as a mechanism for improving psychosocial outcomes (e.g., quality of life, depression, anxiety, hopelessness, desire for death, and end-of-life despair).

THEORETICAL CONCEPTUAL FRAMEWORK UNDERLYING MEANING-CENTERED PSYCHOTHERAPY

Frankl's Concepts of Meaning

The importance of spiritual well-being, and the role of "meaning" in particular, in moderating depression, hopelessness, and desire for death in terminally ill cancer patients demonstrated by our research group led us to look beyond the role of antidepressant treatment for depression in this population and to focus new efforts on developing nonpharmacologic (psychotherapy) interventions that address issues such as hopelessness, loss of meaning, and spiritual well-being in patients with advanced cancer at the end of life. This effort led to an exploration and analysis of the work of Viktor Frankl and his concepts of logotherapy or meaning-based psychotherapy,[3–6] which serve as the core theoretical conceptual framework of MCP and MCGP. Although Frankl's logotherapy was not designed for the treatment of cancer patients or those with life-threatening illness, his concepts of meaning and spirituality clearly had applications in psychotherapeutic work with advanced cancer patients, many of whom seek guidance and help in dealing with issues of sustaining meaning, hope, and understanding cancer and impending death in the context of their lives.

Frankl's main contributions to human psychology have been to raise awareness of the spiritual component of human experience and the central importance of meaning (or the will to meaning) as a driving force or instinct in human psychology. Frankl's basic concepts related to meaning include the following:

1. Meaning of life: Life has meaning and never ceases to have meaning, from the very first moment of life to the last moment of life. Meaning may change in this context, but it never ceases to exist. When we believe our lives have no meaning, it is because we have become disconnected from meaning in our lives, not because it no longer exists. For the purposes of MCP, we have modified this concept based on clinical experience and our desire to present a secular intervention that relied less on dogma and more on rationality. We offer this concept: The creation or experience of meaning is always possible (in a sentient human being), even in the last months, days, or moments of life.
2. Will to meaning: The desire to find meaning in human existence is a basic, primary motivating force in human behavior. Human beings are creatures who innately search for and create meaning in their lives. We are "meaning-making" creatures.
3. Freedom of will: We have the freedom to find meaning in our existence and to choose our attitude toward suffering, limitations, and uncertainty. Ultimately, if we are unable to control events that are externally or internally impacted on our bodies and our freedom, we still have the last vestige of freedom, which is to choose how we think about the situation and to choose the attitude we take in response to the situation. We have the responsibility to create an existence of meaning, direction, and identity. We must respond to the fact of our existence and create the "essence" of what makes us human. Our "attitude" is a critical element of what comprises our human "essence."
4. Sources of meaning: Meaning in life has specific and available sources (Table 2.1).

TABLE 2.1 SOURCES OF MEANING: EACH

Sources of Meaning	Description
*E*xperiential sources	Connecting with life via relationships, beauty, nature, and humor
*A*ttitudinal sources	Turning personal tragedy into triumph via the attitude taken toward given circumstances (e.g., physical suffering, personal adversity, and one's mortality), transcendence
*C*reative sources	Actively engaging in life via roles, work, deeds, and accomplishments
*H*istorical sources	Legacy that has been given (past) Legacy one lives (present) Legacy one will give (future)

> The four main sources of meaning in life are derived from creativity (work, deeds, and dedication to causes), experience (love, relationships, roles, art, beauty, and humor), attitude (the attitude one takes toward suffering and existential problems), and legacy (meaning exists in a historical context; thus, legacy—past, present, and future—is a critical element in sustaining or enhancing meaning). We created an acronym for the experiential, attitudinal, creative, and historical sources of meaning: EACH. Most of us live lives imbued with a sense of meaning quite natural and unintentionally. We are not conscious of acting in specific ways in order to create a sense of meaning. However, when one is overwhelmed with the emotions of an existential crisis created by the diagnosis of advanced cancer and a confrontation with the finiteness of life, we hypothesized that patients might benefit from learning the sources of meaning and bring them up to a more conscious level in order for them to be able to intentionally "reach for EACH source of meaning" when they feel disconnected from meaning in their lives.

Drawing from these principles, MCGP helps to enhance patients' sense of meaning by helping them to understand and capitalize on the various sources of meaning in their lives. Enhanced meaning is conceptualized as the catalyst for improved psychosocial outcomes, such as improved quality of life, reduced psychological distress, and despair. Specifically, meaning is viewed as both an intermediary outcome and a mediator of changes in these important psychosocial outcomes.

Meaning: Focused Coping

Relatively recently, investigators such as Park and Folkman[38] described conceptual models for meaning in relation to traumatic events and coping, which seem relevant to the theoretical framework of MCP and MCGP. They describe meaning as a general life orientation, as personal significance, as causality, as a coping mechanism, and as an outcome. Critically important to the theoretical conceptual model of MCP is Park and Folkman's concept of a form of "meaning-focused coping." Meaning has also been assessed in terms of re-evaluating an event as positive; answering the question of why an event occurred, or "Why me?"; enumerating ways in which life changed, sometimes for the positive, because of an event; and stating the extent to which one has "made sense of" or "found meaning" in an event.[3–6,39–42] Park and Folkman[38] also describe two levels of meaning: global meaning and situational meaning. Unlike Park and Folkman's conceptualization of meaning as global or situational, Frankl viewed meaning as a state: Individuals can move from feeling demoralized and as if their lives hold no value (see Kissane et al.[37]) to recognizing their personal sense of meaning and purpose, which allows them to value even more intensely the time remaining. Conceptualizing meaning as a state subject to change suggests its potential responsiveness to intervention. Frankl also viewed suffering as a potential springboard, both for having a need for meaning and for finding it.[3,4] Hence, the diagnosis of a terminal illness may be seen as a crisis in the fullest sense of the word—an experience of distress or even despair that may in itself offer an opportunity for growth and meaning. Either one has a loss of sense of meaning and purpose in life or one has a sustained or even heightened sense of meaning, purpose, and peace, which allows one to value more profoundly the time remaining and positively appraise events.

Concepts Central to Existential Philosophy and Psychology Used in Meaning-Centered Psychotherapy

Underlying the development and delivery of MCP and MCGP are concepts central to existential philosophy, psychology, and psychiatry, developed by such pioneers as Kierkegaard, Nietzsche, Heidegger, Sartre, and Yalom.[7,43–46] Although concerns relating to meaning and meaninglessness are central to existential philosophy and psychology, MCP and MCGP have benefitted from the incorporation of a number of important existential concepts that do not directly involve meaning but are interrelated and serve as a critical framework for conducting the psychotherapeutic work of MCP. Therefore, although the emphasis of MCP is on meaning and sources of meaning, clearly much of the psychotherapeutic work is richer when the therapists are well grounded in the basic conceptual framework and theories of existential philosophy and psychotherapy. Important existential concepts that are utilized and incorporated into the theoretical framework of MCP include freedom, responsibility, choice, creativity, identity, authenticity, engagement, existential guilt, care, transcendence, transformation, direction, being unto death, being and temporality, and existential isolation. These existential concepts inform the intervention and are utilized primarily to reinforce the goals of MCP related to the search, connection, and creation of meaning.

TARGET GROUPS OF PATIENTS

MCGP is targeted toward advanced cancer patients with stage IV solid tumor cancers, or stage III solid tumor cancers, excluding breast and prostate cancer. Patients with physical limitations sufficient to preclude participation in outpatient group psychotherapy (i.e., as indicated by a Karnofsky performance rating <50[47]) are not suited for this intervention. The efficacy of MCGP in improving patients' spiritual well-being and sense of meaning, and decreasing anxiety and desire for death, makes it particularly appropriate for patients who are experiencing at least moderate distress (as indicated by a score of 4 or higher on the National Comprehensive Cancer Network's Distress Thermometer[48]), predominantly in the areas of emotional problems and spiritual/religious concerns.

OVERVIEW OF EVIDENCE ON EFFICACY

Prior to the development of MCGP, few interventions specifically focused on existential or spiritual domains in treatment or measured the impact of treatment on such outcomes, particularly in patients with advanced cancer. Early research by Yalom, Spiegel, and colleagues demonstrated that a 1-year supportive group psychotherapy that included a focus on existential issues decreased psychological distress and improved quality of life.[49–51] Relatively recent studies have described short-term interventions that included a spiritual or existential component, including individually based approaches.[36,52–54] However, the results of these studies are inconsistent in terms of their effects on psychological outcomes such as depression, anxiety, and desire for death. More important, specific aspects of spiritual well-being and meaning were not consistently targeted as outcomes. Thus, despite the seeming importance of enhancing one's sense of meaning and purpose, few clinical interventions have been developed that attempt to address this critical issue. MCGP was developed in response to the need for interventions that focused on enhancing spiritual well-being.

Two randomized controlled trials of MCGP[55,56] demonstrated the efficacy of MCGP in significantly improving quality of life, spiritual well-being, and a sense of meaning, as well as in decreasing depression, anxiety, hopelessness, desire for hastened death, and diminished symptom burden distress. These beneficial effects are mediated through the enhancement of meaning. These studies provide support for the effectiveness of MCGP as a novel intervention for improving spiritual well-being, a sense of meaning, and psychological functioning in patients with advanced cancer. Large treatment effects emerged after a short-term intervention, and these benefits appeared to increase even in the weeks after treatment ended. MCGP appears to be a highly effective intervention for the enhancement of quality of life for patients at the end of life. A treatment manual for MCGP was published in 2014 and is widely available.[57] MCGP has recently been approved by the National Cancer Institute as an evidence-based intervention with significant benefit to be included and disseminated via the Research-tested Intervention Program website (http://rtips.cancer.gov/rtips/index.do).

MAIN THEMES AND FORMAT OF THE THERAPY

MCGP is an 8-week (1½-hour weekly sessions) group psychotherapy intervention that uses a mix of didactics, discussions, and experiential exercises that are centered around particular themes related to meaning and advanced cancer (Table 2.2). The intention of this intervention is to sustain or enhance a sense of meaning and purpose by teaching patients how to use the breadth of possible sources of meaning as coping resources through a combination of (1) instructed teaching of the concept of meaning on which the intervention is based; (2) group experiential exercises meant to enhance the learning process, followed by homework for each individual patient to complete; and (3) group leader-facilitated discussion aimed at reinforcing the importance of reconnecting to sources of meaning and using such sources of meaning as resources in enhancing meaning. Although the focus of each session is on the concept of meaning/peace (and its sources) and purpose in life in the face of advanced cancer, other existential concepts, such as freedom, responsibility, authenticity, existential guilt, transcendence, and choice, are also incorporated into session content. Elements of support and expression of emotion are inevitable in each session (but are limited

TABLE 2.2 OUTLINE OF MEANING-CENTERED GROUP PSYCHOTHERAPY SESSIONS

Session Topics	Themes
Session 1: Concepts and Sources of Meaning	Introductions and meaning
Session 2: Cancer and Meaning	Identity before and after cancer diagnosis
Session 3: Historical Sources of Meaning	Life as a legacy that has been given
Session 4: Historical Sources of Meaning	Life as a legacy that one lives and will give
Session 5: Attitudinal Sources of Meaning	Encountering life's limitations
Session 6: Creative Sources of Meaning	Creativity, courage, and responsibility
Session 7: Experiential Sources of Meaning	Connecting with life through love, beauty, and humor
Session 8: Transitions	Final reflections and hopes for the future

by the focus on experiential exercises, didactics, and discussions related to themes focusing on meaning).

The following is an overview of each session, including the experiential exercises used to facilitate discussions and greater understanding of meaning. See Appendix 1 for a complete, de-identified, transcript of an entire eight-session MCGP intervention to illustrate in greater detail the procedures, processes, and techniques of MCGP.

Session 1: Concepts and Sources of Meaning

The first session involves introductions of each group member and an overall explanation of the group's goals. Patient introductions include biographical/demographic information, as well as their expectations, hopes, and questions relating to the group. The session concludes with a discussion of what *meaning* means to each participant. The experiential exercise helps patients to discover how they find a sense of meaning and purpose in general, as well as specifically in relation to having been diagnosed with cancer. As an adjunctive to the group, all patients are given a copy of Frankl's *Man's Search for Meaning*[4] as a means of facilitating each patient's understanding of the main themes of the intervention. The experiential exercise for the first session explores meaningful moments identified by the patient from his or her own life (Box 2.1).

The following MCGP excerpt exemplifies the type of interaction that occurs between group members and leaders during the Session 1 experiential exercise:

Therapist 1: If you remember, one of the things I was talking about, to be fully alive means to be creating meaning in your life, identity, direction, hope, love, relationships, and it makes sense that if you are feeling alive, it's those moments that you create meaning that make you feel most alive. And that's the subject of our experiential exercise for today.

Therapist 2: Would someone like to read the experiential exercise on the next page? What I'd like you to do is write down one or two experiences when life felt particularly meaningful to you, or a moment when you felt really alive, and take a few moments and right down your thoughts, and then we'll share it.

Therapist 2 (after 5 minutes of writing): OK, so maybe in the interest of time we'll get started, as I'm noticing that our session is moving quickly towards the end. Would anyone like to volunteer to go first?

L: I'll go first. I've been told by friends and family that I have the "gift of helps." I guess because of my nursing background I help folks. So I had a

BOX 2.1 SESSION 1 EXPERIENTIAL EXERCISE: "MEANINGFUL MOMENTS"

List one or two experiences or moments when life has felt particularly meaningful to you—whether it sounds powerful or mundane. For example, it could be something that helped get you through a difficult day, or a time when you felt most alive. And say something about it.

group of seniors. My dad is 98, my mom lived to 92. I have a group of seniors in my community. I help them navigate the health care system. I feel like a highlight for me has been helping them to navigate the health care system, getting them services, helping them to get the help they need to stay healthy.

Therapist 1: So you have provided help. Compassion.

L: Yes, compassion.

Therapist 1: When you've been compassionate, how did that make you feel?

L: Useful, that I'm using a talent I have, using knowledge I have.

Therapist 1: Using your talents, living to your full potential . . .

L: Thank you.

Therapist 1: It's interesting, you're giving, not taking.

L: Yes, I have difficulty taking.

Therapist 1: Thanks, L. P?

P: The birth of each of my three children. I remember each time. The sense of elation I felt was unparalleled to anything else, but also, the sense of dread. The first one, how do I diaper the baby? How do I take care of it? I guess maybe the middle one, not so much. My kids are 18, 16, and 4. So, clearly we had a "whoopsy" baby, which was unbelievable, since I was a parent of teenagers, and that just, what doesn't kill you makes you stronger. On one hand we couldn't go to sleep because the teenager was out, or we were up because the baby was up. Anyway, so that's the first, personal thing that I'm most happy about.

Professionally, it's a client I had. He was a 30 something man who was retarded and lived with his parents, on Staten Island, and he was their boy. He fell down the steps in their home and he went to the ER, and he had 3 different surgeries on his neck due to previous issues with his spine, and when the doctor in the ER took an x-ray that showed a problem, the doctor just sent him home. Unbelievable. Anyway, he's quadriplegic now, and I represented him, and we sued the hospital and I met this guy several times and he was actually . . . he should be a model for everyone. He's one of the happiest men I've ever met. I got him enough money that they would be able to make it accessible for him, and enough money to have a caretaker. So he can come home and be with his parents.

Therapist 1: Let me make a quick comment, and people feel free to step in. L, you were talking about compassion, but it's also an example of love. And so, really, your story, your example of a meaningful moment was really a source of meaning that we would identify as experiential, love, connectedness with people you care about. You had several sources of meaning, P, love of your children and wife. Very often, important life events are profoundly meaningful, because they have such an impact on so many aspects of our lives, like having children. You became a father. It's very important to your identify, and all this love came into your life. And then you talk about work, and how meaningful work is. And an example of work that is, a case that is, so meaningful. What was so remarkable about him was that despite the fact that he was quadriplegic, he was happy. He controlled the attitude towards his suffering experience. Your life is made up of all these moments when we have choices. . . . This guy chose to have hope, he chose to have a life despite suffering. Hope, this was a choice.

C, you want to go?

C: I didn't have a connection to my children because of my drug history. But, a number of years ago my daughter sent me a note, saying that I'm the greatest dad in the world. That was the happiest moment I can remember, other than the time that I first picked her up. And I looked at her and it scared the crap out of me, and now, I finally got her back. And now, every Wednesday, no matter what happens, we talk, and about everything. I've been alive ever since. It's given me a sense of purpose. And the other thing, I don't have a formal college education. I don't have a paper like you guys have on your walls, I'd love to have that. I don't have something on the wall that says I graduated from . . . but I did pass an exam to become a certified counselor. But, the doctor I work for now came into my office and told me to come in and run the detox group, and I said I don't have any formal training, and she said, "C, you have 20 years of experience of working with people and I believe in you." And that's . . . now I have doctors calling me and asking me what I think!

P: My job, I know an awful lot of lawyers, and I've sued an awful lot of doctors, and none of them are really smarter than you are. I mean, they have degrees on their walls, and some are just brilliant academically, but in terms of being life smart? No, no they're not smarter than you.

C: But you can understand the importance of my passing that test, for my certification? I can't wait to go to work each day . . .

P: Of course.

Therapist 1: You know, people think that you only get meaning in life from happy things, like the birth of children or winning some prize, but it also comes out of suffering experiences, experiences that you might think were shameful, or you might be insecure about, failings, C, your story, your meaningful moment comes out of overcoming limitations, not having an education, not being ... not believing in yourself, but there it was, you had done enough, you experienced redemption, right? And it didn't just come to you out of the blue, you did something to deserve these doctors believing in you, you did something right with your daughter, that led her to write that letter and re-establish that relationship. S, you want to go?

S: Yeah, one of the sweetest moments ... I couldn't have children of my own due to my liver problems. My niece, who's 7, means the world to me. One of the happiest moments was being able to swim with her, and be her playmate, and have her run into my arms and hug me, and at that time last summer, I had enough substance not to be knocked over by her, and to feel the weight of her and her energy and her love and her enthusiasm and her positivity. ... I was enfolded in it. And at the same time, getting so much pleasure, drinking in nature, nature is so spiritual for me, so meaningful. So being outdoors, and connecting with her, and with nature, it's just been such a gift.

And then, because I had a pretty good attitude when I went back after my liver transplant, I went on rounds with the doctors and saw the patients because I could talk to them one way, in a different way than the doctors. I didn't have that piece of paper, but having been through it, I was on the other side, and we all have bumps in a serious operation, there were certain things I was able to say to them about the bumpy road ... just specific things I said due to my experience ... about the healing process, and it was really good. I hadn't been a nurse or a doctor, but now, when I go to see my doctor, I usually try to take an afternoon and see patients who are having problems pre or post transplant.

Therapist 1: Thank you S. Which sources of meaning do you think your two stories tap into?

S: Love, absolutely.

Therapist 1: And what else?

S: Well, experiential, all the senses. And compassion ...

Therapist 1: And creativity. ... It was almost like a job, it was a cause, that you were dedicated to, and you were doing something valuable with your life, seeing these patients. It was unpaid work, but took dedication. A really great example of the creative source of meaning.

Session 2: Cancer and Meaning

Session 2 is a continuation of sharing meaningful experiences, as well as a detailed explanation of what, or who, made these experiences particularly meaningful to patients. In addition, each patient is asked to impart something about his or her identity by answering the question, "Who am I?" This exercise provides the opportunity to discuss how cancer has affected each patient's identity, as well as how cancer has affected what each patient considers to be meaningful in his or her life. The emphasis of this session is the linking of identity as a central element of meaning. The experiential exercise for Session 2 explores what makes the individual who he or she is and how cancer has impacted his or her identity (Box 2.2).

The following MCGP excerpt exemplifies the type of interaction that occurs between group members and leaders during the Session 2 experiential exercise:

Patient A: I am a daughter, a mother, a grandmother, a sister, a friend, and a neighbor. I attempt to respect all people in their views, which sometimes can be difficult. I represent

BOX 2.2 SESSION 2 EXPERIENTIAL EXERCISE: "IDENTITY AND CANCER"

1. Write down four answers to the question, "Who am I?" These can be positive or negative, and include personality characteristics, body image, beliefs, things you do, people you know, etc. For example, answers might start with, "I am someone who ________," or "I am a ________."
2. How has cancer affected your answers? How has it affected the things that are most meaningful to you?

myself honestly and frankly without being offensive, or at least I try. And my philosophy is to do unto others as they would have done unto you. I'm somebody who can be very private and not always share all my needs and concerns. I also have been working on accepting love and affection and other gifts from other people. I'm more of a caregiver than someone who gets care from others, I don't like to receive care, but I'm beginning to, … actually … this may be the one thing that my illness has caused me to mull over. That I'm more accepting of people wanting to do things.

Therapist 1: Thank you. That's really interesting. I want to make some comments, but first let's hear from someone else. Patient B, would you like to go?

Patient B: Well in terms of pre-cancer, I'm my niece's loving aunty who she currently adores … she's seven, I'm not sure how long that will last, but right now, that's really important to me, and it's brought my brother and me closer. I'm active and am always ready for an adventure. All my friends knew I was a "yes let's do it person," enthusiastic, open. I'm a young adult librarian, with a real connection to the teens. I really loved working with them, especially on the advisory council; I really just loved it, and oftentimes would stay very late with them, into the night. I was just, really … connected. … I ran around a lot and I was rarely home before 11 pm. … My friends always asked why I wasn't home more. It wasn't that I didn't like home, it's just that I wanted to be out, experiencing life. I also love concerts, and I danced. And I dated; I was the essence of positive, a very good friend, I'm really proud of that.

Therapist 2: Thanks guys. Do you have any questions for each other about the things that you said? Were there any commonalities that you noticed?

Patient A: I guess the commonality, that most of us spoke about, is being a member of a unique group, a family, and for most of us, that was in the top position. That was most important.

Patient B: I have a comment but I don't know if it's what you're asking for. Patient A was talking about being a giver, but that it's basically hard for her to receive. I've had friends who are like that and it's frustrating to want to give to a person like you, but you also don't want to take people's wishes lightly. … I know I'm probably speaking out of turn for all of your friends, who want to be generous back to you.

Patient A: Most of them have been, … because they, you know, sit me down and do what they want to do. I guess most of my good friends are very strong-willed people like me and they listen and do for the most part what they want. And I don't get offended for the most part.

Therapist 1: It was actually quite striking … that there were many similarities in what you shared about your identities pre-cancer. For many people, the first, the most important source of your identify, had to do with your love relationships, family relationships, your role in a family, being a daughter, father, an aunt, being a member of immediate family. So it's from these connections that we derive meaning in life, through our connectedness with people we love. And often they are members of our family. And, often, these are our sources of identify, as a member of a family, as a father, an aunt …

Patient A: These roles are also source of pain.

Therapist 1: Yes, but also a source of meaning. Do you remember which source of meaning? It's the experiential source of meaning. Through love, connectedness with people. … Someone made a comment that Patient C didn't mention this source of meaning. Patient C, you said something interesting. You said you've been alone too long. But you also said that you're a loyal friend, loyal as a puppy, and a good lover. So for you, love is very relevant for you too. You derive a sense of meaning through friendship and romantic love. Those are all similar, all love, right? Let me ask you something, Patient C, did you leave out being a son, or a family member, for a specific reason?

Patient C: Well, I never knew my dad. I didn't really know my mother until I was older. And I have a brother and a sister, but I'm not close to either of them. So, in a way, my job became more of my family, the people I worked with, people in recovery, they were my family. Because I became more connected to them. But outside of that, no … no real family. So in a sense, family has been a disappointment, pain. So everyone talks about family reunions, I don't have that. That's not a part of my life.

Therapist 1: So again this idea comes up that the things that give us meaning are the sources of pain. The other thing I heard that was common for other people, besides love and connectedness to other people, is connectedness to other kinds of experiences in life, like dancing, and Patient D, you were talking about baking, cooking … so it's not just relationships with people, it's relationships to the world, and being in nature, and engaging in pleasurable things, like dancing and eating. And in addition to that, several people talked about their identify coming from what they did for work, being a nurse, a lawyer, a librarian . . . your work, these are creative sources of meaning, because we derive meaning through things we create, the work we do in our lives. And you added something interesting, Patient A, that had to do with . . . I think I used the word compassion. . . . It had to do with caring for other people?

Patient A: Well, you know, you talked about our professions, but I didn't actually talk today about my professional life, I didn't say anything about being a nurse or a health care provider, but I talked about being a caretaker. A caretaker in general, to the people in my life.

Therapist 1: Exactly. So this creative source of meaning doesn't just come from a job you get paid to do, but from the person you create in the world. You've created a person who is loving, giving, and caring. You've created a virtue, a value, compassion is important, caring for others is important. So it's not just the job you do, but the kind of person you become and create in the world, and what values that represents, that is meaningful to you.

Sessions 3 and 4: Historical Sources of Meaning

Sessions 3 and 4 focus on giving patients a chance to share their life story with the group, which helps them to better appreciate past accomplishments while still elucidating future goals. The theme of Session 3 is "Life as a legacy that has been given" via the past, such as legacy given through one's family of origin. The facts of our lives that have been created by our genetics and the circumstances of our past are discussed in terms of how they have shaped us and perhaps motivated us to transcend limitations. Session 4 focuses on "Life as a legacy that one lives and will give," in terms of patients' living legacy and the legacy they hope to leave for others. The Session 3 experiential exercise helps patients to understand the ways in which their pasts have shaped what they find meaningful, and the Session 4 experiential exercise fosters a discussion of future goals, no matter how small. As a homework assignment after Session 4, patients are asked to tell their life story to a loved one(s) in their life, highlighting experiences that have been a source of meaning and pride for them and things they wished they might have accomplished but have yet to do. The experiential exercise for Session 3 allows the patient the opportunity to explore and express meaningful past experiences in order to uncover the historical context of his or her living legacy (Box 2.3).

The following MCGP excerpt exemplifies the type of interaction that occurs between group members and leaders during the Session 3 experiential exercise:

Therapist 2: Why don't you take a few minutes to review the questions about life as a legacy that has been given, and then we'll go around and listen and discuss your answers.

A, can we start with you today?

Patient A: Ok. So, when I look back on my life and upbringing . . . my family offers me the most significant memories. One being, I'm much younger than my brother and two sisters, so at one point I felt like an only child, they're 3 years apart each, and then there's a 6-year gap, and then me. So in some ways I felt like an only child. And I do remember the recurring theme that I was "too young," too young to go bike riding, to go to the movies, not old enough to join them . . . so I felt excluded.

BOX 2.3 SESSION 3 EXPERIENTIAL EXERCISE: "LIFE AS A LEGACY" THAT HAS BEEN GIVEN

1. When you look back on your life and upbringing, what are the most significant memories, relationships, traditions, etc., that have made *the greatest impact on who you are today?*

For example: Identify specific memories of how you were raised that have made a lasting impression on your life (e.g., your relationship with parents, siblings, friends, teachers, etc.). What is the origin of your name? What are some past events that have meaningfully touched your life?

And then I wrote down about my name. I know how I got my name. My father didn't want an Irish name, like my siblings . . . so he chose T. Although ironically, it actually is Irish, but he didn't know. I have read about the meaning of my name a long time ago, and if I remember correctly, it has something to do with harvesting crops, or something like that.

And events that touched my life? The major events I'd say, the first was going away to boarding school at age 13, and then the second was when I was 16. I just sort of, I contracted a very rare circulation disorder that came out when I was at boarding school that almost killed me. I was taken to the children's hospital of Philadelphia and they thought I wouldn't survive and I was the first person to survive that in the US.

Therapist 1: Thank you, T. I'm going to wait to comment until a few more people have gone. B?

Patient B: I considered myself to be a cross-breed, a product of an African American woman and Afro-Caribbean man. They married in 1939, very unusual for those cultures to be together, but it was a very proud Black household. I was raised in an extended family-type situation. My grandmother raised 6 children on her own. We all lived together in a four-story brownstone, where my dad still lives. At times there were 13 of us there. My cousins were more like brothers and sisters to me. As the oldest girl child in my generation, I got a lot of opportunities that most African American children didn't get. At age 9 I spent the summer in Europe and got to visit 10–13 countries. My uncle was in the service and could bring his family there. So that started my wanderlust for travel. I was very close to my family, my father. As an adult, they were also my best friends, very supportive. Education very important to them, my dad is 101. Still a doctor. One of the oldest living Black doctors. Which is rare. Productivity, responsibility, both were very important to them. So, yeah, I think that's it.

Therapist 1: That's very rich. Can I say a few things? That's really interesting that A and B, your stories, they almost represented the opposite ends of a certain spectrum. From the perspective of the kinds of things that I think about when I think about sources of meaning and how meaning in your life forms. A, you talked about being the only child, felt like the only child, and the more powerful events in your life were about being sent away, being on your own, and so I got the sense that being disconnected from everyone else, those moments were moments of meaning. And for B, your moments were all about family and connecters, and family being supportive and resources for each other. You, A, you talked about being the youngest, and you B, the oldest, roles which have different sets of expectations. What you talked about B was being the oldest child in a family with high standards and expectations, and you A were talking about being "too young," not being able to do very much. "You aren't even baked yet!" That was the message you got. The ingredients were raw. So you wonder how those two sets of expectations affected how you both went about creating a life. Would you say they did?

Patient B: Oh yes, burdensome at times, even, such high expectations. I was supposed to be a mentor, supposed to be a teacher, someone the younger children looked up to, not an easy road necessarily.

Therapist 1: And T how'd that feel?

Patient B: Lonely. I was left alone.

Therapist 1: Were you burdened by that?

Patient B: I don't think so . . .

Therapist 1: So the issue of having this family history, experiences you had as a child, for you, sometimes they're burdensome, and sometimes, not, they can be gifts.

Patient B: Yes, I see the general experience as a gift, I had many gifts, I was very blessed, but at the same time a lot was expected of me, I *could not* fail.

Therapist 1: So do you think being alone was a burden, T?

Patient A: Yes and no. I learned how to entertain myself, so I didn't get bored. And I don't now.

Therapist 1: So you developed that ability to be on your own. Sometimes good things become burdensome, sometimes negative things become gifts, right? They encourage you to grow in other ways.

Session 4 explores the present and future components of legacy in the second experiential exercise (Box 2.4).

The following MCGP excerpt exemplifies the type of interaction that occurs between group members and leaders during the Session 4 experiential exercise:

Therapist 2: Today the focus is really on the present and future—the legacy that you live and

BOX 2.4 SESSION 4 EXPERIENTIAL EXERCISE: "LIFE AS A LEGACY" THAT YOU LIVE AND WILL GIVE

1. As you reflect upon who you are today, what are the meaningful activities, roles, or accomplishments that you are most proud of? As you look toward the future, what are some of the life lessons you have learned along the way that you would want to pass on to others?
2. What is the legacy you hope to live and give?

will give, the one you are actively creating now, and the one that you will leave for others.

Therapist 1: So today, yes, it's really about ... when we asked you all last session to define "legacy" for us, many of you, most of you shared thoughts that really had to do with this notion of legacy. The second part, what you hope to leave for others when you are no longer here. Which, I know, is a difficult thought. So, we started a bit late today and for time sake, I want to jump right in to the experiential exercise, which is really focused on the ways in which you are actively, currently, creating your legacies, and those things which you hope to pass on to others.

Therapist 2: A, would you like to go first?

Patient A: Sure. In 1975, 30 years ago, when I found out that I was sick with a very serious liver problem, despite the fact that I didn't drink or anything. They were already wondering about my life span, if I should work, and I already knew that I couldn't have children. My greatest accomplishment? I've lived my life despite being ill, I've held a career, had two marriages, close relationships, been self-sufficient, and was really into sports and dance. Despite what the doctors were saying, I contained that someplace and did everything I wanted to do, and maybe even more, because life was already precious. And in terms of my career, I really loved my career, and in terms of a legacy that I might leave, it's the message to the teens that I work with that they can really make a difference. I've never thought of myself as creative in the artistic sense, and I've always rationalized it by saying that everyone needs an audience, but in my career, I was incredibly creative, thinking out of the box so often. Another key aspect of my legacy is my perseverance. I persevered when I got divorced the first time, I realized that I couldn't just keep my house by the work I did as a librarian, and so I took out a loan and bought my husband out of the house, and that took a lot of time and energy, to get the money together, but I did, so that I could have some stability in my life. More importantly, in terms of perseverance, is seeking what I desperately need. Of course that's been getting a very good doctor at MSKCC, and so in terms of legacy and medicine, I would say, teaching others to not always accept what one doctor says to you. It took me a long time to learn to defend myself and seek info elsewhere. And of course, being an active part of my niece's life is a key aspect of my legacy, and I hope those things that I deem important, she will too.

Therapist 1 : I hope that you'll still have something to say about the second part of the exercise, A, but what's interesting about what you're saying, B and C were talking about family and creative sources of meaning in terms of work, and experiential sources of meaning in terms of love, and you spoke about creative sources of meaning as well in the less traditional ways, but also, what you spoke about is the importance of the attitude that you took towards the circumstances you were in, in the face of suffering and limitations—with the house, for example—that attitude was something that you're quite proud of in terms of how you've lived your life. Is that correct?

Patient A: Yeah, you've put it in a nutshell.

Session 5: Attitudinal Sources of Meaning

This session examines each patient's confrontation with limitations in life and the ultimate limitation—our mortality and the finiteness of life. This session focuses on our freedom to choose our attitudes toward such limitations and find meaning in life, even in the face of death. In discussing the experiential exercise, group leaders emphasize Frankl's core theoretical belief that by choosing our attitude toward circumstances that are beyond our control (e.g., cancer and death), we may find meaning in life and suffering, which will then help us to rise above or overcome such limitations. One of the more critical elements of this session involves the experiential exercise in which patients are asked to discuss their thoughts, feelings, and concepts of what constitutes a "good" or meaningful death. Common issues that have arisen include where patients prefer to die (e.g., at home in their own bed), how they want to die (e.g., without pain and surrounded by family), and what patients expect takes place after death—funeral fantasies, family issues, and the afterlife. This exercise is designed to detoxify the discussion of death and to allow for a safe examination of the life they have lived and how they may be able to accept that life. Inherent in these discussions are issues of tasks of life completion, forgiveness, and redemption. At the end of Session 5, patients are presented with the "Legacy Project," which integrates ideas presented in treatment (e.g., meaning, identity, creativity, and responsibility), in order to facilitate the generation of a sense of meaning in light of cancer. Some examples of Legacy Projects include creating a legacy photo album or video, mending a broken relationship, or undertaking something the patient has always wanted to do but has not yet done. The experiential exercise for this session allows the patient to reflect on times when he or she has faced obstacles and limitations in the past (Box 2.5).

The following MCGP excerpt exemplifies the type of interaction that occurs between group members and leaders during the Session 5 experiential exercise:

Therapist 1: Today's focus is on what we call the attitudinal source of meaning, which really refers to the situations in our lives where we've encountered some kind of limitation and as human beings, we're often driven to create a life and a trajectory or direction, forward, up, and so when you encounter limitations that prevent this movement, it can cause us to stress or suffer. There are all sorts of limitations—the ones that you all are experiencing now in terms of cancer and your physical capabilities, fatigue, stamina, pain—and for all of us, the ultimate limitation is the finiteness of life, the fact of death. And so what this attitudinal source of meaning is about is, no matter what situation you find yourself in, your sense of control and loss, what is it that you do still have the ability to control? And this boils down to the attitude that you take towards your situation. The idea is that you're trying to transcend or overcome the limitations, live fully within the limitations.

Sometimes it's a difficult concept to really grasp, but through the experiential exercise I think we'll be able to flesh this all out. We're all confronted by the same limitations of the finiteness of life, and this is made all the more real with cancer. So that's the focus of today's exercise.

Therapist 2: There are really three exercises to do today, and we'll try to get through them all. The first has to do with losses, limitations or obstacles you faced in the past, how you dealt with them, coped with them in the past, what did you do? How did you overcome them?

Therapist 1: A, you seem ready, you want to start?

Patient A: I guess so. Life's limitations. When I first looked at that question, the current

BOX 2.5 SESSION 5 EXPERIENTIAL EXERCISE: "ENCOUNTERING LIFE'S LIMITATIONS"

1. What are some of the life limitations, losses, or obstacles that you have faced in the past, and how did you cope or deal with them at the time?
2. Since your diagnosis, what are the specific limitations or losses you have faced, and how are you coping or dealing with them now? Are you still able to find meaning in your daily life despite your awareness of the limitations and finiteness of life? (If yes, please briefly describe.)
3. What would you consider a "good" or "meaningful" death? How can you imagine being remembered by your loved ones? (For example, what are some of your personal characteristics, the shared memories, or meaningful life events that have made a lasting impression on them?)

situation is so much bigger than any past trauma I've had to think about. It just is. But, looking back, I guess, the first major limitation I encountered was when I was a teenager my parents split up. When I look back now, it's decades ago . . .

Therapist 1: And you had shared that you've begun to reconcile with your dad . . .

Patient A: But you know, at the time, divorce I guess was coming into fashion, but as a kid I was the only one I knew who had parents who were getting divorced and so I felt in that way like an outsider. The way I dealt with it was in some degree, I rebelled. I know I hung out with kids who my mother definitely didn't approve of, I smoked and drank and did a lot of stereotypical things that teenagers do, and ultimately, it took going to college and putting some distance between myself and my family situation to start feeling better. And I dealt with the anger, and I got over it.

The second limitation was about a year before my cancer diagnosis, I was not getting along with my wife. I just, and, um, I'm not a particularly vocal person about my feelings, I felt like she would criticize me when I shared feelings and so I stopped, I just became passive aggressive. It lasted for 6 months. And I went to her eventually and I told her that I didn't feel anything anymore. And once I said it, I realized that that wasn't the case. I guess what I learned was that I have to say things before I internalize them so much that I end up saying things that are just blatant lies. So, yeah, those are the two major ones.

Therapist 1: So A, one was about your family of origin and a lot of emotion, and the second was about feeling an absence of emotion. And so both situations were challenges that involved losses, the loss of your family, and your parents splitting up, and the other was a sense of loss that you were feeling with your wife, loss of connection. When you said the way you dealt with your anger, it sounds like you had to think about the feelings you were having in order to really believe them? To accept them as true?

Patient A: Yes, I did. With my wife, you know, I'm not perfect, neither is she. And there are certain things about her. She's not the most observant, of, things, which may be part of the reason why I ended up repressing things and doing what I did. But it's not for lack of caring, but it's just a capability that she doesn't have. And either you accept it or you don't.

Therapist 2: So it's about change or acceptance?

Patient A: Well, did she change? It was a change in my attitude.

Therapist 1: Exactly. Did that change your marriage at all?

Patient A: It did.

Therapist 1 : For the worse? For better?

Patient A: For the better, completely. We transformed as a couple. It went from my being monosyllabic to being a couple again.

Therapist 2: Ok. Before we run out of time, let's try to tackle this third question here. This one's a hard one, I'm not going to pretend it's not. But another limitation, the ultimate limitation, is death. Everyone is aware of that, even before cancer, but with cancer, we all become more aware of it. So the last question is really asking you to think your death and what would be the ideal way, the best way, what would be the circumstances, how would you want to be remembered. I know this is hard, but let's see if we can get through this last one. Who wants to start?

Patient C: Um, I hope I'll be remembered lovingly as a good role model and as a person who had values and standards that were clear for others to see. That I cared and gave to others, helped when I could. And that, you know, my attempt was to steer the young people in a positive direction, talk about things that were meaningful, give them standards that were important for them to achieve. With education being important, meaningful work, doing the right thing.

Therapist 1: In terms of a good or meaningful death?

Patient C: A good or meaningful death? I don't know how to answer that. One without too much pain, hopefully! I don't fear dying, per se. I believe in an afterlife. But I do fear the process. The discomfort, pain, whatever. If that gets to be a part of the process, I won't have control but that's what I fear.

Patient D: I wrote, dying with dignity and on my own terms, no matter where I may be. But ideally, at home, as opposed to the sterile hospital or hospice. And I want to be remembered for the person I am, nothing glorified, nothing more. I don't want people to say about me things they wouldn't say to me now. So nothing more or less, that I'm a good person, a friend, a family member. I know they all realize this. I want them to say these things to me now, just like they will then. I mean, they already say them so I know them to be true. So basically, I just want to have a little bit of control. Dying with dignity and on my own terms. That's what's important to me.

Therapist 2: Thanks, D. E?

Patient E: In terms of a good death, the dying part of it, I would very much like it to be painless, and I've already arranged with long-term care to try to die at home, not at the hospital, and not have extraordinary measures be taken. A good death would be if I achieved something by dying. If I could save someone's life in the process of dying, that would be a good death.

Therapist 1: A heroic death?

Patient E: Yeah. One of the things I was thinking was maybe I should do something really adventurous and daring, where I could potentially die, like hang-gliding, but someone said to me when I suggested that, that I could just break every bone and be in pain, so I revised that, but if I knew I could just die, I would be scared, but would be great to do something really daring, really take a risk. So, that was about dying. I actually think it's good that I've given this thought, in terms of a living will, I want to be near a window near the air, I'm so afraid of being in an airless room, a tank, and that was even before I had trouble breathing. I really just want to be by fresh air, I want to be by nature until the end. And I certainly agree with L, I'd like to leave with integrity and standards and have people think that I've done the right thing.

Therapist 1: So these virtues are important to you, passing those on?

Patient E: Yes, for them to remember everything that I've added to their lives, in terms of laughter and fun and adventure.

Session 6: Creative Sources of Meaning

Session 6 focuses on "creativity" as a source and resource of meaning in life. One important element of the experiential exercises deals with the issue of "responsibility" (our ability to respond to the fact of our existence—to answer the question, "What life have we created for ourselves?"). Patients are asked to discuss what their responsibilities are, as well as for whom they are responsible. Any unfinished business or tasks patients may have are also examined. This discussion forces group members to focus on the task at hand, as opposed to focusing only on their suffering. In addition, by attending to their responsibility to others, meaning may be enhanced by the realization that their lives transcend themselves and extend to others. The experiential exercise for this session allows patients to explore the concepts of creativity, courage, and responsibility in their own lives (Box 2.6).

The following MCGP excerpt exemplifies the type of interaction that occurs between group members and leaders during the Session 6 experiential exercise:

Therapist 1: Today, we're going to focus on creativity, our engagement in the world. So, basically our job is, when we're born, the question is, how do you respond to this fact that you're alive? You find the world calling to you to pursue something. And that is part of what we mean by creating a life. So in simplistic terms, it's meaning that comes from creating your life, your life's work, although it could be other commitments in your life, could be a cause you're dedicated to, a value that's so important to you. What's really interesting is

BOX 2.6 SESSION 6 EXPERIENTIAL EXERCISE: "ACTIVELY ENGAGING IN LIFE"

1. Living life and being creative requires courage and commitment. Can you think of a time(s) in your life when you have been courageous, taken ownership of your life, or made a meaningful commitment to something of value to you?
2. Do you feel you have expressed what is most meaningful to you through your life's work and creative activities (e.g., job, parenting, and causes)? If so, how?
3. What are your responsibilities? Who are you responsible to and for?
4. Do you have unfinished business? What tasks have you always wanted to do but have yet to undertake? If so, what do you think is holding you back?

that this notion of having to create your life, if you're religious, you might say God created and determined this for you, but if you're not, the responsibility for creating your life lies on you. So this issue of responsibility and creativity are very much linked, the idea that how you respond to being alive, by creating a life that's unique to you, and trying to live that life to its fullest potential, and that's your responsibility. I like to play on the word responsibility. Responsibility is really your ability to respond to life, to being alive. So I find the notion of responsibility interesting, as it relates to this exercise.

So there are four questions today, the first two have to do with ways in which you've been creative, ways in which you've engaged in life fully, and as you can probably tell, it takes a little bit of courage . . .

Patient A: To live?

Therapist 1: Yes, to live. To live with adversity, with cancer, and threat of cancer and all that it can do to you. It takes courage to keep wanting to live, to keep loving people you might lose. So I thought maybe we'd first select one question from the first group, and one then from the second group of questions. How does that sound?

Patient A: That works.

Patient B: Yeah, that's fine.

Therapist 1: How would you feel about doing the courage one? Living life and being creative requires courage and commitment. Can you think of times in your life when you've been courageous, taken ownership of your life, and made a meaningful commitment to something of value to you?

Patient A: Something that you said, about the word despite, despite the absolute of cancer, and the limitations that cancer has. When first getting cancer, and other blows from cancer, like the mets, I'm not good for a while. I don't seem courageous, I'm dissolving in a puddle of tears, or I'm frantic, or I'm wondering how I'd ever cope, and then it's eventually getting used to the idea, getting to the new normal. People ask me how I cope and I don't cope at all, really. I completely drown in fear, thinking about how much worse it could get, it's the opposite of what you're talking about, I feel like I have no courage. It's eventually getting to the point of responding, eventually learning to pick myself up. So, there's no continuum here, there are peaks and valleys, I mean I don't know if that's been your experience, B, that there's been a process of pulling together to cope, B, but I know that I'm just going through that right now, knowing that one of my cancer markers skyrocketed. I don't feel courageous at all right now.

Patient B: I'm just hoping that the progress is slow. People keep saying to me "Well, once you get better . . .". And I keep saying, "I hope," but I don't have that much control, I only have a certain amount of control, I certainly think lifestyle and diet contribute, and I'm doing my best to eat well, healthfully, and do alternative therapies and drinking all these different types of tea that are supposed to cut off oxygen to tumors.

Therapist 1: So on one level, courage is incredibly important when coping with cancer, and like S, do you feel like you have moments when you can sum up some courage and others when you're very frightened?

Patient B: Yeah, definitely. I remember when I first learned of the recurrence, every test was coming back with more and more bad news, and it was crushing me, I felt like I couldn't take all of it. And then I started psych meds, the psych team started showing up in my room.

Therapist 1: Ha Ha, It's always a bad sign when that happens!

Therapist 1: I think one more exercise fits in nicely with what we're been talking about. The third question is about responsibilities. What are your responsibilities? Who are you responsible to and for?

Patient B: I wrote down that I'm just responsible for myself, right now. It's a relatively easy answer for me. Honestly, I'm just responsible for me.

Therapist 2: That's living authentically, that's your life right now. Just like when you were 16 you took care of yourself, and now, you're doing the same.

Patient B: And I'm doing an ok job.

Therapist 2: It sounds like you're doing more than an ok job.

Patient C: I was also going to say that I'm mostly responsible to myself. And I guess my brother and sister-in-law and my niece as well, but I think they could all live without me. I mean, my niece is very attached to me and would be devastated without me, but they would all live just fine, I think.

Therapist 1: So you both are number one on your list as being responsible to yourselves. But what does that actually mean to you guys?

Patient B: I'm responsible for feeding, clothing, getting medical care, having a roof over my head, taking care of all things, which is not easy, and you know I still need help sometimes, I can't really work and do very much outside of taking care of the cancer. And I'm in a lot of pain.

Patient C: I've been responsible for myself for many decades now.

Therapist 1: So you would have answered the question in the same way 10–15 years ago?

Patient C: No, things were different then. I felt there was more potential then.

Therapist 1: Meaning?

Patient C: I wasn't as sick, my illness didn't limit so much of what I did. I delight in doing better than what the doctors would think. My whole life I've always tried to do beyond what on paper I was supposed to do. But now I'm feeling more of the restrictions.

Therapist 1: So would you have said you're responsible for other people?

Patient C: Yeah, an entire department at work, and now I just cover one desk. I was someone who was taking care of others, close friends and cousins. I didn't need as much help as I do now.

Therapist 1: When we were first developing this, I used to do the exercise with the patients, and so when it came to this exercise, I wrote down my own answer, and I would right down everyone in my world, but not myself, not me, I left that off. So it's really amazing that both of you have come to this place of knowing that you're responsible to yourselves. One after the other, my patients had themselves on their list, but I didn't. So at first, I said to myself, this must be some selfish thing that you're all putting that down . . .

Patient B: No, it's unselfish.

Therapist 1: Right, a patient said to me, Dr. B., that's unselfish for you to take care of yourself. If you don't take care of yourself, you can't take care of others. They said, cancer teachers you that right away. And it will burden those who take care of you, if you don't also take care. You said it's unselfish, what does that mean?

Patient B: If I take responsibility and have my needs met, then I'm not burdening others.

Therapist 1: So being a burden is a concern?

Patient B: I mean, I am a bit of a burden, and I do feel badly that they have to come here since I can't travel down to the Bahamas to see them, but just so that I don't have to increase their burden, it's a big thing. I don't want anyone to have to pay for anything, that's the biggest thing, that my medical costs are taken care of.

Session 7: Experiential Sources of Meaning

Session 7 focuses on discussing experiential sources of meaning, such as love, beauty, and humor. Whereas creative and attitudinal sources of meaning suggest more of an *active involvement with life*, experiential sources embody more of a *passive or even sensory engagement with life*. Patients explore moments and experiences when they have felt connected with life through love, beauty, and humor. Often, the discussions highlight how these sources of meaning become particularly important for patients since their cancer diagnosis. Feelings concerning the group's upcoming termination are discussed in preparation for the final session. During the experiential exercise for this, patients are invited to provide examples of ways they connect to these sources of meaning (Box 2.7).

The following MCGP excerpt exemplifies the type of interaction that occurs between group members and leaders during the Session 7 experiential exercise:

Therapist 2: Take a few moments to write a few answers down to the question about how you connect to life and feel alive through the experience of love, beauty, and humor.

Patient A: Sometimes I just sit back, with my brothers and sisters and family, and sit back and listen to them, whatever they're doing, whether they're fighting or having a good

BOX 2.7 SESSION 7 EXPERIENTIAL EXERCISE: "CONNECTING WITH LIFE"

List three ways in which you connect with life and feel most alive through the experiential sources of

1. Love
2. Beauty
3. Humor

time. I'm just content with having them around me, just receiving, just being in the moment.

Therapist 1: You said something really beautiful B to me outside of group that I'd like to repeat if that's ok. You were walking on the grounds of XYZ hospital and you saw this building, and its beauty stood out to you, and you felt, I think the word you used was, exhilarated?

Patient B: I was just really excited by the prospect of seeing such an interesting and different and beautiful building, it was Frank Gehry architecture. I was in awe. Finding it was amazing.

Therapist 1: And in that moment, did you lose a sense of the present?

Patient B: Yes, everything else just dissipated. Time, space, everything.

Therapist 1: You were connected to everything.

Patient B: I was pretty thrilled.

Therapist 1: Did you write down anything else?

Patient B: In terms of love, I of course put my niece, and I haven't really mentioned my brother, and my cousins in England, and my friends. And then I put water and great music. There are times when I hear a note of music and I can almost just start to cry. It takes you beyond your situation. I forget everything else when that happens.

Therapist 1: Do you have a favorite piece of music?

Patient B: I don't know. It can be anything. The other day I was really struck by an opera piece, and I'm not really into opera, but I heard one aria and I couldn't believe how beautiful it was and I was so transported, so taken away by it. It was the tone that connects you to the universe.

Therapist 1: And what about humor?

Patient B: Definitely. My friends at the library usually go out about once a month, we went out a few weeks ago and were laughing the entire night, before we even got to the table. We had our own jokes and had such a good time. Just such good moments.

And I also seek out TV shows that have humor in them, because they also transport me. Sometimes when I feel upset I'll just go to YouTube and try to find something funny to watch.

Therapist 1: D?

Patient D: Love, of my children and grandchildren, nieces and nephews. Their sense of awe, they look at me as if I know everything, or at least did when they were little. But yes, there is great love there. Museums and concerts. And I have a love of worship, I love liturgical music. There's nothing more beautiful than hearing the songs of the Church.

In terms of beauty, I feel calm and peace near a body of water. I love the sound of the waves, it's just the calmest. I always thought of myself as a New Yorker, I would never move anywhere if it was far from water. But when I think about vacations, it's always about water.

Therapist 1: Do you have a favorite place?

Patient D: I guess it is Barbados. I mean, there's the cultural connection.

And I see beauty in the faces of children of different cultures. I love looking at books or TV documentaries where you see children of different ethnic groups.

I also love flowers and plants, although I'm not talented like T in that respect. I'm not a farmer or gardener, but I do admire them. I love fresh flowers.

In terms of humor, years ago when I was feeling down I would always put on the movie, *Too Wong Foo*? Or something like that? They're all dressed in drag there? It always made me laugh, always made me feel better. And then, I hope this is not misunderstood, coming from a Caribbean culture, I grew up in a community where most of my friends were Barbadian Americans, so we would have fun mocking the speech patterns, the nuances of the natives. One of the funniest experiences was going to court in Barbados and seeing all these black folk dressed up as the English, with white wigs.

Patient B: They take it very seriously!

Patent D: I know!

Patient E: And that's even funnier!

Therapist 1: And F, I bet that's one thing about being a lawyer in the US. I bet you don't mind not having to do.

Patient F: That's true, I don't have a powdered wig.

Session 8: Transitions

The final session provides an opportunity to review patients' Legacy Projects, as well as to review individual and group themes. In addition, the group is asked to discuss topics such as the following: (1) How has the group been experienced? (2) Have there been changes in attitudes toward your illness or suffering? and (3) How do you envision continuing what has been started in the group? The experiential exercise that ends this session focuses on answering the question, "What are your hopes for the future?" The experiential exercise for the final session facilitates discussion of transitions and the future (Box 2.8).

The following MCGP excerpt exemplifies the type of interaction that occurs between group members and leaders during the Session 8 experiential exercise:

Therapist 2: So, welcome everyone. All of a sudden we're here at Session 8, or at least it seems like all of a sudden, and there's a lot to reflect on today and talk about today. And I had spoken to a few of you in the interim about the Legacy Projects, so we will want to take some time to see if anyone came in with projects this week. I know E, you had mentioned to me that you were going to bring something in, would you like to go first?

Patient E: Sure. Well, I just brought in a series of pictures, and all of them except for one, I took of myself by myself of me. The first is me and my dog in Cape May . . .

Group: He's so cute!

Therapist 2: Great picture!

Patient D: And you look great!

Patient E: Thanks guys. I love him so much, and I'm excited because I just booked my ticket to go home in 2 weeks to see him, and my family. So I'll have to get some treats and other things for him. And then the other picture is just this last weekend, this is me and my college roommate, she and I went to the Walk for the Cure. I didn't walk but I registered and we went and just watched. And the third, that's me and C, my niece. Last Christmas, so she's important.

Therapist 1: So what do these pictures represent?

Patient E: They all represent important things to me . . . people, places, time. I love my niece and my college roommate. All of them are recent, maybe all except for the dog.

Therapist 2: Thanks for sharing these meaningful pictures.

Therapist 1: Are you going to share them with anyone else?

Patient E: My mother, many people have seen them, just not all together at once.

Therapist 1: That's a beautiful set of pictures, and what I think is beautiful, aside from having you in them, is that they represent all the people that you love and your passions in life.

Therapist 1: So they represent experiential and creative sources of meaning . . . so it's a meaningful legacy project.

Therapist 1: So what has it been like to be in this group?

Patient A: I wrote, it's been a positive experience to find meaning, it makes my life feel lighter.

Therapist 2: It makes you feel lighter?

Patient A: It's a joyful experience, not a sorrowful one. It's not like you're doing it all the time. And I guess I've realized that if you look for it, it's always there. All you need to do is look. If you look, you'll find it. Just my looking at the squirrels out my window, I can find meaning in that. So before I might not have said that, and I guess now I realize that my life really does have a lot of meaning. If you say there is no meaning, then you're really just not looking.

Therapist 1: So there's a choice to find meaning, to see it?

Patient A: Yeah, totally.

Therapist 1: It's a little like what E said, about choosing to find it, to look for it, it's always there.

Patient A: I mean, I never thought my life was meaningless, but I never sat down and looked for specific meanings, either. So I've found this a positive experience that's made me feel lighter, because there's an awful lot of stress

BOX 2.8 SESSION 8 EXPERIENTIAL EXERCISE: "REFLECTION AND FEEDBACK"

1. What has it been like for you to go through this learning experience over these past seven sessions? Have there been any changes in the way you view your life and cancer experience having been through this process?
2. Do you feel like you have a better understanding of the sources of meaning in life, and are you able to use them in your daily life? If so, how?
3. What are your hopes for the future?

and strain when you're sick, and it changes from week to week and day to day and so it's nice to be able to figure out what's meaningful to you, and what you give meaning to, because you can then have that with you no matter what type of week or day you're having.

Therapist 1: What do you guys think about what A just shared?

Patient F: I think it makes a lot of sense. And what I hear her saying, and I guess for me, meaning translates into a connectedness. Whether it's with people, or nature, or animals, or whatever, the things that you enjoy doing, that you get pleasure and comfort out of, I think it can be very simple, like the last few weeks, I was really just communicating with nature, just watching the lake, and being outside. Just simple, a little bit of nothing, but looking at God's love and let go of the stress or feel connected through my belly, on a gut level, is usually for me in nature, watching the sunset, or the water, it's always different. So I think it's interesting to find that that connectedness is life, you know, it's life at its best. And what you're saying is that you may have cancer, but, you can still connect, and still find meaning. And I think that's the point of this intervention you call this.

Therapist 1: That's so well said! I hope we're recording this.

Therapist 2: We are . . .

Therapist 1: This is really, this is exactly what we had hoped you guys would have come away with from this intervention.

Therapist 1: The second question has to do with whether you have a better understanding of these different sources of meaning and if you're better able to put them to work in your life. And I think you've all already addressed some of this, begun to talk about this. I would imagine in the beginning when we talked about meaning, it was a very abstract concept, right?

Patient E: It was. At first, I was searching to come up with something, but now, it's just right there. Once I thought about it, it was easier, it was right there.

Therapist 2: You know, the language that you're using, that's changed as well. It's really very striking.

Patient F: You should actually be sending us these tapes! So that we have a record of this! We maybe could continue to learn from them, learn phrases we didn't fully get at first.

Therapist 1: Do you guys want to add anything to your answers? Did you get a notion from the 8 weeks that we wanted you to understand that there were very available and understandable sources of meaning in life, and all you have to do is recognize that they're there, and know that a lot of it has to do with connectedness, to people, causes, work, history, values, and also, overcoming and choosing your attitude towards your suffering? And did you also get the idea that it was helpful to know these different sources of meaning so that you could move around from one to another if you had to?

Group: Yes, yes.

Therapist 1: Which brings us to the last exercise. If you can take a few minutes and write down some thoughts about your hopes for the future . . .

Patient B: Well my hopes for the future are to get better and live life to the fullest physically, given all that cancer has limited for me. I've been limited physically much more so than mentally. But they're, the symptoms, they're getting better. So I'm hoping they'll get so better that I don't have them anymore. And also, to make as much as I can with what limitations I'm feeling. Not let the physical stuff consume me, and not wallow in self-pity. It's ok to do that once in a while, but to stay there is not good. So to do the best that I can, given whatever is going on, on a given day. To keep my mind in a positive place. To choose to be hopeful, not hopeless. So, to be as light as I can to fill each day, is what I hope to gain.

Therapist 1: A lightness.

Patient B: Yes. To have my mind as free of anxiety and worry as possible.

Therapist 1: That was really beautiful. You've really become a meaning-centered therapist.

Patient D: My hope is to try to stay in some kind of good shape for as long as I can and take advantage of the fact that I feel pretty ok most of the time. I also want to work on being less intimidating, and be easier to get along with. And there are people who I've offended, and so I want to make some amends.

Therapist 1: Amend friendships.

Patient D: Yes. And to be more open to people's imperfections.

Therapist 1: Forgiving?

Patient D: To be more tolerant. And not always have to be jumping in and doing things on my own. And also, to accept offers and love from others without feeling like I'm being a burden. And I want to share my family experiences with my grandchildren.

Therapist 2: So your legacy is important to pass on.

Therapist 1: And all those things are particularly meaningful given all that you said the first week. Those things were all so hard for you.

Patient D: Yeah. They were. I hadn't come here as the most open person.

Therapist 1: Are those tears of sadness, D? Joy? Mixture?

Patient D: They're just . . . emotions.

Therapist 1: Emotions. Ok. Thank you, that was beautiful.

Therapist 1: So it's hard to realize, but we've come to the end of our eight sessions. Today was a very beautiful session. It's hard to end things when they're so beautiful. Maybe better to end when you're happy?

Patient F: Well, it's hard to end something that's been so helpful.

Therapist 1: Let me just say on my behalf, it's always this great privilege, as a physician, to become this intimate with people. It's an honor and on some level this has felt like a sacred experience, because you've all shared so many meaningful experiences in here. You've shared sadness and hopes and dreams and for that I'm extremely grateful. I'm grateful to you for sharing with us and with each other. It's always sad for me to see these things end, but I'm sure we'll see each other again, even if it's just in the hallway.

Therapist 2: I just want to add to what B has just said. This has been . . . I have felt equally as honored to sit with you, and just as you've shared with us these really intimate experiences and stories of how cancer has impacted you. . . . One of the things about these groups is that we mutually learn. You have all really impacted me by my sitting here. Last week we were talking about courage, and some of you shared that you didn't feel courageous. I can't imagine how much courage it took to sit here and share what you did and for that you are my heroes.

Therapist 1: We will not forget you.

Patient E: Well you all created an environment that made it comfortable. So thank you.

Therapist 1: Thank you so much everyone.

KEY THERAPIST TECHNIQUES IN THE APPLICATION OF MCGP

Group Process Skills and Techniques

MCGP is essentially a group intervention, and as such, attention to basic tenets of group process and dynamics remains important. Co-facilitators must be cognizant of group etiquette, especially in terms of working together as co-facilitators, attending to and promoting group cohesion, and facilitating an atmosphere that is conducive to productive exchanges between patients. Although MCGP is not intended to be primarily a supportive group intervention, elements of support are in fact quite inevitable but are not intentionally promoted or specifically fostered.

Psychoeducational Approach: Didactics and Experiential Exercises to Enhance Learning

MCGP is also essentially an educational intervention. The goal of MCGP is to have patients understand the concept of meaning, and its importance, particularly as one faces a terminal illness and the ultimate limitation of death. In addition, MCGP strives to have patients learn about sources of meaning in order for these to become resources in coping with advanced cancer. This educational or learning process is achieved primarily through a set of brief didactics that introduce each session, followed by an experiential exercise designed to link learning of these abstract concepts with patients' own emotional experiences. Patients each share the content of their experiential exercises, and the process of experiential learning is reinforced through the comments of co-facilitators and patients, as well as through the identification of commonalities among patients' responses.

A Focus on Meaning and Sources of Meaning as Resources

MCGP is designed to have patients learn Frankl's concepts of meaning and to incorporate these sources of meaning as resources in their coping with advanced cancer. In each session, the co-facilitators listen carefully for and highlight content shared by patients that reflect sources of meaning. Co-facilitators identify "meaningful moments" described by patients and also draw attention to "meaning shifts" when patients begin to incorporate the vocabulary and conceptual framework of meaning into the material they share. An emphasis is also placed on the importance of the patient's ability to shift from one source of meaning to another, as selected sources of meaning become unavailable due to disease progression. A specific technique used to facilitate this process is called *moving from ways of doing to ways of being*. This refers to helping patients become aware that meaning can be derived in more passive ways. For example, patients can still be good fathers even if they cannot go out to the backyard and play ball with their sons; they can be good fathers in more passive ways, such as sitting and talking about their son's life goals and fears and also through expressing affection. In MCGP, it is also important for co-facilitators to be aware of the "co-creation of meaning" between co-facilitators and patients and also between group members. Co-facilitators and patient participants are "witnesses" or repositories of meaning for each other and thus are part of a meaningful legacy created by each of the patient participants in MCGP.

Incorporating Basic Existential Concepts and Themes

A central concept in MCGP is that human beings are creatures. We create values and, most important, we create our lives. In order to live fully, human beings must create a life of meaning, identity, and direction. Important existential concepts that are utilized by the co-facilitators in responding to the content of patient experiential exercise responses include freedom, responsibility, choice, creativity, identity, authenticity, engagement, existential guilt, care, transcendence, transformation, direction, being unto death, being and temporality, and existential isolation. For example, creative sources of meaning are directly related to such existential concepts as responsibility, transformation, authenticity, and existential guilt. "Detoxifying death" through the therapeutic stance and attitude of the co-facilitators is an important technique utilized throughout MCGP. Co-facilitators speak openly about death as the ultimate limitation that causes suffering and for which meaning can be derived through the attitude that one takes toward suffering (e.g., transcendence and choice). Another technique, the "existential nudge," occurs when co-facilitators gently challenge the resistance of patients to explore difficult existential realities, such as the ultimate limitation of death or existential guilt.

Case Example

Allen is a 56-year-old gay man who has worked in the advertising field for 30 years. His work is fast-paced, taxing, and consuming at times. He reported that although he enjoyed his work, he had begun to think of doing other things in recent years that may be more fulfilling. However, such feelings where usually overtaken by fears of what he would do with his life and what identity he would subsequently have. He has had a long and satisfying relationship with his partner of many years—a relationship in which Allen finds great solace and comfort.

His initial battle with cancer began 16 years ago when he was diagnosed with thyroid cancer. The subsequent surgeries for this cancer left him with significant scarring of his neck, which significantly impacted his self-image and sense of self. He stated, "I felt like a fish that had been filleted." Despite this, he related that he believed he had overcome cancer and that the "battle was won." However, a routine examination 3 years ago revealed advanced prostate cancer. Allen stated that this discovery "completely overwhelmed me. I felt crushed." He began to experience significant anxiety and depression and to question the value of fighting this battle once again. He also reported that his current life felt empty and meaningless in the face of his new cancer, and that he felt alone and "singled out" by having to face this challenge again. Allen began seeing a staff psychiatrist in order to help him with his mood symptoms, who immediately referred him for MCGP.

After the first session, Allen later reported that he felt "overwhelmed by all these other people with cancer." He considered ending the group, but he discussed this with his psychiatrist and decided to stick it out. He was relieved when other group members began to share similar feelings, and he began to feel more connected to them. He no longer felt as alone, and now, in addition to the support of his psychiatrist, he had people who understood the unique experience of facing cancer and possible death.

As the group progressed, Allen began to alter his worldview significantly. He began to view the pressures of work, which had seemed so compelling and all-consuming, as being secondary to his own needs and quality of life. His long-standing desire to leave his work began to take on a new intensity. Session 6, which focuses on patients' feelings of responsibility to themselves and others, as well as any unfinished business, was an important turning point for Allen. "I used to be so afraid of what I would do and who I would be. But I've battled cancer twice! If I can fight these kind of fights, those fears really seem to pale. My work was important for me. But it's the 'me' that counts here. Me and my partner count so much more." Such a change is a good example of the type of cognitive restructuring in the face of illness that often occurs in the groups. Allen's shift of taking into account not only himself but also his partner illustrates this session's goal of enhancing patients' sense of meaning through the realization that their lives transcend themselves and extend to others as well.

For his Legacy Project, Allen resolved to accomplish two goals. The first was to finish his employment and put his available resources into his relationship. The second was to begin the process of renovating his home, something he and his partner had wanted to do but his illness had up until now prevented from occurring. Allen related that he used to think, "I'm dying. Why bother?" His new outlook on life and his illness allowed him to view his remaining time as precious and worthy of investment. In addition, he came to the realization that despite the anxieties and pain his illness caused, he still lived and therefore he should carry on living to the end. "Until I go, I'm still here. Why should I stop experiencing the simple joy of still existing? I won't let it rob me of that."

At the conclusion of the group, Allen reported that he believed it to have been of great value to him. "I would not have seen the purpose or even the possibility of making these changes without this group and all of you." At the 2-month follow-up we conduct with patients, Allen had indeed carried out the twin goals of his Legacy Project. He felt an enhanced sense of meaning in his life, and he was finding it easier to cope with his illness.

KEY CHALLENGES IN APPLICATION OF MCGP

Occasionally, challenging situations are encountered in delivering MCGP. We have selected a few such scenarios and summarized how we have dealt with them. In addition, the problem of attrition in conducting weekly group sessions in advanced cancer patients is discussed.

Problems Encountered in Using Frankl's Book, *Man's Search for Meaning*

Patient speaks about reading Frankl, discussing her negative reactions to the text, and subsequently feeling "unheard" when she brought this up in group. Patient is offended that the Holocaust is being compared to the experience of having cancer. She further notes that she understands that the therapists have to go along with the "protocol" but wishes they were more understanding about this issue. The therapist acknowledges the patient's complaint and highlights that all members of the group had strong reactions to Frankl, which in its own way is a unifying and meaningful process: Each member has his or her own unique perspective on the reading, which parallel's each participant's unique meaning in life. In addition, this experience has changed how the therapists introduce giving Frankl's book, *Man's Search for Meaning*, as a resource to utilize in MCGP. We overtly state that we are not comparing having cancer to the Holocaust. We describe that Frankl's experience is an example of a human being's experience in choosing to find meaning and his attitude toward a suffering experience. We also tell patients that at one point in the book, Frankl describes that those patients who were not indiscriminately killed in the camps but were left alive did better if they had "reason" to stay alive. We make a point of saying that we are not implying that any particular attitude is more likely to lead to survival with cancer but only that meaning can enhance the quality of one's life.

Concerns About Not Finding Meaning: Pressure That There Is a Right and Wrong Way to Die

Patient speaks about the pressure to search for meaning at the end of life and her feeling that there is a "right way" to die, which includes suffering gracefully. Patient questions, What if you do not find it?—"It feels like I'm searching for the Holy Grail and that you have to hurry up and find it before you die." Patient notes that this process feels burdensome. The therapist explains that there is no "right way" to die but, rather, that the group is meant to highlight what is meaningful in each patient's life and the ability to continue to choose to search for meaning up until the very end, despite limitations and suffering. The point is also made that it is the "search" for meaning that is most rewarding and uplifting, not the ultimate finding of meaning. In other words, the journey is more important than the destination. And if one engages in the journey, that is what living life truly is about.

Patient Focuses on Religion, Alienating Group Members

Patient describes seeing the World Trade Center the day before the towers fell and noticing that the clouds over it looked like angel's wings coming out of the sky. She came to the conclusion that there is meaning to life and that a higher power indeed exists: "There is a higher god or person influencing us. We just have to be open enough to hear it." Group members are silent. The therapist responds by saying that one of the amazing things about the group is hearing the variety of interpretations one could have of meaningful events and observing how an individual's personal meaning takes shape. The therapist highlights that we have the freedom to choose our own perspective and attitude when something meaningful occurs: "Some people find meaning in spirituality, while others don't." The therapist further states that meaning is there for *you* to make it. She brings it back to the patient in the end, stating that she sees how special, spiritual, and meaningful this moment was for her as a person.

Patient Already Has Meaning?

Patient explains that she feels she already has meaning. She notes that she wanted to come to group not because she is struggling with her illness but, rather, because she feels she could be of service to others. She highlights that she is a positive person who finds meaning in her daily life, noting that she views her cancer as a gift. The therapist responds that people come to group experiencing various degrees of meaning. Some are already in touch with their meaning, whereas others feel they are in an existential vacuum. She elaborates, stating that it is important to remember that meaning is infinite: If a patient believes he or she already has meaning, the group is there to help the patient further tap into those sources and even enhance them.

Difficulty with Concept of Legacy You Live and Give

Patient is having difficulty identifying the legacy she lives and gives. Patient harps on how she has not done enough in her life. The group responds by pointing out her accomplishments, including writing various articles for magazines. Patient states that these magazines are subpar and do not compare to the publications to which her friends submit their articles. The therapist notes that each person's legacy is unique and that comparing one's legacy to another's is a challenge many patients face. Therefore, it would be advantageous to examine what the patient brings to the table, what is uniquely hers, in order to tap into the power of her own individual legacy.

Attrition

The key challenge in applying MCGP in an advanced cancer population is related to inflexibility that is innate to a weekly group intervention that requires regular weekly attendance at a specified day and time. MCGP also has specific themes that are covered weekly, and there is a logical progression of content as the sessions unfold that focus on the various sources of meaning. Therefore, it is ideal for patients to attend all sessions in order to theoretically obtain the optimal response. All intervention research with advanced cancer or palliative care populations experiences the problems of attrition and missed sessions. Attrition is primarily the result of episodes of illness, conflicts with scheduling of chemotherapy, diagnostic tests, other doctor appointments, and even brief hospitalizations, in addition to progression of disease. Our clinical trials of MCGP have typically struggled with attrition rates as high as 30% (interestingly, rates of attrition for MCGP groups vs. supportive psychotherapy groups are essentially the same). Despite these attrition rates, our clinical trials have been able to demonstrate that if patients attend a minimum of three or four sessions, they derive almost the same benefit as those who have attended six to eight sessions.[56] This lack of flexibility and high rates of attrition have led us to develop a more flexible individual format of MCP that we call individual meaning-centered psychotherapy, which is described in Chapter 3.

REFERENCES

1. Breitbart W, Rosenfeld B, Pessin, H, et al. Depression, hopelessness, and desire for hastened death in terminally ill cancer patients. *J Am Med Assoc.* 2000;284:2907–2911.
2. Breitbart W, Rosenfeld B, Gibson C, et al. Impact of treatment for depression on desire for hastened death in patients with advanced AIDS. *Psychosomatics.* 2010;51:98–105.
3. Frankl VF. *The Doctor and the Soul.* New York, NY: Random House; 1955/1986.
4. Frankl VF. *Man's Search for Meaning.* 4th ed. Boston, MA: Beacon; 1959/1992.
5. Frankl VF. *The Will to Meaning: Foundations and Applications of Logotherapy, Expanded Edition.* New York, NY: Penguin; 1969/1988.
6. Frankl VF. *Man's Search for Ultimate Meaning.* New York, NY: Plenum; 1975/1997.
7. Yalom ID. *Existential Psychotherapy.* New York, NY : Basic Books; 1980.
8. Breitbart W, Bruera E, Chochinov H, et al. Neuropsychiatric syndromes and psychiatric

symptoms in patients with advanced cancer. *J Pain Symptom Manage.* 1995;10:131–141.
9. Breitbart W, Chochinov HM, Passik SD. Psychiatric aspects of palliative care. In: Doyle D, Hanks GW, MacDonald N, eds. *Oxford Textbook of Palliative Medicine.* 2nd ed. New York, NY: Oxford University Press; 1998:216–246.
10. Chochinov HM, Breitbart W. *The Handbook of Psychiatry in Palliative Medicine.* New York NY: Oxford University Press; 2000.
11. Rousseau P. Spirituality and the dying patient. *J Clin Oncol.* 2000;18:2000–2002.
12. Puchalski C, Romer AL. Taking a spiritual history allows clinicians to understand patients more fully. *J Palliat Med.* 2000;3:129–137.
13. Portenoy R, Thaler HT, Kornblith AB, et al. The Memorial Symptom Assessment Scale: An instrument for evaluation of symptom prevalence, characteristics and distress. *Eur J Cancer.* 1994;30A:1326–1336.
14. Pulchalski C, Ferrell B, Virani R, et al. Improving the quality of spiritual care as a dimension of palliative care: The report of the consensus conference. *J Palliat Med.* 2009;12:885–904, p. 887.
15. Brady MJ, Peterman AH, Fitchett G, et al. A case of including spirituality in quality of life measurement in oncology. *Psycho-Oncology.* 1999;8:417–428.
16. Karasu BT. Spiritual psychotherapy. *Am J Psychother.* 1999;53:143–162.
17. Baider L, Russak SM, Perry S, et al. The role of religious and spiritual beliefs in coping with malignant melanoma: An Israeli sample. *Psycho-Oncology.* 1999;8:27–35.
18. Koenig HG, Cohen HJ, Blazer DG, et al. Religious coping and depression among elderly, hospitalized medically ill men. *Am J Psychiatry.* 1992;149:1693–1700.
19. Koenig HG, George LK, Peterson BL. Religiosity and remission of depression in medically ill older patients. *Am J Psychiatry.* 1998;155:536–542.
20. McCullough ME, Larson DB. Religion and depression: A review of the literature. *Twin Res.* 1999;2:126–136.
21. Sloan RP, Bagiella E, Powell T. Religion, spirituality, and medicine. *Lancet.* 1999;353:664–667.
22. Brady MJ, Peterman AH, Fitchett G, et al. A case of including spirituality in quality of life measurement in oncology. *Psycho-Oncology.* 1999;8:417–428.
23. Nelson C, Rosenfeld B, Breitbart W, et al. Spirituality, depression and religion in the terminally ill. *Psychosomatics.* 2002;43:213–220.
24. McCullough ME, Larson DB. Religion and depression: A review of the literature. *Twin Res.* 1999;2:126–136.
25. Sloan RP, Bagiella E, Powell T. Religion, spirituality, and medicine. *Lancet.* 1999;353:664–667.
26. Singer PA, Martin DK, Kelner M. Quality end-of-life care: Patients' perspective. *J Am Med Assoc.* 1999;281:163–168.
27. Moadel A, Morgan C, Fatone A, et al. Seeking meaning and hope: Self-reported spiritual and existential needs among an ethnically diverse cancer patient population. *Psycho-Oncology.* 1999;8:1428–1431.
28. Morita T, Tsunoda J, Inoue S, et al. An exploratory factor analysis of existential suffering in Japanese terminally ill cancer patients. *Psycho-Oncology,* 2000;9:164–168.
29. Meier DE, Emmons CA, Wallerstein S, et al. A national survey of physician-assisted suicide and euthanasia in the United States. *N Engl J Med.* 1998;338:1193–1201.
30. Brady MJ, Peterman AH, Fitchett G, et al. A case of including spirituality in quality of life measurement in oncology. *Psycho-Oncology.* 1999;8:417–428.
31. McClain C, Rosenfeld B, Breitbart W. The influence of spirituality on end-of-life despair among terminally ill cancer patients. *Lancet.* 2003;361:1603–1607.
32. Yanez B, Edmondson D, Stanton AL, et al. Facets of spirituality as predictors of adjustment to cancer: Relative contributions of having faith and finding meaning. *J Consult Clin Psychol.* 2009;77:730–741.
33. Watson M, Haviland JJ, Greer S, et al. Influence of psychological response on survival in breast cancer population-based cohort study. *Lancet.* 1999;354:1331–1336.
34. Breitbart W, Rosenfeld B. Physician-assisted suicide: The influence of psychosocial issues. *Cancer Control.* 1999;6:146–161.
35. Chochinov HM, Wilson K, Enns M, et al. Prevalence of depression in the terminally ill: Effects of diagnostic criteria and symptom threshold judgments. *Am J Psychiatry.* 1994;51:537–540.
36. Chochinov HM, Wilson KG, Enns M, et al. Desire for death in the terminally ill. *Am J Psychiatry.* 1995;152:1185–1191.
37. Kissane D, Block S, Miach P, et al. Cognitive existential group therapy for patients with primary breast cancer—Techniques and themes. *Psycho-Oncology.* 1997;6:25–33.
38. Park C, Folkman S. Meaning in the context of stress and coping. *Rev Gen Psychol.* 1997;1:115–144.
39. Andrykowski MA, Brady MJ, Hunt JW. Positive psychosocial adjustment in potential bone marrow transplant recipients: Cancer as a psychosocial transition. *Psycho-Oncology.* 1993;2:261–276.

40. Folkman S. Positive psychological states and coping with severe stress. *Social Sci Med.* 1997;45:1207–1221.
41. Taylor SE. Adjustment to threatening events: A theory of cognitive adaptation. *Am Psychologist.* 1983;38:1161–1173.
42. Taylor EJ. Factors associated with meaning in life among people with recurrent cancer. *Oncol Nursing Forum.* 1993;20:1399–1405.
43. Kierkegard S, Hong H, Hong E. *Fear and Trembling/Repetition.* Princeton, NJ: Princeton University Press; 1983.
44. Heidegger M. *Being and Time.* Translated by Joan Stambaugh. Albany, NY: State University of New York Press; 1996.
45. Nietzsche F. *Human, All Too Human: A Book for Free Spirits.* Cambridge, UK: Cambridge University Press; 1986.
46. Sartre JP. *Being and Nothingness.* New York, NY: Citadel Press; 1984.
47. Schag CC, Heinrich RL, Ganz PA. Karnofsky performance status revisited: Reliability, validity, and guidelines. *J Clin Oncol.* 1984;2:187–193.
48. National Comprehensive Cancer Network. NCCN distress management clinical practice guidelines. *J Natl Comprehensive Cancer Network.* 2003;1:344–374.
49. Spiegel D, Yalom I. A support group for dying patients. *Int J Group Psychotherapy.* 1978;28:233–245.
50. Spiegel D, Bloom J, Yalom ID. Group support for patients with metastatic breast cancer. *Arch Gen Psychiatry.* 1981;38:527–533.
51. Yalom I, Greaves C. Group therapy with the terminally ill. *Am J Psychiatry.* 1977;134:396–400.
52. Lee V, Cohen SR, Edgar L, et al. Meaning-making and psychological adjustment to cancer: Development of an intervention and pilot results. *Oncol Nursing Forum.* 2006;33:291–302.
53. Kissane DW, Bloch S, Smith GC, et al. Cognitive existential group psychotherapy for women with primary breast cancer: A randomised controlled trial. *Psycho-Oncology.* 2003;12:532–546.
54. Coward DD. Facilitation of self-transcendence in a breast cancer support group: II. *Oncol Nursing Forum.* 2003;30:291–300.
55. Breitbart W, Rosenfeld B, Gibson C, et al. Meaning-centered group psychotherapy for patients with advanced cancer: A pilot randomized controlled trial. *Psycho-Oncology.* 2010;19:21–28.
56. Breitbart W, Rosenfeld B, Pessin H, et al. Meaning-centered group psychotherapy: An effective intervention for improving psychological well-being in patients with advanced cancer. *J Clin Oncol* 2015;33(7):749–754.
57. Breitbart W, Poppito S. *Meaning Centered Group Psychotherapy Treatment Manual.* New York, NY: Oxford University Press; 2014.

3

Individual Meaning-Centered Psychotherapy for Advanced Cancer Patients

WILLIAM BREITBART, WENDY G. LICHTENTHAL, ALLISON J. APPLEBAUM, AND MELISSA MASTERSON

INTRODUCTION

Physical, psychological, and spiritual domains of end-of-life care have been identified as priorities by both medical professional organizations and cancer patients. Two milestone Institute of Medicine reports—"Approaching Death: Improving Care at the End of Life" (1997) and "Improving Palliative Care for Cancer" (2001)—as well as the National Consensus Project for Quality of Palliative Care clinical practice guidelines (2004) and the National Quality Forum recommendations for preferred practices for palliative and hospice care (2006) identified spiritual well-being (psychological, psychiatric, spiritual, and existential domains of care) as core domains of quality end-of-life care.

Facing a diagnosis of advanced cancer is challenging for even the most resilient individuals. Distress associated with this diagnosis can manifest in many ways, including physical symptoms, psychological symptoms, and spiritual/existential symptoms.

Existential concerns are a major issue among the advanced cancer population as feelings regarding one's mortality are brought to the forefront. A consensus conference on improving the quality of spiritual care as a dimension of palliative care was held in 2009.[1] This conference was formed under the central premise that spiritual care is a fundamental component of end-of-life support. Importantly, the consensus panel explicitly recommended psychotherapy approaches that focus on meaning to address spiritual/existential issues for end-of-life care.

THEORETICAL BACKGROUND FOR MEANING-CENTERED PSYCHOTHERAPY

Approximately 15 years ago, our research group at Memorial Sloan Kettering Cancer Center began to understand that a meaning-centered approach to psychosocial care was imperative to alleviate distress among advanced cancer patients. For those patients who are in fact facing death, meaning and the preservation of meaning are not only clinically and spiritually/existentially important but also central concepts to therapeutic intervention. Individual meaning-centered psychotherapy (IMCP) was conceived at the intersection of a baffling clinical problem and inspiration. Clinically, we witnessed despair and hopelessness take hold of our advanced cancer patients and, consequently, the emergence of the desire for hastened death. What we found most surprising was that although 45% expressing a desire for hastened death were struggling with a clinical depression,[2] a significant percentage were not clinically depressed but, rather, facing an existential crisis encompassing a loss of meaning, value, purpose, and hope.

When our research group as well as others demonstrated the central role that meaning plays in diminishing psychosocial distress and despair at the end of life, we were inspired to develop a meaning-centered intervention. This effort led us to the work of Viktor Frankl, his concepts of logotherapy,[3–6] and pioneers in existential philosophy and psychiatry. We found Frankl's concepts of meaning and spirituality to be powerful tools that could be utilized in our psychotherapeutic work with advanced cancer patients facing existential issues at the end of life. Frankl's main contributions have been increased awareness of the spiritual component of human experience and the central importance of meaning (or the will to meaning) as a motivating force in human psychology. Frankl's basic concepts include the following:

1. Meaning of life: Life has meaning and never ceases to have meaning even up

to the last moment of life, and although meaning may change in this context, it never ceases to exist. When we believe our lives have no meaning, it is because we have become disconnected from meaning in our lives, not because it no longer exists. For the purposes of meaning-centered psychotherapy (MCP) we have modified this concept based on clinical experience and our desire to present a secular intervention that relied less on dogma and more on rationality. We offer this concept: The creation or experience of meaning is always possible (in a sentient human being) even in the last months, days, or moments of life.

2. Will to meaning: The desire to find meaning in human existence is a primary instinct and basic motivation for human behavior. Human beings are creatures who innately search for and create meaning in their lives. We are "meaning-making" creatures.
3. Freedom of will: We have the freedom to find meaning in existence and to choose our attitude toward suffering, limitations, and uncertainty. Ultimately, if we are unable to control events that are externally or internally impacted on our bodies and our freedom, we still have the last vestige of freedom, which is to choose how we think about the situation and to choose the attitude we take in response to the situation. We have the responsibility to create an existence of meaning, direction, and identity. We must respond to the fact of our existence and create the "essence" of what makes us human. Our "attitude" is a critical element of what comprises our human "essence."
4. The three main sources of meaning in life are derived from creativity (work and deeds), experience (art, nature, humor, love, and relationships), and attitude (the attitude one takes toward suffering and existential problems).
5. Meaning exists in a historical context, and thus, legacy (past, present, and future) is a critical element in sustaining or enhancing meaning.

Model of Individual Meaning-Centered Psychotherapy

Based on Viktor Frankl's logotherapy and his principles of meaning, we developed IMCP to help patients with advanced cancer sustain or enhance a sense of meaning, peace, and purpose in their lives even as they approach the end of life.[7–10] This intervention is based on a theoretical model in which the enhancement of meaning results in improved quality of life and reduced distress, despair, and suffering. Figure 3.1 depicts the empirically-supported model underlying our IMCP intervention, in which enhanced meaning is conceptualized as the catalyst for improved psychosocial outcomes.

Specifically, meaning is viewed as both an intermediary outcome and a mediator of changes in these important psychosocial outcomes. Religious faith is not expected to directly impact

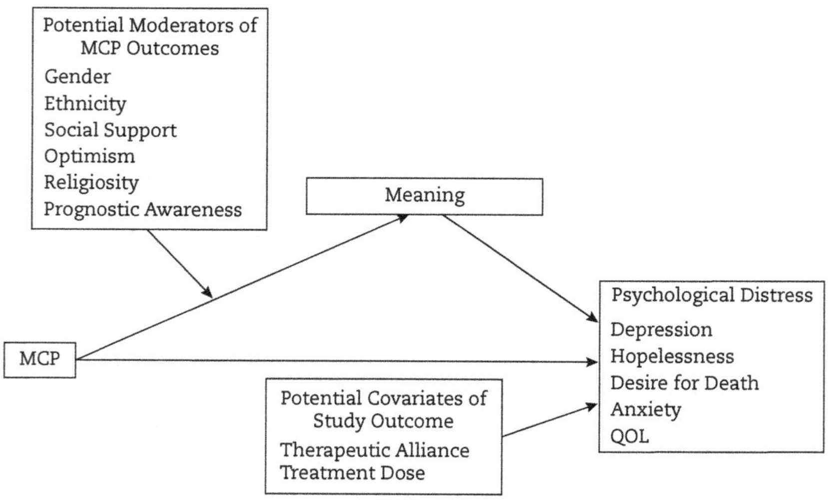

FIGURE 3.1 Model of individual meaning-centered psychotherapy.

psychosocial outcomes, but it may moderate the intermediary outcome of meaning (indicating that religious faith does not provide a unique contribution to enhanced psychosocial outcomes after controlling for spirituality).[11] This model also presumes that other factors will impact response to a meaning-based intervention, including prognostic awareness, psychosocial treatment preference, and therapeutic alliance. We recognize many of the variables included in this model could potentially have bidirectional influence; however, we present the model we believe underlies the intervention.

In order to target the despair and hopelessness driving the desire for hastened death observed in advanced cancer patients, a number of existential concepts were called upon that do not directly involve meaning but serve as a critical framework for conducting the therapeutic work of IMCP. Although the IMCP intervention is literally centered on meaning and sources of meaning, the richness of the therapeutic content is due to the integration of meaning and the theories of existential philosophy and psychotherapy. The therapeutic value of IMCP would be limited without the contribution of existential concepts such as death anxiety, freedom, responsibility, choice, creativity, identity, authenticity, existential guilt, transcendence, transformation, mortality, and existential isolation.

These concepts inform the intervention and are utilized to reinforce the goals of MCP related to the search, connection, and creation of meaning.

Appropriate Participants for Individual Meaning-Centered Psychotherapy

Although the majority of advanced cancer patients could benefit from participation in IMCP, the intervention is best suited for individuals with moderate to extreme distress, as indicated by a score of 4 or higher on the National Comprehensive Cancer Network's Distress Thermometer. The Distress Thermometer is a brief screening tool that assesses the patient's level of current distress by asking, "Please note your current distress on a scale from 0 to 10," where 0 is "No distress" and 10 is "Extreme distress." When the source of the patient's distress is emotional or spiritual/religious in nature, IMCP may be a particularly efficacious intervention. Furthermore, IMCP is currently delivered in the outpatient setting; therefore, patients with physical limitations sufficient to preclude participation in the outpatient setting are not suited for this intervention. The patient's physical limitations are assessed using the Karnofsky Performance Rating Scale (KPRS). KPRS scores range from 0 ("Dead") to 100 ("Normal, no complaints: no evidence of disease"). Scores less than 60 ("Requires considerable assistance and frequent medical care") deem a participant inappropriate for study participation in the outpatient setting.

INDIVIDUAL MEANING-CENTERED PSYCHOTHERAPY

IMCP is a seven-session individual intervention that utilizes didactics, discussions, and experiential exercises that focus on specific themes related to both meaning and advanced cancer. IMCP serves three major purposes: (1) to promote a supportive environment for cancer patients to explore personal issues and feelings surrounding their illness on a one-to-one therapeutic basis, (2) to facilitate a greater understanding of possible sources of meaning both before and after a diagnosis of cancer, and (3) to aid patients in their discovery and maintenance of a sense of meaning in life during illness. The ultimate goal of this intervention is to optimize coping through the pursuit of an enhanced sense of meaning and purpose. As Frankl points out, the possibility of creating or experiencing meaning exists until the last moment of life.

In a randomized controlled trial of IMCP for patients with advanced cancer, 120 patients with stage III or IV cancer were randomly assigned to seven sessions of either IMCP or therapeutic massage.[8] Participants were assessed for spiritual well-being and quality of life, as well as anxiety, depression, hopelessness, and symptom burden. Post-treatment, cancer patients in the IMCP group reported significantly greater improvement in the primary study outcomes: depression, anxiety, hopelessness, desire for death, meaning, spiritual well-being, and quality of life.[8] Furthermore, IMCP patients demonstrated greater improvements in symptom burden and symptom-related distress than patients in the therapeutic massage group. The benefits of IMCP are mediated through enhancement of meaning. Our group recently completed recruitment of a randomized controlled trial of IMCP in 320 advanced cancer patients comparing IMCP to individual supportive psychotherapy and to enhanced usual care. We hope to soon publish the results of this larger randomized controlled trial funded by the National Cancer Institute.

The IMCP intervention is intended to help broaden the scope of possible sources of meaning through the combination of (1) didactic teaching of the philosophy of meaning on which the intervention is based; (2) session exercises and homework for each participant to complete; and (3) open-ended discussion, which may include the therapist's interpretive insights and comments. However, it is important for clinicians to understand that meaning-making is an individualized process and, therefore, it is the individual patient's responsibility to use these sessions to actively explore and discover the sources of meaning in their own right. In this format, patients are not passive recipients of the intervention but, rather, active participants in the process itself, bringing to the table their own experiences, beliefs, and hopes that shape their journey to enhanced meaning and purpose. Although session topics remain the same within both individual and group formats, IMCP includes seven sessions, whereas meaning-centered group psychotherapy (MCGP) is an eight-session intervention. The additional session in MCGP allows for ample time to cover the third topic, historical sources of meaning and legacy, and to have each group member participate in the often lengthy discussion of one's legacy. A list of session topics for the individual format of MCP (seven-session format) is provided in Table 3.1.

Next, an overview of each session is provided. For a comprehensive guide to session content, refer to the book, *Individual Meaning-Centered Psychotherapy for Patients with Advanced Cancer: A Treatment Manual*, by Breitbart and Poppito.[12]

Session 1: Concepts and Sources of Meaning

The initial session of IMCP includes a series of introductions. During this session, introductions between the patient and therapist occur in addition to an introduction of the intervention to the patient. IMCP is a therapeutic program drastically different from traditional forms of psychotherapy; therefore, it is imperative that the therapist spend time in the first session orienting the patient to the structure, logistics, and goals of the intervention. Following introductions, the therapist welcomes the patient to share his or her cancer story, beginning at the time of diagnosis and continuing to the present day. The therapist should encourage the patient to describe how he or she has been affected physically, emotionally, and socially. The remainder of the session focuses on the concept of meaning. Patients are asked to provide their own definition of meaning to help the therapist better understand how the patient connects to and defines meaning in his or her own life. Following this exercise, the therapist presents a definition developed by our research team to offer the patient additional ways to think about the concept of meaning.

See Appendix 2 for a complete, de-identified, transcript of two entire seven-session IMCP patient interventions to illustrate in greater detail the procedures, processes, and techniques of IMCP.

The experiential exercise for the first session explores meaningful moments identified by the patient from his or her own life (Box 3.1).

During completion of this exercise, the therapist begins to develop a deeper understanding of what the patient finds to be meaningful and rapport begins to build. The following IMCP excerpt from Session 1 exemplifies the type of interaction that can occur:

Interventionist: I'm going to ask you to write down a few thoughts and experiences of moments life, when bottom line, when you felt most

TABLE 3.1 INDIVIDUAL MEANING-CENTERED PSYCHOTHERAPY SESSION TOPICS AND THEMES

Session Topics	Themes
Session 1: Concepts and Sources of Meaning	Introductions and meaning
Session 2: Cancer and Meaning	Identity before and after cancer diagnosis
Session 3: Historical Sources of Meaning	Life as a legacy that has been given Life as a legacy that one lives and will give
Session 4: Attitudinal Sources of Meaning	Encountering life's limitations
Session 5: Creative Sources of Meaning	Creativity, courage, and responsibility
Session 6: Experiential Sources of Meaning	Connecting with life through love, beauty, and humor
Session 7: Transitions	Final reflections and hopes for the future

BOX 3.1 SESSION 1 EXPERIENTIAL EXERCISE: "MEANINGFUL MOMENTS"

List one or two experiences or moments when life has felt particularly meaningful to you—whether it sounds powerful or mundane. For example, it could be something that helped get you through a difficult day or a time when you felt most alive. And say something about it.

alive, some of the most meaningful moments in your life. You can list one, two, three, you may have, seems like a very rich life. Write down a few experiences, moments when you felt your life was particularly meaningful, when you felt the most alive. Take a few moments to write that down and then we'll discuss that a little bit, and then we'll be able to wrap up.

Patient: Okay.

Interventionist: Okay? Why don't you share that with me?

Patient: Okay, well the first is my daughter's wedding. I couldn't believe how great I felt, how wonderful everyone looked, it was a perfect day, I mean it rained, but it seemed to stop raining when it needed to. And it was just a, everyone from the family was there. It was just um, it was a celebration of life.

Interventionist: Right, and what we find are that milestones in life are often very meaningful moments.

Patient: Mm-hmm.

Interventionist: Because they often represent progress along this trajectory, this life that you are hoping to create and fulfilling your life to its full potential and I suppose for you being a mother and being a grandmother is one of the things that you saw as fulfilling your full potential.

Patient: Right, yeah, I mean it was.

Interventionist: So, that gives meaning to your life also. And in terms of sources of meaning right, it relates to, it relates to who you are, you're identity. I'm all these things, but I'm also a parent, a mother, and now a grandmother. And it falls into these creative sources of meaning through uh, through experiences the joys of life.

Patient: Uh-huh.

Interventionist: Through the joys of love, and family. And is also related to this historical legacy, sources of meaning, right?

Patient: Mm-hmm.

Interventionist: You know, it's a continuation of the chain of events and traditions uh that started long ago, and your grandparents and parents. Your parents were there for your wedding.

Session 2: Cancer and Meaning

In Session 2, the main goal is to explore the topic of "cancer and meaning" in light of the guiding theme, "identity—before and after diagnosis." In order to reflect upon the origins of meaning in each person's life, it is important to start with each person's own understanding of who he or she is. This session helps to reveal the patient's authentic sense of identity and what made his or her personal experiences meaningful. The experiential exercise for Session 2 explores what makes this individual who he or she is and how cancer has impacted his or her identity (Box 3.2).

BOX 3.2 SESSION 2 EXPERIENTIAL EXERCISE: "IDENTITY AND CANCER"

1. Write down four answers to the question, "Who am I?" These can be positive or negative, and include personality characteristics, body image, beliefs, things you do, people you know, etc. For example, answers might start with, "I am someone who ________," or "I am a ________."
2. How has cancer affected your answers? How has it affected the things that are most meaningful to you?

What the patient is most likely to discover through this exercise is that the core aspects of his or her identity after cancer are strikingly similar to those of the patient's identity prior to cancer. Furthermore, it is the role of the clinician to attend to these themes and highlight them as characteristics that have persevered despite a life-altering diagnosis of advanced illness.[12] The following IMCP excerpt from Session 2 exemplifies the type of interaction that can occur:

Patient: I am someone who loves her family and friends. I am an optimistic person. I am someone who was comfortable in their own skin. I am someone who loves to explore New York City.

Interventionist: Tell me a little more about being optimistic and how that characterizes who you are.

Patient: I think I'm always a hopeful person in general, like glass half full and I guess when I was reading this I noticed personality characteristics, so I knew also that I had to compare it and so that's where I wrote that down because I feel like the cancer is kind of eating away at that optimistic thing because of the worry and the fear I try to stay strong to my true self, but this other angle creeps in. But on the positive side, cancer has really intensified my relationships with people and has also made me aware and reminded me to be a more generous person. It is just mind blowing the amount of people who want to bring us meals, and ask me how I'm doing and ask my husband how he is doing and people have given us monetary donations. And I keep telling people don't worry I'm fine, I don't need a meal, I'm functioning, feed your own family, but they all insist and want to do something. So it's always in my head that I need to pay it forward, and it really is a wonderful thing.

Interventionist: Absolutely.

Patient: It's something wonderful to come out of a really shitty thing.

Interventionist: Yes it is, and recognizing that and taking that approach is attitude.

Patient: Yes, yes, it is.

Interventionist: Out of something so negative, but out of it something so beautiful that the things that are most important to you have become more intense and more meaningful, and it has given you the opportunity, the illness has, to see the world as a more wonderful place than you thought it was before your illness.

Patient: I think I took it for granted and I don't take it for granted anymore.

Interventionist: And that is a great thing that has come out of this, this after cancer identity. What strikes me is that you said you were kind of surprised when you look at this after cancer part and thought, wow, three out of these four things aren't affected by cancer, or at least aren't affected by cancer in a bad way. It goes to show that from such a profound challenge that can challenge you physically and psychologically, the core of who you are and the things that make you, you, haven't changed. And in fact you are now someone who argues less and loves more, who sees the world and people as being caring and generous and wants to give back to the world. I think that is incredible.

Patient: Yes, I agree. It is nice to be reminded of that, these, almost the positives that have come out of cancer.

Session 3: Historical Sources of Meaning—"Life as a Living Legacy"

The main goal for Session 3 is to introduce and explore the topic of "historical sources of meaning" and the guiding theme, "life as a living legacy." Following the discussion of identity in the previous session, Session 3 serves as an opportunity to explore the context in which identity developed through the exploration of legacy. In IMCP, we present the idea of legacy through three temporal parts: (1) the legacy that has been given from the past, (2) the legacy that one lives in the present, and (3) the legacy one will give in the future.[12] The first question in the experiential exercise for Session 3 allows the patient the opportunity to explore and express meaningful past experiences in order to uncover the historical context of his or her living legacy (Box 3.3).

The following IMCP excerpt exemplifies the type of interaction that occurs during the Session 3 experiential exercise:

Patient: My mother taught me always to be self-sufficient. Her beliefs in loyalty, freedom, and conscience are her legacy to me. My father's kindness, sweet personality, and liberal politics are always with me. My parents were very left leaning in a time, well always, I don't know how to explain it but I'll tell you this, in 1948, when apartheid became the law in South Africa, I came home from school, I was 6 years

BOX 3.3 SESSION 3 EXPERIENTIAL EXERCISE: "LIFE AS A LEGACY" THAT HAS BEEN GIVEN

1. When you look back on your life and upbringing, what are the most significant memories, relationships, traditions, etc., that have made *the greatest impact on who you are today?*

For example: Identify specific memories of how you were raised that have made a lasting impression on your life (e.g., your relationship with parents, siblings, friends, teachers, etc.). What is the origin of your name? What are some past events that have meaningfully touched your life?

old. And my mother sat me down in the living room and said to me, "I have something to tell you." And she explained to me what apartheid was and she said, "That is a shame before God and we should never allow it." So, in the 50s and 60s I took up what she said and I started carrying and advocating for voters rights, I marched against Vietnam. I did what my parents did in the 30s and 40s, I carried that tradition on, and that's my legacy. But I have no one to leave it to.

Interventionist: But it sounds like you made an impact on the world though?

Patient: I don't know about that. But I did what I thought was right, and that is what counted. Whether I impacted or not, I don't know, but I had a sense of satisfaction that I did fight against it.

For some patients, discussion of the "legacy given" will be a pleasant trip down memory lane, whereas for others it may include difficult experiences related to unmet needs, losses, or disappointments. Whether memories are awesome or dreadful, it is undeniable that this legacy is a part of who our patients are. Our role as therapist is to bear witness to the patient's story; the experience of telling the story may be comforting and transformative for a patient who is struggling physically and emotionally.[12]

Furthermore, this session explores the present and future components of legacy in the second question of the experiential exercise (Box 3.4). Through this process, the patient can begin to witness his or her living legacy as a cohesive whole by integrating past memories with present accomplishments and future contributions.[12] The therapist should help the patient find the thread that weaves through his or her past, present, and future legacy while listening for themes of hardship, loss, and adversity that can be reflected upon in the next session discussing life's limitations.

The following IMCP excerpt exemplifies the type of interaction that occurs during the second part of the Session 3 experiential exercise:

Patient: How do I want to be remembered? I don't know. I guess as someone who was uh thoughtful, um and patient, um not too opinionated, uh you know someone who loved them. I want them to think of me in loving terms.

Interventionist: Yeah, some combination actually of your great grandmother, and grandmother, and your mother and your father.

Patient: Yeah, when I think of them . . .

Interventionist: And the lessons that you've learned from them, the good ones. . . .

Patient: And the not so good ones you know um, you know I jokingly would tell my girls, um when they wanted to discuss something,

BOX 3.4 SESSION 3 EXPERIENTIAL EXERCISE: "LIFE AS A LEGACY" THAT YOU LIVE AND WILL GIVE

1. As you reflect upon who you are today, what are the meaningful activities, roles, or accomplishments that you are most proud of? As you look toward the future, what are some of the life lessons you have learned along the way that you would want to pass on to others? What is the legacy you hope to live and give?

that they're something as a mother, I run a benevolent dictatorship, and I wanted them to understand that, that they're some things that we are not going to discuss, or you know so that. I guess I guess what I'd want them to know is that I had a strong sense of myself, and that I was true to who I . . . I, you know how I interacted with them was really who I was.

Interventionist: Yeah you mentioned that you lived a life that was true to yourself.

Patient: Right, yeah, you know that the essence of who I am . . .

Interventionist: And that's what you want for them too.

Patient: That's what I want for them too. I want them to be themselves.

Interventionist: Yeah so you want them to remember you as someone who lived the life that they wanted to live for themselves.

Session 4: Attitudinal Sources of Meaning—"Encountering Life's Limitations"

The main goal for Session 4 is to explore the topic of "attitudinal sources of meaning" and the guiding theme, "encountering life's limitations." Session 4 is centered on Viktor Frankl's core theoretical belief that the last vestige of human freedom is our capacity to choose our attitude toward suffering and life's limitations in any given situation. Furthermore, the session focuses on Frankl's belief that meaning and suffering are not mutually exclusive but that one has the potential to find meaning in life through suffering. The attitudinal source of meaning is offered to patients as a way in which they can take control of their life in a meaningful way during a time in which the illness has likely stripped from them their sense of peace and control. The experiential exercise for this session allows the patient to reflect on times when he or she has faced obstacles and limitations in the past (Box 3.5).

It is the role of the therapist to point out how the patient has chosen his or her attitude in the past and how he or she can continue to use this source of meaning to face the challenges presented by illness.[12] The review of how the patient has turned tragedies into triumphs in the past bolsters strength and self-efficacy, highlightingthe patient's ability to combat the obstacles and limitations that lie ahead.

The following IMCP excerpt exemplifies the type of interaction that occurs during the Session 4 experiential exercise:

Patient: I think the tragic loss of both my parents shortly after I graduated from college. My father passed away when I was 19½ and my mom 1 year later. I had two brothers who were a great support to me and 1 year before my mom passed, I met my dear husband, who I married 1 month after her death. I gathered the strength to bear the loss of my parents drawing on the values and love passed on to me by my dear mom and dad. They left a whole lifetime of values with me and that is what helped me get through this. That and my husband coming into my life just a year previous, so I was very lucky in that respect. I don't know what would have happened if I hadn't met him at that point, life

BOX 3.5 SESSION 4 EXPERIENTIAL EXERCISE: "ENCOUNTERING LIFE'S LIMITATIONS"

1. What are some of the life limitations, losses, or obstacles that you have faced in the past, and how did you cope or deal with them at the time?
2. Since your diagnosis, what are the specific limitations or losses you have faced, and how are you coping or dealing with them now? Are you still able to find meaning in your daily life despite your awareness of the limitations and finiteness of life? (If yes, please briefly describe.)
3. What would you consider a "good" or "meaningful" death? How can you imagine being remembered by your loved ones? (For example, what are some of your personal characteristics, the shared memories, or meaningful life events that have made a lasting impression on them?)

would have went a very different way maybe, but I was able to gather a lot of strength then and I got through it. It was really balanced by a wonderful time in my life, during a tragic situation.

Interventionist: It sounds like you fell in love in the wake of grief.

Patient: Exactly, when I think back I think it is an amazing thing that happened. He never met my father, but met my mother when she was not herself. I fell in love with my husband the second he opened the door for a blind date, that was a gift from God. I have had a lot of gifts from God.

Interventionist: So meeting him and the love that you experienced with him certainly gave you strength and it sounds like your brothers were also pillars of strength for you during that time. It really seems that the way you have always been able to cope with losses and limitations in the past is through the support of your family. When I came in today, I saw your children all around your chemo suite and I think it is such a touching and beautiful example of how you continue to utilize the strength found in your family to face the current limitations presented by your illness.

Patient: I couldn't get through this without them, they are so amazing.

The homework assigned in Session 4 is a long-term homework assignment intended to build on the work done thus far and further explore the concept of "life as a legacy." Additional information on this long-term homework assignment can be found in *Individual Meaning-Centered Psychotherapy for Patients with Advanced Cancer: A Treatment Manual.*[12]

Session 5: Creative Sources of Meaning—"Actively Engaging in Life Via Creativity and Responsibility"

The main goal for Session 5 is to introduce and explore the topic of "creative sources of meaning" and the guiding theme, "actively engaging in life via creativity and responsibility."

It is the role of the clinician in this session to provide psychoeducation regarding the relationship between creativity, courage, and responsibility. As humans, our existence calls us to create, and our ability to respond to this creative calling forms the basis for taking responsibility for our lives. Creativity and responsibility, therefore, are inextricably linked. Whereas creativity requires action, the beauty of this source of meaning is that it continually gives us second chances to start over, make amends, forge new paths, traverse uncharted territories, and transcend our given bounds.

The challenge of creativity is that it takes substantial courage, tenacity, and inner fortitude to continually risk putting oneself out there in the face of uncertainty and doubt. For example, it takes a great deal of courage to confront an advanced-stage cancer diagnosis and find the energy and inner resolve to move ahead despite an uncertain future. Patients may feel existential guilt when they ignore this creative calling and fail to respond to life. It is imperative to normalize the guilt that patients may experience as well as to foster strength by helping patients to acknowledge their day-to-day ability to create as courageous. The experiential exercise for this session allows patients to explore the concepts of creativity, courage, and responsibility in their own lives (Box 3.6).

BOX 3.6 SESSION 5 EXPERIENTIAL EXERCISE: "ACTIVELY ENGAGING IN LIFE"

1. Living life and being creative requires courage and commitment. Can you think of a time(s) in your life when you have been courageous, taken ownership of your life, or made a meaningful commitment to something of value to you?
2. Do you feel you have expressed what is most meaningful to you through your life's work and creative activities (e.g., job, parenting, and causes)? If so, how?
3. What are your responsibilities? Who are you responsible to and for?
4. Do you have unfinished business? What tasks have you always wanted to do but have yet to undertake? If so, what do you think is holding you back?

By the end of Session 5, the patient should have a solid understanding of the significance of "creativity and responsibility" as important sources of meaning in life.[12] The following IMCP excerpt exemplifies the type of interaction that occurs during the Session 5 experiential exercise:

Interventionist: The courage to create in a time when life is uncertain is truly profound. We spoke in our last session about the greatest limitation in life is the fact that it is finite, so just the courage to invest in a life that we know is limited is something that we must acknowledge. You have demonstrated this courage throughout your battle with cancer by pursuing new treatments and dedicating yourself to this fight regardless of knowing what the outcome will be.

Patient: Yeah I guess so, you're right. I never really thought of myself as courageous, but I think sometimes just having cancer and being able to smile takes courage.

Interventionist: Absolutely, it does. When life is really hard and throws you a curveball, like cancer, it can be challenging to want to create, and therefore the ability to move forward in spite of that and to smile is courageous.

Session 6: Experiential Sources of Meaning—"Connecting with Life"

The main goal for Session 6 is to introduce and explore the topic of "experiential sources of meaning" by way of the guiding theme, "connecting with life." Thus far, the sources of meaning introduced have required active involvement in life; experiential sources embody more passive engagement with life. Such creative and attitudinal sources ask us to *give to life*, whereas experiential sources call us to *give ourselves over* to the lightness of being alive.[12] There are three major ways in which we connect to life—through love, beauty, and humor. During the experiential exercise for Session 6, patients are invited to provide examples of ways they connect to these sources of meaning (Box 3.7).

> **BOX 3.7 SESSION 6 EXPERIENTIAL EXERCISE: "CONNECTING WITH LIFE"**
>
> List three ways in which you connect with life and feel most alive through the experiential sources of
>
> 1. Love
> 2. Beauty
> 3. Humor

Following engagement in this exercise, it is the role of the therapist to reflect on the fact that experiential sources of meaning remain accessible despite limited physical capabilities or emotional hardship.[12] As the illness progresses, patients may find comfort in these sources of meaning that require little activity to access. By the end of Session 6, the patient should have a solid understanding of the significance of connecting with life through experiential sources of meaning. The following IMCP excerpt exemplifies the type of interaction that occurs during the Session 6 experiential exercise:

Patient: With regard to beauty, I wrote down, the everyday sunrise from my bedroom window. By my bed there are two big mountains and every morning when I wake up I can see the sunrise over the mountains. So everyday now, I open my eyes and I say, "Wow, the sun is up, and it is a beautiful day." I think it's especially beautiful when the sun reflects on the snow.

Interventionist: Yes.

Patient: You know everyone is complaining this winter, I work in an office and everyone is complaining about the weather. All they do is complain about the weather. One girl in the office said the other day, "Ugh, summer is never coming." And I just think, it isn't even spring yet.

Interventionist: Right.

Patient: I don't know, I think the older I get, you can't control the weather; you just have to enjoy it, whatever it is. I don't like shoveling it either, but there is beauty in everything and I think that every snowfall is really beautiful.

Interventionist: And that is attitude, to choose your response to the cards you are dealt and to choose to find the beauty instead of the burden in snow.

Patient: And spring will come, and summer will come. You just have to be patient.

Session 7: Transitions and Hopes for the Future

The final seventh session allows for time to reflect upon the experience of engaging in this intervention during the previous six sessions. The patient's thoughts and feelings surrounding the finality of this therapeutic experience in light of facing important transitions and endings in his or her own life should be explored.[12] Furthermore, these themes can be explored through the sharing of the meaningful experiences within the treatment process. The experiential exercise for Session 7 facilitates discussion of transitions and the future (Box 3.8).

The following IMCP excerpt exemplifies the type of interaction that occurs during the final session:

Patient: I never thought that I was a strong person, but I think you made me realize that I am.

Interventionist: You have overcome so much. Not only have you overcome obstacles, but you have gone the extra mile to create the life that you want despite the limitations you have faced. You have showed me that when life wasn't really giving you what you wanted and what you needed you went out and found it, you went out and created it. That is attitude.

Patient: Did I tell you that my boss and dear friend had adopted a baby from China?

Interventionist: Yes, and you were asked to be her godmother?

Patient: Yes. I was there yesterday, and this baby that we brought over together is now 17 years old. I forgot the joy the child brought me and she came trotting down the lobby and started hugging and kissing me and I thought, I am so lucky. Even if I don't see her that often, I am so lucky. She brought great joy to my life.

Interventionist: That is wonderful and I am so struck by that because in our last session we talked about these experiential sources of meaning and of love.

Patient: And I didn't put that down! I needed to realize how much I love that child.

Interventionist: So in thinking about some of the themes we have discussed such as love, in general, what was this experience going through meaning-centered psychotherapy like for you?

Patient: You know what is interesting, I never really talked about my husband until these sessions, but at my last memoir class the prompt was about looking at a painting, and looking through the painting. The bottom line is that I have a picture of the shore near where we met and for the first time in my life I wrote about him. My class and instructor were so struck that I had never mentioned him, and I think that I did that because I was able to open up with you.

Interventionist: So what did it feel like to write about him and to have the story of you and him witnessed by others?

Patient: It felt so good that they loved it. Professionally, I love having the ability to write and be appreciated for it, but emotionally, I loved writing that story.

Interventionist: It is so wonderful that you were able to open up to others and connect that way.

Patient: It was so rewarding. I think overall, over these seven sessions, I have opened up.

Interventionist: I have certainly noticed. Which is why I think we have made some progress and I encourage you to explore how opening up and connecting to others can provide you with freedom and take you on a unique journey through the rest of your life.

BOX 3.8 SESSION 7 EXPERIENTIAL EXERCISE: "REFLECTION AND FEEDBACK"

1. What has it been like for you to go through this learning experience over these past six sessions? Have there been any changes in the way you view your life and cancer experience having been through this process?
2. Do you feel like you have a better understanding of the sources of meaning in life and are you able to use them in your daily life? If so, how?
3. What are your hopes for the future?

DIFFICULT SCENARIOS

Occasionally, challenging situations are encountered in delivering IMCP. We have selected a few such scenarios and summarized how we have dealt with them.

No Legacy to Leave Behind

Patient speaks about feeling she has no legacy to leave behind. She is divorced with no children and believes her nieces will only vaguely remember her and do not make an effort to spend time with her. Patient feels that she is alone and that no one came to her aid during a previous illness and during her cancer treatment. Therapist explains that perhaps that is the legacy she can live and leave behind, to be selfless and give back to others. She believes this is useless as she has no one to leave these values behind. Therapist encourages her to tell her story to her nieces and write about it in her memoirs, which she has started writing prior to therapy. An additional concept is introduced and that is the concept of "significance." Significance is related to meaning in the sense that we human beings often feel the need to have had our lives, as well as our suffering, witnessed—the idea that there was a "sign" (*sign*ificance) that they lived and had an impact on the world and people in some way. What is explored with patients is the fact that they have always been the one constant witness to their own lives. And they are the recipient of the legacy of the life they have lived: They are the judge of whether they have lived an authentic life—a life they can accept as "good enough" as they face the possibility of death. The legacy that is left behind is not knowable to them, but what is knowable is the legacy they are living—the life they are living and witnessing, a life of significance.

Resistance to Meaning-Centered Material

Patient is very resistant to listening about MCP concepts and particularly learning about Frankl. He says he searches for meaning on his own. He does not want to learn about meaning. He does enough of that work at his synagogue, where he is the director. Patient is very ambivalent about learning about Frankl. He knows a lot about the Holocaust and does not believe he needs to learn further about it. The therapist lets him vent his feelings about the material, and eventually the patient allows the therapist to introduce meaning and Frankl.

Resistance to the Idea of Suffering

Patient feels he is not suffering. He is very angry and very resistant to the idea that he is suffering. He believes he brought the disease on himself, having hepatitis. He believes that you are here and then you die. He is not afraid of dying and does not believe he is suffering. He opens up eventually with regard to his attitude toward suffering, explaining that he has struggled with not feeling in control with what is happening to him. He believes he has made the choices he has in life, and he has to live with them now. The patient eventually opens up that he feels he has had a good life and has done what he has wanted in life. He believes that the existential quest for meaning never ends, and he works on these principles at his synagogue. The therapist explains that they will work on taking this foundation that he already has and dial it up—to take the principles that he already has and expand on them.

Unfocused Patient

Patient is introduced to sources of meaning, creativity, courage, and responsibility. Patient becomes tangential frequently, and the therapist works to redirect her to the topic of the session and the exercise to be completed. Eventually, the patient engages in the material but is very resistant and preoccupied at first.

Patient frequently interrupts while the therapist explains the layout of each session. When the patient interrupts, he frequently goes on lengthy tangents about his attitude toward cancer and that he does not think about it at all. The therapist works to listen to the patient and his thoughts while working to redirect him back to the overview of the layout of each session. Frequently, the patient rejects the overview of each session, its concepts and line of thought being presented to him, and continues on another tangent. Each time, the therapist works to redirect him back to the material.

SUMMARY

Individual meaning-centered psychotherapy has been demonstrated, in randomized clinical trials, to be an effective intervention to diminish despair in patients with advanced cancer. IMCP is efficacious in decreasing anxiety, depression, hopelessness, desire for hastened death, and symptom burden distress while improving quality of life and spiritual well-being. This is all mediated through the enhancement of meaning. IMCP, the individual format of MCP, has some advantages over the group format of MCP (MCGP) in that there is greater flexibility in scheduling and an ability to have more intensive sessions with an individual patient. Readers are referred to Appendix 2 for a full transcript of an exemplar course of IMCP treatment of two patients with advanced cancer. In addition, for a comprehensive guide to session content, refer to *Individual Meaning-Centered Psychotherapy for Patients with Advanced Cancer: A Treatment Manual*.[12]

REFERENCES

1. Puchalski C, Ferrell B, Virani R, et al. Improving the quality of spiritual care as a dimension of palliative care: The report of the consensus conference. *J Palliat Med*. 2009;12(10):885–904.
2. Breitbart W, Rosenfeld B, Pessin H, et al. Depression, hopelessness, and desire for hastened death in terminally ill patients with cancer. *J Am Med Assoc*. 2000;284(22):2907–2911.
3. Breitbart W. Spirituality and meaning in supportive care: Spirituality and meaning-centered group psychotherapy interventions in advanced cancer. *Supportive Care Cancer*. 2002;10(4):272–280.
4. Frankl VF. *The Doctor and the Soul*. New York, NY: Random House; 1955/1986.
5. Frankl VF. *Man's Search for Meaning*. 4th ed. Boston, MA: Beacon; 1959/1992.
6. Frankl VF. *The Will to Meaning: Foundations and Applications of Logotherapy, Expanded Edition*. New York, NY: Penguin; 1969/1988.
7. Frankl VF. *Man's Search for Ultimate Meaning*. New York, NY: Plenum; 1975/1997.
8. Breitbart W, Gibson C, Poppito SR, et al. In review. *Can J Psychiatry*. 2004;49:366–372.
9. Breitbart W, Poppito S, Rosenfeld B, et al. A pilot randomized controlled trial of individual meaning-centered psychotherapy for patients with advanced cancer. *J Clin Oncol*. 2012;30(12):1304–1309.
10. Breitbart W, Rosenfeld B, Gibson C, et al. Meaning-centered group psychotherapy for patients with advanced cancer: A pilot randomized controlled trial. *Psycho-Oncology*. 2010;19:21–28.
11. Nelson CJ, Rosenfeld B, Breitbart W, et al. Spirituality, religion, and depression in the terminally ill. *Psychosomatics*. 2002;43(3):213–220.
12. Breitbart W, Poppito S. *Individual Meaning-Centered Psychotherapy for Patients with Advanced Cancer: A Treatment Manual*. New York, NY: Oxford University Press, 2014.

4

Meaning-Centered Group Psychotherapy for Breast Cancer Survivors

WENDY G. LICHTENTHAL, KAILEY E. ROBERTS, GRETA JANKAUSKAITE, CARALINE CRAIG, DAWN WIATREK, KATHERINE SHARPE, AND WILLIAM BREITBART

INTRODUCTION

The 2005 Institute of Medicine (IOM) report, "From Cancer Patient to Cancer Survivor," highlighted the psychosocial challenges of survivorship, especially psychiatric disorders and existential distress.[1] Among cancer survivors, the majority of research on psychosocial distress has focused on those with a history of breast cancer because of the size of this subpopulation. Specifically, several studies have documented the unique challenges that breast cancer survivors (BCS) face in finding a sense of meaning, identity, and purpose in their lives after treatment completion.[2–8] Having confronted their own mortality, the desire to live meaningful lives is often intensely heightened. However, a significant subset of BCS feel "stuck"[8] and struggle with reorganizing their sense of meaning, identity, and purpose.[6] A decreased sense of meaning has been associated with depression, anxiety, and lower quality of life among cancer survivors.[4,9–12] In addition, studies have shown that having a sense of meaning in life actually mediates the relationship between depression and physical symptoms (e.g., fatigue and pain) that BCS commonly experience.[9,13–15]

There has been a clear need to develop empirically supported, conceptually sound interventions that directly address post-treatment adjustment issues in BCS. This need is compounded by the disproportionate lack of psychotherapeutic interventions targeting psychosocial issues after cancer treatment is completed,[16–18] a time when distress has been shown to peak for many survivors. Furthermore, existing interventions have only demonstrated small effects.[19] This may be in part because interventions are not focusing on issues about which BCS are most concerned.

BCS have voiced that their greatest unmet need is support for existential issues.[7] Despite the central role that finding meaning and purpose plays in their adjustment, there is an absence of empirically supported interventions that focus on enhancing meaning as a means of addressing the psychosocial challenges that BCS often face. Meaning-centered group psychotherapy for breast cancer survivors (MCGP-BCS), which has been adapted from meaning-centered group psychotherapy for advanced cancer patients, addresses this need.[20,21] We believe MCGP-BCS has the therapeutic potential to address the challenges in finding meaning that many BCS face. It represents a response to the unmet need of survivors for support targeting existential issues.[7] This chapter describes our efforts, in collaboration with the American Cancer Society (ACS), to adapt and pilot test MCGP-BCS, which is being delivered "virtually" through a web-conferencing application to facilitate connections among survivors who may not be able to return to the cancer treatment facility at which they were treated for support.

Rationale for Initially Focusing on Breast Cancer Survivors

BCS comprise the largest cohort of survivors of any cancer.[22,23] Of the 2.8 million BCS in the United States, 89%—that is, approximately 2.5 million—will live at least 5 years.[22] Several studies have reported the challenges that many BCS face in finding a sense of meaning, purpose, and identity following the threat to their mortality and the physical health changes that result from the cancer experience.[3,4,8,24–27] Survivors often express a heightened desire to live authentic and meaningful lives, but a significant subset struggle with their altered sense of identity and values and report feeling "stuck."[8] A decreased sense of meaning can have substantial negative consequences, including heightened depression and anxiety, and reduced quality of life.[9,10,28–30] Furthermore, studies have demonstrated that a lower sense of meaning actually mediates the relationship between depression and common physical symptoms that BCS face (e.g., fatigue and pain).[9,14] BCS are twice as likely as the general population to suffer from depression or anxiety within the first year of diagnosis,[31] and depression in BCS has been associated with greater functional impairment[32] and reduced return to work.[33] Thus, targeting decreased meaning in life—a risk factor for depression—in BCS is an important priority in psycho-oncology.

Breitbart et al.[28] demonstrated the buffering role of meaning, suggesting that interventions focusing on enhancing meaning may reduce depression. Among BCS, an increased sense of meaning has been associated with reduced depression 5–8 years post-diagnosis.[11] In addition, given that the relationship between depression and physical symptoms is accounted for in part by decreased meaning in life,[9,14] researchers have suggested that the impact of common physical symptoms (e.g., fatigue) may be mitigated by fostering meaning in survivors.[9,13] Psychosocial interventions may be particularly important for individuals with less severe but still impairing psychological symptoms; a meta-analysis demonstrated that antidepressants are relatively ineffective with less severe depressive symptoms.[34] Although individuals who do find meaning and growth after cancer have received much attention,[4,35,36] those who struggle with finding meaning must not be neglected. Furthermore, as stated above, BCS have reported that their most common unmet need is help with existential issues.[7]

Of note, our work has started with a more homogenous survivor population—those with a history of breast cancer—in order to make initial modifications to MCGP and to promote group cohesion. In the future, using our BCS adaptation as a model, we intend to tailor the intervention for survivors of other cancers who share similar existential concerns.[37–39]

The Need for Interventions for Post-treatment Survivors

The World Health Organization has emphasized that as the number of survivors continues to increase, health care providers must find ways to address long-term psychosocial and quality-of-life issues that emerge in the wake of survivors' illness.[40] Yet, as noted previously, there is a dearth of empirical support for psychosocial interventions targeting the post-treatment period.[16] In his 2009 article defining clinical practice guidelines for the psychosocial care of cancer survivors, Jacobsen[16] highlighted that only 8% of trials recruited cancer patients who completed treatment. The majority of psychotherapy trials have focused on patients actively receiving treatment[41–43] rather than targeting the large population of survivors post-treatment, who the IOM aptly refers to as "lost in transition."[1] Furthermore, interventions that have been tested have not been particularly efficacious.[19,44] Those with stronger effects (e.g., cognitive–behavioral therapy[17]) have not targeted post-treatment survivors nor addressed or assessed existential issues, such as loss of meaning. There is a compelling need to develop and empirically validate theoretically driven, acceptable psychosocial interventions for BCS that directly address their unique survivorship issues.

Developing empirically supported interventions that target the existential distress that a significant subset of BCS has reported is critical to the improvement of their quality of life. The efficacy of a variety of interventions (e.g., mindfulness, cognitive–behavioral stress management, and writing about illness benefits)[17–19,37,41,45,46] in reducing psychological distress among early stage breast cancer patients currently receiving treatment has been examined. Despite the empirically demonstrated relationship between meaning and adjustment following cancer, and frequent recommendations by researchers, to our knowledge, few interventions have focused specifically on fostering meaning as a means of reducing psychological distress in cancer survivors.[47,48] MCGP-BCS directly addresses the struggles that many BCS face in finding meaning in their lives.

ADAPTATION OF MEANING-CENTERED GROUP PSYCHOTHERAPY FOR BREAST CANCER SURVIVORS

In order to adapt MCGP into MCGP-BCS, we conducted three focus groups composed of BCS recruited from Memorial Sloan Kettering Cancer Center (MSK) and ACS to obtain feedback on the approach and to help shape the adapted MCGP-BCS intervention manual. We recruited 16 participants for each of the three focus groups, and 12 BCS ultimately participated. The use of focus groups provided us with an opportunity to identify survivorship issues that may not have been reported in the existing psychosocial literature and helped us to determine survivors' preferences for communication about these issues.[49] We obtained important feedback through the focus groups to ensure the intervention is comprehensive and appropriately tailored to BCS' unique issues, needs, and preferences. The focus groups also enabled us to determine additional survey questions and outcomes that might be important to include in evaluating MCGP-BCS.

The three focus groups each lasted 2 hours and were facilitated by W.L. through a virtual meeting platform, using both a phone and a computer. A focus group guide was used to engage participants in discussion about the existing intervention. Focus group discussions were transcribed by a professional transcription service and analyzed using thematic content analysis—a well-established, systematic qualitative method in health research—to derive meaning from participants' discussion.[50] We followed Morse's[50] guidelines for conducting rigorous qualitative research (e.g., use of an audit trail and saturation). Four coders, including W.L. and K.R., independently reviewed each focus group transcript; identified themes; and synthesized and interpreted BCS' views regarding the content, feasibility, and acceptability of MCGP-BCS. After independent review, the coding team had several meetings to reach consensus on a final set of thematic findings from all three focus groups.[51,52]

Overall, focus group participants provided positive feedback on the applicability and utility of a meaning-centered approach for addressing their existential concerns. However, they offered a number of suggestions to better tailor the therapy to their experiences. Although they valued the meaning-centered approach, the majority of the participants expressed that there should be a reduced emphasis on the past and an increased focus on the present and future. Exercises were modified accordingly. For example, the identity exercise, *Who Am I?* which is conducted in Session 2, now includes a more explicitly future-oriented experiential question, "Who do you want to be?" In addition, BCS provided feedback on other experiential exercises and suggested they be modified to provide more opportunities to develop short-term meaning-centered goals. Accordingly, several exercises now draw on cognitive–behavioral techniques for developing short-term goals and identifying barriers to completing those goals in order to promote change and reduce "stuckness." For example, in Session 4, BCS are asked not only to reflect on the story they would like to create but also to identify three specific changes they would make to create this story. In Sessions 5 and 6, group members are encouraged to problem solve around potential obstacles they may face in engaging with a meaningful attitude or task. In addition, some BCS expressed that Viktor Frankl's[53] work, which is discussed in MCP, did not seem relevant to their experience; for others, Frankl's principles and Holocaust narrative resonated. Finally, the analysis identified several suggestions for altering the language used in MCGP-BCS to reduce associations with death, including replacing the word "legacy" with "story" and the word "limitations" with "challenges," adding "survivor" as an example of identity, and adapting language to be less abstract overall.

OVERVIEW OF MEANING-CENTERED GROUP PSYCHOTHERAPY FOR BREAST CANCER SURVIVORS

MCGP is a novel, manualized, 8-week, nonpharmacologic intervention developed by Dr. William Breitbart and colleagues at MSK and designed to enhance a sense of meaning and purpose among advanced cancer patients.[54–56] Based largely on Frankl's work,[57] MCGP addresses existential issues using didactics and experiential exercises. MCGP, as well as an individual version of meaning-centered psychotherapy, have both demonstrated efficacy in reducing existential suffering and improving psychosocial functioning among advanced cancer patients.[54–56] However, the existential issues that advanced cancer patients, who are approaching death, face are very different than those of cancer survivors, who face an uncertain but promising future. Thus, as noted previously, in order to meet the unique existential and survivorship issues of cancer survivors, it was necessary to first modify MCGP.

MCGP-BCS, the resulting adapted manualized intervention, uses psychoeducation, experiential exercises, and homework focusing on themes related to meaning, cancer, and survivorship. Like MCGP, MCGP-BCS is based on Frankl's principles of logotherapy and concepts, including (1) the consistency of meaning in life and one's authentic identity; (2) the will to meaning; (3) freedom of will and choosing one's attitude in the face of suffering; and (4) sources of meaning, derived from creativity and experience.[57] The MCGP-BCS manual outlines eight, 90-minute sessions. Within the MCGP-BCS framework, cognitive techniques[58,59] such as those suggested by Kissane et al.[60,61] can be incorporated to enhance meaning-making and reframe maladaptive thinking. Behavioral strategies, as described here, are also employed. Based on the feedback we received from our focus groups, the therapy was modified to have an increased emphasis on the future, identifying "unsought gifts"[62] as a result of the cancer experience and taking small steps toward continuing to create their story based on the sources of meaning identified by the BCS throughout the group.

Application of the Meaning-Centered Theoretical Model in MCGP-BCS

Cancer survivorship can result in a crisis in meaning. "Meaning" is a complex construct that has been defined in many ways,[26,36,63,64] including the conceptual model suggested by Viktor Frankl[57] that underlies MCGP. Frankl defined meaning as the conviction that one has successfully created a life with meaning, purpose, and identity through connectedness with valued relationships and roles in the world.[53] This model assumes that, based on empirical literature,[36,65–67] cancer can positively or negatively impact one's sense of meaning. Applying MCGP-BCS is believed to enhance meaning, facilitating a process that, for some survivors, comes naturally.[36,65–67] Meaning is hypothesized to be both an intermediary outcome (a construct to be enhanced in its own right) and a mediator, driving improvement in multiple psychological distress outcomes (e.g., by redirecting attention toward meaningful activities).[68] Studies have shown several unique ways in which components of meaning may be impacted among BCS. The following are examples:

- *Identity*: One's sense of identity is intimately connected to one's sense of meaning and purpose in life. Challenges to BCS' sense of identity may include alterations in body image,[69] physical limitations,[70] and choosing the extent to which a "survivor identity" is meaningful.[2,27] An altered sense of self is associated with heightened psychological distress.[5,8] Self-transformation, in contrast, has been associated with well-being in BCS.[8]
- *Existential isolation*: Changes in one's identity and a heightened awareness of mortality may result in disconnection and existential isolation. This has been referred to as "survivor loneliness" in BCS and has been associated with an altered sense of identity and a desire to lead a more authentic life.[5]
- *Disconnection from sources of meaning*: During treatment, there may be a disconnection from sources of meaning, such as meaningful relationships and responsibilities. After treatment, survivors may similarly feel disconnected from their health care providers, as well as the structure provided by their treatment regimens, and they may be less likely to follow up for survivorship care.
- *Fear of cancer recurrence*: Cancer survivors may also become preoccupied with fears that their disease will recur and threaten their existence. Among BCS, fear of recurrence is associated with increased distress, poorer psychological adaptation, and decreased quality of life.[1,71,72]
- *Meaning of the illness*: The meaning of the illness in the context of BCS' lives also plays an important role in adjustment. BCS who ascribe a more negative meaning of their illness (e.g., as punishment) have higher levels of depression and anxiety and lower quality of life than women who find positive meaning in their illness.[3,4]
- *Benefit-finding and posttraumatic growth*: In contrast, identifying the positive consequences and meaning of the cancer experience (e.g., increased appreciation of life),[4,24–26] referred to as benefit-finding, and resulting posttraumatic growth[25,73] has been associated with decreased depression and improved physical functioning.[35,74–76]

MCGP-BCS Session Overview

MCGP-BCS addresses each of these facets of meaning, applying Frankl's[57] recommendation to reconnect with valued sources of meaning. The intervention is designed to facilitate this process of reconnecting with or enhancing meaning and also integrates other components of meaning, such as identity and reducing isolation. The eight sessions are as follows:

1. Concepts and Sources of Meaning
2. Identity, Cancer Survivorship, and Meaning
3. Historical Sources of Meaning: The History that Has Been Given
4. Historical Sources of Meaning: Life as a Story One Creates
5. Attitudinal Sources of Meaning: Encountering Life's Challenges
6. Creative Sources of Meaning: Actively Engaging in Life

7. Experiential Sources of Meaning: Experiencing and Connecting with Life
8. Hopes for the Future: Opportunities and New Beginnings

Table 4.1 provides an overview of the sessions. Each session includes an experiential exercise to which group members respond both in writing, ideally as a homework assignment in advance of the next session, and verbally. Although homework is not required of group members, engagement with the material outside of the group setting is strongly encouraged to facilitate regular application of meaning-centered principles in their daily lives. When members have not written out their responses in advance of the group, the group facilitators can designate time during the session for members to reflect on and briefly write out their responses.

In Session 1, members are introduced to the intervention, including the sources of meaning and the definitions of meaning underlying the intervention. In addition, members are invited to engage in the first experiential exercise through which they describe one or two meaningful moments in their lives. These meaningful moments vary from the mundane to the extraordinary (e.g., taking a walk and noticing the sunset or the birth of a child). As members describe their meaningful moments, the therapist makes note of how the moments reflect one or more sources of meaning and draws connections between sources of meaning held by members to promote group cohesion. Although Frankl's work is not as strongly emphasized in MCGP-BCS as it often is in MCGP for advanced cancer patients, the first chapter of *Man's Search for Meaning* is assigned as a first homework activity to highlight how one can reconnect with sources of meaning despite extremely challenging circumstances.[53] Members are also encouraged to complete the experiential exercise, "Identity and Cancer Survivorship," in preparation for the second session.

The second session focuses on identity and survivorship, highlighting the link between valued sources of meaning and one's sense of self. Members are invited to share their responses to questions about their sense of identity before cancer, after cancer, and who they would like to be in the future. In addition to drawing connections between members, the group facilitator attempts to identify the ways in which each member has maintained core aspects of her identity despite cancer. Changes to members' sense of self that appear to be valued by the individual and adaptive, such as identifying as someone who "appreciates the moment," are also highlighted. Members are asked to respond to the experiential exercise for the next session, which explores participants' past as an introduction to historical sources of meaning.

Session 3 is the first of two sessions focusing on historical sources of meaning, which are explored through conceptualizing "life as a story" that one can author in any way she chooses. In this session, members are invited to discuss the story that they were given by reflecting on significant memories, relationships, and traditions

TABLE 4.1 MEANING-CENTERED GROUP PSYCHOTHERAPY–BREAST CANCER SURVIVORS (MCGP-BCS) SESSION OVERVIEW

Session Topics	Themes
Session 1: Concepts and sources of meaning	Introductions and meaning
Session 2: Identity, cancer survivorship, and meaning	Identity before and after cancer diagnosis
Session 3: Historical sources of meaning	The history that has been given (past)
Session 4: Historical sources of meaning	"Life as story" that one creates (present and future)
Session 5: Attitudinal sources of meaning	"Encountering life's challenges" (choosing one's attitude toward life)
Session 6: Creative sources of meaning	"Actively engaging in life" (through creativity and responsibility)
Session 7: Experiential sources of meaning	"Experiencing and connecting with life" (through love, beauty, and humor)
Session 8: Hopes for the future	Opportunities and new beginnings

that have made the greatest impact in their lives. A focus group member described this as a discussion of the "good, the bad, and the ugly." It often helps elucidate why members' valued sources of meaning came to be that way. Session 4 continues the theme of "life as a story" by asking members to reflect on the meaningful activities, roles, and accomplishments of which they are most proud. Connections between the past and present may demonstrate that a member has maintained the story she was given or that she worked to create a new story, even prior to cancer. A core concept highlighted is that each moment one is alive offers another opportunity to author one's story as one would like it to be. Session 4 concludes with an opportunity for members to consider the story they are currently living and how it compares to the story they would like to create. Members are asked to identify three changes they would like to make in their lives to help create the life they would like to live. They are also asked to consider the extent to which they would like their cancer experience to be a part of this story. To assist with creating a coherent narrative and increase their sense of connection to others, members are invited to share their story with a loved one and observe the feelings they experience from having others hear them.

The fifth session opens with a chance for members to reflect on their experiences sharing their stories. When members are unable to identify someone with whom they could share their story, their courage in sharing with the group thus far might be reinforced. The choice in *how* members have told their stories often provides a useful segue into Session 5, which focuses on attitude as a source of meaning. This is a central meaning-centered principle described by Frankl as a way to find meaning in the face of suffering.[53] For cancer survivors, suffering may take the form of, for example, post-treatment side effects, body image concerns, and fear of disease recurrence. How BCS face these challenges can be a choice they value—in other words, a source of meaning in and of itself. Members are asked to reflect on how they have faced past challenges. The choices they have had in coping with prior stressful situations are highlighted. At the conclusion of Session 5, the "Putting the Me in Meaning" project is introduced. This is similar to the Legacy Project in MCGP for advanced cancer patients, encouraging members to pursue something they have been wanting to do but have not yet done (e.g., a hobby, job, mending a relationship, and traveling). Facilitators help members focus on goals that may help them get "unstuck."

The focus of Session 6 is creativity as a source of meaning, exploring how members actively engage in life. Similar to MCGP-BCS, the facilitator emphasizes the significant role that courage and commitment play in creative pursuits.[53] The existential concept of responsibility is highlighted as members respond to the experiential exercise questions about instances when they have been courageous and made a commitment to something meaningful. The facilitator highlights how even seemingly mundane actions can be viewed as courageous. Members are also invited to reflect on whether they have expressed what is most meaningful through their work and creative activities (e.g., job, parenting, hobbies, and causes). They are then asked to consider to and for whom they are responsible. The theme of self-care often emerges for cancer survivors, who may have realized the importance of taking care of themselves through the cancer experience but struggle to attend to their own needs. Finally, the group considers tasks they have wanted to accomplish and barriers to doing so. Members are encouraged to problem-solve together and to activate one another.

Session 7 is nearly identical to the corresponding session in MCGP.[21] The didactic portion of this session communicates the idea that experiential sources of meaning enable one to connect with life and can assist individuals with transcending difficult times. Members discuss the ways in which they experience and connect with life through receiving love, appreciating beauty, and through humor. During this session, feelings about the group coming to a close are also explored. Members are reminded to attend to the Putting the Me in Meaning project, which they present in Session 8.

The eighth and final session focuses on hopes for the future, framed as opportunities and new beginnings. Much of the session is devoted to reflecting on the experience of the therapy, sources of meaning, and the opportunities for growth that it may have provided. Members also share their Putting the Me in Meaning projects. If a project has not been completed, the facilitator may highlight ways the group member has engaged in the group and should encourage her to pursue her project after the group has finished. Other hopes for the future are explored, and potential obstacles to achieving goals are discussed. The group concludes with expressions of appreciation for the ways in which members have been meaningfully touched by their connections with one another.

CURRENT EFFORTS TO EVALUATE MCGP-BCS

In order to initiate a larger scale randomized controlled trial (RCT) of MCGP for BCS, we are currently conducting a pilot RCT in collaboration with ACS to demonstrate the feasibility and preliminary efficacy of this intervention. The study has consisted of two phases. The first phase was the adaptation phase using focus groups described in this chapter. In the second phase, currently underway, we are recruiting BCS who indicate at least a moderate level of distress (Distress Thermometer score of 4 or greater)[77,78] related to their breast cancer or survivorship experience, have completed active treatment for their cancer (may be receiving hormonal treatment), and do not have metastatic disease. Participants are randomly assigned, stratified by surgery type, to receive eight sessions of MCGP-BCS or eight sessions of a standardized supportive group psychotherapy (SGP), a standardized, manualized intervention developed by the MSK Psychiatry Service and utilized in our completed RCTs of MCGP.[79] SGP is based on supportive psychotherapy models described by Rogers[80] and Bloch,[81] with a focus on here-and-now topics relevant to BCS (e.g., maintaining and eliciting social support, financial strains, return to work, and physical symptom management). Both MCGP-BCS and SGP are delivered "virtually" through a secure, web-based audio conferencing system. Assessments of feasibility, acceptability, and psychosocial outcomes are being conducted pre-intervention, mid-intervention, post-intervention, and 3 months post-intervention. Measures are completed online to increase convenience for participating survivors.

Group Case Example

The following case example illustrates the progression of one MCGP-BCS group that participated in our study. The group included four women ranging in age from 44 to 70 years and was facilitated by W.L. and W.B. In Session 1, members were provided with introductions to the therapy and invited to share their cancer stories. The process of sharing their cancer stories enabled members to begin an initial connection to each other, as well as understand their unique stories. Shared themes included loneliness, fear of disease recurrence, and a legacy of cancer in the family.

Toward the end of the first session, group members were asked to share meaningful moments in their lives. In the following excerpt from the first session, one member, Beverly, describes her struggle with a profound sense of loneliness and disconnection from sources of meaning:[1A]

W.L.: Any challenges you want to share with the group in terms of meaning?

Beverly: Yeah, well my challenge is ... I am very lonely, I feel ... cut off from society ... and I really do feel a bit my life is meaningless.

W.L.: Well, that's certainly something that we've heard from a lot of breast cancer survivors ... this disconnection that happened feeling different through the cancer experience because even treatment itself or whatever one is suffering from ... they call this "survivor loneliness." So it takes a lot of courage to speak about that, and so thank you so much for sharing that with us. ... But I do want to point out just in your story that you ... bestowed upon yourself to the same care that you if you did professionally ... and that speaks to what Dr. Breitbart was saying about taking responsibility for oneself. I think that was really, really powerful.

Despite her disconnection from sources of meaning, this member described two meaningful moments—her relationship with God and the feeling of love she receives when she comes home from work to her dog—that illustrated she has maintained a connection to meaning through allowing herself to experience love.

As a second member, Mary, shared her sense of disconnection from sources of meaning such as her book club, poetry, and her daughters, an opportunity arose to reflect on the idea of choosing one's attitude as a source of meaning. Highlighting how group members' choice to participate in the group is a form of self-care can facilitate discussion about other ways in which they are choosing to engage in self-care or in their lives in general. The following excerpt illustrates how the therapists identify feelings of disconnection and highlight sources of meaning, including the attitude chosen, early on in the therapy:

Mary: I kind of lost everything, and then cancer really threw me. But I was trying to come back and ... I said this might even help me more. I

[1A] Names and other personal details have been changed to protect privacy.

was in the book club, I had dropped out of that, but I think I might go back now, you know, in the church. Oh, and I used to write poetry, and I stopped that . . . I just couldn't think, I couldn't focus . . .

W.B.: So this is what you meant by feeling disconnected, right?

Mary: Oh, right. I was feeling disconnected before the cancer, you know so I wasn't sure if I should belong in this group. . . . But I am always afraid that it is going to come back . . . my mother had it, so there's a history; my aunt had it . . . so I am a little afraid here. . . . I am very afraid . . . and I shouldn't live my life like this, but . . . being alone you keep thinking about it, and I don't want to burden my daughter, she is close by. My other daughter lives far, she has four kids now. . . . I'm trying to be independent, that's the biggest thing . . . and I'm having a hard time (laughs) . . . so I'm almost—not giving up, I guess I can't give up—but I do regress, I go backwards. And I try to hide it from my daughter because I think she is picking up that I'm a little . . . down.

W.B.: So, you know what I'm hearing is there are many sources of meaning in your life—your daughters, your work, poetry . . . all sorts of things that give you pleasure. . . .

Mary: But I haven't done any of that.

W.B.: . . . But you have just become disconnected from them.

Mary: I forgot about the "drawers," I knew they were there, and I forgot. I just didn't think about them, I don't know why.

W.B.: Right. So, we've got to help you identify the drawers and fill them up a little bit (laughs).

Mary: Yeah, I just realized when you said that, I thought, wow, there are a lot of things . . .

W.B.: I see.

W.L.: And I heard you say "I can't give up" . . .

Mary: . . . Yeah, I can't give up because of my children. I feel like I can't give up. I wonder if I was alone if that would be the same, I don't know . . .

W.L.: Well, I think when you say that, when someone says, "I can't give up," what that says to us is about the attitude you have, and of course it's complicated by feeling this disconnection to other sources of meaning, but wrapped up in there is something about the attitude you have in terms of life. And you know, that will be part of the work that we do is recognizing that more, calling it out more, and giving yourself credit for—despite these challenges—the fact that you have been, you know, keeping your head up of water and trying to figure out a way. And . . . something important to acknowledge while we are all in this group together is that by virtue of participating in this group, when you are approached about it, saying, you know, "I'm going to go ahead and do this"—that's extremely courageous . . .

As the group progressed from session to session, each of the four members' connections with sources of meaning, many of which were already present in their lives, and the meaningful choices in attitude they had made were brought to their attention. The idea that they could choose their attitude toward situations that were beyond their control resonated with the members. They expressed a desire to focus more on self-care and an increased appreciation of life following their cancer experience. Members also described ways in which their past experiences impacted how they approached their illness and cancer survivorship. As some members struggled to acknowledge their achievements, the facilitators and other group members highlighted these and the possibilities that their future could hold. Movement toward valued goals was encouraged and supported.

Beverly's Putting the Me in Meaning project illustrated this as, by the final, eighth session, she demonstrated a striking shift in attitude, mood, and level of motivation. In the following excerpt from Session 8, she describes her intention to write a memoir and how engaging in the project had pushed her to begin the process. She shared the title of the book she planned on writing, as well as its core idea, which reflected a meaningful and powerful new attitude she had adopted:

Beverly: I always wanted to write a book.

W.L.: Okay.

Beverly: I read extensively, and I used to write short stories as a child and—because I have this very wild imagination . . . and I have started a few times to write this book, but I just could not decide exactly what I'm going to write. So I shelved that idea for awhile. But through this group, I decided that I am going to write the book, and this book will be called, "Finding Myself Again." [2B]

[2B] The book title has been changed to protect privacy.

Similarly, Mary used the group and the Putting the Me in Meaning project as an impetus to focus on self-care through engagement with meaningful connections and creative activities:

Mary: My main project will consist of me nurturing myself first, so that I'll be able to help my family and friends in need. I will look in to massage, yoga, trying to exercise more, eat right, lose weight. I'll try to concentrate on mending relationships, especially with my brother. I do want to play an instrument. I mean, these are all things that I am like really going to think about now because we talked about it. Most likely guitar, and I'll try to get back to writing. I was writing poetry for a while, and then I stopped a long time ago, and so I might do that again. And then with retirement in sight, I said I hope to have more time to do all of these projects, as well as fixing up my home, and hopefully going out with friends and that ... that's something to look forward to in the future.

Of note, Mary remarked how she got many of the ideas about what she could do for herself from other members of the group. Later in Session 8, the members were invited to reflect on their experience within the group and engaging with the meaning-related material. By this final session, Beverly, who had expressed a deep sense of disconnection and loneliness in the first group session, described how she had chosen to reconnect with others by reaching out to others who had experienced cancer:

Beverly: This has been a very valuable experience for me, and I just want to, you know, let you all know how much I appreciate what we have shared throughout, you know, these sessions. And, for me, I have opened up so much. I never spoke about my feelings as I did here. And after speaking here, I have begun to speak elsewhere, and it has made the world of difference to myself and to other people. And I have been getting a lot of feedback from people that say that I have become an inspiration for them ... you know, I did a project in October, it being cancer month, and it was just to reach out to people who had someone who they cared for who was going through cancer or had been through cancer. And I tried to just do little mini seminars on, you know, what people who go through cancer feel and what they would like from other people, because we hear so often, you know, "I don't know what to say," "I don't know what to do," you know, "How can I help?" ... so I tried to make it as a little easier for them. And it has worked, and I feel so empowered, you know, by this. And I think I have only to thank you guys for encouraging me to speak up and to speak out, and I just want to say thank you very much and God bless you.

W.L.: That was beautiful ... I am so touched by the courage—thinking back to our very first group, and the challenges you shared, and the fact that you were so saddened about "not feeling" ...

Beverly: I was so disconnected.

W.L.: So disconnected, and we talked about the courage it takes to engage in life and to create a life, and you responded to that. You took responsibility for your life and started responding and engaging in a way, giving people the opportunity to then respond to you authentically ... I think what happened in the group and their responses to you ... was inspiring.

Mary also reflected on the importance of engaging with others and shared the significance of her newfound awareness that she can choose her attitude toward different situations. Although she reflected on how she would like to have a calmer and less depressive attitude in the face of challenges, she also noted that simply the idea of having the freedom to choose her attitude was empowering:

Mary: Well, for me, it's been very enlightening. I've always had, like, this "defeatist" attitude, but now I'm aware that I have this attitude, and I have the choice to react differently, so now I have to, you know, I'm aware of it now. So, I have to stop and say, "Wait, I can change ... this is not the end of the world." And I think that's what I have learned.

W.L.: What's so striking about that to me ... is ... no one ever said, no one in this group, obviously, ever said that you've had a defeatist attitude.

Mary: Well, I've known it, I probably didn't share that (laughs). I've been down, I get overwhelmed ... you know, I guess depressed, that's the word, I hate to use it, but I get depressed very easily, and down. And I have to just say something—my daughter noticed that I wasn't down ... she was driving me somewhere, and she goes, "Are you okay?" And

I said, "Yes," and she goes, "Well, you sound ... you seem very "'uppity,'" like she noticed a difference in me. And I just said, "I wonder if it's the group" (laughs). You know, because of the group. I tell my brother all about it, and he is so happy that I am doing this. So I'm trying to connect slowly.

After W.L. highlighted how Mary is now recognizing the freedom she has to choose her attitude, Mary expanded upon this idea:

Mary: I never thought about that before ... to react differently. I just thought, you just go downhill, but I don't have to go downhill (laughs). I can go down a little bit, but come back up slowly ... so that's what I have to keep remembering.

As Mary described current challenges she was facing with her health, the therapist then reiterated a core meaning-centered principle:

W.L.: Suffering is inevitable, Frankl would say, but how you face it is what we have the freedom to choose ... that's what we have. It's not that you're not going to have more down times. You know, this is not a group designed to "prevent suffering." It's designed to help with something that is believed to transcend suffering, which is finding meaning. Finding meaning in the things you do, the things you experience, the attitude you take, and the life you've lived, and the story you're telling, writing, and will continue to live.

In summary, Beverly and Mary moved from feeling stuck and a sense of meaninglessness to taking responsibility for their lives and a deeper sense of connection to others after eight sessions of MCGP-BCS.

SUMMARY

After completing treatment for cancer, existential issues commonly rise to the fore. MCGP-BCS has the potential to address these issues, reducing the sense of isolation that may develop through feeling different than others who have not faced a life-threatening illness by bringing cancer survivors together. We have used direct input from BCS to adapt MCGP into an intervention that is more future-oriented and behavioral in nature to help members get "unstuck" post-treatment. The intervention assists survivors with identifying sources of meaning in their lives and bringing these to the forefront of their consciousness. It highlights the choices survivors have in how they face the sequelae of their disease. We have successfully been using web conferencing to bring survivors, who often are unable to regularly return in person to their treating institution or providers, together virtually. We will continue to refine MCGP-BCS and, in collaboration with ACS, to evaluate its potential in enhancing survivors' sense of meaning in the wake of the cancer experience.

ACKNOWLEDGMENTS

We are grateful for the input of the breast cancer survivors who participated in our research. The study described in this chapter is funded by American Cancer Society Contract 11656 (Lichtenthal/Breitbart).

REFERENCES

1. Hewitt ME, Greenfield S, Stovall E; National Cancer Policy Board (US), Committee on Cancer Survivorship: Improving Care and Quality of Life. *From Cancer Patient to Cancer Survivor: Lost in Transition.* Washington, DC: National Academies Press; 2006.
2. Kaiser K. The meaning of the survivor identity for women with breast cancer. *Soc Sci Med.* 2008;67(1):79–87.
3. Degner LF, Hack T, O'Neil J, et al. A new approach to eliciting meaning in the context of breast cancer. *Cancer Nurs.* 2003;26(3):169–178.
4. Park CL, Edmondson D, Fenster JR, et al. Meaning making and psychological adjustment following cancer: The mediating roles of growth, life meaning, and restored just-world beliefs. *J Consult Clin Psychol.* 2008;76(5):863–875.
5. Rosedale M. Survivor loneliness of women following breast cancer. *Oncol Nurs Forum.* 2009;36(2):175–183.
6. Park CL, Zlateva I, Blank TO. Self-identity after cancer: "Survivor," "victim," "patient," and "person with cancer." *J Gen Intern Med.* 2009;24(Suppl 2):S430–S435.
7. Hodgkinson K, Butow P, Hunt GE, et al. Breast cancer survivors' supportive care needs 2–10 years after diagnosis. *Support Care Cancer.* 2007;15(5):515–523.
8. Carpenter JS, Brockopp DY, Andrykowski MA. Self-transformation as a factor in the self-esteem and well-being of breast cancer survivors. *J Adv Nurs.* 1999;29(6):1402–1411.
9. Simonelli LE, Fowler J, Maxwell GL, et al. Physical sequelae and depressive symptoms in gynecologic cancer survivors: Meaning in life as a mediator. *Ann Behav Med.* 2008;35(3):275–284.

10. Salsman JM, Yost KJ, West DW, et al. Spiritual well-being and health-related quality of life in colorectal cancer: A multi-site examination of the role of personal meaning. *Support Care Cancer.* 2011;19(6):757–764.
11. Carver CS, Antoni MH. Finding benefit in breast cancer during the year after diagnosis predicts better adjustment 5 to 8 years after diagnosis. *Health Psychol.* 2004;23(6):595–598.
12. Tomich PL, Helgeson VS. Five years later: A cross-sectional comparison of breast cancer survivors with healthy women. *Psycho-Oncology.* 2002;11(2):154–169.
13. Thompson P. The relationship of fatigue and meaning in life in breast cancer survivors. *Oncol Nurs Forum.* 2007;34(3):653–660.
14. Jim HS, Andersen BL. Meaning in life mediates the relationship between social and physical functioning and distress in cancer survivors. *Br J Health Psychol.* 2007;12(Pt 3):363–381.
15. Lethborg C, Aranda S, Cox S, et al. To what extent does meaning mediate adaptation to cancer? The relationship between physical suffering, meaning in life, and connection to others in adjustment to cancer. *Palliat Support Care.* 2007;5(4):377–388.
16. Jacobsen PB. Clinical practice guidelines for the psychosocial care of cancer survivors: Current status and future prospects. *Cancer.* 2009;115(18 Suppl):4419–4429.
17. Osborn RL, Demoncada AC, Feuerstein M. Psychosocial interventions for depression, anxiety, and quality of life in cancer survivors: Meta-analyses. *Int J Psychiatry Med.* 2006;36(1):13–34.
18. Lengacher CA, Johnson-Mallard V, Post-White J, et al. Randomized controlled trial of mindfulness-based stress reduction (MBSR) for survivors of breast cancer. *Psycho-Oncology.* 2009;18(12):1261–1272.
19. Duijts SF, Faber MM, Oldenburg HS, et al. Effectiveness of behavioral techniques and physical exercise on psychosocial functioning and health-related quality of life in breast cancer patients and survivors: A meta-analysis. *Psycho-Oncology.* 2011;20(2):115–126.
20. Breitbart W, Rosenfeld B, Gibson C, et al. Meaning-centered group psychotherapy for patients with advanced cancer: A pilot randomized controlled trial. *Psycho-Oncology.* 2010;19(1):21–28.
21. Breitbart W, Rosenfeld B, Pessin H, et al. Meaning-centered group psychotherapy: An effective intervention for improving psychological well-being in patients with advanced cancer. *J Clin Oncol.* 2015;33(7):749–754.
22. Ries L, Melbert D, Krapcho M, et al. SEER cancer statistics review, 1975–2005. Bethesda, MD: National Cancer Institute. Retrieved from http://seer.cancer.gov/csr/1975_2005, based on November 2007 SEER data submission, posted to the SEER website in 2008.
23. American Cancer Society. What are the key statistics about breast cancer? August 25, 2014. Retrieved from http://www.cancer.org/cancer/breastcancer/detailedguide/breast-cancer-key-statistics; accessed January 7, 2016.
24. Ferrell BR, Smith SL, Juarez G, et al. Meaning of illness and spirituality in ovarian cancer survivors. *Oncol Nurs Forum.* 2003;30(2):249–257.
25. Jim HS, Jacobsen PB. Posttraumatic stress and posttraumatic growth in cancer survivorship: A review. *Cancer J.* 2008;14(6):414–419.
26. Sears SR, Stanton AL, Danoff-Burg S. The yellow brick road and the emerald city: Benefit finding, positive reappraisal coping and posttraumatic growth in women with early-stage breast cancer. *Health Psychol.* 2003;22(5):487–497.
27. Shapiro CL, McCabe MS, Syrjala KL, et al. The LIVESTRONG Survivorship Center of Excellence Network. *J Cancer Surviv.* 2009;3(1):4–11.
28. Nelson CJ, Rosenfeld B, Breitbart W, et al. Spirituality, religion, and depression in the terminally ill. *Psychosomatics.* 2002;43(3):213–220.
29. McClain CS, Rosenfeld B, Breitbart W. Effect of spiritual well-being on end-of-life despair in terminally-ill cancer patients. *Lancet.* 2003;361(9369):1603–1607.
30. Bauer-Wu S, Farran CJ. Meaning in life and psycho-spiritual functioning: A comparison of breast cancer survivors and healthy women. *J Holist Nurs.* 2005;23(2):172–190.
31. Burgess C, Cornelius V, Love S, et al. Depression and anxiety in women with early breast cancer: Five year observational cohort study. *BMJ.* 2005;330(7493):702.
32. Pirl WF, Greer J, Temel JS, et al. Major depressive disorder in long-term cancer survivors: Analysis of the National Comorbidity Survey Replication. *J Clin Oncol.* 2009;27(25):4130–4134.
33. Spelten ER, Verbeek JH, Uitterhoeve AL, et al. Cancer, fatigue and the return of patients to work—A prospective cohort study. *Eur J Cancer.* 2003;39(11):1562–1567.
34. Fournier JC, DeRubeis RJ, Hollon SD, et al. Antidepressant drug effects and depression severity: A patient-level meta-analysis. *J Am Med Assoc.* 2010;303(1):47–53.
35. Bellizzi KM, Blank TO. Predicting posttraumatic growth in breast cancer survivors. *Health Psychol.* 2006;25(1):47–56.
36. Park CL. Making sense of the meaning literature: An integrative review of meaning making and its effects on adjustment to stressful life events. *Psychol Bull.* 2010;136(2):257–301.

37. Cruess DG, Antoni MH, McGregor BA, et al. Cognitive-behavioral stress management reduces serum cortisol by enhancing benefit finding among women being treated for early stage breast cancer. *Psychosom Med.* 2000;62(3):304–308.
38. McGregor BA, Antoni MH, Boyers A, et al. Cognitive-behavioral stress management increases benefit finding and immune function among women with early-stage breast cancer. *J Psychosom Res.* 2004;56(1):1–8.
39. Antoni MH, Ironson GH, Scheiderman N. *Cognitive-Behavioral Stress Management.* New York, NY: Oxford University Press; 2007.
40. World Health Organization. *Cancer Control: Knowledge Into Action: WHO Guide for Effective Programmes. Module 4: Diagnosis and Treatment.* Geneva, Switzerland: World Health Organization; 2008.
41. Antoni MH, Lehman JM, Kilbourn KM, et al. Cognitive-behavioral stress management intervention decreases the prevalence of depression and enhances benefit finding among women under treatment for early-stage breast cancer. *Health Psychol.* 2001;20(1):20–32.
42. Antoni MH, Lechner SC, Kazi A, et al. How stress management improves quality of life after treatment for breast cancer. *J Consult Clin Psychol.* 2006;74(6):1143–1152.
43. Andersen BL, Shelby RA, Golden-Kreutz DM. RCT of a psychological intervention for patients with cancer: I. Mechanisms of change. *J Consult Clin Psychol.* 2007;75(6):927–938.
44. Meyer TJ, Mark MM. Effects of psychosocial interventions with adult cancer patients: A meta-analysis of randomized experiments. *Health Psychol.* 1995;14(2):101–108.
45. Fillion L, Gagnon P, Leblond F, et al. A brief intervention for fatigue management in breast cancer survivors. *Cancer Nurs.* 2008;31(2):145–159.
46. Stanton AL, Danoff-Burg S, Sworowski LA, et al. Randomized, controlled trial of written emotional expression and benefit finding in breast cancer patients. *J Clin Oncol.* 2002;20(20):4160–4168.
47. Vos J. Meaning and existential givens in the lives of cancer patients: A philosophical perspective on psycho-oncology. *Palliat Support Care.* 2015;13(4):885–900.
48. van der Spek N, Vos J, van Uden-Kraan CF, et al. Effectiveness and cost-effectiveness of meaning-centered group psychotherapy in cancer survivors: Protocol of a randomized controlled trial. *BMC Psychiatry.* 2014;14(1).
49. Vogt DS, King DW, King LA. Focus groups in psychological assessment: Enhancing content validity by consulting members of the target population. *Psychol Assess.* 2004;16(3):231–243.
50. Morse JM. Designing funded qualitative research. In: Denzin NK, Lincoln YS, eds. *Handbook of Qualitative Research.* Thousand Oaks, CA: Sage; 1994:220–235.
51. Hill CE, Knox S, Thompson BJ, et al. Consensual qualitative research: An update. *J Counseling Psychol.* 2005;52(2):196–205.
52. Charmaz K. Premises, principles, and practices in qualitative research: Revisiting the foundations. *Qual Health Res.* 2004;14(7):976–993.
53. Frankl VE. *Man's Search for Meaning: An Introduction to Logotherapy.* 3rd ed. New York, NY: Simon & Schuster; 1984.
54. Breitbart W. Spirituality and meaning in supportive care: Spirituality- and meaning-centered group psychotherapy interventions in advanced cancer. *Support Care Cancer.* 2002;10(4):272–280.
55. Gibson CA, Lichtenthal W, Berg A, et al. Psychologic issues in palliative care. *Anesthesiol Clin.* 2006;24(1):61–80, viii.
56. Yalom ID. *Existential Psychotherapy.* New York, NY: Basic Books; 1980.
57. Frankl VE. *Man's Search for Meaning.* Rev. ed. New York, NY: Washington Square Press; 1959/1984.
58. Tatrow K, Montgomery GH. Cognitive behavioral therapy techniques for distress and pain in breast cancer patients: A meta-analysis. *J Behav Med.* 2006;29(1):17–27.
59. Butler AC, Chapman JE, Forman EM, et al. The empirical status of cognitive-behavioral therapy: A review of meta-analyses. *Clin Psychol Rev.* 2006;26(1):17–31.
60. Kissane DW, Bloch S, Smith GC, et al. Cognitive-existential group psychotherapy for women with primary breast cancer: A randomised controlled trial. *Psycho-Oncology.* 2003;12(6):532–546.
61. Kissane DW, Bloch S, Miach P, et al. Cognitive-existential group therapy for patients with primary breast cancer—Techniques and themes. *Psycho-Oncology.* 1997;6(1):25–33.
62. Lichtenthal WG, Neimeyer RA. Directed journaling to facilitate meaning-making. In: Neimeyer RA, ed. *Techniques of Grief Therapy: Creative Practices for Counseling the Bereaved.* New York, NY: Routledge; 2012:165–168.
63. Park CL, Blumberg CJ. Disclosing trauma through writing: Testing the meaning-making hypothesis. *Cogn Ther Res.* 2002;26(5):597–616.
64. Janoff-Bulman R, Frantz CM. The impact of trauma on meaning: From meaningless world to meaningful life. In: Power MJ, Brewin CR, eds. *The Transformation of Meaning in Psychological Therapies: Integrating Theory and Practice.* Hoboken, NJ: Wiley; 1997:91–106.
65. Andrykowski MA, Brady MJ, Hunt JW. Positive psychosocial adjustment in potential

bone marrow transplant recipients: Cancer as a psychosocial transition. *Psycho-Oncology.* 1993;2:261–276.

66. Andrykowski MA, Lykins E, Floyd A. Psychological health in cancer survivors. *Semin Oncol Nurs.* 2008;24(3):193–201.
67. Cordova MJ, Cunningham LL, Carlson CR, et al. Posttraumatic growth following breast cancer: A controlled comparison study. *Health Psychol.* 2001;20(3):176–185.
68. Vickberg SM. The Concerns About Recurrence Scale (CARS): A systematic measure of women's fears about the possibility of breast cancer recurrence. *Ann Behav Med.* 2003;25(1):16–24.
69. Sundquist K, Yee L. Sexuality and body image after cancer. *Aust Fam Physician.* 2003;32(1–2):19–23.
70. McWayne J, Heiney SP. Psychologic and social sequelae of secondary lymphedema: A review. *Cancer.* 2005;104(3):457–466.
71. Mast ME. Survivors of breast cancer: Illness uncertainty, positive reappraisal, and emotional distress. *Oncol Nurs Forum.* 1998;25(3):555–562.
72. van den Beuken-van Everdingen MH, Peters ML, de Rijke JM, et al. Concerns of former breast cancer patients about disease recurrence: A validation and prevalence study. *Psycho-Oncology.* 2008;17(11):1137–1145.
73. Tedeschi RG, Calhoun LG. The Posttraumatic Growth Inventory: Measuring the positive legacy of trauma. *J Trauma Stress.* 1996;9(3):455–471.
74. Katz RC, Flasher L, Cacciapaglia H, et al. The psychosocial impact of cancer and lupus: A cross validation study that extends the generality of "benefit-finding" in patients with chronic disease. *J Behav Med.* 2001;24(6):561–571.
75. Bellizzi KM. Expressions of generativity and posttraumatic growth in adult cancer survivors. *Int J Aging Hum Dev.* 2004;58(4):267–287.
76. Barskova T, Oesterreich R. Post-traumatic growth in people living with a serious medical condition and its relations to physical and mental health: A systematic review. *Disabil Rehabil.* 2009;31:1709–1733.
77. Roth AJ, Kornblith AB, Batel-Copel L, et al. Rapid screening for psychologic distress in men with prostate carcinoma: A pilot study. *Cancer.* 1998;82(10):1904–1908.
78. National Comprehensive Cancer Network. Distress management: Clinical practice guidelines. *J Natl Comprehens Cancer Network.* 2003;1(3):344–374.
79. Breitbart W, Rosenfeld B, Gibson C, et al. Meaning-centered group psychotherapy for patients with advanced cancer: A pilot randomized controlled trial. *Psycho-Oncology.* 2009;19:21–28.
80. Rogers CR. *Client-Centered Therapy: Its Current Practice, Implications, and Theory.* Boston, MA: Houghton Mifflin; 1951.
81. Bloch S. *An Introduction to the Psychotherapies.* 3rd ed. New York, NY: Oxford University Press; 1996.

5

Meaning-Centered Group Psychotherapy for Cancer Survivors

NADIA VAN DER SPEK AND IRMA VERDONCK-DE LEEUW

INTRODUCTION

This chapter describes the adaptation and evaluation of meaning-centered group psychotherapy for cancer survivors (MCGP-CS). First, the background is described, followed by a four-step adaptation process. Finally, the results of a multicenter randomized trial on the efficacy of MCGP-CS are presented.

BACKGROUND

Although cancer is still a leading cause of death worldwide, increasing numbers of people are being treated successfully.[1–3] Nowadays, more than half of cancer patients in developed countries recover from cancer and become long-term survivors.[3]

For many survivors, a cancer diagnosis turns their world upside down. The diagnosis leads to an intense confrontation with their own mortality,[4] and often existential questions are triggered, such as "Why me?" "What is the purpose of my life?" "Who am I?" and "What is fundamentally important to me?" Some patients suddenly realize that they might not live long enough to participate in important, meaningful life events in the future, such as the graduation or marriage of one's child or the birth of grandchildren.

Many cancer survivors seem to experience the diagnosis of cancer as a challenge in perceiving life as meaningful, for instance, due to shifted priorities in life or physical hindrances in achieving goals. Lee[4] refers to the so-called "existential plight of cancer" as the "search for meaning" following the cancer experience. Some survivors derive meaning from the cancer experience, feel more resilient, experience life more fully in the present, or reprioritize their lives. Others, however, struggle with existential issues such as fear of death, isolation, rejection, meaninglessness, life questions, and threats to self-identity.[5–9]

Park and Folkman[10] proposed an integrated framework, "the meaning making model," which was recently further adjusted,[11] to explain how people find meaning in response to stressful events. This model proposes that people's perception of discrepancies between their appraised meaning of a particular situation and their global meaning (i.e., what they believe and desire) creates distress, which in turn gives rise to efforts to reduce the discrepancy and resultant distress, resulting in what is called a meaning-making process or search for meaning. This process appears to be beneficial only when meaning is found.

Several studies among cancer patients show that finding meaning is associated with psychological well-being, greater social adjustment, and less distress, whereas a continued search for meaning (without finding meaning) is negatively related to well-being, leads to higher levels of distress, and is maladaptive.[12–15]

To date, the literature on meaning in cancer patients has focused mostly on patients with advanced cancer in the palliative phase of the disease, who face meaning-related existential issues such as demoralization and desire for hastened death.[16–18] However, sense of meaning is also an important issue in survivorship[12,19]

Cancer survivors encounter fundamental uncertainties that they have to deal with, such as possible recurrence and negative effects of treatment. Also, the diagnosis is often accompanied by losses in different domains in life (e.g., physical, work, and relationships), which can challenge the experience of meaning in life.[4,19] Among cancer survivors, meaning is strongly related to successful adjustment and better quality of life up until years after cancer diagnosis.[12,20–23] In total, 24% of cancer survivors express a need for help regarding existential issues and meaning.[24] Psychological interventions that focus on enhancing meaning can be beneficial for cancer patients to increase adequate adjustment to life after cancer and prevent and decrease psychological distress.[25–27]

MCGP was developed to help advanced cancer patients in the palliative phase of the disease enhance or sustain a sense of meaning in their lives in order to cope with the consequences of cancer.[28,29] Several studies have provided evidence of the effectiveness of MCGP targeting advanced cancer patients,[26,30] and these studies are described elsewhere in this book. This chapter describes the adaptation and evaluation of MCGP-CS.

ADAPTATION OF MCGP FOR CANCER SURVIVORS

The goal was to adapt the MCGP manual so that it would correspond with the needs of cancer survivors in the Netherlands. To achieve this, the following four steps were taken: (1) a focus group study on meaning-making issues in Dutch cancer survivors, (2) expert meetings on meaning-making in cancer survivorship, (3) adaptation of the MCGP manual, and (4) a pilot study to test the feasibility of the adapted MCGP-CS manual. All four steps are described in the following sections.

Step 1: A Focus Group Study on Meaning-Making Issues in Dutch Cancer Survivors

As a first step, a focus group study on meaning-making processes in cancer survivors was conducted. The results of this study are summarized here but were fully published by Van der Spek and colleagues.[19] The aim was to identify meaning-making themes that play a role in cancer survivors, how patients experience and talk about meaning-making, and the perceived needs for help in this particular area. Four focus groups were conducted with 23 cancer survivors (<5 years after diagnosis), who were treated with curative intend. Participants responded to questions about their experiences with meaning-making, perceived changes in meaning-making after cancer, and the perceived need for help in this area.

From the focus group discussions, it became clear that meaning is a difficult concept to grasp for Dutch patients, and the term is not often used in daily Dutch language. Patients gave suggestions for other terms, calling meaning "a thrill," "a sense of fulfillment," "a kick," or "the important things in life." This was relevant information for the adaptation of the manual, as well as the phrasing of the study recruitment brochures.

Patients reported experiencing meaning mostly through *relationships* and *experiences* (e.g., enjoying nature more and feeling more at ease). For instance, one 47-year-old female bone cancer survivor reported enhance meaning through experiences:

> I enjoy the little things in life more and I live more in the present. I do not look as far ahead anymore, as it is of no use.

Some people indicated that they became more goal-oriented, live life more consciously, and that they know better now what they find important in life:

> I used to be a true workaholic, working 60, 70 hours a week. But I don't do that anymore, it's not worth it. Really, there are so many things I want to do. So many things I could spend my precious time on.

In general, cancer survivors experienced enhanced meaning after cancer through relationships, experiences, resilience, goal-orientation, and leaving a legacy.

Some participants, however, said they also experienced a loss of meaning in their lives because they were not able to continue their meaningful activities due to physical impairments, such as not being able to work, not being able to have children, or not being able to do specific recreational, enjoyable activities anymore:

> I have an invisible prosthesis in my leg. I can't run anymore and lift heavy things anymore. I cannot make long walks. The treatment left me with neuropathy. That's something you're confronted with for every minute of your life.

Most losses of meaning were experienced through experiences, social roles, relationships, and uncertainties about the future.

In general, participants tried to keep sources of meaning the same as they were before diagnosis, but in some cases they felt forced to search for other sources of meaning:

> I can do less things now, but the intensity has been shifted to other things. For example, things which used to give me satisfaction or purpose, it has been shifted from doing sports to. . . . to, like, enjoying the moment.

Others said they were still searching for a new meaning:

> I used to get ideas and then I would just start. I can't do that anymore. My artwork in the

field, in the moment, that was where I got my thrill. And I don't have that back yet. I can't find it. I think I find it hard to accept that I can't do as much physically.

The results of this study showed that there is a group of cancer survivors that has succeeded in meaning-making efforts and sometimes experienced even more meaning in life than before diagnosis, whereas there is also a considerable group of survivors that struggled with meaning-making and has an unmet need for help with meaning-making. These results indicated that there is a basis for MCGP for cancer survivors, and they were an encouragement to take the next step in this project.

Step 2: Organizing Expert Meetings

In the literature, knowledge on meaning-making in cancer survivorship is scarce, especially with respect to psychological interventions targeting meaning for this population. Therefore, in addition to conducting a qualitative study among the target group, we decided to obtain the (clinical) experience of experts as well. Involving experts—who will deliver the intervention eventually—from the beginning also helps to create broader support in the field early on, which will help implementation in a later phase. We organized two expert meetings. The first one included experts from multiple backgrounds (i.e., researchers, an MCPG expert, a religion scientist, a philosopher, and psychologists with clinical experience with cancer survivors) and aimed to bundle knowledge on meaning in cancer survivorship.

In the second meeting, we focused on the content of the MCGP manual to be adapted for cancer survivors (MCGP-CS), and we invited two experienced psychotherapists to brainstorm about potential adjustments to the manual. The outcomes of the two meetings provided very useful input for the adaptation of the manual (Step 3).

Step 3: Adaptation of the Treatment Manual

Adaptations for Survivors

Overall, the adjustments made in MCGP-CS were limited, and the core stayed the same (Table 5.1). All themes and topics addressing meaning-making issues and sources of meaning appeared to be as relevant for survivors as for patients in the palliative phase. There were some adaptations because compared to MCGP, MCGP-CS involves a more future-oriented approach. The discussion topics and homework assignments more often have a focus on looking forward to the future and continuing one's life narrative despite limitations and uncertainties. An example of an adjustment made in this context is in the exercise "encountering one's limitations," in which the question "What do you consider a good or meaningful death?" was replaced by "How can you carry on in life, despite limitations?" Another example of a future-oriented approach is that participants create a life's lessons portfolio, which is a collection of their homework assignments, and use these lessons to set future goals.

Cultural Adaptations

Based on the focus group outcomes and expert meetings, the tone of voice in the manual was adjusted. Less direct emphasis was placed on Viktor Frankl, and more attention was paid to clearly explaining the theoretical concepts. An important cultural difference between the Netherlands and the United States is that in the Netherlands, more cancer survivors are nonreligious. The Netherlands is a much more secular country. This was borne in mind when adjusting the manual and explaining the theories of

TABLE 5.1 SESSION TOPICS COVERED IN MCGP-CS

Session No.	Themes
1	Concept and sources of meaning
2	Meaning before and after cancer, sharing each other's cancer stories
3	The story of our life as a source of meaning: What made us who we are today
4	The story of our life as a source of meaning: Things we have done and want to do in the future
5	Attitudinal sources of meaning: Encountering life's limitations
6	Creative sources of meaning: Responsibility, courage, and creativity
7	Experiental sources of meaning
8	Termination: Presentations of our life lessons and goodbyes

meaning (e.g., meaning is often considered to be a religious concept), to make the Dutch manual more suitable for a nonreligious population.

In addition to the adaptations for survivors and the cultural adaptations, a few more adaptations were made based on the preferences of the researchers and therapists involved in the adaptation process. The order of some topics and themes was changed—for instance, the telling of everyone's cancer stories was moved to Session 2 instead of being done in the first session. Also, a brief mindfulness exercise was added before each experiental exercise to enhance a sense of introspection. The experts involved in Step 2 of the adaptation process commented on the final draft.

Step 4: Pilot Study

After adapting the MCGP treatment manual for cancer survivors (MCGP-CS), based on the input of patients and experts, the next step was to evaluate the adapted treatment manual. Before conducting a large-scale randomized controlled trial (RCT), a pilot study was conducted to determine acceptability and feasibility of MCGP-CS for a Dutch cancer survivor population.[31] We performed MCGP-CS in two groups, and a total of 11 cancer survivors participated. The research procedures were tested, participant's satisfaction with the MCPG-CS was evaluated, and the efficacy of MCGP-CS was investigated among the participants of this (nonrandomized) pilot study. The results of this pilot study showed that participants found MCGP-CS overall as acceptable, they were highly satisfied with the intervention and with the therapists, and the compliance was high. The following research procedures were tested: recruitment strategy, filling out the informed consent, screening process, and baseline and follow-up assessments. The most important lesson for recruitment was to include multiple hospitals in the study and to approach patients directly through mailings instead of via a research nurse recruiting patients when visiting the outpatient clinic. The first outcome results of this (nonrandomized) pilot study were overall positive and encouraging to start a multicenter RCT. After MCGP-CS, some participants were interviewed about their experiences. Box 5.1 presents some quotes on what participants valued the most about MCGP-CS.

EFFICACY OF MCGP-CS

Between August 2012 and September 2014, an RCT was conducted to assess the efficacy and cost utility of MCGP-CS.[32,33] A total of 170 cancer survivors (40 male and 130 female) diagnosed with cancer in the past 5 years were randomly assigned to one of the three study arms: MCGP-CS (n = 57), supportive group psychotherapy

BOX 5.1 WHAT PARTICIPANTS VALUED THE MOST ABOUT MCGP-CS

"This training gave me new insights, a nice experience with meaningful conversations. I would not want to miss it."

"This training made me realize how many areas of my life are impacted by the cancer. The most important thing I learned were to discriminate those areas, or sources . . . that I have a different story to tell on all those areas, was so inspiring. To ask ourselves the question, 'What does really matter to me? Where do I gain strength from?' It helped me realize that there are also still meaningful and beautiful things in life. And it gave me especially strength to see this in the lives that have experienced such adversities."

"It was interesting to talk about meaning in life in a broader way, not just religion. I learned that you always have a choice in each situation. . . . That gave me a sense of freedom. Some sessions were heavy though, emotional, for instance sharing each other's cancer stories. After these emotional discussions, we did a meditation exercise, which was really helpful and calming."

"Most helpful to me were, I think, your own life lessons, writing down your own story and learn your own lessons for the future. Also, I realized how important nature and creativity are to me. I want to be more creative. Realizing this, writing it down, makes you think: Ah, these things really matter to me. And the training also helps you to commit to this for the future."

(SGP) (n = 56), or care as usual (CAU) (n = 57). Common cancer diagnoses were breast (65%) and colon (20%). Baseline assessment took place before randomization, with follow-up assessments post-intervention and at 3- and 6-month follow-up.

Mixed model analyses (intention to treat) showed significant differences between MCGP-CS, SGP, and CAU on the course of personal meaning, purpose in life, personal growth, positive relations, environmental mastery, goal-orientedness, spiritual change, distress, depression, fighting spirit, and helplessness/hopelessness.

Post hoc analyses showed significantly stronger treatment effects of MCGP-CS compared to CAU for personal meaning, positive relations, purpose in life, goal-orientedness, distress, depression, fighting spirit, and helplessness/hopelessness. They also showed significantly stronger effects of MCGP-CS compared to SGP for environmental mastery and personal growth. A significantly stronger treatment effect of SGP compared to CAU was observed for goal-orientedness.

Effects on positive relations, purpose in life, personal meaning, goal-orientedness, and fighting spirit were only observed post-intervention. Effects of MCGP-CS were observed on personal growth and helplessness/hopelessness at 3-month follow-up and on depression, distress, and environmental mastery at 6-month follow-up. The effect of SGP on goal-orientedness compared to CAU was only observed post-intervention.

The effect size of MCGP-CS was large on personal meaning (0.81), goal-orientedness (1.07), and helpless/hopeless (–0.87). Other significant effects of MCGP-CS were mostly moderate (<0.80).

In summary, the results of this RCT provide evidence for the efficacy of MCGP-CS, showing that cancer survivors benefit from MCGP-CS not only by enhanced sense of meaning but also by improving adjustment to cancer and decreasing distress and depressive symptoms in the longer term.[33]

Client Satisfaction of MCGP-CS

In addition to efficacy, client satisfaction is important, especially for successful implementation of the intervention in clinical practice. Therefore, client satisfaction was also evaluated during the RCT. The results of this evaluation showed that 86% of the participants were (very) satisfied with MCGP-CS, 10% had mixed feelings, and 6% were unsatisfied. In addition, 65% would definitely recommend the MCGP-CS to other patients, 31% were not sure, and 4% would not recommend it. More than half of the participants (67%) stayed in touch with the other group participants after MCGP-CS.

Case Example

Mrs. Y is a 44-year-old woman who was diagnosed with colorectal cancer 1½ years ago. She underwent colorectal surgery and chemotherapy, which she completed 9 months before she engaged in MCGP-CS. She is married to Mr. X, who is her high school sweetheart, and they have a 15-year-old son. Mrs. Y is a housewife with no paid job. As a young mother, she found it difficult to combine her job with her role as a mother and a wife; therefore, she quit her job as a nurse at a local hospital when her son was 4 years old. Mrs. Y had been bullied in her childhood and described herself as insecure and with low self-esteem; the cancer had increased her feelings of insecurity about the future, her life, and her role as a wife and a mother. Since the cancer treatment, she suffered from neuropathy and fatigue, which made it more difficult for her to carry out her regular household tasks. Her husband was not very understanding of this. In the telephone interview before the start of the training, she said that she felt lonely, left out, and unsupported. Furthermore, she stated that she experienced fear of cancer recurrence and therefore did not dare to make plans for the future, such as planning a summer holiday for the family.

In the group discussions about historical sources of meaning and life's lessons, she realized that there are many things in her life that she had overcome: She was able to cope with severe bullying in primary school; she dealt with several losses of loved ones in her life; and she had always managed to be a good mother—even when she was in the hospital for chemotherapy, she made sure that her son was looked after and cared for. Also, when she reflected on her life, she realized that she had always been a kind and loving person who was there for people in need—in her previous work as a nurse but also in volunteer work she had done—even when times were difficult for her. Realizing this and being acknowledged for this by the other group members gave her a sense of self-worth and meaning, and this gave her more confidence in her ability to cope with the challenge of cancer as well. She realized that she cannot change her life story, but she can change how she looks back on it and whether she learns from it. She also learned that she can choose how she wants to continue her life story. She became more content with who she was and who she had become. She realized that taking care of others was an important source of meaning for her and that she wanted to focus more on this, now and in the future. She signed up for volunteer work in an elderly home, even though she was afraid her husband would not agree; she felt supported by the group members to make this decision.

In the session about attitudinal sources of meaning, it became even more clear to Mrs. Y that even though the cancer experience was horrible and dreadful for her, she could derive meaning from the way that she dealt with it, and that she, even in the most hopeless moments, did not lose faith and did not abandon her values of caring for others. She also experienced an enhanced sense of meaning through responsibility and courage because of the fact that she, with the help of the training and of the group members, was learning about herself and taking care of herself as well.

During the session about creativity as a source of meaning, Mrs. Y shared that embroidery had always been an important creative source of meaning, something she had practiced her whole life since childhood, and that she has lost this joy because the neuropathy she experiences made this impossible. She felt like she had lost an important meaningful activity in her life for good. A group member suggested that she consider teaching others about this handicraft. Mrs. Y thought this was an excellent idea, and she immediately placed an ad for free embroidery lessons. By the end of the training, she had two "students," and she enjoyed passing on her knowledge to others and leaving a legacy.

In the session about experiences as a source of meaning, Mrs. Y shared that she enjoyed the little things in life much more than she did before being diagnosed with cancer. She enjoyed sitting in her garden for hours and just looking at the flowers and listening to the birds sing. She never used to do this before she was diagnosed with cancer, but now it gave her a sense of peace. Mrs. Y also realized that spending time with her son, doing adventurous things with him, made her feel alive. She and her husband used to take their son camping when he was little; they would build their own camp and make their own fire. These were truly meaningful experiences for her and her family. Mr. X used to plan and arrange camping trips, but for the past several years he had not done so, which Mrs. Y regretted. With support of the group members, Mrs. Y decided that if her husband would not do it, she would plan a camping trip for her family, even though she felt insecure as to whether she was capable of planning it well and finding all the right equipment. She wanted to re-create this meaningful experience for her family and herself.

The group training had given Mrs. Y much more confidence to commit to the things that are important to her in life, as she stated at the final session, in which all survivors presented their life's lessons. She believed that the exercises helped her to discover the common thread in her life; the experience taught her more about who she is and about the things that are fundamentally important and meaningful to her. She said that the most important lesson she had learned was that no matter what happens to her in her life, she will have a choice with regard to how to cope with it, and that she has much more resilience and worth than she had ever thought.

RECOMMENDATIONS FOR FUTURE STEPS

Our findings showed that a meaning-centered group psychotherapy benefits cancer survivors not only by enhancing a sense of meaning but also by improving adjustment to cancer and decreasing distress in the longer term. Therefore, we recommend implementation of MCGP-CS in psycho-oncology health care settings. Developing and conducting a train-the-trainer program for oncology psychologists, and subsequently including MCGP-CS in the mental health care offer of centers of psychosocial oncology care, are important next steps to take. To make MCGP-CS better accessible for all cancer survivors with existential concerns, MCGP-CS could be adapted to be used via an eHealth application. There is convincing evidence of the effectiveness of self-help interventions and online treatment of mental disorders[34–36] and also for people with physical health problems.[37] It is plausible that adapting MCGP-CS into an eHealth application can be beneficial for cancer survivors as well. Based on the findings of the conducted RCT,[33] it is recommended to include a peer support element in the application. In addition, assessing the feasibility of a meaning-centered online self-help intervention, and actively involving patients in the development process, is an important first step to take.

Meaning-making processes are important aspects of adjustment not only in patients but also in caregivers.[38] In our focus group study, patients expressed a need for help for their caregivers. Moreover, experiencing meaning in the role of caregiving and social support are associated with lower levels of burden for caregivers.[39] Future research is needed to investigate the effectiveness of MCGP-CS among informal caregivers of cancer survivors.

SUMMARY

Cancer survivors, defined as cancer patients treated with curative intent, have to deal with a number of meaning-making and other existential issues in the years following diagnosis and treatment.[4,5,9,40] A substantial group of survivors experiences problems with meaning-making and existential issues and expresses a need for help.[19] The literature extensively describes the importance of meaning-making in cancer patients in relation to psychological well-being and successful adjustment to the disease. The goal of MCGP is to enhance or maintain a sense of meaning in order to cope better with the sequelae of their disease. MCGP, initially developed for patients with advanced cancer, was adjusted for cancer survivors (MCGP-CS). The MCGP-CS manual was developed in close collaboration with both cancer survivors and health care providers in the psycho-oncology field. The results of our feasibility study showed good acceptability of MCGP-CS and high treatment satisfaction.[31] An RCT was conducted that compared MCGP-CS with supportive group psychotherapy and care as usual, with assessments at baseline, post-intervention, and 3- and 6-month follow-up.[32] We found strong support for the efficacy of MCGP-CS, showing effects on personal meaning, psychological well-being, distress, depression, and adjustment to cancer up to 6 months after participation in the intervention.[33]We recommend implementation of MCGP-CS in psycho-oncology health care settings; the cultural adaptations made to the manual may be applicable in other northern European countries. In addition, we recommend further adaptation of MCP for novel target groups.

This chapter provided a brief overview of existential concerns of cancer survivors, a description of the four steps that were taken to adapt MCGP for cancer survivors, and a summary of the results of an RCT providing evidence on the efficacy of MCGP-CS. Cancer survivors struggle with meaning-making issues, and an evidence-based intervention such as MCGP-CS is an important and welcomed addition to psycho-oncological health care.

REFERENCES

1. Brenner H. Long-term survival rates of cancer patients achieved by the end of 20th century: A period analysis. *Lancet*. 2002;360:1131–1135.
2. Richards MA, Stockton D, Bapp P, et al. How many deaths have been avoided through improvements in cancer survival? *Br Med J*. 2000;320:895–898.
3. Siegel R, Naishadham D, Jemal A. Cancer statistics, 2013. *CA Cancer J Clin*. 2013;63:11–30.
4. Lee V. The existential plight of cancer: Meaning making as a concrete approach to the intangible search for meaning. *Support Care Cancer*. 2008;16(7):779–785.
5. Henoch I, Danielson E. Existential concerns among patients with cancer and interventions to meet them: An integrative literature review. *Psycho-Oncology*. 2009;18(3):225–236.
6. Tedeschi RG, Calhoun LG. Posttraumatic growth: Conceptual foundations and empirical evidence. *Psychol Inq*. 2004;15(1):1–18.
7. Thornton AA. Perceiving benefits in the cancer experience. *J Clin Psychol Med Settings*. 2002;9(2):153–165.
8. Helgeson VS, Snyder P, Seltman H. Psychological and physical adjustment to breast cancer over 4 years: Identifying distinct trajectories of change. *Heal Psychol*. 2004;23(1):3–15.
9. Tomich PL, Helgeson VS, Vache EJN. Perceived growth and decline following breast cancer: A comparison to age-matched controls 5-years later. *Psycho-Oncology*. 2005;1029:1018–1029.
10. Park CL, Folkman S. Meaning in the context of stress and coping. *Rev Gen Psychol*. 1997;1(2):115–144.
11. Park CL. Making sense of the meaning literature: An integrative review of meaning making and its effects on adjustment to stressful life events. *Psychol Bull*. 2010;136(2):257–301.
12. Tomich PL, Helgeson VS. Five years later: A cross-sectional comparison of breast cancer survivors with healthy women. *Psycho-Oncology*. 2002;11(2):154–169.
13. Park CL, Edomondson D, Fenster JR, et al. Meaning making and psychological adjustment following cancer: The mediating roles of growth, life meaning, and restored just-world beliefs. *J Consult Clin Psychol*. 2008;863–875.
14. Thompson SC, Pitts J. Factors relating to a person's ability to find meaning after a diagnosis of cancer. *J Psychosoc Oncol*. 1994;11:1–21.
15. Jaarsma TA, Pool G, Ranchor AV, et al. The concept and measurement of meaning in life in Dutch cancer patients. *Psycho-Oncology*. 2007;16(3):241–248.
16. Nelson CJ, Rosenfeld B, Breitbart W, et al. Spirituality, religion, and depression in the terminally ill. *Psychosomatics*. 2002;43(3):213–220.
17. McClain CS, Rosenfeld B, Breitbart W. Effect of spiritual well-being on end-of-life despair in terminally-ill cancer patients. *Lancet*. 2003;361(9369):1603–1607.

18. Lethborg C, Aranda S, Cox S, et al. To what extent does meaning mediate adaptation to cancer? The relationship between physical suffering, meaning in life, and connection to others in adjustment to cancer. *Palliat Support Care.* 2007;5(4):377–388.
19. van der Spek N, Vos J, van Uden-Kraan CF, et al. Meaning making in cancer survivors: A focus group study. *PLoS One.* 2013;8(9):e76089.
20. Bower JE, Meyerowitz BE, Desmond KA, et al. Perceptions of positive meaning and vulnerability following breast cancer: Predictors and outcomes among long-term breast cancer survivors. *Ann Behav Med.* 2005;29(3):236–245.
21. Zika S, Chamberlain K. On the relation between meaning in life and psychological well-being. *Br J Psychol.* 1992;83(1):133–145.
22. Debats DL. Sources of meaning: An investigation of significant commitments in life. *J Humanist Psychol.* 1999;39(4):30–57.
23. Lee V, Cohen SR, Edgar L, et al. Clarifying "meaning" in the context of cancer research: A systematic literature review. *Palliat Support Care.* 2004;2(3):291–303.
24. Jansen F, Van Uden-Kraan CF, Van Zwieten V, et al. Cancer survivors' perceived need for supportive care and their attitude towards self-management and e-health. *Support Care Cancer.* 2015;23(61):1679–1688.
25. LeMay K, Wilson KG. Treatment of existential distress in life threatening illness: A review of manualized interventions. *Clin Psychol Rev.* 2008;28:472–493.
26. Breitbart W, Rosenfeld B, Gibson C, et al. Meaning-centered group psychotherapy for patients with advanced cancer: A pilot randomized controlled trial. *Psycho-Oncology.* 2010;19(1):21–28.
27. Lee V, Cohen SR, Edgar L, et al. Meaning-making intervention during breast or colorectal cancer treatment improves self-esteem, optimism, and self-efficacy. *Soc Sci Med.* 2006;62(12):3133–3145.
28. Breitbart W. Spirituality and meaning in supportive care: Spirituality- and meaning-centered group psychotherapy interventions in advanced cancer. *Support Care Cancer.* 2002;10(4):272–280.
29. Greenstein M, Breitbart W. Cancer and the experience of meaning: A group psychotherapy program for people with cancer. *Am J Psychother.* 2000;54(4):486–500.
30. Breitbart W, Rosenfeld B, Pessin H, et al. Meaning-centered group psychotherapy: An effective intervention for improving psychological well-being in patients with advanced cancer. *J Clin Oncol.* 2015;33:749–754.
31. van der Spek N, van Uden-Kraan CF, Vos J, et al. Meaning-centered group psychotherapy in cancer survivors: A feasibility study. *Psycho-Oncology.* 2014;23(7):827–831.
32. van der Spek N, Vos J, van Uden-Kraan CF, et al. Effectiveness and cost-effectiveness of meaning-centered group psychotherapy in cancer survivors: Protocol of a randomized controlled trial. *BMC Psychiatry.* 2014;14(1):22.
33. van der Spek N, Vos J, van Uden-Kraan CF, et al. Efficacy of meaning-centered group psychotherapy for cancer survivors: A randomized controlled trial. Submitted for publication.
34. Griffiths KM, Farrer L, Christensen H. The efficacy of Internet interventions for depression and anxiety disorders: A review of randomised controlled trials. *Med J Aust.* 2010;192(11 Suppl):S4–S11.
35. Spek V, Cuijpers P, Nyklicek I, et al. Internet-based cognitive behaviour therapy for symptoms of depression and anxiety: A meta-analysis. *Psychol Med.* 2007;37(03):319.
36. Andrews G, Cuijpers P, Craske MG, et al. Computer therapy for the anxiety and depressive disorders is effective, acceptable and practical health care: A meta-analysis. *PLoS One.* 2010;5(10):e13196.
37. Cuijpers P, van SA, Andersson G, et al. Internet-administered cognitive behavior therapy for health problems: A systematic review. *J Behav Med.* 2008;31:169–177.
38. Tan JYS, Lym HA, Kuek NMY, et al. Caring for the caregiver while caring for the patient: Exploring the dyadic relationship between patient spirituality and caregiver quality of life. *Support Care Cancer.* 2015;23(12):3403–3406.
39. Delalibera M, Presa J, Barbosa A, et al. Sobrecarga no cuidar e suas repercussões nos cuidadores de pacientes em fim de vida: Revisão sistemática da literatura. *Rev Ciência Saúde Coletiva.* 2015;20(9):2731–2747.
40. Helgeson VS, Reynolds KA, Tomich PL. A meta-analytic review of benefit finding and growth. *J Consult Clin Psychol.* 2006;74(5):797–816.

6

Meaning-Centered Psychotherapy for Cancer Caregivers

ALLISON J. APPLEBAUM

INTRODUCTION

There is growing recognition that comprehensive care for cancer patients involves attending to the psychosocial needs of their informal caregivers.[1,2] Informal caregivers (ICs) are defined as any relative, friend, or partner who has a significant relationship with and provides assistance (i.e., physical and emotional) to a patient with a life-threatening, incurable illness.[3] In 2009, 65.7 million people in the United States served as ICs for medically ill relatives, including 4.6 million cancer patients.[4] This number may be a reflection of the rising costs of health care, which have placed the responsibility of caring for the chronically medically ill—including cancer patients—on ICs.[5] Because the number of ICs will likely continue to increase in the future, special attention should be paid to the unique burden of ICs, not only for the benefit of the caregiver but also for that of the patient.

CAREGIVER BURDEN

Providing care to a patient with cancer has been described as a full-time job.[6] When family/friends become caregivers, they take on the responsibilities of the patient and the household, in addition to their own, which often leads to caregiver burden.[7–13] Given and colleagues[14] describe such burden as a "multidimensional biopsychosocial reaction resulting from an imbalance of care demands relative to caregivers' personal time, social roles, physical and emotional states, financial resources, and formal care resources given the other multiple roles they fulfill." ICs are often unprepared to take on all the aspects that this new role entails,[14–20] and they often have a wide range of unmet needs.[8,11,21–25] Not only do ICs face the physical and emotional demands associated with caregiving but also the patients for whom they provide care may no longer be able to provide them with the emotional support that they once did.[26] Therefore, ICs are not only often unprepared to provide instrumental support (i.e., the "doing" of caregiving) but also often may be in great need of emotional support themselves. Perhaps not surprisingly, ICs experience a range of psychological complications,[8,11,27–37] including fear, hopelessness, and mood disturbances.[38,39] Studies have reported rates of anxiety and depression among family caregivers that are comparable to[40–46] and even surpass[44,47–52] those of the patients for whom they provide care. For example, rates of depression between 12% and 59%[53,54] and rates of anxiety between 30% and 50%[53] have been reported in samples of family caregivers, in comparison to rates of depression between 10% and 25%[55] and rates of anxiety between 19% and 34%[56] in patient samples.

In addition to mental health issues, ICs also experience a range of physical health complications as a result of their role,[41,57,58] including sleep difficulties,[59–61] fatigue,[62,63] cardiovascular disease,[64,65] poor immune functioning,[66,67] and increased mortality.[68,69] Studies have also reported an increase in alcohol and tobacco use, lack of exercise, and decreased health service utilization among ICs.[70,71] In addition, caring for a patient with cancer places a major financial and temporal demand on those providing care.[54,72] Data from a national survey of caregivers showed that, on average, cancer caregivers provide care for 8.3 hours each day for 13.7 months,[73] and that this care includes providing emotional, instrumental, tangible, and medical support. Moreover, the annual economic value of caregiving in the United States was recently estimated at $375 billion.[4] Therefore, the burden experienced by ICs is multifaceted and includes the potential for significant psychological, physical, temporal, and financial demands.

EXISTENTIAL DISTRESS AMONG CANCER CAREGIVERS

A critical, potential driving, element of caregiver burden is existential distress. Although no one definition of existential distress exists, it has been described as including feelings of hopelessness, demoralization, loss of personal meaning and dignity, feelings of burden toward others, and the desire for death or the decreased will to continue living.[74–76] Cherny and colleagues[77] describe existential distress in terms of whether individuals are focused on past (e.g., unfulfilled aspirations and regret), present (e.g., loss of important occupational, social, and familial role functions), and future (e.g., the death of/separation from a loved one) concerns. Included in their description of existential distress are issues related to identity, personal integrity, meaninglessness, hopelessness, death, futility, and religious/spiritual concerns.

Existential distress and suffering experienced by ICs is common and may lead to increased feelings of guilt and powerlessness.[74] For ICs, the competing demands of cancer caregiving, other caregiving responsibilities (i.e., child care), paid employment, and personal life goals have the potential to lead to psychological, spiritual, and existential distress. However, the caregiving experience is also an opportunity for meaning-making and growth.[78] Importantly, finding meaning in the experience of being an IC for a patient with cancer has the potential to buffer against caregiver burden. The addition of meaning-based coping[78] to Lazarus and Folkman's original model of stress and coping was based on the reports of caregivers of men with AIDS,[79] which highlighted their concurrent experience of meaning and suffering in the context of providing care to their terminally ill loved ones. Indeed, a growing number of studies have documented the experience of post-traumatic growth[80,81] as a result of stressful experiences, and finding meaning has been proposed as one mechanism through which positive outcomes can be achieved.[36,82–90]

Meaning-making is rooted in the existential concept of one's ability to find meaning or "make sense" out of suffering. Having a loved one diagnosed with cancer and experiencing the resultant challenges of becoming an IC is a potential source of great anguish. Although this distress may be a transformative experience that ultimately leads to more adaptive coping,[91] it is a process that may also result in feelings of guilt and powerlessness. Frankl[91–94] suggested that we may find meaning through the choices we make (e.g., the attitude an IC takes toward this role), our creative endeavors (e.g., ICs may create new ways to provide care), and experiences (e.g., gaining a new appreciation for their relationship with the patient). Making meaning of suffering, therefore, is one possible mechanism through which ICs may experience growth as opposed to distress.

In a descriptive study of the unmet needs and intervention preferences among cancer ICs,[95] we identified existential concerns—including guilt, issues with role changes, sense of identity, and responsibility to the self—as a critical area of distress. Qualitative analysis of caregiver responses to the study questions highlighted a common theme among participant responses: *An increased sense of meaning would decrease burden.* However, very few caregivers reported at the time of assessment naturally engaging in a process of meaning-making. This study included an assessment of both patients and caregivers, and almost unanimously, patients acknowledged the benefits to their caregivers of finding meaning in this role. These responses corroborated the need for an intervention focused on existential needs.

Limited Interventions for Existential Distress Among Cancer Caregivers

Although a growing number of psychosocial interventions have been developed to target caregiver burden, our review of this literature[96] highlighted the dearth of interventions that attend to existential distress or meaning-making among caregivers. Indeed, of the 49 interventions reviewed, only 1 specifically targeted existential concerns of ICs,[97] although others acknowledged the importance of existential issues, including the importance of finding meaning through the cancer caregiving experience.[32,98–101]

Since the publication of our review in 2013, one additional intervention that attends to caregivers' existential concerns has been reported. Existential behavioral therapy[102] (EBT) was developed to provide support to ICs of palliative care patients (not limited to cancer) through a manualized, six-session group psychotherapy intervention that is described as a "third-wave" behavioral therapy[102] integrating traditional cognitive and behavioral therapeutic techniques with existential themes. Sessions focused equally on existential concerns and mindfulness skills practice; topics included mindfulness, death, bereavement, finding meaning, self-care, stress management, and personal values.[103] A randomized controlled trial comparing the impact of EBT to usual care among 160 caregivers of palliative care patients demonstrated efficacy of the intervention in improving anxiety and quality of life immediately after completion of the program, as well as depression and quality of life 1 year after completion.[103] Notably, participants were caregivers of patients with life expectancies of 6 months or less and included both current and bereaved caregivers.

To date, there are no empirically supported interventions that specifically target meaning-making among informal cancer caregivers. Importantly, the experience of providing care to a patient with cancer varies significantly from the experience of providing care for patients with neurological diseases, such as Alzheimer's or Parkinson's disease; therefore, interventions developed for this population must account for the unique experience of cancer caregiving. In light of previous research indicating that finding meaning in caregiving leads to more positive mental health outcomes among informal caregivers, including enhanced caregiving capacity and improved care for the patient,[104] interventions that foster meaning-making among caregivers have the potential to improve their quality of life and that of the patients for whom they provide care. Although the benefits of such interventions will likely be vast across the caregiving trajectory, when delivered early—such as well in advance of a patient's transition to hospice care—they have the potential to serve a protective role against poor psychosocial outcomes.

MEANING-CENTERED PSYCHOTHERAPY

The 2009 Institute of Medicine report, "Retooling for an Aging America: Building the Health Care Workforce," highlighted the responsibility of health care professionals to prepare ICs for their role and the need to establish programs to assist them with managing their own stress that results from providing care.[2] This includes attention to spiritual and existential distress, which is a critical component of palliative care. Currently, however, very few interventions focus specifically on these needs.

Our group has developed meaning-centered psychotherapy (MCP),[105–107] an existential therapeutic model that addresses the existential issues of suffering, guilt, and death. MCP has demonstrated efficacy in improving spiritual well-being and a sense of meaning and in decreasing symptoms of anxiety in patients with advanced cancer. Secondary analyses from a trial of individual meaning-centered psychotherapy (IMCP)[108,109] indicated that IMCP improved patients' sense of meaning and purpose in life, led to their finding comfort and strength in spiritual beliefs, and led to increases in life productivity. Both individual and group formats of MCP have been developed and tested. Meaning-centered group psychotherapy (MCGP) includes eight 1½-hour-long sessions, whereas IMCP involves seven 1-hour-long session. As an established, efficacious intervention, MCP provides a solid foundation for a meaning-making intervention that is tailored toward the unique needs of individuals caring for a loved one with cancer. Importantly, given the underutilization of psychosocial services by this population,[110–112] it is hypothesized that attention to meaning will be congruent with the IC's experience and thus offer an attractive intervention that promises to ameliorate a critical element of caregiver burden.

MEANING-CENTERED PSYCHOTHERAPY FOR INFORMAL CANCER CAREGIVERS

Numerous studies have documented the experience of post-traumatic growth[80,81] as a result of stressful experiences, and finding meaning has been proposed as one mechanism through which such positive outcomes are achieved.[36,83–90,113] Meaning-making is rooted in the existential concept of one's ability to find meaning in suffering. Having a loved one diagnosed with advanced cancer and experiencing the resultant challenges of becoming an IC is a potential source of great suffering. Although this suffering may be a transformative experience that ultimately leads to more adaptive coping,[91] it may also result in feelings of guilt and powerlessness. Frankl[92–94] suggested that we may find meaning through the choices we make (e.g., the attitude an IC takes toward this role), our creative endeavors (e.g., ICs may create new ways to provide care), and experiences (e.g., ICs may gain a new appreciation for their relationship with the patient). Making meaning of suffering, therefore, is one possible mechanism through which ICs may experience growth as opposed to distress. For example, suffering may lead to ICs becoming disconnected from elements of their identity that they once prioritized, disconnected from important activities and relationships, and experiencing a decrease in their sense of meaning and purpose generally or specifically as related to caregiving. Such loss of meaning ultimately increases suffering and burden of ICs, and it negatively impacts the quality of care provided to patients. Such suffering, however, may exist concurrently with positive emotions, connectedness, and growth. Through an exploration of the unique experience of providing care for a patient with cancer—including ICs' previous experiences of illness, loss, and care, the manner in which ICs respond to the limitations of the caregiving role, how providing care for another may serve as a catalyst for improved self-care, and the relationship with oneself and the care recipient—ICs may find great meaning in caregiving, which ultimately will improve their quality of life and protect them from the burden commonly associated with the caregiving role. These outcomes serve as the impetus for the adaptation of meaning-centered psychotherapy for cancer caregivers (MCP-C).

The goal of MCP-C is to help ICs connect—or reconnect—to various sources of meaning in their lives. The four sources of meaning addressed in MCP-C are historical, attitudinal, creative, and experiential. Table 6.1 outlines these sources of meaning and their relevance to the experience of providing care to a patient with cancer.

Historical sources of meaning refer to critical elements of ICs' past, present, and future legacies, many of which may be connected to the caregiving role. Past legacy refers to components of the ICs' upbringing that they did not choose, but that had a significant impact on who they are, including the family into which they were born and the cultural, religious, and spiritual values of their family of origin. Particularly critical elements of past legacy for ICs include previous experiences of providing care or watching others (i.e., parents and grandparents) provide care to friends and family members; past experiences of illness or loss; and religious, spiritual, or familial traditions that promoted commitment to the family. Present legacy refers to the legacy the IC is currently living and creating, including engaging in caregiving. Future legacy refers to the impact the IC has on others, and it includes how others view the IC in this role and, importantly, the ways in which this role sets an example for future generations, family members, and friends.

Attitudinal sources of meaning refer to the ways in which ICs choose to face limitations and challenges, many of which are endemic to the caregiving role. Reflecting on how one faces challenges can be an incredibly meaningful

TABLE 6.1 SOURCES OF MEANING AND CAREGIVING

Source	Content
Historical	Legacy given (past), lived (present), and to give (future): Examples include previous experiences of providing or watching others provide care, of illness or loss, and family values associated with an ethic of care; taking pride in caregiving; and setting examples for future generations.
Attitudinal	Choosing how one faces limitations associated with caregiving: Reflection on challenges faced before caregiving and previous modes of facing such challenges, such as achievements in the face of adversity and rising above or transcending difficult circumstances. Discussion of choosing new ways to respond and taking pride in one's attitude. Examples include the choice one makes to provide care, how one faces the limitations that result from the caregiving role, and choosing to engage fully in the relationship with the patient despite the possibility of its ending.
Creative	Engaging in life and taking responsibility for one's life through creative acts, such as through work, causes, family, artistic endeavors, and self-care: Examples include courageously engaging fully in the caregiving role and taking responsibility for oneself through improved self-care, and discussion of existential and neurotic guilt as indicators of deficient self-care.
Experiential	Connecting with life through love, relationships, nature, art, and humor: Examples include feeling and expressing love for the care recipient via a tight hug or handhold, finding humor in dark moments, and deriving hope for the future from a sense of belonging to something greater than oneself.

experience. Critically, becoming an IC is not generally perceived as a choice. However, helping ICs to recognize how they came to decide to engage in this role—and specifically how and to what extent they do so—may serve as a catalyst for improved self-efficacy. In addition, highlighting how caregivers choose to face limitations due to caregiving, such as the inability to make advanced plans, interruptions to personal goals and employment, and often a limited amount of time remaining with the patient for whom they are providing care, can be a source of great meaning and strength and can foster the development of new skills, clarified values, and resilience.

Creative sources of meaning refer to the ways in which ICs create and take responsibility for their lives, including how they engage in the caregiving role. Creating one's life requires courage and commitment, and engaging fully in caregiving for a loved one who is terminally ill is an example of an act that requires courage and commitment. In addition, a critical area of creativity is responsibility to the self and how one may continue to create one's life fully and attend to one's own needs while providing care to a patient with cancer.

Finally, experiential sources of meaning include ways in which ICs connect with the world through their five senses. Experiential sources of meaning, unlike those discussed previously, are derived in a more passive manner. For example, through a tight handhold or hug, ICs may feel connected through love for the patient; may be transported from present suffering merely through listening to their favorite music or sharing a laugh at a difficult moment with the patient; or may feel a sense of tranquility through experiencing the beauty of nature, which often serves as a reminder of the longevity of the world around them and the connectedness of humans and nature.

MCP-C may be delivered in group (eight sessions) and individual (seven sessions) formats. The outline for these sessions is presented in Table 6.2.

TABLE 6.2 MEANING-CENTERED PSYCHOTHERAPY FOR CANCER CAREGIVERS WEEKLY TOPICS[a]

Session	Session Title	Content
1	Concepts and Sources of Meaning	Introductions; review of concepts and sources of meaning; "Meaningful Moments" experiential exercise; copies of *Man's Search for Meaning* distributed for optional reading
2	Cancer Caregiving, Identity, and Meaning	Discussion of sense of identity before and after becoming a cancer caregiver; "Who Am I?" experiential exercise; homework reflection on Session 3 experiential exercise
3	Historical Sources of Meaning (Past Legacy)	Discussion of life as a legacy that has been given (past); "Historical Sources of Meaning—Past" experiential exercise; homework reflection on Session 4 experiential exercise
4	Historical Sources of Meaning (Present and Future Legacy)	Discussion of life as a legacy that one lives (present) and gives (future); "Historical Sources of Meaning—Present and Future" experiential exercise; homework reflection on Session 5 experiential exercise and optional sharing of one's story
5	Attitudinal Sources of Meaning: Encountering Life's Limitations	Discussion of confronting limitations associated with caregiving; "Encountering Life's Limitations" experiential exercise; introduction to Legacy Project; homework reflection on Session 6 experiential exercise
6	Creative Sources of Meaning: Engaging in Life Fully	Discussion of creativity, courage, and responsibility; "Creative Sources of Meaning" experiential exercise; homework reflection on Session 7 experiential exercise
7	Experiential Sources of Meaning: Connecting with Life	Discussion of experiential sources of meaning, such as love, nature, art, and humor; "Love, Beauty, and Humor" experiential exercise; homework is planning/completion of Legacy Project for presentation in Session 8
8	Transitions: Reflections and Hopes for the Future	Review of sources of meaning, reflections on lessons learned; "Hopes for the Future" experiential exercise; goodbyes

[a] When delivered individually, the materials from group Sessions 3 and 4 are combined into one session on legacy.

The first two sessions are an introduction to the concept of meaning and meaning-making and the identity of the IC. The next five (or four, in the individual format) sessions are each focused on one of the four sources of meaning and how the IC may connect or reconnect with each one of these so that they become resources at various points in the caregiving trajectory. The final session is an opportunity for ICs to reflect on goals for the future, which in some cases may include preparation for the loss of their loved one and the creation of a new life in the future. Each session includes didactics and experiential exercises through which ICs begin to understand the relevance and importance of sustaining, reconnecting with, and creating meaning in their lives and caregiving through the sources of meaning previously described.

Case Example

Mr. X is the 64-year-old husband and primary caregiver of his wife, a 60-year-old retired high school teacher who was diagnosed with advanced endometrial cancer with metastases to the brain 9 months before he engaged in MCP-C. He and his wife have two adult daughters in their early twenties, both of whom live outside of the New York metropolitan area, where the couple reside. Mr. X had previously worked full-time in real estate development, but he reduced his hours dramatically when his wife was diagnosed, and recently he was forced to take an unpaid leave from work in order to attend to her growing needs. By the time he engaged in MCP-C, Mrs. X was experiencing several neurocognitive changes associated with brain metastases, including seizures, dizziness, and balance and visual disturbances. She also was beginning to have occasional speech difficulties and incontinence. As a result of these symptoms, she was no longer able to complete all activities of daily living, such as dressing and feeding herself, and neither she nor her husband believed that it was safe for her to spend much time on her own. Importantly, Mr. X described his wife as someone who, for their 28 years of marriage, was self-sufficient, independent, took care of him, and was even-tempered but recently had become verbally aggressive, irritable, forgetful, and had a significant growing number of needs. Mr. X had no notable psychiatric history and had never before received professional psychological services. At the time that he enrolled in MCP-C, he was experiencing chronic worry about his wife and his future. This worry interfered with his sleep and ability to concentrate, and it was associated with somatic symptoms such as nausea and muscle tension. He also reported at times feeling hopeless about the future, fearful of living life without his wife, and abandoned by his daughters for not being present to help care for their mother.

Historical Sources of Meaning

Mr. X identified as a first-generation American, having been raised in a small family of Jewish immigrants from Russia. These key elements of his past legacy had a significant impact on his sense of identity and values. As a young man, he worked in his parents' dry cleaning store, a business they started the year they arrived in the United States. He was taught at an early age an unquestionable devotion to family and the need to support one's family in order to survive. The identification of this element of his past legacy helped Mr. X to clarify why, in part, having his daughters live far away and not involved with helping him to care for his wife was so upsetting to him. He also described watching his mother take care of his father through his progressive deterioration due to Alzheimer's disease and, through this, reported holding an old-fashioned belief in the responsibility of women to provide care, which also contributed to feelings of frustration with and resentment toward his daughters. Through a discussion of current and future legacy, Mr. X became open to the possibility that the legacy he was creating in that moment and the one he would give to others, including his daughters, could be accomplished in a manner different from that of earlier generations. Specifically, Mr. X recognized that his past legacy had significantly impacted the value he placed on unquestionable support for family and his desire to have his daughters more involved but, concurrently, that he could set a new example for future generations of a more flexible approach to traditional gender roles of care.

Attitudinal Sources of Meaning

Mr. X felt strongly that he had no choice in becoming a caregiver. His adult daughters lived in Michigan and California, and both his and his wife's parents were deceased, although his wife's sister and brother-in-law were local. Despite this fact, he reported having a very difficult time asking friends and extended family for help or agreeing to receive help when it was offered to him. Instead, he tended to take on all of the responsibilities of caregiving, in part because he believed that as a "real man" he should be able to handle the challenges he faced on his own.

Through an exploration of the ways in which Mr. X responded to limitations and losses in the past, such as his parents' deaths and a layoff from a previous job, it became clear that he had a history of coping through isolating himself and hiding his emotions. He never allowed himself to cry, and when sad or scared he would remember his father saying to him as a young child to "keep a stiff upper lip," which he did. However, he also reported being a problem-solver. For example, when he was laid off from a job due to budget cuts, he immediately put himself on the job market, networked, and used all of his professional and personal resources to learn about new potential opportunities.

The discussion of attitude allowed for the possibility of a more flexible view of the caregiving role to emerge. In many ways, Mr. X had indeed chosen the extent to which he was engaging in this role, had chosen to be his wife's primary caregiver, and repeatedly refused offers of assistance from family members and friends. Although he was proud of his ability to do everything for his wife at the present time (and specifically as a man taking on what he had historically believed was a role meant for women)—an element of attitude that he identified as a source of meaning and strength and one that would continue to be a resource for him throughout the caregiving trajectory—he also recognized his role in making his current situation more challenging and the possibility that he could respond to caregiving differently. For example, whereas previously he had accepted his daughters' lack of involvement in his wife's care, he recognized in session that his frustration with their limited involvement was an opportunity to address his desire to have them more engaged in her care and family life generally, an attitude very much influenced by his past legacy. He also recognized that he could choose to allow more extended family to be involved in caring for his wife and that, through problem-solving, he could activate additional support networks, such as professional support through the help of social workers and in-home skilled nursing aides and also his sister-in-law and her family. He also recognized the benefit he could derive from beginning to speak openly about his feelings. Keeping a "stiff upper lip" was no longer a strategy that would serve either him or his wife well, particularly because as her disease would progress and her neurocognitive capacity become increasingly compromised, he would have to take on increased responsibility for decision-making. Mr. X had kept his concerns of his wife's passing to himself for fear of upsetting her and in so doing had isolated them both from one another. Through the session on attitude, Mr. X realized that although speaking about his fears openly with his wife would be painful, it would allow for increased connectedness between them, allow for more shared responsibility in decision-making while it was possible, and facilitate improved communication with her physicians moving forward. Indeed, whereas his previous approach of concealing emotions had left him chronically worried and contributed to somatic complaints such as insomnia and gastrointestinal distress, the conversation about choosing one's attitude underscored new ways in which Mr. X could respond to limitations he was currently facing, which would have a more positive impact on his mental and physical health.

Creative Sources of Meaning

The session on creative sources of meaning was a particularly powerful one for Mr. X. The discussion of creating and using one's life led to the emergence of several important themes, with which Mr. X had likely struggled for many years long before his wife's cancer diagnosis. First, he described feeling that he had not fulfilled his dreams or used his life to its fullest. As a young adult, he had aspirations to travel the world and spend time cultivating his musical talents. However, the need to work from a young age to help contribute financially to his family prevented him from what Mr. X described as "indulging" in these interests. He and his wife married in their early twenties, and as soon as their first child arrived, the demands of working full-time and being an active husband and father led to what he described as "shoving those dreams away." Through an exploration of creativity, Mr. X was able to identify how critical these dreams had been for him and to recognize that he had the capacity to continue to create his life, despite his current challenges. This discussion helped Mr. X to acknowledge that despite the pain and difficulties associated with the inevitable loss of his wife due to cancer, he would have a future that was open to new possibilities for growth and renewal, one that he could shape in a manner that would meet his own needs. He also realized that despite the limitations of caregiving, he did not need to wait until his wife's passing to re-engage in his life and could, for example, spend time practicing the guitar while he was spending time with his wife. Through this conversation, Mr. X began to embrace the possibility of concurrently feeling intense pain and sadness as well as hope.

A second important theme that emerged was Mr. X's acknowledgment of the courage it had taken him to continue to engage fully in his marital relationship. He described his 28-year marriage as "solid" and "loving." He reported that, similar to himself, his wife rarely verbalized her emotions, the couple said "I love you" to one another on only rare occasions, and their manner of solving or resolving arguments in the past was to "let things go" with time. Despite this, there was always a feeling of love and connectedness between them, a connectedness that became particularly important when their daughters moved away from home. Mr. X reported that since his wife's diagnosis, he felt an urgency to discuss important issues, such as her wishes for end-of-life care. He also reported the conflict he felt regarding his desire to engage more than ever emotionally with his wife but fear of doing so when their time together was becoming more limited and the inevitability of her passing a reality. The group members helped to highlight the courage Mr. X possessed in acknowledging his desires to be more open, in his taking steps to do so, and engage more fully in his relationship, despite the challenges associated with doing so. This conversation also helped Mr. X to recognize that the courage he was demonstrating and improved emotional engagement would likely prevent future feelings of guilt and regret after his wife's passing.

Finally, the session on creativity highlighted Mr. X's general difficulty in taking responsibility for his own needs. Like other group members, he had great difficulty in clearly identifying what specifically his own needs were and asking others for help. This difficulty was particularly clear at the time of the group meeting, after a year of Mr. X's intense caregiving, repeated rejection of others' help, and increasing burden. Discussion with group members helped Mr. X recognize that he would be unable to continue to provide the level of care his wife required if he continued to neglect his basic needs for sleep, exercise, and engaging in activities that could bring brief moments of pleasure. The group also reminded him that over time, as his wife's disease would progress and her needs increase, he would be required to involve others in her care. In addition, Mr. X recognized that his tendency to take full responsibility for his wife's care was, in part, a means of coping with the uncertainty of her illness and their future, similar to how he had coped with challenges and limitations in the past.

Experiential Sources of Meaning

The session on experiential sources of meaning highlighted this source of meaning as one that Mr. X had engaged at various times throughout his life and one that had the potential to become an even more significant resource for him at the present time, when the demands of caregiving were great. Mr. X identified that in the past, he had found peace and contentment through playing the guitar and through participating in religious services. Since his childhood, he had experienced a sense of connectedness to something much greater than himself through prayer, along with a sense of awe, hope, and peace. In addition, through music, he would often find the hours "flying by" and would get lost in the present moment. When asked about more recent experiences of connectedness through love, beauty, and humor, Mr. X shared that before her illness, he and his wife often attended sporting events together, during which they would get "lost in the moment," cheering for their favorite team and becoming energized by the crowds. Discussion with group leaders and members encouraged Mr. X to think more flexibly about how to continue to engage in this type of activity, despite his wife's limitations, such as through watching sports games together on television. The discussion also highlighted the sense of peace Mr. X felt at night when he fell asleep holding his wife's hand, something he had done almost every night of their marriage. Despite his wife's limitations, in those moments Mr. X felt cared for, deeply loved, safe, and connected. He recognized that this connectedness was a gift, a feeling that he could experience despite the difficult circumstances and one that, though time-limited, was very much present at the time of this session.

DISCUSSION

A large and growing body of literature identifies existential distress as a critical, but often overlooked, component of caregiver burden. Existential distress may underlie many related psychological elements of burden and frame unique opportunities for intervention for ICs at their causal origin through an exploration of meaning. Indeed, meaning-making has been described as a potential mechanism for positive growth and buffering against such burden. Despite these facts, the state of the science of intervention development for ICs of patients with cancer remains in its infancy, and only a limited number of investigations have explored interventions that attend to various elements of existential well-being.[97,102]

MCP-C is a novel, therapeutic approach intended to address the existential concerns commonly experienced by ICs of patients with cancer. Based on an empirically supported intervention that has demonstrated efficacy in improving the quality of life of patients with advanced cancer, breast cancer survivors, and bereaved parents,[106,114–116] MCP serves as a robust basis on which to develop a targeted psychotherapy to address the existential needs of ICs. Critically, the delivery of such an intervention early in the caregiving trajectory has the potential to mitigate burden and, eventually, to protect against poor bereavement outcomes, including prolonged grief disorder.

Although psychiatric diagnoses, such as anxiety and depression, are not discussed directly in the course of MCP-C, such symptoms are conceptualized in the context of caregivers becoming disconnected from various sources of meaning in their life. Helping caregivers to derive a new understanding of, or reconnection with, various sources of meaning has the potential to mitigate depressive and anxious symptomatology often associated with caregiver burden. MCP-C leaders help caregivers to understand the benefits of connecting with meaning in their lives and how these sources of meaning may serve as resources and buffer common symptoms of burden and diminish despair, especially as loved ones transition to end-of-life care.

The case example provided highlights various ways in which the exploration of four sources of meaning in life—legacy, attitude, creativity, and connectedness—may serve as resources for caregivers who feel burdened by the caregiving role and are struggling to attend to their own needs. The exploration of legacy gives context to ICs' experience of caregiving and helps them to recognize the historical factors that contributed to their engaging in and experience of this role, as well as how their caregiving work will form a key element of the legacy they will give to others in their lives. The discussion of attitude—and specifically the ability of ICs to choose their attitude in the face of the suffering they experience in their caregiving role—can be an incredibly transformative experience for those who believe that they have no choice in their role and little efficacy in their daily life. Responsibility to care for oneself and the desire to continue to create one's life, despite the limitations of caregiving, are common themes that emerge when discussing creative sources of meaning. Through an exploration of creativity, courage, responsibility, and guilt, ICs are afforded the opportunity to reflect on ways in which they are taking responsibility for their own lives, in addition to the life of their loved one with cancer, and how within the limitations of the caregiving role they may continue to create their lives. Although the experiential source of meaning can serve as a resource throughout the caregiving trajectory, it is particularly salient for ICs who are overwhelmed by the demands of caregiving and for those whose loved ones are no longer eligible for curative treatment. Indeed, ICs' recognition of their ability to experience the world through their five senses and through love, beauty and humor despite the challenges of caregiving can promote moments of peace and transcendence, and lead to positive transformative experiences.

SUMMARY

Randomized controlled trials are currently underway to evaluate the preliminary efficacy of MCP-C in enhancing spiritual well-being and meaning and decreasing burden, anxiety, and depression among ICs of patients with cancer. Previous studies have documented the many challenges of enrolling and maintaining ICs in in-person psychotherapy trials.[96] Highlighted in the literature are the benefits that may be derived from interventions delivered in alternate modalities, such as over the telephone or Internet. In addition to the in-person intervention, our group is currently investigating the efficacy of MCP-C delivered over the Internet. If successful, the web-based version of MCP-C will have the potential to reach ICs throughout the country and the world who, for a variety of reasons, are unable to access high-quality face-to-face mental health care. In addition, a recent systematic review by our group[117] highlighted existential distress as a particularly critical source of suffering among ICs of patients with brain tumors, whose loved ones often experience significant personality and neurocognitive changes and a rapid disease course. Hence, the delivery of MCP-C to ICs of brain tumor patients—and possibly an adaptation of MCP-C to meet the unique existential needs of these particularly burdened ICs—is another important application of this work.

Our hope is that through the development and dissemination of MCP-C, an intervention developed specifically to address the existential distress experienced by cancer caregivers, the unique needs of this underserved and highly vulnerable group can be better met by the psycho-oncology and palliative care communities.

ACKNOWLEDGMENT

We thank Allison Marziliano, M.A., for her assistance with the preparation of this manuscript.

REFERENCES

1. Breitbart WS, Alici Y. Psycho-oncology. *Harv Rev Psychiatry.* 2009;17:361–376.
2. Institute of Medicine. *Retooling for an Ageing America: Building the Healthcare Workforce.* Washington, DC: Institute of Medicine; 2008.
3. Hudson P, Payne S. The future of family caregiving: Research, social policy and clinical practice. In: Hudson P, Payne, S, eds. *Family Carers in Palliative Care: A Guide for Health and Social Care Professionals.* Oxford, UK: Oxford University Press; 2015.
4. National Alliance for Caregiving in collaboration with AARP. *Caregiving in the U.S.* Bethesda, MD: National Alliance for Caregiving; 2009.
5. Pasacreta JV, McCorkle R. Cancer care: Impact of interventions on caregiver outcomes. *Annu Rev Nurs Res.* 2000;18:127–148.
6. Rabow MW, Hauser JM, Adams J. Supporting family caregivers at the end of life: "They don't know what they don't know." *J Am Med Assoc.* 2004;291:483–491.
7. Vess JD, Moreland JR, Schwebel AI. A follow-up study of role functioning and the psychological environment of families of cancer patients. *J Psychosoc Oncol.* 1985;3:1–13.
8. Northouse L. A longitudinal study of the adjustment of patients and husbands to breast cancer. *Oncol Nurs Forum.* 1989;16:511–516.
9. Siegel K, Raveis VH, Houts P, et al. Caregiver burden and unmet patient needs. *Cancer.* 1991;68:1131–1140.
10. Schott-Baer D. Dependent care, caregiver burden, and self-care agency of spouse caregivers. *Cancer Nurs.* 1993;16:230–236.
11. Kissane DW, Bloch S, Burns WI, et al. Psychological morbidity in the families of patients with cancer. *Psycho-Oncology.* 1994;3:47–56.
12. Boyle D, Blodgett L, Gnesdiloff S, et al. Caregiver quality of life after autologous bone marrow transplantation. *Cancer Nurs.* 2000;23:193–203.
13. Kuijer RG, Buunk BP, Ybema JF, et al. The relation between perceived inequity, marital satisfaction and emotions among couples facing cancer. *Br J Soc Psychol.* 2002;41:39–56.
14. Given B, Kozachik S, Collins, C, eds. *Caregiver Role Strain.* St. Louis, MO: Mosby; 2001.
15. Hinds C. The needs of families who care for patients with cancer at home: Are we meeting them? *J Adv Nurs.* 1985;10:575–581.
16. Morse SR, Fife B. Coping with a partner's cancer: Adjustment at four stages of the illness trajectory. *Oncol Nurs Forum.* 1998;25:751–760.
17. Northouse LL, Mood D, Templin T, et al. Couples' patterns of adjustment to colon cancer. *Soc Sci Med.* 2000;50:271–284.
18. Carlson LE, Ottenbreit N, St. Pierre M, et al. Partner understanding of the breast and prostate cancer experience. *Cancer Nurs.* 2001;24:231–239.
19. Nijboer C, Tempelaar R, Triemstra M, et al. The role of social and psychologic resources in caregiving of cancer patients. *Cancer.* 2001;91:1029–1039.
20. Bishop MM, Beaumont JL, Hahn EA, et al. Late effects of cancer and hematopoietic stem-cell transplantation on spouses or partners compared with survivors and survivor-matched controls. *J Clin Oncol.* 2007;25:1403–1411.
21. Hileman JW, Lackey NR, Hassanein RS. Identifying the needs of home caregivers of patients with cancer. *Oncol Nurs Forum.* 1992;19:771–777.
22. Laizner AM, Yost LM, Barg FK, et al. Needs of family caregivers of persons with cancer: A review. *Semin Oncol Nurs.* 1993;9:114–120.
23. Covinsky KE, Goldman L, Cook EF, et al. The impact of serious illness on patients' families: SUPPORT Investigators. Study to Understand Prognoses and Preferences for Outcomes and Risks of Treatment. *J Am Med Assoc.* 1994;272:1839–1844.
24. Hodgkinson K, Butow P, Hobbs KM, et al. After cancer: The unmet supportive care needs of survivors and their partners. *J Psychosoc Oncol.* 2007;25:89–104.
25. Kim Y, Given BA. Quality of life of family caregivers of cancer survivors: Across the trajectory of the illness. *Cancer.* 2008;112(11 Suppl):2556–2568.
26. Francis LE, Worthington J, Kypriotakis G, et al. Relationship quality and burden among caregivers for late-stage cancer patients. *Support Care Cancer.* 2010;18:1429–1436.
27. Ell K, Nishimoto R, Mantell J, et al. Longitudinal analysis of psychological adaptation among family members of patients with cancer. *J Psychosom Res.* 1988;32(4–5):429–438.
28. Johnson J. Cancer: A family disruption. *Recent Res Cancer.* 1988;108:306–310.
29. Pederson LM, Valanis BG. The effects of breast cancer on the family: A review of the literature. *J Psychosoc Oncol.* 1988;6:95–118.
30. Oberst MT, Thomas SE, Gass KA, et al. Caregiving demands and appraisal of stress among family caregivers. *Cancer Nurs.* 1989;12:209–215.

31. Sales E. Psychosocial impact of the phase of cancer on the family: An updated review. *J Psychosoc Oncol.* 1991;9:1–9.
32. Toseland RW, Blanchard CG, McCallion P. A problem solving intervention for caregivers of cancer patients. *Soc Sci Med.* 1995;40:517–528.
33. Toseland RW, McCallion P, Gerber T, et al. Use of health and human services by community-residing people with dementia. *Soc Work.* 1999; 44:535–548.
34. Weitzner MA, McMillan SC, Jacobsen PB. Family caregiver quality of life: Differences between curative and palliative cancer treatment settings. *J Pain Symptom Manage.* 1999;17:418–428.
35. Emanuel EJ, Fairclough DL, Slutsman J, et al. Understanding economic and other burdens of terminal illness: The experience of patients and their caregivers. *Ann Intern Med.* 2000;132:451–459.
36. Manne S, Ostroff J, Winkel G, et al. Posttraumatic growth after breast cancer: Patient, partner, and couple perspectives. *Psychosom Med.* 2004; 66:442–454.
37. Murray SA, Kendall M, Boyd K, et al. Archetypal trajectories of social, psychological, and spiritual wellbeing and distress in family care givers of patients with lung cancer: Secondary analysis of serial qualitative interviews. *Br Med J.* 2010;340:c2581.
38. Dumont S, Turgeon J, Allard P, et al. Caring for a loved one with advanced cancer: Determinants of psychological distress in family caregivers. *J Palliat Med.* 2006;9:912–921.
39. Oldham L, Kristjanson L, Ng C, et al. Female relatives' experience of testicular cancer. *Aust J Cancer Nurs.* 2006;7:18–24.
40. Given CW, Stommel M, Given B, et al. The influence of cancer patients' symptoms and functional states on patients' depression and family caregivers' reaction and depression. *Health Psychol.* 1993;12:277–285.
41. Given B, Wyatt G, Given C, et al. Burden and depression among caregivers of patients with cancer at the end of life. *Oncol Nurs Forum.* 2004;31:1105–1117.
42. Kornblith AB, Herr HW, Ofman US, et al. Quality of life of patients with prostate cancer and their spouses: The value of a data base in clinical care. *Cancer.* 1994;73:2791–2802.
43. Baider L, Kaufman B, Perez T. Mutuality of fate: Adaptation and psychological distress in cancer patients and their partners. In: Baider L, Cooper L, De-Nour AK, eds. *Cancer and the Family.* New York, NY: Wiley; 1996.
44. Cliff AM, MacDonagh RP. Psychosocial morbidity in prostate cancer: II. A comparison of patients and partners. *BJU Int.* 2000;86:834–839.
45. Kris AE, Cherlin EJ, Prigerson H, et al. Length of hospice enrollment and subsequent depression in family caregivers: 13-Month follow-up study. *Am J Geriatr Psychiatry.* 2006;14:264–269.
46. Rivera HR. Depression symptoms in cancer caregivers. *Clin J Oncol Nurs.* 2009;13:195–202.
47. Baider L, Kaplan De-Nour A. Adjustment to cancer: Who is the patient—the husband or the wife? *Isr J Med Sci.* 1988;24:631–636.
48. Baider L, Perez T, De-Nour AK. Gender and adjustment to chronic disease: A study of couples with colon cancer. *Gen Hosp Psychiat.* 1989;11:1–8.
49. Ey S, Compass BE, Epping-Jordan JE. Stress response and psychological adjustment in patients with cancer and their spouses. *J Psychosoc Oncol.* 1998;16:59–77.
50. Gallagher J, Parle M, Cairns D. Appraisal and psychological distress six months after diagnosis of breast cancer. *Br J Health Psychol.* 2002;7:365–376.
51. Braun M, Mikulincer M, Rydall A, et al. Hidden morbidity in cancer: Spouse caregivers. *J Clin Oncol.* 2007;25:4829–4834.
52. McLean LM, Walton T, Matthew A, et al. Examination of couples' attachment security in relation to depression and hopelessness in maritally distressed patients facing end-stage cancer and their spouse caregivers: A buffer or facilitator of psychosocial distress? *Support Care Cancer.* 2011;19:1539–1548.
53. Grunfeld E, Coyle D, Whelan T, et al. Family caregiver burden: Results of a longitudinal study of breast cancer patients and their principal caregivers. *Can Med Assoc J.* 2004;170:1795–1801.
54. Hauser JM, Kramer BJ. Family caregivers in palliative care. *Clin Geriatr Med.* 2004;20:671–688.
55. Pirl WF. Evidence report on the occurrence, assessment, and treatment of depression in cancer patients. *J Natl Cancer Inst Monogr.* 2004:32–39.
56. Traeger L, Greer JA, Fernandez-Robles C, et al. Evidence-based treatment of anxiety in patients with cancer. *J Clin Oncol.* 2012;30:1197–1205.
57. Burton LC, Newsom JT, Schulz R, et al. Preventive health behaviors among spousal caregivers. *Prev Med.* 1997;26:162–169.
58. Given B, Given CW. Patient and family caregiver reaction to new and recurrent breast cancer. *J Am Med Womens Assoc.* 1992;47:201–206, 212.
59. Carter PA. Family caregivers' sleep loss and depression over time. *Cancer Nurs.* 2003;26:253–259.
60. Cho MH, Dodd MJ, Lee KA, et al. Self-reported sleep quality in family caregivers of gastric cancer patients who are receiving chemotherapy in Korea. *J Cancer Educ.* 2006;21:S37–S41.
61. Hearson B, McClement S. Sleep disturbance in family caregivers of patients with advanced cancer. *Int J Palliat Nurs.* 2007;13:495–501.

62. Jensen S, Given BA. Fatigue affecting family caregivers of cancer patients. *Cancer Nurs.* 1991;14:181–187.
63. Teel CS, Press AN. Fatigue among elders in caregiving and noncaregiving roles. *West J Nurs Res.* 1999;21:498–514.
64. Lee S, Colditz GA, Berkman LF, et al. Caregiving and risk of coronary heart disease in U.S. women: A prospective study. *Am J Prev Med.* 2003;24:113–119.
65. von Kanel R, Mausbach BT, Patterson TL, et al. Increased Framingham Coronary Heart Disease Risk Score in dementia caregivers relative to non-caregiving controls. *Gerontology.* 2008;54:131–137.
66. Kiecolt-Glaser JK, Glaser R, Shuttleworth EC, et al. Chronic stress and immunity in family caregivers of Alzheimer's disease victims. *Psychosom Med.* 1987;49:523–535.
67. Rohleder N, Marin TJ, Ma R, et al. Biologic cost of caring for a cancer patient: Dysregulation of pro- and anti-inflammatory signaling pathways. *J Clin Oncol.* 2009;27:2909–2915.
68. Schulz R, Beach SR. Caregiving as a risk factor for mortality: The Caregiver Health Effects Study. *J Am Med Assoc.* 1999;282:2215–2219.
69. Christakis NA, Allison PD. Mortality after the hospitalization of a spouse. *N Engl J Med.* 2006;354:719–730.
70. Riess-Sherwood P, Given BA, Given CW. Who cares for the caregiver: Strategies to provide support. *Home Health Care Manage Practice.* 2002;14:110–121.
71. Sherwood PR, Given BA, Donovan H, et al. Guiding research in family care: A new approach to oncology caregiving. *Psycho-Oncology.* 2008;17:986–996.
72. Grov EK, Fossa SD, Sorebo O, et al. Primary caregivers of cancer patients in the palliative phase: A path analysis of variables influencing their burden. *Soc Sci Med.* 2006;63:2429–2439.
73. Yabroff KR, Kim Y. Time costs associated with informal caregiving for cancer survivors. *Cancer.* 2009;115(18 Suppl):4362–4373.
74. Chochinov HM, Krisjanson LJ, Hack TF, et al. Dignity in the terminally ill: revisited. *J Palliat Med.* 2006;9:666–672.
75. Henery N. Constructions of spirituality in contemporary nursing theory. *J Adv Nurs.* 2003; 42:550–557.
76. Henoch I, Danielson E. Existential concerns among patients with cancer and interventions to meet them: an integrative literature review. *Psycho-Oncology.* 2009;18:225–236.
77. Cherny NI, Coyle N, Foley KM. Suffering in the advanced cancer patient: A definition and taxonomy. *J Palliat Care.* 1994;10:57–70.
78. Folkman S, Chesney MA, Christopher-Richards A. Stress and coping in caregiving partners of men with AIDS. *Psychiatr Clin North Am.* 1994;17:35–53.
79. Lazarus RS, Folkman S. *Stress, Appraisal and Coping.* New York, NY: Springer; 1984.
80. Hudson PL, Hayman-White K, Aranda S, et al. Predicting family caregiver psychosocial functioning in palliative care. *J Palliat Care.* 2006;22:133–140.
81. Pinquart M, Sorensen S. Differences between caregivers and noncaregivers in psychological health and physical health: A meta-analysis. *Psychol Aging.* 2003;18:250–267.
82. Ayres L. Narratives of family caregiving: The process of making meaning. *Res Nurs Health.* 2000;23:424–434.
83. Bauer-Wu S, Farran CJ. Meaning in life and psycho-spiritual functioning: A comparison of breast cancer survivors and healthy women. *J Holist Nurs.* 2005;23:172–190.
84. Calhoun LG, Tedeschi RG. *Handbook of Posttraumatic Growth: Research and Practice.* New York, NY: Erlbaum; 2006.
85. Farran CJ, Keane-Hagerty E, Salloway S, et al. Finding meaning: An alternative paradigm for Alzheimer's disease family caregivers. *Gerontologist.* 1991;31:483–489.
86. Pargament KI, Ano GG. Spiritual resources and struggles in coping with medical illness. *South Med J.* 2006;99:1161–1162.
87. Park CL, Folkman S. Stability and change in psychosocial resources during caregiving and bereavement in partners of men with AIDS. *J Pers.* 1997;65:421–447.
88. Pearlin LI, Mullan JT, Semple SJ, et al. Caregiving and the stress process: An overview of concepts and their measures. *Gerontologist.* 1990;30:583–594.
89. Rhoades DR, McFarland KF. Caregiver meaning: A study of caregivers of individuals with mental illness. *Health Soc Work.* 1999;24:291–298.
90. Thornton AA, Perez MA. Posttraumatic growth in prostate cancer survivors and their partners. *Psycho-Oncology.* 2006;15:285–296.
91. Frankl VE. *Man's Search for Meaning.* New York, NY: Washington Square Press; 1963.
92. Frankl VE. *Psychotherapy and Existentialism.* New York, NY: Washington Square Press; 1967.
93. Frankl VE, ed. *Meaninglessness: A Challenge to Psychologists.* Philadelphia: Saunders; 1973.
94. Frankl VE. *The Unheard Cry for Meaning.* New York, NY: Washington Square Press; 1978.
95. Applebaum AJ, Farran CJ, Marziliano AM, et al. Preliminary study of themes of meaning and psychosocial service use among informal cancer caregivers. *Palliat Support Care.* 2014;12:139–148.

96. Applebaum AJ, Breitbart W. Care for the cancer caregiver: A systematic review. *Palliat Support Care.* 2013;11:231–252.
97. Duggleby W, Wright K, Williams A, et al. Developing a living with hope program for caregivers of family members with advanced cancer. *J Palliat Care.* 2007;23:24–31.
98. Kozachik SL, Given CW, Given BA, et al. Improving depressive symptoms among caregivers of patients with cancer: Results of a randomized clinical trial. *Oncol Nurs Forum.* 2001;28:1149–1157.
99. McLean LM, Jones JM, Rydall AC, et al. A couples intervention for patients facing advanced cancer and their spouse caregivers: Outcomes of a pilot study. *Psycho-Oncology.* 2008;17:1152–1156.
100. Northouse L, Kershaw T, Mood D, et al. Effects of a family intervention on the quality of life of women with recurrent breast cancer and their family caregivers. *Psycho-Oncology.* 2005;14:478–491.
101. Scott JL, Halford WK, Ward BG. United we stand? The effects of a couple-coping intervention on adjustment to early stage breast or gynecological cancer. *J Consult Clin Psychol.* 2004;72:1122–1135.
102. Hayes S. Acceptance and commitment therapy, relational frame theory, and the third wave of behavioral cognitive therapies. *Behav Ther.* 2003;35:639–665.
103. Fegg MJ, Brandstatter M, Kogler M, et al. Existential behavioural therapy for informal caregivers of palliative patients: A randomised controlled trial. *Psycho-Oncology.* 2013;22:2079–2086.
104. Park CL. Making sense of the meaning literature: An integrative review of meaning making and its effects on adjustment to stressful life events. *Psychol Bull.* 2010;136:257–301.
105. Breitbart W, Rosenfeld B, Gibson C, et al. Meaning-centered group psychotherapy for patients with advanced cancer: A pilot randomized controlled trial. *Psycho-Oncology.* 2010;19:21–28.
106. Breitbart W, Poppito S, Rosenfeld B, et al. Pilot randomized controlled trial of individual meaning-centered psychotherapy for patients with advanced cancer. *J Clin Oncol.* 2012;30:1304–1309.
107. Breitbart W, Rosenfeld B, Pessin H, et al. Meaning-centered group psychotherapy: An effective intervention for improving psychological well-being in patients with advanced cancer. *J Clin Oncol.* 2015;33:749–754.
108. Lichtenthal WG, Poppito S, Olden M, et al. *Effects of Meaning Centered Psychotherapy on Facets of Meaning Among Advanced Cancer Patients: A Closer Look at the FACIT-Sp.* Montreal, Ontario, Canada: Society of Behavioral Medicine; 2009.
109. Lichtenthal WG, Poppito S, Olden M, et al. *Facets of Meaning: Differential Effects of Meaning Centered Psychotherapy Among Advanced Cancer Patients.* Montreal, Ontario, Canada: Association for Death Education and Counseling; 2008.
110. Hart T, O'Neil-Pirozzi TM, Williams KD, et al. Racial differences in caregiving patterns, caregiver emotional function, and sources of emotional support following traumatic brain injury. *J Head Trauma Rehabil.* 2007;22:122–131.
111. Lichtenthal WG, Nilsson M, Kissane DW, et al. Underutilization of mental health services among bereaved caregivers with prolonged grief disorder. *Psychiatr Serv.* 2011;62:1225–1229.
112. Shelby RA, Taylor KL, Kerner JF, et al. The role of community-based and philanthropic organizations in meeting cancer patient and caregiver needs. *CA Cancer J Clin.* 2002;52:229–246.
113. Ayres L. Narratives of family caregiving: Four story types. *Res Nurs Health.* 2000;23:359–371.
114. Lichtenthal WG, Breitbart W. The central role of meaning in adjustment to the loss of a child to cancer: Implications for the development of meaning-centered grief therapy. *Curr Opin Support Palliat Care.* 2015;9:46–51.
115. Lichtenthal WG, Tuman M, Corner G, et al. *Development of a Meaning-Centered Group for Breast Cancer Survivors (MCG-BCS): Focus Group Findings and Preliminary Effects.* Tampa, FL: American Psychosocial Oncology Society; 2014.
116. Lichtenthal WG, Sweeney C, Roberts K, et al. *Meaning-Centered Grief Therapy: Theory, Practice and Promise.* San Antonio, TX: Association for Death Education and Counseling; 2015.
117. Applebaum A, Kryza-Lacombe M, Buthorn J, et al. Existential distress among caregivers of patients with brain tumors: A review of the literature. *Neuro Oncol Pract.* 2015; 29((2):105–120.

7

Meaning-Centered Grief Therapy

WENDY G. LICHTENTHAL, STEPHANIE NAPOLITANO, KAILEY E. ROBERTS, CORINNE SWEENEY, AND ELIZABETH SLIVJAK

INTRODUCTION

The loss of a child is the most painful, intense, and devastating type of bereavement, and parents who lose a child to cancer, specifically, face unique challenges in making meaning of their loss. As they relinquish their role of caregiver fighting tirelessly against the illness, they may struggle with their sense of identity and purpose, meaning in their child's life, and finding sense and significance in the loss.[1,2] The 2003 Institute of Medicine (IOM) report, "When Children Die: Improving Palliative and End-of-Life Care for Children and Their Families," highlighted how challenges in finding meaning of such an untimely loss are related to bereaved parents' severe and protracted grief responses.[3] Not surprisingly, bereaved parents are at increased risk for pathological grief reactions, including prolonged grief disorder (PGD), a syndrome that has been associated with numerous negative physical and mental health outcomes.[4,5] Despite their increased risk, however, there is an absence of empirically supported interventions for this highly vulnerable population.

There has been a strong, unmet need to develop empirically supported, conceptually sound interventions for bereaved parents. Grief researchers have long argued that finding meaning in and after a loss is key to adaptation, thus suggesting the therapeutic value of facilitating meaning-making to reduce PGD symptoms and improve overall adjustment.[6–8] Given this, meaning-centered psychotherapy (MCP), which has demonstrated efficacy in enhancing meaning and purpose among advanced cancer patients,[9,10] has the potential to address the challenges in finding meaning that bereaved parents frequently report.[11] This chapter discusses the development and evaluation of an innovative application of MCP, which we have adapted into meaning-centered grief therapy (MCGT) for a new but critically important and underserved population: parents bereaved by cancer. We believe MCGT has the potential to improve bereaved parents' sense of meaning and to reduce their PGD symptoms.

The adaptation of MCP into MCGT was based on data from a formative National Cancer Institute-funded study of parents bereaved by cancer, which provided essential information from surveys and interviews on parents' PGD symptoms, meaning-making challenges, and intervention use preferences and barriers. Importantly, we also found in this study that access to mental health services is impeded by financial and time constraints and not knowing where to go for help, suggesting that parents' underutilization of services may be addressed through outreach and use of convenient, low-cost delivery mediums such as videoconferencing.[12] Thus, we are currently conducting a trial of MCGT delivered through videoconferencing to further reduce barriers to accessing support that parents frequently face, evaluating the feasibility, acceptability, and preliminary effects of the intervention.[12]

RATIONALE FOR FOCUSING ON BEREAVED PARENTS

Cancer is the leading cause of death by disease in children.[13] The IOM has emphasized that bereavement care is part of comprehensive emotional and spiritual care for family members and is a public health priority.[3] Bereaved parents are at heightened risk for numerous detrimental mental and physical health outcomes, including psychiatric illness, existential suffering, marital problems, and even mortality.[14–16] They are also at increased risk for prolonged grief disorder (PGD), a syndrome characterized by separation distress and loss of meaning.[5] PGD occurs in approximately 10–20% of the general population and has been associated with life-threatening conditions including cancer, depression, suicidality, heart disease, and adverse health behaviors (tobacco and alcohol consumption), and it may persist for years if left untreated.[17] In a recent study, we found that 12% of parents who lost a child to cancer met diagnostic criteria for PGD (according to self-report; not formal clinical diagnoses), although a much larger proportion (77%) reported persistent yearning for their child.[12]

Psychotherapeutic interventions have the potential to reduce PGD symptoms and counter bereaved parents' increased risk of physical and psychological health morbidity, including their elevated risk of mortality.[18] However, empirically supported interventions for bereaved parents are lacking. Furthermore, despite their distress and heightened risk for adverse outcomes, bereaved parents appear to underutilize existing mental health services.[3,12] We have found that bereaved caregivers suffering from PGD, specifically, underutilize services, despite a heightened risk of suicidality.[19] Furthermore, nearly half (47%) of parents bereaved by cancer indicated they would like assistance with their coping, but 40% of those in this group were not accessing mental health services.[12] Among those who were not using services, the most common barriers to mental health service use were that it was too painful to speak about their loss, too difficult to find help, too financially challenging, and believing it was too difficult to find help.[12] In addition, parents have reported that existing interventions are not helpful.[12,20,21]

The 2003 IOM report on death in children highlighted the challenges that bereaved parents face in making meaning of their loss,[3] and a large body of research suggests that finding meaning in a loss and restoring a sense of purpose may be therapeutic. A meaning-centered intervention may be especially beneficial for parents bereaved by cancer who are suffering from PGD, whose sense of identity and meaning in life are often challenged by the additional loss of the caregiver role, because of its potential to assist them with restoring a sense of purpose in their lives.[22,23]

ADDRESSING BARRIERS TO INTERVENTION USE

Our research with bereaved parents suggested that it is not sufficient to simply develop a conceptually sound intervention—it must also be accessible and reach underserved populations. Parents who lose a child to cancer often wish to continue the relationship with the institution where their child was treated to avoid yet another loss.[24,25] However, it is often not practical for them to participate in bereavement care in person because of logistical and emotional barriers (e.g., geography, time, and the pain of being in the hospital where memories of their child may be too raw). Telemental health approaches such as videoconferencing, which has been shown to be as efficacious as in-person delivery in several studies,[26–28] can address these barriers by offering convenience while facilitating continuity of care with the treating institution. Several randomized controlled trials (RCTs) targeting post-traumatic stress disorder[26,27] and depression[28] have shown that telemental health and in-person services yield equivalent outcomes and patient satisfaction, attendance, and dropout levels. In our current study, we additionally offset financial barriers by offering the interventions free of charge and by providing tablet computers. Thus, we have tried to reduce barriers to accessing mental health services through videoconferencing while reaching out to underserved groups, including minorities and fathers.

ADAPTATION OF MEANING-CENTERED GRIEF THERAPY FOR PARENTS BEREAVED BY CANCER

Our current study of MCGT has involved execution of key intervention development and evaluation activities as part of stage I of the stage model of behavioral therapies (manual writing, pilot testing, and adherence/competence measure development).[29] There have been four phases in this process. Phase 1 involved adaptation of the MCP manual, adding relevant grief-focused sessions and exercises, resulting in a 16-session treatment. We obtained feedback on the manual using a modified Delphi method with key informants. The Delphi method involves gathering opinions from a group of experts, keeping feedback anonymous, and circulating it back to the group in rounds until consensus is reached.[30] Because selection of key informants for a Delphi method should not be random and should involve nomination of individuals,[30] our team selected 13 bereaved parents who completed a previous study on psychosocial needs of bereaved parents, demonstrated insight about mental health services, and agreed to be contacted for future research. Psychotherapists ($n = 3$) with expertise in intervention manual development and grief were also recruited. We conducted two feedback rounds in phase 1, first providing the parents and therapists with a copy of the MCGT treatment workbook or manual and requesting feedback on content, format, and language through interview or in writing. Nine parents and three therapists completed the study, providing qualitative feedback that was analyzed using thematic content analysis—a well-established, systematic qualitative analysis approach in health research[31]—to identify themes in participants' feedback.[31] We followed Morse's[31] guidelines for conducting rigorous qualitative research (e.g., audit trail, member checking, and saturation) using Atlas.ti software and meeting until consensus on a final set of thematic findings to tailor the manual was reached.[32,33] After modifications were made based on feedback, the experts received the revised treatment materials and a summary of changes along with a survey to provide any further feedback based on the comments of the other experts. Key changes resulting from this feedback included suggestions for improving the accessibility and emotional sensitivity of the language, reducing the emphasis on the theoretical background of the intervention, increasing the focus on the child and loss, and emphasizing the transformation of reflections to actions within sessions. To increase active engagement with the reflections on meaning, several experiential exercises (e.g., imaginal dialogue and letter writing) were added to the manual based on the expert feedback. Feedback on formatting, language, and content was synthesized and guided the revision of the manual in preparation for an open trial of MCGT.

Phase 2 of the study was a brief open trial of MCGT delivered in person with five bereaved parents who reported elevated PGD symptoms (PG-13 scores ≥34) to further refine the treatment through active participant feedback and to identify ways to improve therapeutic alliance to maximize the impact of delivery via videoconferencing. Treatment sessions took place at an outpatient counseling center affiliated with the institute where their child was treated but physically situated in a different location from the main hospital. Assessments were conducted at baseline, mid-intervention, post-intervention, and 3 months post-intervention. Participants also provided their feedback about MCGT through a post-treatment exit interview, in which they commented on specific aspects of the intervention they found helpful, areas for potential change or modification, and provided other suggestions to make the intervention more accessible. All parents who completed reported an overall positive experience with the intervention, as well as reduced PGD symptoms at post-treatment. Notably, due to intense, painful emotions associated with the main hospital where their child was treated, several of the parents indicated that attending in-person sessions would not have been feasible if they took place at that location. These interviews were used to help further refine the MCGT manual.

Phase 3 was another brief open trial with three bereaved parents delivering MCGT via videoconferencing, which, as mentioned previously, numerous studies have shown is as efficacious as in-person delivery.[26–28] This small trial helped us to resolve logistical challenges, such as improving Internet connectivity and audiovisual issues, in advance of our planned pilot RCT. All parents were provided with instruction sheets containing information about connecting to the videoconferencing session and troubleshooting help. Explicit instructions, training, and technical support for videoconferencing were provided by our trained staff and therapists, with more in-depth training for parents who had limited computer experience.

During the open trial exit interviews, we also obtained parent testimonials to help address barriers to accessing mental health services that were identified by Lichtenthal et al.,[12] such as that it is too painful to discuss their loss and will not be helpful. Parents were given the opportunity to convey what they wished other bereaved parents considering seeking treatment to know. These testimonials are being used to recruit for phase 4 of the study, which is an RCT comparing MCGT to supportive psychotherapy.

MEANING-CENTERED GRIEF THERAPY OVERVIEW

MCGT is adapted from MCP, a manualized intervention developed by Dr. William Breitbart and colleagues that was designed to enhance a sense meaning in advanced cancer patients.[34–36] Based on the work of Viktor Frankl,[37] MCP addresses existential issues using didactics and experiential exercises and has demonstrated efficacy in reducing existential suffering and improving psychosocial functioning among advanced cancer patients.[34–36] However, the existential issues that advanced cancer patients, who are approaching death, face are very different from those of parents bereaved by cancer.

The resulting grief intervention, MCGT, addresses bereaved parents' unique meaning-making challenges in order to assist with improving PGD symptoms. MCGT is a manualized, one-on-one intervention that uses psychoeducation, experiential exercises, and homework focusing on themes related to meaning, identity, purpose, and legacy. Within the MCGT framework, cognitive schemas and techniques[38,39] and grief psychoeducation for parents and their primary supporters are incorporated to enhance meaning-making and reframe maladaptive thinking. Adaptive continuing bonds are cultivated through discussion of legacy. Adaptations for various cultural and ethnic meaning systems are incorporated to assist with making MCGT more acceptable to minority bereaved parents.

We are using a one-on-one rather than a couples approach because our prior research showed that PGD symptom levels were not significantly correlated in mothers and fathers from the same household ($p > 0.10$). This suggested that an individualized framework is most appropriate, although MCGT explores relational sources of meaning in couples and provides PGD psychoeducation to partners or other social support providers, who are invited to attend a therapy session. Connections with other bereaved parents through, for example, support groups, are also encouraged.

APPLICATION OF THE MEANING-CENTERED THEORETICAL MODEL IN MCGT

Bereaved parents often face a profound crisis in meaning.[40] Meaning is a complex term that has been defined in many ways.[41–44] Prior studies and our own research have demonstrated that there are several facets of meaning that may be impacted by the loss of a child.[45] These are discussed next.

Sense-Making

The untimely loss of a child challenges assumptions about the way the world works, leaving bereft parents struggling to make sense of their loss.[36,37,46] They may wonder if they, as their child's caregivers, could have prevented the death, often resulting in self-blame or guilt.[22] Although some parents who lose their child to an expected cause, such as cancer, focus on how their child is no longer suffering, many parents vehemently express that sense-making is not possible when it comes to losing a child.[2,22,47] In fact, one study found that 35% of parents who had lost a child to cancer found it problematic when attempting to merge their view of the world with the experience of losing their child.[48] Furthermore, we have found that the struggle to make sense of the loss of a child is highly prevalent and is associated with greater levels of PGD symptoms.[2,22]

Benefit-Finding and Post-traumatic Growth

Following their loss, parents may recognize positive ways in which they or their families have grown or changed, a process referred to as benefit-finding.[49] For example, parents who have lost a child to cancer have described changes in their priorities and an enhanced outlook on life.[50] These positive consequences, referred to as posttraumatic growth,[51–53] such as a family becoming closer as a result of the illness, may give a greater significance to the death within the larger context of their lives.[49] Posttraumatic growth has been associated with better mental and physical adjustment[51–53] and, among bereaved parents, with less intense grief symptoms.[54] We have demonstrated that benefit-finding is associated with decreased PGD symptoms.[22,55] Notably and justifiably, discussion of positive consequences arising from the tragic loss of a child is a sensitive issue, and some parents find it too challenging to consider making meaning in this way.[2,22]

Identity

A parent's sense of meaning and purpose is inextricably linked to his or her sense of identity.[22] Parents bereaved by cancer lose not only their beloved child but also their sense of identity as devoted caregiver.[31] Their identity as parents to their child may also be challenged[45,46] as they struggle to preserve a bond with their child. In a study of parents who had lost their child to cancer 6 months prior, 40% reported challenges to their sense of identity.[48] The concept of identity disintegration,[57] "in which establishing a new purposeful life after the child's death is equated to denying the deceased child's existence and the parental role" (p. 405), was found at 6, 12, and 18 months post-loss when exploring parents' sense of identity.[22,58] Notably, more parents expressed qualities of identity disintegration at 18 months (vs. 6 or 12 months), which suggests that challenges to parents' sense of identity may exacerbate over time.[58]

Disconnection from Sources of Meaning

According to Frankl,[37] a person's will to live is often linked to sustaining a connection to sources of meaning, such as work, hobbies, love, and beauty.[22] Disconnection often begins while parents are providing care to their ill child as they focus increasingly more of their time on caregiving and less on other meaningful activities, roles, relationships, and experiences.[59,60] Parents' sense of purposelessness may be intensified following the child's death because they are left with an empty space that caregiving once filled and isolated from friends and family, who may have difficulty grasping their profound pain.[60] Parents may also feel disconnected from their child's medical team, which is often a significant source of support during their child's illness but is less available to them after their child's death.[22,24] In two-parent homes, parents may feel disconnected from their partners as they grieve their child differently and exhibit different needs at different times.[61,62]

Legacy and Meaning of the Child's Life

Bereaved parents often struggle to find meaning in the life of their deceased children, whose early death robs them of opportunities to further develop their own identities and meaning.[22] They report a deep fear that their children will be forgotten.[63] Parents may continue their bond with their children, which in most cases is viewed as adaptive,[64] by becoming active in causes and learning from the way their children lived.[40] However, for some parents, this is a challenge because reminders of their child are too painful.[12,65]

To address these challenges to parents' sense of meaning, MCP applies the conceptual model suggested by Viktor Frankl,[37] who maintained that meaning and purpose can be found through connectedness with valued relationships and roles in the world. Central to this model is the principle that individuals have the freedom to choose their attitude toward their suffering, and that this attitude (i.e., the way they face their tragic circumstances) can be a source of meaning in and of itself. Our research has not only confirmed the presence of key meaning-related themes but also suggested a complex relationship between these various aspects of meaning that has significant clinical implications. Based on qualitative interviews we conducted with parents bereaved by cancer, this "reciprocal pathway theory of meaning-making" highlights the reciprocal relationship between the meaning constructs described here, suggesting that enhancing one domain may positively impact another (e.g., facilitating sense-making through benefit-finding, and reconciling one's sense of identity by exploring the child's legacy and choosing one's attitude).[22] This suggests that there are multiple "clinical entry points" at which a therapist can intervene to enhance meaning.[45,66]

Built on the foundation of MCP, MCGT also incorporates principles of Neimeyer's meaning reconstruction,[67] fostering creation of a coherent narrative of the loss to facilitate sense-making and benefit-finding; cognitive–behavioral therapy,[55] assisting parents with challenging unhelpful thoughts based on their preexisting cognitive schemas[55] and engaging in adaptive behaviors; and attachment theory,[68] helping parents to transform the caregiving role to continue their bond to their deceased child in new, adaptive, and meaningful ways (Figure 7.1).[68,69] This model assumes that, based on empirical literature,[7,70] the loss of a child can positively or negatively impact one's sense of meaning through meaning-making (i.e., cognitive processes that result in a sense of meaning of the loss and about one's

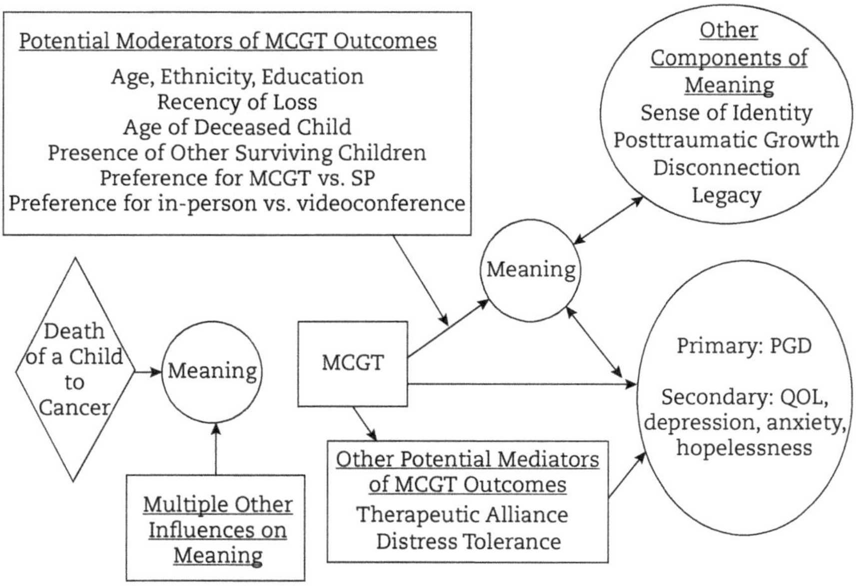

FIGURE 7.1 Conceptual model of meaning-centered grief therapy.

Note. MCGT = Meaning-Centered Grief Therapy. SP = Supportive Psychotherapy. PGD = Prolonged Grief Disorder. QOL = Quality of Life.

life). We believe that MCGT can enhance meaning, facilitating a process that, for some parents, occurs naturally.[71] Meaning is both an intermediary outcome (a construct to be enhanced in its own right) and a mediator, driving improvement in multiple psychosocial outcomes, including PGD symptoms (e.g., by redirecting attention toward meaningful activities),[72] which in turn may further enhance meaning in a bidirectional relationship.

MCGT SESSION OVERVIEW

Table 7.1 summarizes the content of the 16 MCGT sessions. MCGT initially begins with a focus on the child, gradually shifts to the parent's own history, and then integrates both, with

TABLE 7.1 MEANING-CENTERED GRIEF THERAPY SESSION OVERVIEW

Session No.	Session Title	Session Content
1	Introductions and Overview of MCGT	Focuses on the basic concepts and sources of meaning, both in general and how it may relate specifically to loss and grief
2	Managing Challenging Emotions Through Meaning: Permission to Grieve	Centers on parent's own evaluation of emotional responses to losing a child, with a focus on helping the parent give him- or herself permission to grieve
3	Your Child's Living Legacy: Continuing Bonds	Explores continuing bonds—that is, the continued connection between the parent and the child and the link between the parent's legacy and the child's legacy
4	Telling Your and Your Child's Story: Choosing a Narrative	Focuses on "choosing one's life narrative" and how to keep the child an active part of the parent's story
5	Identity Before and After Loss	Centers on "loss and identity," focusing on sense of identity before and after the loss of a child
6	Your Story as a Source of Meaning: The Past	Explores "your story as a source of meaning," reflecting on one's life story as the parent's past is considered
7	Your Story as a Source of Meaning: The Present	Explores "your story as a source of meaning," reflecting on one's life story as the parent's present is considered
8	Your Story as a Source of Meaning: The Future	Explores "your story as a source of meaning," reflecting on one's life story as the parent's future is considered
9	Meaningful Connections: Identifying Support and Meaningful Relationship	Focuses on the importance of support providers in the face of loss; support provider invited to this session
10	Attitude as a Source of Meaning: Encountering Life's Limitations	Addresses "attitude as a source of meaning" by way of "encountering life's limitations" and how choosing one's attitude in the face of limitations may be a source of meaning to some
11	Creating as a Source of Meaning: Creativity, Courage, and Responsibility	Discusses "creating as a source of meaning" through ways parents have created and taken responsibility for their lives via the world of family, work, community, etc.
12	Experiencing as a Source of Meaning: Experiencing and Connecting with Life	Explores "experiencing as a source of meaning" and ways of "connecting with life" through, for example, love, beauty, and humor
13	Revising Your Story: Reconstructing Emotional Events and Thoughts	Focuses on persistent challenging emotions or events related to their child's illness and death
14	Creating Significance: Reactions to Moving Forward	Centers on the topic of meaning and significance, considering reactions to moving forward
15	Living Legacies: Presentation of the Living Legacy Project	Focuses on presentation of the Living Legacy Project and discussion of continuing the parent's bond to his or her child
16	Reflections: Hopes for the Future	Gives the parent a chance to reflect on their experience, as well as to explore hopes for the future

a focus on the intertwining of the child's and parent's stories. Sources of meaning are then explored, and the intervention culminates with the Living Legacy Project. Specifically, in Session 1, parents discuss their child and their loss experience, as well as learn about basic concepts related to meaning. In Session 2, parents begin to explore their own emotional reactions to the loss and their grief experience. Session 3 focuses on continuing bonds, linking both parent and child stories together. In Session 4, parents learn to keep their child an active part of their own story. Session 5 transitions to discussions of parents' identity and how this has changed following their loss. In Sessions 6–8, parents examine their story as a source of meaning through examination of their past experiences, present life, and future goals. Session 9, during which a support provider (e.g., partner or family member) is invited to join, emphasizes the importance of supportive relationships in the face of loss. In Sessions 10–12, parents explore additional sources of meaning, including attitude, creating, and experiencing. In Session 13, parents continue reconstruction of their story with a focus on emotions or events that seem persistently difficult to adaptively integrate. Session 14 focuses on parents' reactions to moving forward. In Session 15, parents present the Living Legacy Project and discuss continuing bonds with their child moving forward. In Session 16, parents reflect on their MCGT experience and discuss hopes for the future.

CURRENT EFFORTS TO EVALUATE MCGT

Currently, we are completing phase 4 of our study, which involves evaluation of MCGT through an RCT. As described in this chapter, MCGT is being compared to supportive psychotherapy, with both interventions delivered through videoconferencing to assist with reducing access to care barriers. We are using supportive psychotherapy (SP) based on Parker and Fletcher's[73] recommendation to compare specific interventions (i.e., MCGT) to interventions that use only nonspecific factors (e.g., support and empathy) for psychotherapy RCTs. SP is a manualized intervention based on supportive psychotherapy models described by Rogers[74] and Bloch.[75] The essential components include reassurance, explanation, guidance, encouragement, and permission for catharsis.[75] The process emphasizes nonspecific and nondirective Rogerian[74] concepts (e.g., empathic understanding) and avoids techniques that are not exclusively supportive (e.g., MCGT).

In phase 4 of the study, we are acquiring information about the feasibility, tolerability, and acceptability of MCGT. This phase will also allow us to determine effect size estimates to assist in planning a larger, efficacy RCT. We are enrolling biological, adoptive, and step-parents who lost a child aged 6 months to 39 years to cancer between 6 months and 6 years ago, who are age 18 years or older, who are English speaking, and who score at least 34 on the PG-13.[4] This cutoff score was selected based on prior studies of PGD interventions, our qualitative interview cutoff score of at least 34 to identify parents experiencing greater grief challenges, and our research demonstrating that parents with scores of 34 or higher have significantly more mental health and adjustment problems than those scoring less than 34 ($p < 0.05$). Participating parents are at least 6 months post-loss to avoid pathologizing acute bereavement distress in the immediate wake of the death. We are aiming to recruit an ethnically/racially diverse sample. Only one parent of a child is eligible to participate. Enrolled participants are assessed pre-intervention, mid-intervention, post-intervention, and 3 months post-intervention. Weekly evaluations of prolonged grief, meaning, and the therapy are also being collected.

Case Example

Danielle is a 39-year-old woman whose 3-year-old son, Ryan, died of neuroblastoma almost 3 years ago.[1A] During her first MCGT session, Danielle appeared sullen and despairing. She expressed her profound grief, describing Ryan as her "everything" and expressing her sense of hopelessness. She stated that she felt lost and angry, and that if it was not for her 16-month-old son Jonathan, who was conceived after Ryan died, she would have no reason to live. She had become disconnected from her husband, her family of origin, her religion, and her career as a social worker, which previously provided her with a great sense of meaning. She also reported challenges to her sense of identity, noting how prior to her son's death, she would have described herself as calm, cool, collected, and positive and now is anxious about "everything." Her score on the PG-13 following this first session was 44. Her score on the McGill

[1A] Names and other personal details have been changed to protect privacy.

Quality of Life Questionnaire item assessing current meaning in life (0–10 scale, with 10 reflecting the highest sense of meaning)[76] was 5.

In Session 2, which explores the parent's beliefs about experiencing and expressing emotion in an effort to foster a sense of permission to grieve, Danielle described the importance of remaining strong and needing to maintain a "poker face" for others. She also expressed concern that she was too dependent on her surviving son, Jonathan, as a sole source of meaning. The therapist explored the idea that her son was too central a source of meaning, asking why this was so anxiety-provoking for her. Danielle replied that she did not want Jonathan to think that if he was not available, she and her husband would not "be okay." She went on to say that she does not want him feeling pressure "because throughout my whole life I felt pressure," describing the pressure she felt to "be the best at everything" and the one who has to "keep it together for everybody" in her family. The therapist encouraged exploration of this theme as she and Danielle explored what it means to "keep it together" and the impact of that on experiencing her grief and related emotions. The therapist then facilitated Danielle's completion of the mindfulness guided imagery exercise in the session, supporting her expression of emotion, encouraging acceptance of the strong feelings that emerged, and providing an opportunity to connect to Ryan. Danielle engaged in the exercise, tearfully reporting that she has difficulty finding time to grieve Ryan in her busy day-to-day life and that she fears "that he will start fading away." Given Danielle reported that she was able to visualize and feel connected to Ryan through this exercise, the therapist encouraged identification of quiet times for Danielle to regularly practice this exercise.

During the next several sessions, MCGT involved engagement in an imaginal dialogue with Ryan and writing a letter to him, as well as one from him to her. These sessions focused on how Danielle's and Ryan's legacies were deeply intertwined and ways Danielle could continue to nurture Ryan and preserve her sense of identity as his mother, all of which highlighted her deep connection and continued bond with her son. This helped Danielle to maintain her meaningful connection to Ryan, drawing on her faith that he was an angel present in her life and her belief that he wished for her to be happy again. Also emphasized was the choice Danielle had in how she faced each day, including the way she made meaning of her grief and the ways she connected with important sources of meaning from which she had become disconnected.

The first "sudden gain" in therapy for Danielle occurred at her seventh session. She arrived to the session with a transformed affect, smiling and enthusiastic, expressing that for the first time since Ryan died, she was feeling *hope*. She shared that during that past week, she found herself creating a space in her home for some of Ryan's items, and although at first surprised by her actions, upon further reflection she tearfully expressed, "Of course I'm still taking care of him, why wouldn't I be? I'm still his mommy." Her PG-13 was 38, decreasing 6 points, but her meaning score remained 5. She arrived at her eighth session describing how, in the past week, she rejoined an organization through which she donates her professional services to community crises and was feeling empowered and excited about doing this volunteer work—something she was *choosing* to do, something that previously gave her a great sense of meaning but from which she became disconnected after Ryan became ill. Her PG-13 score had decreased to 29 that week, a 15-point reduction from her first session, and her meaning score increased to 6. Specific improvements were seen in yearning; avoidance; feeling stunned, shocked, or dazed by her loss; feeling confused about her role in life; trouble accepting the loss; difficulty trusting others; bitterness over the loss; difficulty moving on; and feeling that life is meaningless. One of the most significant symptom reductions was in emotional numbness, which went from 5 ("overwhelmingly") to 2 ("slightly") as she re-engaged in life.

As the sessions continued, the therapist continued to highlight the choices Danielle made and her ability to remain connected to Ryan. She encouraged Danielle to give herself permission and space to grieve. Danielle began doing this more regularly as she sought out ways to feel closer to Ryan, allowing the waves of grief without judging herself harshly or trying to "hide it" from others. Danielle also began looking at, in her words, "the positive" side of challenging situations—something she had expressed was a very important part of her sense of identity prior to Ryan's cancer diagnosis from which she had become disconnected since his death. The therapist noted that the goal of MCGT is not to encourage parents to "be more positive," which could be viewed as highly insensitive, but rather to meet parents wherever they are at and help them focus on the most important aspects of their lives. For Danielle, an important source of feeling was her sense of self and identity.

In Session 15, during which the Living Legacy Project is discussed, Danielle described four efforts she had made to honor Ryan. The first was to share cartoons that Ryan enjoyed with her son Jonathan—something she had avoided doing because being reminded of Ryan was so painful. She described how she wanted Jonathan to experience the same joy that Ryan had experienced. The second was to place meaningful photos of Ryan that she had deleted because they were too painful to look at back onto her cell phone. During this session, Danielle shared these photos with her therapist, who expressed her appreciation of Ryan's special characteristics and highlighted the many ways in which he seemed to positively affect others in his life. Third, Danielle reached out to volunteer for a nonprofit organization that provides support to families with children affected by serious illness. Finally, Danielle presented a journal she had created that detailed dreams that family and friends had had about Ryan. She described one of her own dreams that was particularly meaningful because she viewed it as Ryan's effort to communicate with her. The therapist highlighted the powerful sources of meaning present in these efforts: the meaning of being a mother to Ryan and Jonathan, the meaning of giving to others, the meaning of Ryan's messages and influence in her current day-to-day life, and the meaning in Danielle's choice to interpret the dreams in ways that preserved her connection to Ryan. These sources of meaning helped encourage Danielle's engagement in life despite the persistent presence of grief.

By the end the 16 sessions of therapy, Danielle's PG-13 score had decreased to 25, a 19-point reduction from her first session, with a meaning score of 9. In an exit interview at the conclusion of therapy, Danielle expressed the following:

> I feel like I, believe it or not, I got closer to my son, and it's weird to say that because he's not physically here, so how do you get closer to a child that's not here? Well, with the works and how to involve him even though he's physically not here, which is what I have learned, I do—I got closer to him. And not only that, I also got . . . even if was a little bit of . . . "me" back. And that's what a lot of parents miss, and I know I missed it dearly. I missed the person that I was before I lost my son. And with the therapy, I got that little bit of "me" back, which was me being positive.

She described how, despite her continued grief over Ryan, she "now finally" realized she has control over her story, recognizing her ability to choose the way she views her grief and the way she faces each day.

SUMMARY

Parents who lose a child to cancer often face challenges to their sense of meaning, identity, and purpose. MCGT attempts to systematically address these common existential issues, providing multiple pathways to enhancing meaning and coping with intense grief symptoms. Efforts are made to minimize pathologizing grief. Instead, the focus is on parents' ability to choose their attitude—that is, the way they think about and respond to situations—in the face of circumstances beyond their control and to connect with sources of meaning in their lives. This includes strengthening the connection they have to their deceased child.

Although efforts to develop and evaluate MCGT have focused on bereaved parents, the concepts and principles have the potential to assist those who have experienced other types of losses. Future endeavors will help extend the application of MCGT to additional bereaved populations, tailoring it as needed while keeping a meaning-centered approach.

ACKNOWLEDGMENTS

We are indebted to the bereaved parents who have shared so much as part of the research to develop and evaluate meaning-centered grief therapy. We are grateful for the invaluable mentorship of William Breitbart, MD. We also thank David Kissane, MD, Janice Nadeau, PhD, Robert Neimeyer, PhD, Holly Prigerson, PhD, and Lori Wiener, PhD, as well as Geoffrey Corner, BA, for their invaluable contributions to this work. The research described in this chapter was funded by National Cancer Institute grants R03 CA139944 (Lichtenthal) and K07 CA172216 (Lichtenthal).

REFERENCES

1. Davies R. New understandings of parental grief: Literature review. *J Adv Nurs.* 2004;46(5):506–513.
2. Lichtenthal WG, et al. Sense and significance: A mixed methods examination of meaning making after the loss of one's child. *J Clin Psychol.* 2010;66(7):791–812.
3. Institute of Medicine. *When Children Die: Improving Palliative and End-of-Life Care for Children and Their Families.* Field MJ, Behrman RE, eds. Washington, DC: National Academies Press; 2003.

4. Prigerson HG, et al. Prolonged grief disorder: Psychometric validation of criteria proposed for DSM-V and ICD-11. *PLoS Med.* 2009;6(8):e1000121.
5. Rando TA. *Parental Loss of a Child.* Champaign, IL: Research Press; 1986.
6. Neimeyer RA. Reauthoring life narratives: Grief therapy as meaning reconstruction. *Isr J Psychiatry Relat Sci.* 2001;38(3-4):171-183.
7. Neimeyer RA. Searching for the meaning of meaning: Grief therapy and the process of reconstruction. *Death Stud.* 2000;24(6):541-558.
8. Neimeyer RA, Sands DC. Meaning reconstruction in bereavement: From principles to practice. In: Neimeyer RA et al., eds. *Grief and Bereavement in Contemporary Society: Bridging Research and Practice.* New York, NY: Routledge; 2011:9-22.
9. Breitbart W, et al. Pilot randomized controlled trial of individual meaning-centered psychotherapy for patients with advanced cancer. *J Clin Oncol.* 2012;30(12):1304-1309.
10. Breitbart W, et al. Meaning-centered group psychotherapy for patients with advanced cancer: A pilot randomized controlled trial. *Psycho-Oncology.* 2010;19(1):21-28.
11. Wheeler I. The role of meaning and purpose in life in bereaved parents associated with a self-help group: Compassionate friends. *Omega J Death Dying.* 1993;28(4):261-271.
12. Lichtenthal WG, et al. Mental health services for parents who lost a child to cancer: If we build them, will they come? *J Clin Oncol.* 2015;33(20):2246-2253.
13. Trends in childhood cancer mortality—United States, 1990-2004. *Morbid Mortal Weekly Rep.* 2007;56(48):1257-1261.
14. Li J, et al. Hospitalization for mental illness among parents after the death of a child. *N Engl J Med.* 2005;352(12):1190-1196.
15. Li J, et al. Mortality in parents after death of a child in Denmark: A nationwide follow-up study. *Lancet.* 2003;361(9355):363-367.
16. Oliver LE. Effects of a child's death on the marital relationship: A review. *Omega J Death Dying.* 1999;39(3):197-227.
17. Lichtenthal WG, Cruess DG, Prigerson HG. A case for establishing complicated grief as a distinct mental disorder in DSM-V. *Clin Psychol Rev.* 2004;24(6):637-662.
18. Grimby A, Johansson AK. Does early bereavement counseling prevent ill health and untimely death? *Am J Hosp Palliat Care.* 2007;24(6):475-478.
19. Lichtenthal WG, et al. Underutilization of mental health services among bereaved caregivers with prolonged grief disorder. *Psychiatr Serv.* 2011;62(10):1225-1229.
20. Lichtenthal WG, et al. *Barriers to mental health service use among parents who lost a child to cancer.* Paper presented at the annual meeting of the American Psychosocial Oncology Society, Anaheim, CA, 2011.
21. Arnold J, Gemma PB, Cushman LF. Exploring parental grief: Combining quantitative and qualitative measures. *Arch Psychiatr Nurs.* 2005;19(6):245-255.
22. Lichtenthal WG, Breitbart W. The central role of meaning in adjustment to the loss of a child to cancer: Implications for the development of meaning-centered grief therapy. *Curr Opin Support Palliat Care.* 2015;9(1):46-51.
23. Calhoun LTR. *Trauma and Transformation: Growing in the Aftermath of Suffering.* Thousand Oaks, CA: SAGE; 1995.
24. Lichtenthal WG, et al. Bereavement follow-up after the death of a child as a standard of care in pediatric oncology. *Pediatr Blood Cancer.* 2015;62(Suppl 5):S834-S869.
25. D'Agostino NM, et al. Bereaved parents' perspectives on their needs. *Palliat Support Care.* 2008;6(1):33-41.
26. Frueh BC, et al. A randomized trial of telepsychiatry for post-traumatic stress disorder. *J Telemed Telecare.* 2007;13(3):142-147.
27. Germain V, et al. Assessment of the therapeutic alliance in face-to-face or videoconference treatment for posttraumatic stress disorder. *Cyberpsychol Behav Soc Netw.* 2010;13(1):29-35.
28. Ruskin PE, et al. Treatment outcomes in depression: Comparison of remote treatment through telepsychiatry to in-person treatment. *Am J Psychiatry.* 2004;161(8):1471-1476.
29. Rounsaville BJ, et al. A stage model of behavioral therapies research: Getting started and moving on from stage I. *Clin Psychol Sci Pract.* 2001;8:133-142.
30. de Meyrick J. The Delphi method and health research. *Health Educ.* 2003;103(1):7-16.
31. Morse JM. Designing funded qualitative research. In: Denzin NK, Lincoln YS, eds. *Handbook of Qualitative Research.* Thousand Oaks, CA: Sage; 1994;220-235.
32. Hill CE, et al. Consensual qualitative research: An update. *J Counsel Psychol.* 2005;52(2):196-205.
33. Charmaz K. Premises, principles, and practices in qualitative research: Revisiting the foundations. *Qual Health Res.* 2004;14(7):976-993.
34. Breitbart W. Spirituality and meaning in supportive care: Spirituality- and meaning-centered group psychotherapy interventions in advanced cancer. *Support Care Cancer.* 2002;10(4):272-280.
35. Gibson CA, et al. Psychologic issues in palliative care. *Anesthesiol Clin.* 2006;24(1):61-80, viii.

36. Yalom ID. *Existential Psychotherapy*. New York, NY: Basic Books; 1980:xii.
37. Frankl VE. *Man's Search for Meaning: An Introduction to Logotherapy*. 3rd ed. New York, NY: Simon & Schuster; 1984.
38. Tatrow K, Montgomery GH. Cognitive behavioral therapy techniques for distress and pain in breast cancer patients: A meta-analysis. *J Behav Med*. 2006;29(1):17–27.
39. Butler AC, et al. The empirical status of cognitive–behavioral therapy: A review of meta-analyses. *Clin Psychol Rev*. 2006;26(1):17–31.
40. Wheeler I. Parental bereavement: The crisis of meaning. *Death Stud*. 2001;25(1):51–66.
41. Park CL. Making sense of the meaning literature: An integrative review of meaning making and its effects on adjustment to stressful life events. *Psychol Bull*. 2010;136(2):257–301.
42. Janoff-Bulman R. The impact of trauma on meaning: From meaningless world to meaningful life. In: Power M, Brewin CR, eds. *The Transformation of Meaning in Psychological Therapies: Integrating Theory and Practice*. Hoboken, NJ: Wiley; 1997:91–106.
43. Sears SR, Stanton AL, Danoff-Burg S. The yellow brick road and the emerald city: Benefit finding, positive reappraisal coping and posttraumatic growth in women with early-stage breast cancer. *Health Psychol*. 2003;22(5):487–497.
44. Park CL, Blumberg CJ. Disclosing trauma through writing: Testing the meaning-making hypothesis. *Cognit Ther Res*. 2002;26(5):597–616.
45. Lichtenthal WG, Roberts KE, Shuk E. *Meaning in parents bereaved by cancer: A mixed methods study*. Paper presented at the Association of Death Education and Counseling 33rd Annual Conference, Miami, FL, 2011.
46. Janoff-Bulman R. *Shattered Assumptions: Towards a New Psychology of Trauma*. New York, NY: Free Press; 1992.
47. Lichtenthal WG, et al. Cause of death and the quest for meaning after the loss of a child. *Death Stud*. 2013;37(4):311–342.
48. Barrera M, et al. Early parental adjustment and bereavement after childhood cancer death. *Death Stud*. 2009;33(6):497–520.
49. Davis CG, Nolen-Hoeksema S, Larson J. Making sense of loss and benefiting from the experience: Two construals of meaning. *J Personality Soc Psychol*. 1998;75(2):561–574.
50. Gilmer MJ, et al. Changes in parents after the death of a child from cancer. *J Pain Symptom Manage*. 2012;44(4):572–582.
51. Park CL, Cohen LH, Murch RL. Assessment and prediction of stress-related growth. *J Pers*. 1996;64(1):71–105.
52. Tedeschi RCL. Posttraumatic growth: Conceptual foundations and empirical evidence. *Psychol Inq*. 2004;15(1):1–18.
53. Parkes CM. Psycho-social transitions: A field for study. *Soc Sci Med*. 1971;5(2):101–115.
54. Engelkemeyer SM, Marwit SJ. Posttraumatic growth in bereaved parents. *J Trauma Stress*. 2008;21(3):344–346.
55. Boelen PA. Cognitive–behavioral therapy for complicated grief: Theoretical underpinnings and case descriptions. *J Loss Trauma*. 2006;11(1):1–30.
56. Woodgate RL. Living in a world without closure: Reality for parents who have experienced the death of a child. *J Palliat Care*. 2006;22(2):75–82.
57. Talbot K. *What Forever Means After the Death of a Child: Transcending the Trauma, Living with the Loss*. New York, NY: Brunner-Routledge; 2002:.xxxii.
58. O'Connor K, Barrera M. Changes in parental self-identity following the death of a child to cancer. *Death Stud*. 2014;38(6):404–411.
59. Kreicbergs U, et al. Care-related distress: A nation-wide study of parents who lost their child to cancer. *J Clin Oncol*. 2005;23(36):9162–9171.
60. Hinds PS, et al. Key factors affecting dying children and their families. *J Palliat Med*. 2005;8(Suppl 1):S70–S78.
61. Alam R, et al. Bereavement experiences of mothers and fathers over time after the death of a child due to cancer. *Death Stud*. 2012;36(1):1–22.
62. Wijngaards-de Meij L, et al. Couples at risk following the death of their child: Predictors of grief versus depression. *J Consult Clin Psychol*. 2005;73(4):617–623.
63. Capitulo KL. Perinatal grief online. *Am J Matern Child Nurs*. 2004;29(5):305–311.
64. Field NP, Gao B, Paderna L. Continuing bonds in bereavement: An attachment theory based perspective. *Death Stud*. 2005;29(4):277–299.
65. Foster TL, et al. Comparison of continuing bonds reported by parents and siblings after a child's death from cancer. *Death Stud*. 2011;35(5):420–440.
66. Lichtenthal WG, Applebaum A, Breitbart W. *Using mixed methods data to adapt meaning-centered psychotherapy for bereaved parents*. Paper presented at the International Psycho-Oncology Society 13th World Congress, Antalya, Turkey, 2011.
67. Neimeyer RA, ed. *Meaning Reconstruction and the Experience of Loss*. Washington, DC: American Psychological Association; 2001.
68. Bowlby J. *Attachment and Loss*. New York, NY: Basic Books; 1969/1982.
69. Ronen R, et al. The relationship between grief adjustment and continuing bonds for parents who have lost a child. *Omega*. 2009;60(1):1–31.

70. Davis CG, Nolen-Hoeksema S. Loss and meaning: How do people make sense of loss? *Am Behav Scientist*. 2001. **44**(5): p. 726–741.
71. Davis CG, et al. Searching for meaning in loss: Are clinical assumptions correct. *Death Stud.* 2000;24(6):497–540.
72. Vickberg SM. The Concerns About Recurrence Scale (CARS): A systematic measure of women's fears about the possibility of breast cancer recurrence. *Ann Behav Med.* 2003;25(1):16–24.
73. Parker G, Fletcher K. Treating depression with the evidence-based psychotherapies: A critique of the evidence. *Acta Psychiatr Scand.* 2007;115(5):352–359.
74. Rogers CR. *Client-Centered Therapy, Its Current Practice, Implications, and Theory.* Boston, MA: Houghton Mifflin; 1951:xii.
75. Bloch S. *An Introduction to the Psychotherapies.* 3rd ed. New York, NY: Oxford University Press; 1996:xiv.
76. Cohen SR, et al. The McGill Quality of Life Questionnaire: A measure of quality of life appropriate for people with advanced disease. A preliminary study of validity and acceptability. *Palliat Med.* 1995;9(3):207–219.

8

Adapting Meaning-Centered Psychotherapy for Adolescents and Young Adults with Cancer

Issues of Meaning and Identity

JULIA A. KEARNEY AND JENNIFER S. FORD

Keep Me from Fear

Keep me from fear,
that cold paralysis,
the squirming nausea.
I am sick of these half eaten fingernails. No.
I have my whole life to be afraid.
There! With that declaration, the anvil weight of dread
Falls loosely from the chain around my neck.
I have my entire life,
however long it is.
I have my own eternity in a hundred years,
Or in an instant.

BRENDAN OGG[A]

INTRODUCTION

Approximately 70,000 adolescents and young adults (AYAs) are diagnosed with cancer each year, which is six times the number of children diagnosed between birth and 14 years of age.[1] AYAs are an at-risk cohort because of their poorer survival rates compared to those of older and younger patients, unique developmental challenges, and lack of access to clinical trials.[2,3] They experience distress from identity and existential issues[4] and loss of meaning (LOM)[5] at all stages of illness and survivorship. LOM due to loss of independence, disruption of life plans, physical suffering and limitations, boredom, and social isolation is a common and often unavoidable consequence of cancer and treatment in adults.[6–8] Young adults with advanced cancer also report life disruption with increased levels of grief due to losses related to illness.[9] Meaning, LOM, and identity distress have not been fully explored as a target for intervention in AYA patients with cancer, despite the important role that meaning plays in development and identity formation.

Meaning-making is an adaptive cognitive skill and a crucial developmental task of adolescence. It is incorporated into an individual's worldview and is an important part of an integrated, cohesive identity. This loss of meaning during adolescence may both interrupt the developmental task of learning meaning-making, a normal part of identity development,[10–12] and predispose a young person to identity or existential distress. The

[A] Printed with permission, previously published poems from the book *Summer Becomes Absurd* by Brendan Ogg, Finishing Line Press.

developmental tasks of adolescence and young adulthood are particularly sensitive to disruption. Cancer impacts development, and development impacts upon the short- and long-term management of the chronic illness.

The themes of meaning-centered psychotherapy (MCP) may be particularly suited for AYAs, especially after making some adjustments to take into account specific developmental considerations relevant for this age group. The framework of meaning-making complements the issues and concerns that AYAs naturally experience. This stage of development, spanning mid- through late adolescence and into emerging adulthood (this term in developmental psychology is consistent with the *young adult* term in oncology and refers to the early to mid-twenties), is when individuals make significant choices about what is important to them and who they want to be. In this chapter, we explore the recent literature on adolescent and young adult identity development, particularly related to the task of meaning-making, and begin to shape the framework of MCP for this important and underserved developmental stage in order to inform clinical and research applications. Adult clinicians may also be interested in the developmental trajectory of meaning-making to inform their care of patients across the life span.

IDENTITY DEVELOPMENT AND MEANING-MAKING

Meaning-making is a developmental task of adolescence and central to the complex process of identity development. In studies of identity development, meaning-making is described as the ability of an individual to incorporate events and ideas encountered in life into his or her own personal life story, exploring important life events, providing the context about the meaning of those events to the individual, and supporting the individual in building a cohesive, integrated narrative about his or her life.[13–17] To facilitate the identity process, AYAs must ask the very important questions of "Who am I?" and "What am I to become?" Identity formation requires the integration of past and present with an idea about what the future might hold.

In therapy with AYAs, meaning-centered work is identity-development work as well. Defining what is meaningful, to the exclusion of other things that have been ruled out or rejected, is essential in this developmental stage. We therefore summarize the basic principles of identity development to provide the context of the adolescent's stereotypical angst, the importance of allowing space in therapy for the exploration and experimentation with roles and values, and a sense of different trajectories toward identity achievement, which can be disrupted by cancer or serious illness in oneself or a family member. The therapist should be experienced with adolescents and young adults, and be very familiar with all these principles and trajectories, in order to assess readiness of an adolescent for meaning-centered work, to recognize it when it is happening in therapy, and to supportively guide individuals to their own meaningful conclusions.

The field of identity development, within developmental psychology, traces its roots from Erikson's work in the 1950s. In Erikson's *Identity: Youth and Crisis*[10] and other work, adolescents, having established a foundation of trust in their caregivers and a sense of autonomy, initiative, and industry, are prepared to explore the self. Erikson defines adolescence by the effort to navigate a normative "crisis" to achieve a synthesis of identity or, if failing to do so, experience *role confusion* and *identity diffusion*.[18] He defines *ego identity* as "the accrued confidence that one's ability to maintain inner sameness and continuity . . . is matched by the sameness and continuity of one's meaning for others."[19] Through first *commitment to* and then *experimentation with* roles, he or she finds a "niche in some section of his [sic] society."[19] As Josselson and Flum state, "Identity, in Eriksonian terms, is both a structure and a process, both the outcome of developmental progress and a consistent way of being in the world."[20] According to Erikson, identity is a long, complex process of self-definition that provides continuity between past, present, and future and gives direction, purpose, and meaning to life.

IDENTITY STATUS: DEFINING THE PROCESSES OF IDENTITY DEVELOPMENT

The normative *identity crisis* of adolescence became the focus of a developmental theory known as *identity status*, on which was founded a large body of subsequent research classifying and describing stages of identity crisis in adolescence which, ideally, resolve in a stable identity in adulthood. Marcia[21] described the process of how adolescents navigate identity crisis through engaging in *commitment* (strong choices in different developmental domains such as occupation or ideology and the self-confidence that comes from these choices) and *exploration* (actively maintaining commitments through activities such as reflecting on them, seeking information about them, or talking about them with others).[18] One contemporary model has also added a third domain of *reconsideration*, defined as the act of comparing present commitments with possible alternatives, which may or may not lead to revision of commitments.[22] One of the key outcomes of identity status theory is the awareness that adolescence is not, for everyone, a time of "storm and stress" but more commonly marked by consistency and cohesiveness in personality development. Strong commitments may be held even in early adolescence, although the norm is to explore and question during this stage before making choices and commitments in mid- to late adolescence. Multiple studies have upheld that female adolescents often have higher levels of commitment to roles and ideals compared to age-matched males; however, this observation may be explained by an offset timeline of boys and girls. Consistent with earlier female puberty, girls may undergo identity development earlier as well. In a recent large longitudinal study of 1313 Dutch adolescents aged 12–20 years, adolescents experiencing identity statuses low in commitment were also highest in measures of depression and delinquency. Other research has also supported this link between identity distress (distress over the inability to form and explore commitments or the ongoing questioning of them) and internalizing symptoms (depression and anxiety), poor family relationships, poor self-esteem, and avoidant coping styles.[23] In other words, even into emerging adulthood, a strong sense of identity, through identity achievement, is an emotionally stabilizing experience that "serves to guide decisions and actions, fuels one's sense of self-worth in the world, and it provides a sense of meaningful connection between daily activities and long-term goals and broad values."[24]

NARRATIVE IDENTITY DEVELOPMENT: WE ARE BECOMING THE STORIES WE ARE TELLING

The period of adolescence through emerging adulthood is defined by change: physical change through puberty, intellectual change through brain development and education, and social changes in exploration of friendships and romantic relationships as well as a shift toward greater independence in relationships with parents and caregivers. These changes bring challenges in maintaining a sense of personal continuity, which can be bridged by the creation of life narratives and meaning-making. The central idea of narrative identity development is that narrating one's own "life story" to others or oneself is the central process for creating an integrated, stable self. The key narrative mechanism for doing this is known as *autobiographical reasoning*, defined as "a process of thinking or talking about the personal past that involves arguments that link distant elements of one's life to each other and the self in an attempt to relate the present self to one's personal past and future."[17] It is essentially a task of meaning-making, and it is especially relevant at times of biographical upheaval and change, such as a divorce in the family or a diagnosis of a serious life-threatening illness such as cancer.[17]

The cognitive skills and social-motivational context for telling a coherent and meaningful life narrative are also developed in mid-adolescence—at approximately age 14 years, on average (Box 8.1.)

BOX 8.1 COGNITIVE–SOCIAL SKILLS REQUIRED FOR AUTOBIOGRAPHICAL REASONING

- *Temporal sequencing*—ability to tell life events in chronological order
- *Appreciation for cultural concepts of biography*—knowledge of which important details and events to include in a life story
- *Causal coherence*—sense that diverse events may bring about change and development but the self remains the same
- *Thematic coherence*—ability to interpret complex themes from events and integrate them across time

Adapted from Habermas T, Kober C. Autobiographical reasoning is constitutive for narrative identity: The role of the life story of personal continuity. In: McLean KC, Syed M, eds. The Oxford Handbook of Identity Development. New York, NY: Oxford University Press; 2015:149–165.

New attention is paid to biographical themes through required tasks such as applying for jobs and colleges; personal activities such as writing in diaries and reading biographies; and, in current culture, social media activities such as blogging and documenting personal details. The emerging awareness of the facts of one's own life and the context that surrounds it is described further in Box 8.1.[17]

In research interviews studying narrative identity, effective prompts to elicit this type of reflection from adolescents and young adults include questions about "high points," "low points," and "turning points" in a particular life story. Some studies also code entire "life narratives," which consists of essentially asking the subject to tell his or her life story from birth to present. Gifted preadolescent and early adolescent storytellers may be able to tell their "whole life story," but many will have heard these scripts recited countless times by parents and may not have the ability to abstract themes and apply the story to identity development (e.g., through use of high points, low points, and turning points).

In research on narrative identity, narratives about positive (high points) and negative (low points) experiences can reveal how adolescents and young adults view their own personal growth and development. Furthermore, the way they tell the story, resolving negatively or ambivalently (which is anxiety-provoking) versus resolving positively, can impact their personality and adjustment (e.g., anxiety, emotional stability, and conscientiousness). Stories about high points often reinforce identity commitments, unambiguously providing a source of positive self-defining meaning. However, stories of low points can also end positively—if they end with self-affirming (consistent with previously held identity commitments) or self-transforming/turning point (bringing about positive change in identity commitments) interpretations. The ability to make meaning and integrate our personal life narrative may even become a part of our personality, a tool used for coping and creativity, having implications for resilience to disruptive and stressful life events.[17] This begins to shed light on the interaction between AYA identity development, meaning-making, and narratives of negative life experiences.[24]

CANCER AND IDENTITY DISTRESS: A MEANING-CENTERED APPROACH

Cancer is a disruptive life event. Beyond the inconvenience, physical suffering, and uncertainty a cancer diagnosis brings, AYAs describe an assault on their identity. AYAs with cancer may experience a "before self" or a "well self" and an "after self" or a "sick self," which they may individually define as before diagnosis, "off treatment," or just "when I feel well." As clinicians, we cannot assume the exact "breaks" in the story, when and which events are experienced as disconnections from the former self; they will not be the same for each individual. Some feel utterly changed by the diagnosis of being sick, whereas others feel only disconnected from their cohesive self by the experience of feeling sick during treatment or when cancer progresses, and this may be transient or fluctuating depending on their definition and experience.[4,5,25–30]

Many AYAs experience cancer as "wasted time"; a frustrating interruption of their goals and ambitions; and a delay of or theft of important milestones, such as graduations, having an intimate relationship, or moving away from home. Others comment on the "forced dependence" on parents and inability to participate in a "normal social life" and interact with peers at a time in their lives when they are trying to achieve more independence and shift focus from their family of origin to peer relationships. In addition, changes in body image may affect a sense of self as well as interactions with others, both friendships and potential romantic relationships. Cancer also challenges the adolescent/young adult's sense of self-esteem, leading to feelings of "loss of control" at a time of life when self-image is pivotal to normal development. These complaints indicate a readiness and even a need for a meaning-centered approach.

It may help patients experiencing cancer-related identity distress to realize that not all AYAs experience the same changes in "self," but the meaning of the illness may be different for others and may even change over time. The meaning of the time spent in treatment may also be a starting point for exploring these issues; addressing their frustration by identifying specific lost sources of meaning may help them understand their feelings and then focus on still accessible sources of meaning and accepting adjusted plans for the future.

MEANING-CENTERED TECHNIQUES WITH AYAS

Patient Selection

The developmental discussion in the previous sections can inform patient selection for meaning-centered work with AYAs. Patients older than age 14 years will likely be capable of viewing events in their life as having a personalized meaning and feel some sense of ownership over their own life narrative. Asking about identity issues related to illness and cancer, high points, and low points may set the stage and indicate readiness for meaning-centered work. Patients who cannot engage in these types of discussions may not be developmentally ready. Clinical judgment should be used regarding the vocabulary utilized when introducing concepts, as well as care used when utilizing historical or literary examples that are age and developmental stage appropriate.

Therapeutic Approach to Difficult Subjects

Adolescent therapists will be familiar with and have developed their own style toward the general framework and tenor of psychotherapy with this population. The intention of this section is to comment on important differences when applying the principles and practices of meaning-centered psychotherapy (developed for adults) to the population of AYA patients with cancer. Therapists may encounter in medical clinicians, patients' parents and family members, or even in themselves concerns about addressing serious, existential, or "life and death" matters with young patients. The adult meaning-centered psychotherapy manualized treatment suggests using an open, "human-level" of engagement for approaching existential concerns, such as communicating that "we are both human beings in the same existential boat." This allows the therapist and patient of any age to work with the didactic material around meaning concepts in a nonthreatening way, and it works well with AYAs. Indeed, studies have shown that it is not only acceptable but also beneficial for AYAs with cancer to engage in serious discussions around advance care planning. The approach these studies suggest is similar, such as the stating the following:

> Any one of us can die or experience an injury that makes us unable to speak for ourselves. Many young people appreciate being able to understand the kinds of decisions their families might have to make and discuss in advance what they would want their family to do for them. Would you like to have that conversation?

This approach has been shown to be acceptable and tolerable to teens as young as 14 years of age for introducing even detailed discussions about advanced care planning.[31–33]

In our experience, the framework of MCP can be useful with adolescents and young adults at any stage of illness.As described previously, AYAs may feel intense loss of meaning due to the life disruption of treatment, and they do not need to be facing terminal cancer to benefit from a focus on meaning. For this reason, prognostic awareness is not a critical factor for meaningful participation in this type of work. Another important factor to consider is the potential for lack of prognostic awareness among younger adolescent patients. Younger adolescents may have the ability to participate in meaning-centered work with a focus on the present life disruptions, but they may only be partially aware of their true prognosis because they have been protected from a full understanding by parents and clinicians. It is important to understand what the adolescent means by "remission," "good scans," and "doing well" (or "doing poorly") and not to assume the adolescent has full knowledge of his or her medical situation unless the parent or the patient has explained this. Furthermore, classic studies have shown that children's evolving awareness of mortality, prognosis, and anticipated loss waxes and wanes with normal coping. This normal fluctuation should be left intact when it seems adaptive, and the therapy can continue in a supportive manner. As Sourkes states in the classic work on psychotherapy with children with life-threatening illnesses, *The Deepening Shade*, "Most families flow between the two sets of time [real time/reality vs. child time/magical endless time] in a normal and adaptive process of maintaining hope. The therapist need only follow."[34]

Meaning-centered work with AYAs may encounter cognitive and emotional milestones along the way, requiring support and psychoeducation beyond just meaning-centered themes. AYAs benefit from understanding their own increasingly complex psychological selves, with the ability to hold two seemingly contradictory or paradoxical beliefs at once, to be ambivalent in feelings or have mixed feelings about self and others, their body, and their life. Themes drawn from the patients' own narratives can be useful in illustrating these concepts and demonstrating the construction of meaning across time.

Sense of Meaning Develops in Rich Psychosocial Context

When adults participate in MCP, as evidenced by case material elsewhere in this book, they commonly infuse their narratives with the rich context of their life and personal development—family narratives; social narratives such as gender, race, and class issues; and the embodied narratives of their experiences in and with their physical body. The literature referenced here on identity development of AYAs has also looked to these contexts and characteristics for clues on risk and resiliency through adolescence. Clinicians and researchers working with AYAs should be informed about important group differences in adolescent development due to family, social, or physical experience.[35–37] Importantly, AYAs may need explicit permission from clinicians to explore these issues in a meaning-centered format and may not yet understand all the context of their own narratives. A therapists' role in tolerance of ambivalence and support for a sense of meaning that may be in flux may be of great relief.

Potential Role for Parents, Caregivers, or Significant Others

The inclusion of parents or caregivers is standard practice in modern adolescent psychotherapy for facilitating communication, strengthening family support for the adolescent, and advising and guiding parenting decisions and attitudes.[38–40] Indeed, family-centered assessment and intervention is considered an "imperative" in AYA psychosocial care.[1] Narrative identity studies have also identified a role for parents in supporting meaning-making for adolescents, providing narrative "scaffolding," which helps adolescents make meaning of past events.[41,42] In cases in which the AYA patient's development was halted or slowed by physical or psychosocial burdens of illness, the patient–caregiver relationship may be altered or intensified. Especially at the end of life, AYAs may benefit from interventions that facilitate intergenerational relationships and communication. Lyon and colleagues included both private individual sessions for adolescents and joint sessions with parents to promote shared understanding and communication around end-of-life decision-making.[32] Participants showed improved trust in their parents as surrogate decision-makers and ultimately had end-of-life outcomes more consistent with the adolescents' wishes,[32,33] demonstrating the tolerability, feasibility, and effectiveness of family-centered interventions around serious subjects such as decision-making for young people with cancer. We recommend application of this practice to recruit parents in a supportive role. This component should be encouraged (but not mandatory) to allow for some flexibility in the treatment and support the range of autonomy seen in this population.

AYA-Specific Examples, Sources of Meaning, and Themes

Both the manualized individual and group MCP by Breitbart and colleagues[43,44] draw core themes and exemplary quotes from the book *Man's Search for Meaning* by Viktor Frankl,[45] a psychiatrist and survivor of the Holocaust. Frankl's existential approach to meaning-making and resilience around terrible life events were incorporated directly into the intervention.[46–49] Although some young people may be interested in learning about Frankl and his writing as a springboard to a more in-depth discussion of meaning, it may also be useful for therapists to explore with AYAs other sources of inspiration from books, movies, and music for an understanding of meaning-making during difficult times in life. This exploration and use of alternative sources of inspiration may serve to be more developmentally appropriate and accessible, especially for younger AYAs, and enrich the therapeutic encounter.

It can be useful to AYAs to learn about the four sources of meaning in MCP: historical, creative, experiential, and attitudinal. (See Chapters 2 and 3 for further discussion of sources of meaning.) Young patients may need prompts to view their own efforts to seek meaning in their life through these lenses and to understand disruptions as loss of meaning. Thinking developmentally about these issues will also help therapists draw out these themes. An awareness of the importance of peer relationships in adolescence may reveal a profound loss in meaning for a teen in isolation or withdrawn from school because of cancer treatment, for example. Loss of independence for the college-age student, who had previously left home and now must live with and depend on parents for basic needs, may be a deeply troubling loss of meaning.

Loss of Meaning in the Present and the Future

For some patients, it may be that connection (or reconnection) with important sources of meaning is inadequate consolation for the losses incurred. If the patient has had to indefinitely postpone or will never get to experience key developmental milestones such as going away to college, falling in love, having an intimate relationship, or having children, it is possible that explicit grief work will be appropriate.[50] Similar to MCP for bereaved parents, discussed by Lichtenthal and Breitbart,[51] a rush to reframe their suffering as meaningful through the lens of MCP may be experienced as a breach of the therapeutic relationship.

AYA patients, particularly those with advanced disease, catastrophic treatment toxicities, or prolonged treatment courses, may experience profound life disruption and suffering. It can be confusing for young patients to experience feelings of meaninglessness, grief, or suffering coexisting or alternating with feelings of intense value and meaning of life, peace, and even joy. This is perhaps suggested in the following poem by AYA poet and cancer patient, Brendan Ogg[B]:

L'Chaim ("to Life")

Feather rug, soft bed of matted grass
Why did I question this place of endless beauty—
Life—
To my friend, in weakness?
Where was my heart before this time?
Now I feel it in my breast.
Put your hand there, fingers spreading from
the palm.
And feel the warm, insistent pulse.

Ongoing or unaddressed grief, suffering, or loss of meaning may result in the psychological consequences of depression, demoralization, or suicidality. Suicidal ideation is unfortunately not uncommon in AYAs with advanced cancer.[52] These thoughts often are presented in the subtext of a narrative that "this is not a life worth living," but they may also be a passing consideration that belies a search for alternative endings to the narrative of a death from cancer.

In addition to a careful safety assessment and appropriate treatment of emotional and physical symptoms, the psychotherapeutic response to the suicidal patient in this context may start with the question, "What would make today worth living?" Aggressive escalation of symptom management for unrelenting pain or nausea, for example, perhaps with unconventional or alternative therapies previously dismissed, may bring incremental relief and hope. Negotiating with the medical team for compromises in restrictions (e.g. restrictive dietary or protective isolation recommendations for immunocompromised patients) may help restore a sense of meaning and agency. Paradoxically, suicidal ideation, when it stems from loss of meaning or loss of control, may be the opening to a more frank conversation about goals of care and end-of-life wishes, when appropriate, which can give a dying patient some control over his or her circumstances, reduce isolation, and improve communication. When possible, the exploration of meaning-centered and identity themes may help enhance personal continuity and sense of meaning despite overwhelming illness or even death.

Case Example

Eliza,[C] a bright, accomplished pre-med college student, was diagnosed with acute myeloid leukemia (AML) the summer between sophomore and junior year of college. She was stoic and dignified in her initial cycles of a notoriously difficult chemotherapy regimen, and she remained hopeful by focusing on her good chance of cure. She accepted a psychiatry referral when the primary team suggested it, along with the team's observation that some of her unrelenting nausea may be worsened by anxiety. Psychiatric consultation initially focused on aggressive symptom control, general adjustment to the illness, exploration of sources of anxiety, and potential preexisting anxiety history. Unfortunately, Eliza suffered significant toxicity from her next round of chemotherapy, and while in the hospital for more than 1 month in severe pain and nausea, with her treatment on hold until her body healed, she experienced a profound sense of "uselessness," complaining that this was a "huge waste of time"—that "*everything* was on hold." Her sense of meaninglessness, and now depression, persisted even as her medical symptoms improved. Her psychiatrist broached the subject with her of trying some meaning-centered psychotherapy techniques, and she agreed. Loosely using the adult manual, with plenty of time for exploration of how Eliza had experienced the sources of meaning so far in her life, and how her identity had reflected them in her choices and personality, she began to craft a narrative that included her illness. She reported feeling a stronger sense of continuity from her old self to her current self and even allowed the

[B] Printed with permission, previously published poems from the book *Summer Becomes Absurd* by Brendan Ogg, Finishing Line Press.

[C] Identifying details were changed to protect patient privacy. The text of the speech was obtained from the patient with her express permission to reprint.

possibility that her suffering might someday have some meaning in her life. Eliza experienced additional complications, meaning that her planned 6 months of chemotherapy turned into 9 months, with psychiatric support throughout. She slowly healed and regained her energy and returned to college. Two years later, still in remission, she graduated with honors and gave the following keynote address at an awards ceremony. Infused with the language of meaning and identity, her narrative tells of her efforts to transcend suffering and find purpose in the search for meaning in life events:

> Good morning, graduates, esteemed faculty and staff, families and friends. It is my distinct privilege to help welcome you, and further, to walk alongside fellow graduating seniors. The stories I have to share are about people, and kindness. Hopefully they provide you with even a degree of all that you have given me.
>
> I came to college looking for an institution that would accept me not in spite of, but because of my dual interests in science and humanities. From the beginning, I found that my work extended far beyond the classroom. My involvements ranged from volunteering in local children's hospitals, to intramural sports, to mentoring with freshmen. I quickly fell in love with this university, and foremost, its people.
>
> My college experience took a different turn in late May 2012, as I finished my sophomore year at school with severe pain in my thighs and lower back. Exactly one week later, on May 25th, I was diagnosed with AML leukemia. By 7 pm that evening I was admitted into one of the best cancer hospitals in the world. That initial admission lasted seven weeks, and was the first of many inpatient stays. In total I underwent 8 months of chemotherapy, 14 rounds of cranial radiation, and one year away from the school I was so proud to call home.
>
> Surviving cancer and regaining my sense of will and vitality have been the most challenging experiences I have ever endured. I am two years cancer-free, and am certain that my story of struggle changed me in ways that shaped my future. I believe that through suffering, we are presented with the opportunity to find greater meaning and experience new growth. Deep in the trenches of my treatment, I grew acutely aware of what it means to experience a bad day. Pain. Suffering. I am grateful for that. And yet, returning to my work at college after my year away, I came to find my interactions helping other students increasingly difficult. Hearing from others on their struggles to achieve an "A," a disagreement they had with a friend, or just how awful they felt having not received a job, I failed to empathize the way I once used to. I failed to see those experiences as "bad days." I came to find that my own experience with pain isolated me from my peers.
>
> For a while, my default setting was the certainty that the state of my life, and all of the deeply unfair pain I experienced, was incomparable to others. Perhaps some of you have felt the same. Thinking this way is often so automatic that we are hardly cognizant of it happening. However, to do so is to discount all of the personal struggles and experiences of those around us. To see our connections, above our differences, is to consider the possibilities of what we want to pay attention to. It is not impossible that those around us have had cancer, have struggled at their university, or have experienced unimaginable heartbreak. Seeing the world this way, we must be kind, for we are all fighting a hard battle. The work of seeing possibilities is hard, and some days, if you are like me, you will not be able to do it. But it is important all the same. Our college has equipped us with a first-tier education, and with it, the remarkable abilities to problem solve, engineer, compute, create, and study. However with this understanding, it is my hope that we leave this university fully cognizant of our capabilities to do good. To be kind. It is in our power to seek out ways to be caring, and compassionate to others, even those that we do not know.
>
> Several weeks ago I was standing in the check-out line of the nearby grocery store. As I stepped up to the register, I asked the distressed, likely overworked, older man who was bagging groceries how he was doing. He quickly answered "Tired." I nodded, expressed my sympathy, and asked him how long he had been on shift. He sighed, and admitted that he did not know how to say it in English, and went back to his work. I studied him for a moment, unable to discern what language he might speak. Thinking it might be Spanish, a language I studied for nearly a decade, I asked him what language he was fluent in. He told me, "Hindi, Urdu, and Tamil." I smiled, and eagerly asked him, "Aap keisi he?": "How are

> you" in Hindi. He looked up, this time with a wide grin, in dismay at the young white female speaking Hindi in front of him. He asked me how I knew Hindi, and I told him that I studied the language while living in Delhi in my semester abroad. His face lit up and he laughed heartily. He told me that he is from Delhi, told me about his family that still lives there. The Indian woman in the check-out line beside us, who I then understood to be his relative, smiled and nodded knowingly. We exchanged a few more words in Hindi, and then parted ways.
>
> After studying the unique, complex language that is Hindi for two hours a day for two months, nearly all that I have retained are phrases such as hello and how are you. And yet in that moment, all of my effort, hard work and tears in that class finally attained meaning. My education became tangible. Finding meaning from what we have learned at school is now our work. It is our opportunity to delve into what can become beautiful, human interactions.
>
> As honorees today, we represent the most outstanding arts and science students from our university, and across the country. Our academic rigor, pursuit of wisdom, and breadth of intellect allow us the privilege of choice, to do whatever it is that we desire. Further, our education, from our families, experiences, and this university, has given us the power to make an indelible difference in the lives of others. I believe in that. I believe that on the cusp of our graduation, we have the potential to leave this world far better than we found it. Because in true nature, our hearts have, and will always be, in this work.

This patient's own words narrate the journey from the shock of a diagnosis of cancer; the subsequent suffering, disruption, and loss; through a painful time of meaninglessness, disconnection, and doubt; to a triumphant return to connectedness, integrity, and meaning. This can occur even in situations such as Eliza's with good prognoses and ultimate survival. Working with issues of meaning and identity directly allows the patient and therapist an opportunity to create a narrative that transcends these impactful negative experiences, preventing loss of identity, and sometimes even transforming the experience into a meaningful paradigm for the rest of life.

FUTURE RESEARCH

The AYA Progress Review Group, an advisory committee to the National Cancer Institute, convened to develop AYA research priorities, identified as "imperative" the need to strengthen advocacy and support for AYA cancer patients, and devised recommendations for psychosocial research that included the need for the development of AYA-specific evidence-based interventions.[53] Despite the widespread acknowledgment that AYAs experience with cancer is unique and many of their needs remain unmet,[2,54–58] there are no published evidence-based developmentally specific psychosocial interventions. The impact of these unmet needs is that AYA patients may approach end of life with distress, grief, life disruption, and even suicidality without relief or support.[9,31–33,52,59]

In response to this imperative, we are currently working on the adaptation of the MCP manual for the AYA population, including the considerations we have shared here and results of a qualitative narrative study and iterative intervention development study currently underway. We hope this treatment will soon be a much needed, validated treatment to add to the AYA psycho-oncologists' skill set.

SUMMARY

Meaning-making is a core human activity, learned and practiced in childhood and adolescence as we become independent narrators of our own identities, which then manifest in our choices and commitments. Difficult experiences such as cancer may disrupt a sense of continuity of self or result in disconnection from sources of meaning. This is distressing for a patient of any age, but for adolescents and young adults, it may go beyond a sense of loss to actually feeling "lost" and affect the very process of identity development. Through meaning- and identity-centered techniques, psychotherapists working with AYAs with cancer may support the reconstruction of a cohesive, stable sense of meaning and self that transcends illness and even death, the most human of limitations. Developmental considerations and adjustments, based in the understanding of normal and disrupted identity development and recent work with AYAs with cancer, make this work possible and impactful. More research is needed to standardize and validate this developmental adaptation and support dissemination to reach a larger population of AYAs with cancer.

ACKNOWLEDGMENTS

We are deeply grateful to the patients and their families with whom we have been honored to work at Memorial Sloan Kettering Cancer Center. We also offer our sincere thanks to the patient who lent her personal story and her compelling keynote address to this chapter but requested to remain anonymous. We thank Chanelle Mars for editorial support with citations. Finally, to the family of Brendan Ogg, whose work we first encountered in an art installation in Memorial Sloan Kettering's The Lounge (a unique AYA recreational space), we send our gratitude for the use of his astonishing poetry to help illustrate essential themes in the chapter. We are so sorry for your loss.

REFERENCES

1. National Cancer Institute and Lance Armstrong Foundation. *Closing the Gap: Research and Care Imperatives for Adolescents and Young Adults with Cancer.* Bethesda, MD: National Cancer Institute; 2006:06-6067.
2. Smith AW, Parsons HM, Kent EE, et al. Unmet support service needs and health-related quality of life among adolescents and young adults with cancer: The AYA HOPE study. *Front Oncol.* 2013;3:75.
3. Stevens MC. The "lost tribe" and the need for a promised land: The challenge of cancer in teenagers and young adults. *Eur J Cancer.* 2006;42(3):280–281.
4. Parry C. Embracing uncertainty: An exploration of the experiences of childhood cancer survivors. *Qual Health Res.* 2003;13(2):227–246.
5. Jones BL, Parker-Raley J, Barczyk A. Adolescent cancer survivors: Identity paradox and the need to belong. *Qual Health Res.* 2011;21(8):1033–1040.
6. Breitbart W. Reframing hope: Meaning-centered care for patients near the end of life. Interview by Karen S. Heller. *J Palliat Med.* 2003;6(6):979–988.
7. Chochinov HM. Thinking outside the box: Depression, hope, and meaning at the end of life. *J Palliat Med.* 2003;6(6):973–977.
8. Lethborg C. To what extent does meaning mediate adaptation to cancer? The relationship between physical suffering, meaning in life, and connection to others in adjustment to cancer. *Palliat Support Care.* 2007;5(4):12.
9. Trevino KM, Archambault E, Schuster JL, et al. Religiosity and spirituality in military veteran cancer survivors: A qualitative perspective. *J Psychosoc Oncol.* 2011;29(6):619–635.
10. Erikson E. *Identity: Youth and Crisis.* New York, NY: Norton; 1968.
11. Erikson EH. *Youth: Change and challenge.* New York, NY: Basic Books; 1963.
12. Berman SL, Montgomery MJ, Kurtines WM. The development and validation of a measure of identity distress. *Identity.* 2004;4(1):1–8.
13. Habermas T, Bluck S. Getting a life: The emergence of the life story in adolescence. *Psychol Bull.* 2000;126(5):748–769.
14. Habermas T, de Silveira C. The development of global coherence in life narratives across adolescence: Temporal, causal, and thematic aspects. *Dev Psychol.* 2008;44(3):707–721.
15. Habermas T, Ehlert-Lerche S, de Silveira C. The development of the temporal macrostructure of life narratives across adolescence: Beginnings, linear narrative form, and endings. *J Pers.* 2009;77(2):527–559.
16. Habermas T, Hatiboglu N. Contextualizing the self: The emergence of a biographical understanding in adolescence. *New Directions Child Adolescent Dev.* 2014;2014(145):29–41.
17. Habermas T, Kober C. Autobiographical reasoning is constitutive for narrative identity: The role of the life story of personal continuity. In: McLean KC, Syed M, eds. *The Oxford Handbook of Identity Development.* New York, NY: Oxford University Press; 2015:149–165.
18. Hammack PL. Theoretical foundations of identity. In: McLean KC, Syed MU, eds. *The Oxford Handbook of Identity Development*: New York, NY: Oxford University Press; 2015:11–30.
19. Erikson EH. *Identity and the Life Cycle; Selected Papers.* New York, NY: International Universities Press; 1959.
20. Josselson R, Flum H. Identity status: On refinding the people. In: McLean KC, Syed MU, eds. *The Oxford Handbook of Identity Development.* New York, NY: Oxford University Press; 2015:132–146.
21. Marcia JE. Development and validation of ego identity status. *J Pers Soc Psychol.* 1966;3(5):551–558.
22. Meeus W. The study of adolescent identity formation 2000–2010: A review of longitudinal research. *J Res Adolescents.* 2011;21:19.
23. Crocetti E, Meeus W. The identity statuses: Strengths of a person centered approach. In: McLean KC, Syed MU, eds. *The Oxford Handbook of Identity Development.* New York, NY: Oxford University Press; 2015:97–114.
24. Lilgendahl J. The dynamic role of identity processes in personality development: Theories, patterns, and new directions. In: McLean KC, Syed MU, eds. *The Oxford Handbook of Identity Development.* New York, NY: Oxford University Press; 2015:490–507.
25. Di Battista A, Godfrey C, Soo C, et al. "In my before life": Relationships, coping and post-traumatic growth in adolescent survivors of a traumatic brain injury. *J Rehabil Med.* 2014;46(10):975–983.

26. Zebrack B, Isaacson S. Psychosocial care of adolescent and young adult patients with cancer and survivors. *J Clin Oncol.* 10 2012;30(11):1221–1226.
27. Barnett ME, Shuk EM, Conway FP, et al. Cancer-related disclosure among adolescent and young adult cancer survivors: A qualitative study. *J Adolesc Young Adult Oncol.* 2014;3(3):123–129.
28. van der Spek N, Vos J, van Uden-Kraan CF, et al. Meaning making in cancer survivors: A focus group study. *PLoS One.* 2013;8(9):e76089.
29. Woodgate R, McClement S. Symptom distress in children with cancer: The need to adopt a meaning-centered approach. *J Pediatr Oncol Nurs.* 1998;15(1):3–12.
30. Woodgate RL. A different way of being: Adolescents' experiences with cancer. *Cancer Nurs.* 2005;28(1):8–15.
31. Zadeh S, Pao M, Wiener L. Opening end-of-life discussions: How to introduce Voicing My CHOiCES, an advance care planning guide for adolescents and young adults. *Palliat Support Care.* 2014:1–9.
32. Lyon ME, Jacobs S, Briggs L, et al. Family-centered advance care planning for teens with cancer. *JAMA Pediatr.* 2013;167(5):460–467.
33. Lyon ME, Jacobs S, Briggs L, et al. A longitudinal, randomized, controlled trial of advance care planning for teens with cancer: Anxiety, depression, quality of life, advance directives, spirituality. *J Adolesc Health.* 2014;54(6):710–717.
34. Sourkes BM. *The Deepening Shade: Psychological Aspects of Life-Threatening Illness.* Pittsburgh, PA: University of Pittsburgh Press; 1982.
35. Worrell FC. Culture as race/ethnicity. In: McLean KC, Syed MU, eds. *The Oxford Handbook of Identity Development.* New York, NY: Oxford University Press; 2015:249–268.
36. Daniels EA, Gillen MM. Body image and identity: A call for new research. In: McLean KC, Syed MU, eds. *The Oxford Handbook of Identity Development.* New York, NY: Oxford University Press; 2015:406–422.
37. Rote WM, Smetana JG. Parenting, adolescent-parent relationships, and social domain theory: Implications for identity development. In: McLean KC, Syed MU, eds. *The Oxford Handbook of Identity Development.* New York, NY: Oxford University Press; 2015:437–453.
38. Taffel R. *Breaking Through to Teens.* New York, NY: Guilford; 2005.
39. Beyers W, Cok F. Adolescent self and identity development in context. *J Adolesc.* 2008;31(2):147–150.
40. Swartz TT, Kim M, Uno M, et al. Safety nets and scaffolds: Parental support in the transition to adulthood. *J Marriage Family.* 2011;73(2):414–429.
41. McLean KC, Jennings LE. Teens telling tales: How maternal and peer audiences support narrative identity development. *J Adolesc.* 2012;35(6):1455–1469.
42. McLean KC, Mansfield CD. The co-construction of adolescent narrative identity: Narrative processing as a function of adolescent age, gender, and maternal scaffolding. *Dev Psychol.* 2012;48(2):436–447.
43. Breitbart W, Poppito S. *Meaning-Centered Group Psychotherapy Treatment Manual.* New York, NY: Oxford University Press; 2014.
44. Breitbart W, Poppito S. *Individual Meaning-Centered Psychotherapy Treatment Manual.* New York, NY: Oxford University Press; 2014.
45. Frankl VF. *Man's Search for Meaning.* 4th ed. New York, NY: Simon & Schuster; 1959.
46. Breitbart W, Poppito S, Rosenfeld B, et al. Pilot randomized controlled trial of individual meaning-centered psychotherapy for patients with advanced cancer. *J Clin Oncol.* 2012;30(12):1304–1309.
47. Breitbart W, Rosenfeld B, Gibson C, et al. Meaning-centered group psychotherapy for patients with advanced cancer: A pilot randomized controlled trial. *Psycho-Oncology.* 2010;19(1):21–28.
48. Breitbart W, Rosenfeld B, Pessin H, et al. Meaning-centered group psychotherapy: An effective intervention for improving psychological well-being in patients with advanced cancer. *J Clin Oncol.* 2015;33(7):749–754.
49. Frankl VE. Logotherapy. *Isr Annal Psychiatry Relat Discipl.* 1967;5(2):142–155.
50. Trevino KM, Maciejewski PK, Fasciano K, et al. Coping and psychological distress in young adults with advanced cancer. *J Support Oncol.* 2012;10(3):124–130.
51. Lichtenthal WG, Breitbart W. The central role of meaning in adjustment to the loss of a child to cancer: Implications for the development of meaning-centered grief therapy. *Curr Opin Support Palliat Care.* 2015;9(1):46–51.
52. Trevino KM, Abbott CH, Fisch MJ, et al. Patient-oncologist alliance as protection against suicidal ideation in young adults with advanced cancer. *Cancer.* 2014;120(15):2272–2281.
53. National Cancer Institute and Lance Armstrong Foundation. *Closing the Gap: Research and Care Imperatives for Adolescents and Young Adults with Cancer.* Bethesda, MD: National Cancer Institute; 2006.

54. Zebrack B, Mathews-Bradshaw B, Siegel S. Quality cancer care for adolescents and young adults: A position statement. *J Clin Oncol.* 2010;28(32):4862–4867.
55. Coccia PF, Pappo AS, Altman J, et al. Adolescent and young adult oncology, version 2.2014. *J Natl Compr Cancer Netw* 2014;12(1):21–32; quiz 32.
56. Zebrack BJ, Corbett V, Embry L, et al. Psychological distress and unsatisfied need for psychosocial support in adolescent and young adult cancer patients during the first year following diagnosis. *Psycho-Oncology.* 2014;23(11):1267–1275.
57. Zebrack BJ, Block R, Hayes-Lattin B, et al. Psychosocial service use and unmet need among recently diagnosed adolescent and young adult cancer patients. *Cancer.* 2013;119(1):201–214.
58. Palmer S, Patterson P, Thompson K. A national approach to improving adolescent and young adult (AYA) oncology psychosocial care: The development of AYA-specific psychosocial assessment and care tools. *Palliat Support Care.* 2014;12(3):183–188.
59. Trevino KM, Archambault E, Schuster J, et al. Religious coping and psychological distress in military veteran cancer survivors. *J Religion Health.* 2012;51(1):87–98.

9

Adapting Meaning-Centered Psychotherapy in the Palliative Care Setting

Meaning-Centered Psychotherapy—Palliative Care

MELISSA MASTERSON, BARRY ROSENFELD, HAYLEY PESSIN, AND NATALIE FENN

INTRODUCTION

The psychosocial needs of cancer patients are critical components of cancer care across the illness trajectory.[1,2] The need for mental health services that target the unique challenges faced by patients at the end of life is particularly striking because one in three palliative care patients experience clinically significant depression and an equal number experience significant anxiety symptoms.[3] Furthermore, the emotional, psychological, and spiritual needs of palliative care patients greatly impact quality of life.[4] Several psychotherapy approaches have been developed for patients with cancer, covering a range of illness types and disease stages, but surprisingly few have specifically targeted patients in the final weeks or months of life.

Approximately 15 years ago, Breitbart and colleagues Memorial Sloan Kettering Cancer Center began to develop a meaning-centered approach to psychosocial care, aimed to alleviate spiritual despair among cancer patients. Among advanced cancer patients, and particularly those facing the end of life, our research has highlighted the links between spiritual despair, hopelessness, and the desire for hastened death, even in the absence of overt symptoms of depression. A substantial percentage of patients who expressed a desire for hastened death were not clinically depressed[4] but, rather, were facing an existential crisis encompassing the loss of meaning, value, purpose, and hope. For these patients, it was not psychological symptoms that needed to be addressed but, rather, the spiritual and existential concerns that plagued them. After numerous research studies demonstrated the central role that meaning plays in psychosocial distress and despair at the end of life, we began to develop a meaning-centered intervention: meaning-centered psychotherapy (MCP). Grounded in Viktor Frankl's logotherapy,[5,6] MCP was designed to help patients with advanced cancer develop, sustain, or enhance a sense of meaning, peace, and purpose in their lives. Our approach, utilizing MCP to target spiritual and existential issues in patients with advanced cancer has generated strong findings.[7–10]

Several randomized controlled trials of MCP, using both individual and group formats, have demonstrated significant improvement in spiritual well-being, quality of life, depression, hopelessness, and desire for death for patients living with advanced cancer.[8–10] Given the apparent effectiveness of MCP for advanced cancer patients in an ambulatory care setting, and the growing recognition that unmet psychological needs hinder the ability of terminally ill patients to confront death and dying, we adapted this intervention for an inpatient palliative care setting, specifically targeting patients who are rapidly approaching the end of life.

MEANING-CENTERED PSYCHOTHERAPY—PALLIATIVE CARE

Although MCP has demonstrated effectiveness in alleviating existential distress among advanced cancer patients in both group and individual formats, the intervention is not without its challenges, particularly for patients with severe illness. Due to the structure of the MCP

Session One: Experiencing Meaning	Session Two: Sources of Meaning	Session Three: Legacy & Reflections of Meaning
Introductions	Introduction to Sources of Meaning	Introduction to Living Your Legacy Now
Definitions of Meaning	Experiential Exercise: Encountering Life's Limitations	Experiential Exercise: Finding a Sense of Peace
Experiential Exercise: Meaningful Moments	Experiential Exercise: Creativity, Courage, and Responsibility	Experiential Exercise: What you Leave Behind
Experiential Exercise: Cancer & Meaning	Experiential Exercise: Connecting to Life	Experiential Exercise: Reflecting on Meaning
Experiential Exercise: Your History & Meaning		

FIGURE 9.1 Meaning-centered psychotherapy—palliative care session content.

sessions, in which each session builds upon the last, poor attendance is detrimental to the intervention's efficacy. This structure may be particularly problematic for severely ill individuals due to difficulties attending sessions on an outpatient basis. Given these concerns, Meaning-Centered Psychotherapy—Palliative Care (MCP-PC) was designed to address the need for one-on-one flexible care that is critical to patients with very advanced cancer. It represents an opportunity to provide an effective intervention for existential and spiritual suffering that can be delivered in a practical manner, such as at the patient's bedside in the palliative care or hospice setting.

The goals of MCP-PC are to help patients in palliative care and hospice settings understand the importance and relevance of creating, experiencing, reconnecting with, and sustaining meaning in their lives to help diminish despair near the end of life. Furthermore, MCP-PC promotes the belief that the potential for creating or experiencing meaning exists until the last moment of life. The format of MCP-PC is individualized, with each of the three sessions utilizing brief didactics, experiential exercises, and discussions that focus on specific themes of meaning and issues at the end of life (Figure 9.1). These techniques are intended to (1) promote a supportive environment for palliative care patients to explore personal issues and feelings surrounding their illness on a one-to-one therapeutic basis; (2) facilitate a greater understanding of possible sources of meaning in their lives; and (3) aid patients in their discovery and maintenance of a sense of meaning in life during illness. The ultimate goal of this intervention is to optimize coping through the pursuit of an enhanced sense of meaning and purpose. The following sections outline the content of MCP-PC sessions, including some of the exercises used in each session, and provide sample patient–therapist interactions that highlight critical elements of the treatment.

Session 1: Experiencing Meaning

The initial session of MCP-PC includes a series of introductions: introductions between the patient and therapist, introducing the patient to the intervention, and introducing the patient to the concept of meaning. The overarching goal of the initial session is to begin to familiarize the patient with the concept of meaning and its importance. This goal is achieved through the exploration of the definition of meaning and the patient's most meaningful moments, identity, and history. Session 1 includes a series of experiential exercises, one of which is the "Meaningful Moments" exercise. The Meaningful Moments exercise is designed to help concretize the concept of meaning for patients through identifying meaningful moments in their lives.

Experiential Exercise: Meaningful Moments

> Tell me about one or two experiences or moments when life has felt particularly meaningful to you—it can be big or small. It could be something that helped get you through a difficult day or a time when you felt most alive.

Following this exercise, it is the role of the therapist to reframe specific examples provided by the patient utilizing meaning-centered language (i.e., highlighting the sources of meaning). The ability of the therapist to reflect back to the patient his or her own experiences using the intervention terminology helps familiarize the patient with the concepts and apply the concepts to his or her own experiences. The following exchange highlights this process in a case involving a patient who reflected on her time as a teacher prior to her retirement and illness:

Therapist: What do you think it was about your teaching experience that was meaningful for you?

Patient: I was shaping minds for the future. I didn't take it as a clock in, clock out, I saw it as a profession. And I have always been ecologically sensitive, so I really felt that I could use that position to develop children who would be sensitive to the environment and to each other.

Therapist: It sounds like it was really motivating for you.

Patient: Yes, I was interested in the children even though I had 400 of them. I was able to remember their names and to understand them as individuals, so they loved me, the parents loved me, and the administration loved me. And they didn't want to see me leave. Of course I had to leave, I can't be teaching like this.

In addition to serving as an example of an interaction between the therapist and patient, this excerpt demonstrates an important goal of this exercise: to understand what the patient has found meaningful in his or her life. During this exercise, it is often second nature for clinicians to assume that they understand why a patient derives meaning from an experience such as raising children or falling in love. However, we have found that meaning-making is a deeply personal experience that is not always intuitive. In the previous excerpt, the therapist explores the patient's lived experience by asking her to identify what about her teaching experience gave her a sense of meaning rather than prescribing meaning to the experience or assuming that she already understood.

The impact of cancer on one's sense of meaning is also explored in the initial session by allowing patients to describe the qualities, roles, and characteristics that make them unique. Identity is seen as a reflection of meaning, and as a result, this exercise allows the patient to reflect on who he or she is as well as to identify what he or she finds meaningful. During this exercise, the therapist's role is to focus the discussion on qualities that existed prior to admission to the hospice or palliative care facility and to identify those qualities that remain present. The discussion is also intended to be balanced, allowing an opportunity for the patient to describe significant losses and alterations to his or her identity while highlighting characteristics that remain the same and, at times, those qualities that have even been strengthened.

Following the discussion of identity, an exploration of the patient's history serves as an opportunity to explore the context in which his or her identity developed. A critical element of this life review is the exploration of one's legacy. The experiential exercise titled "Your History and Meaning" allows the patient to express meaningful past experiences in order to uncover the historical context of his or her living legacy.

Experiential Exercise: Your History and Meaning

> When you look back on your life and upbringing, what are the most significant memories, relationships, traditions, etc., that have made the greatest impact on who you are today?

It is important to note that for some patients, a discussion of their experiences will be a pleasant experience, whereas for others it may bring up difficult emotions, as themes of hardship, loss, and adversity can emerge. Regardless of the content of the patient's history, it is the role of the therapist to bear witness to the patient's story, knowing that the experience of telling one's story may be transformative for a patient who is struggling and lacks the opportunity to connect with significant others. The following excerpt serves as an example of how the therapist can use him- or herself as a witness to the patient's story:

Therapist: It sounds like you must have impacted her in some way that she felt compelled to respond. I think that says as much about you as it does to her.
Patient: Yeah, the thing is I never found a way to thank her so that she would realize how much it meant to me. You know, I just thanked her and all but . . .
Therapist: [interposing] I would say you're thanking her right now, because you are sharing her kindness with me. You're sharing her story, so it will live on through you sharing it.

Because it facilitates the connection with important others, the importance of sharing one's story cannot be overstated. When clinically appropriate, patients are encouraged to share their story with someone in their lives in order to help the patients connect to those around them in a deeper and more meaningful way.

Session 2: Sources of Meaning

Session 2 of MCP-PC begins with a review of the themes discussed during the first session and gives the patient an opportunity to discuss any thoughts or themes that resonated with him or her. Because cognitive limitations are common among patients with very advanced illness, some repetition of essential topics is a useful element of MPC-PC and helps consolidate the material previously discussed. Following this discussion, the therapist begins to introduce the various sources of meaning that will be explored throughout this session. The main sources of meaning explored in the second session are attitudinal, creative, and experiential, although the balance of time devoted to each source is not necessarily equal; patients are encouraged to spend more time discussing the sources of meaning that are personally relevant to them. For example, whereas attitudinal and creative sources of meaning are more active, experiential sources of meaning are more passive, offering an opportunity for patients to connect to life through things that happen to them rather than actions in which they engage. Although the intervention is structured, considerable flexibility is built into the treatment manual to allow patients to tailor the intervention to their interests and needs rather than dictating the content that should be covered. The following is a sample script for providing the introduction to attitudinal and creative sources of meaning.

Example: Actively Engaging in Meaning

> Throughout life we encounter many limitations and challenges, but facing a serious illness presents its own set of obstacles. Learning to cope with limitations helps us to appreciate those things that we can still engage with despite changes. Not only does attitude help us to face challenges, but the way that we face suffering can be a source of meaning in and of itself.
>
> We have talked about limitations and arguably the greatest limitation in life is that we do not have forever to live. However, the fact that we only have a limited amount of time challenges us to make the most of the time that we do have. You can think of a sculptor who is hammering away at a piece of unshaped stone, knowing that he has a deadline to complete his masterpiece, but is unsure of when that deadline is. The sculptor works to shape the stone so that whenever that deadline strikes, he will be left with the most beautiful piece of art possible. For us, this unshaped piece of stone is our life, and we carve from it our values, meaning, and purpose. The ability to create is what gives us a reason to get up in the morning—a reason to move ahead into the world despite suffering.

Following this introduction, patients participate in one of the pivotal experiential exercises, "Encountering Life's Limitations." During this exercise, it is the role of the therapist to utilize information gained from the patient's life story to validate that the patient was heard while highlighting the ways in which he or she actively sustains meaning.

Experiential Exercise: Encountering Life's Limitations

> What are some of the life limitations, losses, or obstacles that you have faced in the past, and how did you respond to or deal with them at the time?
>
> How are you dealing with the limitations or losses you are facing now?

It is imperative for the patient to reflect on how he or she has faced challenges in the past and for the therapist to identify examples during which the patient consciously chose his or her attitude. Most patients have never considered how their attitude toward a challenging situation may have shaped the meaning that resulted. A skillful therapist will highlight the significance of attitude as a source of meaning and can continue to use this information if the patient encounters obstacles in the future. The following excerpt demonstrates the dialogue that can emerge during this exercise:

Therapist: What has kept you going through this period?

Patient: Well I'd say the Lord Jesus and my Saints. My belief that there is a reason why things happen but we may not know what the reason is. Only God knows, and we can't be arrogant—we must defer to the bigger picture, God's will. This life is temporary for everyone, it's just a matter of how death chooses to take you, but we are all "terminal." No one is getting out of here alive. So I feel that there are reasons why things happen. It's like putting a ceramic in the kiln—you have to go through the fire to get a beautiful piece of pottery.

Therapist: It sounds like your faith has kept you going.

Patient: I think so, and also realizing that there is a reason why all of this happened. I'm not able to see it, but there is a reason and you just have to accept it. Of course in my youth, I was cocky and arrogant and I thought I was in control of my own life, but I've realized that's not the way. You have to defer. You have to listen to life—you can't just do what you want to do, you know? You have to listen to life. Why is something happening? Have I learned from this? Has it changed me? Has it made me a better human being? Has it made me more empathetic? If you come across people who have not had hardship and adversity, they are callous, they can't empathize, but when you have gone through pain you are much more sympathetic to others.

Therapist: So you were able to learn from these experiences in a way that has helped you gain perspective on your life?

Patient: And I still am. Is it what I want? No. I'm not a masochist; it's not what I want but it's what I have right now. There is a saying—that life is playing a bad hand well, and I believe that.

Therapist: It makes me think of one of the things that Nietzsche said: "He who has a why can bear with almost any how."

Patient: That's well put.

Therapist: You have a will that was able to get you through some of the hardest things that anyone has had to deal with and that will is your "why." And you have faith and trust in a larger picture that allows you to transcend your suffering in some ways.

Patient: I think that is a good synopsis of what I said.

These examples can be used later in the sessions as the ideas of creativity, courage, and responsibility are introduced. In many cases, under extreme stress or in the face of devastating loss, simply engaging in life can be viewed (and described) as courageous. Therapists may also wish to underscore how facing an impending death takes tremendous courage for patients. This can be a valuable tactic as these patients fill their toolbox with ways to combat the existential crisis they may be facing. However, we caution against broaching death too directly with all patients. The clinician should ascertain the patient's openness to this line of discussion because pushing a patient to confront death prematurely can be difficult for the patient who is not yet ready.

In addition to discussions of sources of meaning that require substantial effort and initiative, a third source of meaning is presented as a more passive approach. Experiential sources of meaning are important in this intervention, in part because they can be important resources for the patient receiving palliative care or hospice services when physical functioning abilities are often limited. During the experiential exercise "Connecting with Life," patients are encouraged to reflect on ways they can connect to life through the experiences of love, beauty, and humor.

Experiential Exercise: Connecting with Life

List one or more ways in which you "connect with life" through

- Love
- Beauty
- Humor

How can these experiences help you now?

The benefit of the experiential sources of meaning is that they do not have to be present currently in order to have significance for the patient or to help him or her cope with current circumstances. For example, feelings of love remain powerful and important even when the loved one is not physically present. Viktor Frankl wrote about the importance of his love for his wife and how, despite their physical distance, the meaning of that love was paramount throughout his experience in the concentration camp.[5] If patients are struggling to connect with life due to logistical limitations (e.g., hospitalized or bedridden), the therapist might encourage the patient to reflect on the memory of a loved one, as demonstrated in the following exchange:

Therapist: It sounds like a theme throughout what we've talked about so far is that you encountered some really unpleasant people in your life. And then you encountered other people who had a profound impact on you—like the woman you described.

Patient: Oh yes, that's true.

Therapist: And even though you haven't seen her for many years, she is still an important part of your life?

Patient: Yes.

Therapist: So you carry these people with you, and they've had an impact on your life. This sounds like an important source of meaning to you. It's impacted who you are. And when we talk about identity and your ability to choose your attitude in the face of suffering, and you use the word tragedy, I think you're hitting the nail on the head when you say that you can find meaning in these tragic moments. It's not only about the positive things that have happened.

Session 3: Legacy and Reflections of Meaning

The final session covers topics related to legacy, unfinished business, and reflections on the experience of participating in the intervention. Patients are encouraged to reflect on the history they provided in previous sessions and consider how this history has shaped the legacy that they live and will leave to others. One of the defining components of the final session is the opportunity it provides for patients to explore potentially difficult topics related to death, such as unfinished business. The importance of the final session hinges on providing an opportunity for patients to express feelings, fears, and desires regarding the topic of death that they have likely been unable to discuss freely in the past. These themes are explored in the experiential exercise, "Finding a Sense of Peace."

Experiential Exercise: Finding a Sense of Peace

> Are there things that you wish you had done that are still important to you now? Tell me about them.
> Can any of them be accomplished now? Or how can you find a sense of peace for yourself with this now?
> As you reflect on how you have lived your life, what are some of the life lessons you have learned along the way that you would want to pass on to others?

Therapist: Are there things that you reflect on that you wish you had done? Things that are still important to you now?

Patient: I feel that I attempted to do everything as far as personal life. Not as far as marriage and children, but I did sincerely attempt it and you know, I attempted it in good faith.

Therapist: I know.

Patient: So I have no problem walking away from that. I just feel that it wasn't within the scheme of my life for that to happen and I accept that there was another path that was charted for me that did not include conventional marriage and children. And maybe as a substitute, I have these thousands of children.

Therapist: Right, right.

Patient: That way I was able to fully devote myself to them and I accept that because some of them call me mom, you know, so there was kind of a transfer there. I was still a nurturer; it was still maternal. So, you know, the role was still exercised.

Therapist: Right, right. And then so it seems like you have come to a place of acceptance then.

Patient: Yes.

Therapist: You know, you had that need met in a different way, maybe. In a variation and you still had a very meaningful long-term relationship [referring to the patient's long-term partner, who she never married].

Patient: Yes, I did, but in another fashion. I tried my best. I gave it my best shot.

Finally, the session concludes with a discussion about what the experience has been like for the patient, facilitated by the experiential exercise, "Reflecting on Meaning."

Experiential Exercise: Reflecting on Meaning

> What has it been like for you to go through this experience with me? How do you think you can use what we have talked about moving forward?

Following the patient's response, the therapist brings closure to the therapy by reflecting on meaningful experiences, moments, or memories from the shared therapeutic experience. The therapist should ultimately end treatment by expressing his or her gratitude for the legacy created within the therapy and to acknowledge moments of courage and connectedness. It is appropriate during this discussion for the therapist to acknowledge the impact that the patient has had on him or her personally and professionally. The following excerpt depicts the conclusion of therapy:

Therapist: I really appreciate you sharing so much and participating in these conversations. I know that we have covered a lot of ground over three sessions and some of it was very deeply seeded. How has it been for you?

Patient: Definitely . . . and it has given me time to pause and reflect because you know, if you are not being asked specific questions at times you don't pause and reflect as deeply. But I felt like I should tell you as much as I am able to, so it has allowed me that luxury.

Therapist: I wonder if you recognize your own strength . . . because I know sometimes it is hard to see it in yourself, but I am seeing it and I just want to reflect that to you.

Patient: I appreciate that.

Therapist: And even just your ability to structure your day and to participate in all the activities here. I think it's really impressive and I think it demonstrates your courage and commitment, and your ability to face each day with that attitude and that choice to continue to live meaningfully.

The goal of the termination process is to leave the patient with both a greater awareness of the sources of meaning that he or she can continue to draw on and a realization that he or she has the power to impact important others. This awareness can help the patient utilize the tools learned in MCP-PC to bring strength to the challenges that will likely follow.

PILOT STUDY OF MCP-PC

In order to refine and evaluate this brief version of MCP, we conducted a small pilot study of the intervention. The goals of this study were to determine whether MCP-PC could be successfully implemented in an inpatient palliative care facility and to generate preliminary data for additional adaptations or modifications. A secondary goal was to help clarify which aspects of MCP were most salient for terminally ill cancer inpatients and to make necessary modifications to our evolving treatment manual (much of which is described in the session summaries in this chapter). The results of this study are described in more detail elsewhere.[11]

Twelve terminally ill cancer patients with a life expectancy of less than 6 months were recruited from an inpatient palliative care hospital in New York City. Of the 12 patients, 7 were male (58%) and 5 were female (42%), with a mean age of 67 years and an age range of 46–83 years. Six patients (50%) identified as non-Hispanic White, 4 as African American (33%), and 2 as Hispanic/Latino (17%). Patients had a range of primary cancer sites, including gastrointestinal (n = 3; 25%), prostate (n = 2; 17%), lung (n = 2; 17%), and uterine (n = 2; 17%). Pre-treatment levels of psychological distress were equally diverse, with Distress Thermometer[12] scores ranging from 0 to 10 (mean = 3.9, standard deviation (SD) = 3.8), and Hospital Anxiety and Depression Scale (HADS)[13] total scores ranging from 4 to 31 (mean = 13.4, SD = 9.0). Three of the 12 participants had clinically significant levels of depression on the HADS Depression subscale (HADS-D >8).

Of the 12 patients who consented to participate, only 11 initiated treatment (1 patient died before the first session). Eight patients completed the three-session intervention and provided feedback during the post-treatment assessment. Patient responses to treatment were encouraging, with no patients reporting that the intervention was more than "slightly" distressing (mean = 0.25, SD = 0.5) on a 0- to 4-point scale. Furthermore, participants were generally positive about the content of the intervention. In their response to the intervention, 4 of the 8 "completers" indicated that treatment was "quite a bit" or "very much" helpful in finding a sense of meaning (mean = 2.50, SD = 0.9); only 1 patient responded "slightly" to this question, and none responded "not at all."

Although each patient may have found different sources of meaning useful, there were also commonalities evident in our pilot study. Participants strongly connected to experiential sources of meaning, predominantly the concepts of love and connectedness. For some, faith and their relationship to God provided a source of strength during the therapy, particularly in times of discomfort and hardship. For others, relationships to family, friends, or colleagues proved to be significant sources of meaning. Therapists utilized these relationships to highlight the fact that although our friends and family may not be physically present, we can hold them close to our hearts, and the love of these relationships can help us overcome suffering.

Participants also resonated to creative sources of meaning, including themes of responsibility and authenticity. Several participants noted how, despite moments of adversity, their sense of responsibility to family or work pulled them through difficult moments. One participant described a particularly difficult episode during cancer treatment when he was driving and needed to pull off to the side of the road in order to vomit. After sleeping through the day and night, the responsibility he felt to "show up" to his job was the only thing that raised him from bed that day. Similarly, participants responded to the concept of creating life authentically, sometimes even in opposition to what family, friends, or society deemed appropriate for them. Some achieved authenticity by pursuing the career of their choice. For others, it was remaining true to their values or religious beliefs despite outside pressures.

The results of this pilot study suggest that patients were generally satisfied with the content of the intervention, as well as its length and intensity. Of course, these results only summarize some of the trends present in a very small sample. As previously noted, a major benefit of MCP-PC is flexibility, and future implementations of MCP-PC should capitalize on the flexible nature of the treatment by allowing patients to determine which sources of meaning resonate most strongly and warrant the most attention. Nevertheless, these findings provide preliminary support for MCP-PC as a feasible and potentially beneficial approach for helping patients mange the psychological distress associated with terminal illness.

CLINICAL GUIDELINES FOR DELIVERING MCP-PC

Flexibility

One of the key components of MCP-PC is flexibility, both in its structure and in its delivery. Although the treatment is manualized, with structured session content and scripted exercises, it is important to utilize the opportunities for flexibility in order to best serve the individual needs of the patient. In addition to individualizing delivery of the session content (which is critical, given the limited amount of time that palliative care patients can typically sustain their attention and energy), flexibility in scheduling the intervention is imperative. Palliative care and hospice settings present many challenges for delivering psychotherapy, including fatigue, cognitive decline, and frequent interruptions for medical or nursing procedures, visits from family members and friends, and so on. These challenges led us to tailor and dramatically shorten MCP, which although originally designed for outpatient delivery with advanced cancer patients was not intended for those who are so severely ill as to need palliative care.

In addition to shortening the length of each session, maintaining fluidity with session content is critical in order to sustain the patient's attention and offset the many challenges that an inpatient setting presents. Our experience has suggested that the patient's engagement in the experiential exercises is the most influential component of treatment. Therefore, it is necessary to allow the patient to make the most of these exercises. For this reason, the intervention allows patients (and therapists) to "triage" session content at times in order to allow patients to guide the focus within each session (e.g., quickly determining which aspects of the session content are most salient). This allows for a deeper exploration of the most salient topics and facilitates the emergence of the meaning themes that resonate most with each patient. Meaning is a deeply personal construct and, therefore, although these sessions are designed to expose patients to a variety of meaning sources, patients will likely connect more strongly to some sources of meaning than others. The clinician should be alert to these cues in order to guide the treatment toward the most salient topics.

Using Simplification and Repetition

In all modalities of MCP, it is important to repeat key meaning concepts in order to educate and familiarize patients with the terminology. In the palliative care setting, in which symptom burden is high and concentration is often impaired, two techniques have proven critical: simplifying and repeating the content of the treatment. One of the most notable differences between the original design of MCP and MCP-PC is the didactic portion of the intervention. In MCP, lengthy didactics are often used to illustrate concepts that are difficult for some patients to grasp but are central to an existential psychotherapy. However, in the inpatient setting, in which time is limited, interruptions are frequent, and concentration is often impaired, we have found that lengthy explanations are usually ineffective. When delivering MCP-PC, the clinician is given the task of introducing existential concepts in a brief and concise manner to allow for greater focus on the experiential exercises. In this setting, it appears that patients benefit from exploring these topics and applying them to their own experiences more so than from listening to explanations. Second, it is often important to use repetition to help the patient retain and synthesize information that has been provided in order to ensure the patient understands the content. Clinicians must continually assess the patient's physical and mental state during sessions, noting medication administration prior to or during session, increased fatigue, or difficulties with memory, because these can dramatically impact the patient's ability to attend to the session. Although interruptions can be distracting, therapists are encouraged to utilize this time to reflect on what has been said and draw connections to serve as the springboard for the remainder of the session following any interruptions.

Allowing Authentic Reactions and Emotional Expressions

Perhaps the most essential skill needed by any clinician utilizing MCP-PC is the ability to engage a patient on a "human" level. A primary focus of MPC more generally is the emphasis on connectedness, and making a connection between patient and therapist is critical. Hence, the therapist must allow for—and indeed, encourage—the patient's authentic reaction, such as in response to questions posed in the experiential exercises, or more exploration of these difficult concepts more generally. For instance, several patients in our pilot study shared personal histories of hardship and strife, but the majority did not identify themselves as "having suffered" or having faced true limitations. Instead, patients tended to frame these experiences as "facts of life." Nevertheless, the act of exploring these painful memories was identified as beneficial for almost all of our pilot study participants. The patient's ability to share his or her feelings about these painful experiences with the therapist is a way in which they are able to make a meaningful and deep connection through the treatment. Of course, the importance of authenticity is not simply relevant for patients; therapists, too, must be prepared for powerful reactions to the treatment and make determinations about when, how, or if to use disclosures to help facilitate the treatment.

Utilizing Sources of Meaning in the Present

Although MCP-PC prompts patients to call upon meaningful experiences from their past, the intervention also underscores the importance of finding meaning in the present. The palliative care context often places many restrictions on patients (e.g., mobility and the ability to sustain attention for long periods of time), but it is the role of the clinician to help facilitate the meaning-making process despite any limitations imposed by the setting. It is particularly important for clinicians to have familiarity with the treatment setting and to be cognizant of any activities and/or opportunities that are available to their patients in that facility. A therapist can use the patient's participation in available activities and interactions with treatment staff, other patients, and friends and family as an excellent example of how the patient engages in and connects with life. Furthermore, sources of meaning that emerge naturally in session, such as humor, can be used to highlight a patient's continued use of these sources of meaning in the present.

Addressing Suffering

During the pilot study of MCP-PC, many patients discussed experiences of suffering, often arising spontaneously in response to themes of meaning. Some patients reported an enhanced ability to tolerate suffering and, in some cases, even to transcend it. The theme of suffering was particularly salient during many MPC topics, including sharing one's cancer story and identity, choosing one's attitude toward suffering, enhancing courage and facing life's limitations, and the use of meaning to potentially manage symptoms. One patient even noted, "I'm not in pain when I am thinking about this." Although MCP-PC is certainly not intended to be an analgesic, this intervention may help to mitigate the effects of physical suffering. Therapists are encouraged to connect sources of meaning and past experiences, including those that have allowed patients to overcome suffering in the past, as they face challenges in the present.

SUMMARY

MCP-PC is a novel intervention aimed at addressing the emotional, psychological, and spiritual needs of patients receiving palliative care. As described in the chapter, this approach offers a flexible, individualized approach to help patients in the palliative care or hospice setting optimize coping through the pursuit of an enhanced sense of meaning and purpose. Our belief that the potential to create or experience meaning exists until the last moment of life is central to this intervention and is particularly salient among this population because they face many physical, emotional, and temporal limitations. The results of our pilot study of MCP-PC provide preliminary evidence to support the feasibility of this intervention. Patient engagement in the experiential exercises was noted as a particularly influential component of treatment, but many topics and exercises were perceived as helpful. Furthermore, the flexible nature of MCP-PC allows patients to make the most of these exercises by exploring the most salient meaning-centered topics and applying them to their own lived experiences. Our observations and pilot study demonstrate the promise of this flexible and novel intervention to meet the existential needs of patients receiving palliative care.

REFERENCES

1. Carlson LE, Waller A, Mitchell AJ. Screening for distress and unmet needs in patients with cancer: Review and recommendations. J Clin Oncol. 2012;30:1160–1177.
2. Adler NE, Page AEK. *Cancer Care for the Whole Patient: Meeting Psychosocial Health Needs.* Washington, DC: National Academies Press; 2008.
3. Berdine HJ. Anxiety and depression. In: Strickland JM, ed. *Palliative Pharmacy Care.* Bethesda, MD: American Society of Health-System Pharmacists; 2009:57–75.
4. Breitbart W, Rosenfeld B, Pessin H, Kaim M, Funesti-Esch J, Galietta M, ... & Brescia R. Depression, hopelessness, and desire for hastened death in terminally ill patients with cancer. *JAMA*, 2000;284(22), 2907–2911.
5. Frankl VE. *Man's Search for Meaning.* New York, NY: Simon & Shuster; 1959/1985.
6. Frankl VE. *The Doctor and the Soul.* New York, NY: Knopf; 1969/1986.
7. Greenstein M, Breitbart W. Cancer and the experience of meaning: A group psychotherapy program for people with cancer. *Am J Psychother.* 2000;54:486–500.
8. Breitbart W, Rosenfeld B, Gibson C, et al. Meaning-centered group psychotherapy for patients with advanced cancer: A pilot randomized controlled trial. *Psycho-Oncology.* 2010;19:21–28.
9. Breitbart W, Poppito S, Rosenfeld B, et al. Pilot randomized controlled trial of individual meaning-centered psychotherapy for patients with advanced cancer. *J Clin Oncol.* 2012;30:1304–1309.
10. Breitbart W, Rosenfeld B, Pessin H, et al. Meaning-centered group psychotherapy: An effective intervention for improving psychological well-being in patients with advanced cancer. *J Clin Oncol.* 2015;33:749–754.
11. Rosenfeld B, Saracino R, Tobias K, Masterson M, Pessin H, Applebaum A, ... & Breitbart W.Adapting meaning-centered psychotherapy for the palliative care setting: Results of a pilot study. *Palliative Medicine* 2016; 0269216316651570.
12. Roth AJ, Kornblith AB, Batel-Copel L, et al. Rapid screening for psychologic distress in men with prostate carcinoma. *Cancer.* 1988;82:1904–1908.
13. Zigmond AS, Snaith RP. The Hospital Anxiety and Depression Scale. *Acta Psychiatr Scand.* 1983;67:361–370.

10

Cultural and Linguistic Adaptation of Meaning-Centered Psychotherapy for Chinese Cancer Patients

JENNIFER LENG, FLORENCE LUI, ANGELA CHEN, XIAOXIAO HUANG, WILLIAM BREITBART, AND FRANCESCA GANY

BACKGROUND

Cancer Disparities Among Chinese

Asian Americans, generally, and Chinese-speaking immigrants, specifically, are an at-risk group in cancer care. Cancer has been the leading cause of death for female Asian Americans since 1980.[1] Asian American/Pacific Islanders are the only major population group in the United States for whom cancer deaths exceed heart disease deaths. Although Asian Americans are at lower risk for certain cancers, they have higher rates of tumors related to infectious diseases, including gastric, liver, cervical, and nasopharyngeal.[2] Within the Chinese American population, data from California (disaggregated national data on the major Asian ethnic groups are not routinely available) demonstrate that Chinese Americans have higher rates of liver, colorectal, and lung cancer than those of other Asian groups.[2] Liver cancer incidence and death rates among Asian/Pacific Islanders are double those among non-Hispanic whites.[2]

Stark inequalities exist in quality of life (QOL) for minority cancer survivors.[3] Chinese immigrants are a poor, medically underserved population with numerous barriers to good QOL in survivorship.[3] This group is particularly vulnerable because of poor access to culturally and linguistically responsive support, cancer stigma, limited cancer knowledge, lack of health care navigation knowledge, and financial barriers.[4] In the United States, 50% of the Chinese population speaks English less than "very well";[5] in New York City, 45% report speaking English "not well" or "not at all."[6] Language and communication are crucial in effective cancer support, with its complexity and emotional nuance.[7,8] Cultural and language barriers often coexist.[9] Chinese patients may be passive in the health care system. Traditionally, the doctor is not to be challenged,[10] leading to reduced treatment seeking and care participation.[11] Chinese cancer survivors with higher control of negative emotions such as anger, anxiety, and depression are more likely to have higher stress levels and negative coping (hopelessness and anxiety preoccupation) with cancer.[12] Furthermore, Chinese culture is strongly influenced by Buddhism, Taoism, and Confucianism. Cultural differences between Western health care workers and Chinese patients can add difficulty to end-of-life care.[13]

Spiritual Care Needs Among Chinese Cancer Patients

Psychospiritual well-being has been defined as a subjective experience that incorporates both emotional health and meaning-in-life concerns and includes attributes such as self-awareness, coping and adjusting effectively with stress, having satisfying relationships and connectedness with others, sense of faith, sense of empowerment and confidence, and living with meaning and hope.[14] Despite recent findings in the literature suggesting spirituality is associated with health and well-being,[14] few studies have been conducted on spirituality and spiritual care within the context of Chinese culture.[15] Mok et al. explored spirituality among terminally ill Hong Kong Chinese patients and found important themes that included how finding meaning in life was most closely linked to family relationships, the role of a higher power, having a sense of peace, and accepting death.[15] Hsiao et al. examined spiritual needs among

Taiwanese patients with advanced cancer and found similar themes related to learning and fulfilling meanings of life, experiencing reciprocal love, and need for a peaceful mindset and acceptance of death.[13] In a study of Chinese immigrants with breast cancer in the United States, Chiu found that patients' spiritual resources were most related to family closeness; religion; traditional Chinese values; alternative therapy; Chinese support groups; and art, prose, and literature.[16]

Breitbart et al.'s meaning-centered psychotherapy (MCP)[17,18] is an empirically validated treatment based on the principle that humans are motivated by a "will to meaning." Drawn from Victor Frankl's work with Holocaust survivors, MCP is designed to help patients with advanced cancer sustain or enhance a sense of meaning as they approach the end of life.[18] A small but growing body of research has demonstrated that MCP significantly reduces psychological distress (e.g., depression, hopelessness, anxiety, and desire for hastened death) and significantly increases spiritual well-being and a sense of meaning and purpose in life in patients with advanced cancer.[17,19,20] The MCP intervention consists of seven (individual) or eight (group) 90-minute sesssions.[19,20]

The efficacy of MCP was tested in a randomized controlled clinical trial to assess its impact on reducing psychological distress and improving spiritual well-being with an English-speaking, predominantly White (71.2%) sample in which Asian Americans were not included as a demographic category.[20] MCP has not yet been adapted for racial and ethnic minorities who may hold different cultural, spiritual, and religious values, attitudes, and beliefs and for whom the concept of "meaning" may differ from those of their White counterparts.[13] For instance, Mok et al. found that whereas connectedness, faith, and hope were central concepts related to spirituality in Western cultures, among Chinese, the fulfillment of personal responsibilities and acceptance of death as a life process were key spiritual concepts.[15] Researchers have noted that spiritual views and practices among diverse populations are largely an understudied area; thus, there is a paucity of culturally tailored spiritual interventions.[15,21]

The Process of Cultural Adaptation

Although there has been much debate on how to reach and include underserved and minority individuals and groups in evidence-based interventions, the majority have advocated for the cultural adaptation of empirically based treatments for the target community.[22–28] Smith et al. demonstrated that culturally adapted treatments are more efficacious than unmodified treatments, and that interventions implemented with a single minority group are more effective than those delivered to patients with a variety of backgrounds.[29] When evidence-based psychotherapy treatments are specifically adapted for a cultural group, outcomes may exceed those of treatments not specifically adapted.[30,31]

In response to a need for a model of cultural adaptation, Domenech-Rodriguez and Wieling proposed the ecological validity model (EVM), which focuses on cultural adaptations to the content of evidence-based treatments.[22] The EVM consists of eight dimensions of treatment interventions that serve as a framework for adapting psychosocial interventions for minority populations: Language, Persons, Metaphors, Content, Concepts, Goals, Methods, and Context.[22] The dimension of Language refers to the use of culturally appropriate and culturally syntonic language in the intervention to ensure it is received as intended, and it involves cultural knowledge of the expression of emotional experiences and verbal style.[22] Person refers to the racial and ethnic similarities and differences between client and therapist, as well as therapeutic alliance.[22] Metaphors refers to the use of symbols, pictures, concepts, and relevant examples of the population's culture in the intervention program.[22] Content refers to cultural knowledge about clients' values, customs, and traditions, as well as considerations of the cultural, social, economic, and political uniqueness of the group as part of assessment and treatment planning. Concepts refer to the degree to which treatment concepts and theory are consonant with the culture and context of the client.[22] Goals considers the congruence between therapist and client as related to the goals of the intervention—that is, that goals of treatment should be framed within the values, customs, and traditions of the community.[22] Methods refers to the tasks and procedures for achieving intervention goals, which should be compatible and acceptable to the clients' culture.[22] Finally, Context takes into consideration the social, economic, and political context of the intervention, including treatment barriers.[22]

The cultural adaptation process (CAP) was developed to be used together with the EVM.[22] It focuses on the *process* of adaptation and on including the target community. CAP is based on the work of Everett Rogers on the diffusion of innovations;[32] involves important persons in the process of implementing a new intervention, such as change agents (i.e., treatment developers) and opinion leaders (i.e., cultural adaptation specialist); and emphasizes collaboration between such important persons and local communities.[22] This model firmly places community at the center of any dissemination effort.[22] A local community may adopt an intervention in a new way, different from the original intention, and this may lead to positive results.[22] The CAP is structured in three phases: (1) Outline activities to complete pre-intervention, including meeting with community leaders to explore interest and needs and gathering information to inform intervention adaptation; (2) measurement issues and the intervention itself, including selection and review of intervention evaluation metrics, a priori intervention tailoring, and tailoring during the initial pilot testing; and (3) adaptation iterations, to be made as needed.[22] For a detailed review of the CAP model, see Domenech-Rodriguez and Weiling.[22]

Given the unmet need in the Chinese population for spiritual support,[13] the risk of cross-cultural misunderstanding surrounding care at the end of life,[33] a substantial body of literature suggesting that treatments undertaken by minorities are affected by the cultural sensitivity of the treatment,[31] and the interrelatedness between MCP and the themes found in previous studies conducted in this area among Chinese patients,[13,15,16] adapting MCP is a logical and important next step. It will advance the knowledge base to enhance spiritual well-being and quality of life, and it will reduce psychological distress and end-of-life despair in this vulnerable population.

This chapter describes a community needs study of Chinese American advanced cancer patients conducted with key community leaders, corresponding to phase 1 of the CAP model.[22] We sought to determine the needs and issues that are important to the community. Specifically, we inquired about the need for psychosocial interventions in end-of-life care (i.e., the type of end-of-life assistance that is needed and the delivery method that the community prefers for this type of assistance), potential cultural norms and attitudinal barriers to the intervention (i.e., cancer stigmas that might affect the delivery of this care, the role of family members, and the role of religion), and issues that are important to community members with cancer (i.e., spiritual needs, family relationships, standing in the community, etc.) in order to determine how to best adapt the MCP intervention to address the community's needs. The chapter then details strengths that may make MCP especially relevant for the Chinese community, followed by six areas of focus to address in adapting MCP for Chinese cancer patients.

A COMMUNITY NEEDS STUDY

We worked closely with community-based organizations and cancer support organizations serving the Chinese community to identify key community leaders. These individuals included leaders of Chinese-serving community-based organizations and health centers, medical oncologists serving the Chinese population, and palliative care specialists. After the purpose of the MCP intervention and the proposed adaptation process were described, the following areas of inquiry were addressed: (1) Patients' goals for the adapted intervention (relates to the Goals dimension of the EVM), (2) relevance and adaptability of the MCP session themes (relates to the Metaphors, Concept, and Content dimensions of the EVM), (3) relevance of key themes from literature and preliminary work (relates to the Metaphors, Concept, and Content dimensions of the EVM), (4) preference for intervention methods (relates to the Methods dimension of the EVM), and (5) potential impact of contextual barriers on delivery and effectiveness of the intervention (relates to the Context dimension of the EVM).

The 11 interviewees worked in a variety of settings, including in hospitals, hospices, community-based organizations, and community-based private practices. Some provided direct care to patients, whereas others held advocacy/program development roles in the Chinese community. Interviewees were a mix of physicians, nurses, and other health care professionals, and all had direct experience with Chinese patients.

Prominent themes included family, culture, immigration, and end of life.

Family

All interviewees discussed the centrality of the family unit in adapting MCP for the Chinese population. Many specifically emphasized the cultural value of filial piety—that is, a Confucian virtue of respect for one's parents, elders, and ancestors. One interviewee defined filial piety as "You want to honor your primary ancestors and those who came before you." Another observed that filial piety could be interpreted in a variety of ways:

> So one interpretation is that you have to respect your parents, so you don't tell them [their diagnosis] because that would be

> hurting them. Another way to look at it would be, if you respect them as thinking adults who make their own decisions, you should have to tell them. So it depends which way they're spinning it.

Several interviewees described using a family-centric approach in treating their Chinese patients. Interviewees observed that disclosure of medical information and transparency around a patient's diagnosis could be complicated because some patients designated a family member, often an eldest son, to receive information and make decisions about their care:

> In Chinese culture, the family may not even tell the patient their diagnosis, and the patient may not want to know. The patient may not want to bear the psychological stress of knowing their illness and treatment plan. So it's very important to have the family involved.

Interviewees raised the role of the clinician in brokering family dynamics, tensions, and conflicts that arise from a family-centered model of care:

> The adult children or husband or non-sick spouse is saying that you can't [disclose] to the patient. Of course the patient knows she has cancer and says, "Don't tell my kids how much time I have left." But really, when you bridge those gaps is when you can really start to explore meaning, and it becomes a much richer journey.

Others stated that generational differences could impact interactions between clinicians and patients' families because belief systems could differ between first-generation immigrants and their second-generation offspring.

All recommended family participation in the MCP intervention, given the cultural norms around family involvement in medical care: "There's a lot of family support and connection compared to other groups. . . . But it's really hard to have that conversation about reflecting on life and reviewing things. [MCP] would be really powerful [if it could] prompt or engage families [to have that conversation]."

Culture

All interviewees described the unique role of culture in adapting MCP for the Chinese community. Interviewees described traditional views of Chinese patients—for example, guilt, fear of punishment, failure, and fatalism—and superstitious beliefs associated with cancer stigma. One interviewee described how these views might negatively impact spiritual well-being in a hypothetical Chinese cancer patient: "Maybe because I did something wrong, that's why I'm getting this punishment today."

Social norms in Chinese culture were also discussed. One interviewee explained that differences between collectivistic Chinese culture and individualistic Western norms might contribute to Chinese patients' devaluation of interventions such as MCP that focus on the internal psychological processes of the individual: "In Asia generally we're not individualistic, we're more [collectivist]. . . . We hardly live [for] ourselves." Most interviewees also warned that cultural norms of face-saving and privacy could impede treatment:

> A lot of Chinese patients may not ask for help. Sometimes they might feel like it's not appropriate or polite to talk about these issues. It's important to say that it's okay. The idea of therapy [is] foreign for Chinese families and patients and may be seen as a weakness, another misconception that has to be overcome.

However, another interviewee suggested that this norm did not apply to all Chinese individuals and that trust could facilitate treatment. "Trust is number one . . . it's about that relationship. It's an art."

Interviewees suggested incorporating cancer-related education in the adapted intervention to counteract culturally influenced superstitions related to cancer: "In cancer the [cultural perception] is something more mysterious, something bad. Something that seems alienated, not connected to the body." Interviewees discussed how cancer stigma related to fears of contagiousness and contamination. Some described employing indirect references to cancer (e.g., "angry tumor") when treating Chinese cancer patients. Others described the cultural belief some patients held that cancer occurred because of misdeeds the patient had committed in a past life: "They don't want to say they have a disease because the first thing that comes to mind is [cancer is] some kind of payback [for wrongdoing]."

Several interviewees suggested the adapted MCP intervention incorporate Chinese proverbs and terms. The majority of interviewees also endorsed addressing religion in MCP. One observed parallels between Eastern religions and the goals of MCP: "[Many] pay homage to their ancestors, and tradition is really important, [so] in meaning-making it would be good to incorporate that."

Immigration

Interviewees described the significance of Chinese cancer patients' immigration experiences in adapting MCP. Participants discussed Chinese patients' desire to return to their country of origin at the end of life as a common phenomenon that clinicians should be prepared to discuss with patients and their families. Others suggested that immigration presented a challenge in a psycho-spiritual treatment because Chinese immigrant patients have access to fewer practical resources than native-born Whites: "The challenges of [a lack of] social support, of social insulation: Their families are . . . far away, so the caregiving roles are hard. In terms of end-of-life, meaning-making therapy, the loss theme is really big."

Interviewees suggested that clinicians be mindful of the range of immigration histories patients may have experienced, instead of generalizing the experiences of all Chinese immigrants. This heterogeneity extended to religious beliefs ("Older generations or people from Taiwan have more of a religious base. People from China, because of the Cultural Revolution, that's all gone"), language ("Fujianese, Cantonese, Mandarin"), and generational status and education ("The San Francisco area is more Cantonese-speaking, and older. In South Bay [Chinese immigrants are] highly educated").

Interviewees recommended the adapted intervention reframe patients' immigration experiences in discussions about meaning. One interviewee suggested encouraging patients to open up in therapy by referencing the expanded range of cultural norms available to them as immigrants: "Now we're in America. Americans talk about a lot of things openly." Another suggested adopting a strengths-based approach drawing from patients' immigration histories: "Talk about immigrant life, [it's] so powerful. Why did they come here, their history, sacrifices they made [for] their kids."

End of Life

Interviewees identified dying in the family home as a serious cultural taboo that could cause anxiety and negatively impact spiritual well-being among Chinese cancer patients. One interviewee noted that this taboo unfortunately remained unaddressed in a Westernized model of palliative care:

> The whole notion of hospice throughout mainstream US is about being able to die at home for those who want to. But so many Chinese people do not want to die at home. Of course they need the service because they're terminally ill and struggling and suffering, but they don't want to die at home.

In discussing end-of-life concerns for this population, many participants considered the Chinese cultural emphasis on a good death—that is, passing once familial and financial responsibilities have been met and conflicts resolved—and suggested incorporating it into the MCP adaptation. One interviewee provided an example of a community-based workshop focusing on end-of-life issues that could be incorporated into MCP called "Celebrating Life's Journey." This life review included an examination of one's personal history, processing intergenerational concerns (i.e., what will be passed onto the next generation), and making end-of-life care decisions.

Although participants noted that frank discussions about end-of-life concerns would be difficult in this population, the majority believed it presented a valuable opportunity for Chinese patients to resolve family conflicts, make important plans about care, and achieve meaning at the end of life: "Even if life is shortened, even if you are facing the end, you can still have hope. Hope for your children, for your family, not just for yourself."

STRENGTHS OF MCP FOR THE CHINESE COMMUNITY

Drawing from the results of the community needs study, our research team identified several strengths that may make MCP especially relevant to the Chinese community.

Cultural Relevance of Spiritual Well-Being

Several interviewees highlighted the cultural relevance of, and need for, spiritual well-being for this population. They observed the overlap between philosophies held in Eastern religions such as Buddhism and the meaning-enhancing goals of MCP as embodied in the Chinese cultural emphasis on a good death at the end of life. One interviewee described the importance of psychosocial care for attaining the culturally syntonic goal of a "good death": "To die with your heart settled, peacefully—you need to say sorry to the people you [wronged] and to express love to the people you love, and to say goodbye. For Chinese people, this can be very difficult." Another interviewee observed that Buddhists might be more "open" to discussing death as a "part of" life's journey.

Their observations mirror related findings in the literature: The concept of mindfulness, which emphasizes deliberate nonjudgmental attention to present moment experiences, has roots in Buddhism and Asian philosophies, and has been gaining support among mental health professionals as a vital component of mental health care.[34] Mindfulness has been described as a contributor to the development of qualities such as transcendence and interconnectedness that are components of spiritual well-being,[35] and is an important component of acceptance-based therapies that have been demonstrated to reduce self-stigma.[36]

Potential for Family-Centered "Meaning"

Although the cultural value of filial piety may present a stressor to Chinese cancer patients in the realm of diagnosis disclosure and care arrangements, a family-centered version of MCP may have many benefits, especially with regard to spirituality and meaning. In a stratified random national survey of patients, families, physicians, and other care providers examining factors considered important at the end of life, researchers found that among all participants, ensuring that family members were prepared for the patient's death was among the most important factors in end-of-life preparedness,[37] consistent with the notion of a "good" death as including acceptance and closure.[37] Family and social support have been found to contribute to positive spiritual well-being.[38] Another study identifying critical attributes of health-related QOL among terminally ill cancer patients in Taiwan reported that family support was the essential indicator of QOL.[39]

Given the importance of having positive relationships and a sense of connectedness with family and friends to QOL in cancer survivorship, a culturally relevant, family-based intervention model might be especially impactful among Chinese immigrants who, due to culturally influenced obligations to family, participate in the family custom of "white lie" in which bad news is not discussed.[40] One interviewee told the story of a Chinese cancer patient who, despite his advanced stage of cancer and 3-month prognosis, would not consent to a DNR—that is, a legal order of "do not resuscitate," a directive to withhold CPR or advanced cardiac life support out of respect for a terminally ill patient's wishes. It was not until a nurse explored his psychosocial needs that it was discovered that the patient wanted to witness his daughter's wedding before his death but felt too much shame to communicate this need directly to his daughter. By helping to resolve family tensions and miscommunications within the context of an MCP intervention, therapists may greatly impact spiritual well-being in this population. Although the manualized MCP intervention does not specifically account for how to include family members in a family-centered treatment, the protocol could be adjusted for Chinese cancer patients. For instance, family members could be invited to join patients in Session 3, when patients are asked to reflect on their life and identify "the most significant memories, relationships, traditions, etc. that have made the greatest impact on who you are today."

Immigration History and the "Immigrant Paradox"

The literature has documented an "immigrant paradox" whereby, despite the psychological stressors associated with migration and the relatively disadvantaged socioeconomic profile of immigrant families, immigrants are at lower risk for psychiatric disorders compared to non-Hispanic Whites.[41] Mendoza and Fuentes-Afflick proposed a model in which positive cultural health behaviors by the family and its community account for the protective effects of the immigrant paradox, buffering the detrimental effects of poverty.[42] Specifically, when positive cultural health behaviors produce good functional health, the family and community reinforce such behaviors through cultural norms, maintaining the cultural milieu through continued immigration into the community.[42]

These findings echo interviewees' statements that Chinese cancer patients' immigration histories may represent a strength and potential source for spiritual exploration within the context of the MCP intervention. One interviewee suggested Chinese immigrants possess a distinct immigrant culture that may enable them to speak openly about their cancer diagnosis: "You're in the US, you don't have to be restricted. Life doesn't have to be defined by certain parameters." Another suggested that talking specifically about immigrant life would be a "powerful" opportunity to discuss spirituality and meaning: "Why did they come here—what's their history? The sacrifices they made for their kids . . . *Suan tian ku la*, [meaning] what is sweet, what is sour, what is bitter, what is spicy, in their life?" Encouraging the exploration of immigration histories is culturally relevant and may even strengthen the MCP intervention in this population.

AREAS OF FOCUS IN ADAPTING MCP FOR THE CHINESE IMMIGRANT CANCER POPULATION

Drawing from the strengths of MCP for the Chinese community that we determined from the community needs study, we have identified five key areas that should be addressed in adapting MCP for the Chinese population.

Stigma and Shame Around Cancer and Psychotherapy

Interviewees explained how traditional views, social norms, and cancer stigma coalesced to present barriers to delivering mental health care to Chinese immigrant patients with advanced cancer. Given that fear or embarrassment associated with cancer has been linked to delays in seeking help,[43] the prevalence of cancer stigma in the Chinese immigrant cancer population may present a barrier to participation in a psychosocial intervention such as MCP. A National Comprehensive Cancer Care Network-appointed multidisciplinary panel created to address barriers to psychosocial care in cancer suggested that negative meaning and stigma attached to words related to the psychological domain, such as *psychiatric, psychological*, and *psychosocial*, represent a major barrier for both physicians and patients.[44] Moreover, cancer-related stigma can extend to views about the distress experienced by people with cancer,[44] decreasing the probability of accepting psycho-oncology services.[45] This is evidenced by the preponderance of patients who conform with expectations that they must remain "brave" at all times[46] or who fear that discussing their distress will reflect badly on their coping abilities.[47]

Stigma has been identified in the literature as a prominent factor negatively affecting individuals with psychological problems and their families in various cultures.[48–51] The literature further suggests that mental health stigma may be more severe in Chinese culture.[52] Chinese may be more likely to moralize psychological dysfunction (i.e., deem the individual as morally responsible for the illness), further exacerbating self-stigma.[53] Given the high potential for stigma related to a psychosocial intervention, it will be important for MCP therapists treating Chinese cancer patients to raise awareness about spiritual, QOL, and psychosocial needs in cancer care. Therapists might reduce self-stigma by focusing on the psychoeducational aspects of treatment to reduce misconceptions and stigma around help-seeking[54]—a recommendation a number of participants made—and by using alternative words to describe psychological symptoms or concerns, such as *distress*.[44] Other interventions to reduce stigma include verbal confrontation of negative attitudes and public education programs.[55]

Acceptance-based therapies such as acceptance and commitment therapy (ACT), which incorporates acceptance, mindfulness training, and behavioral change strategies, have also been shown to reduce stigmatizing attitudes.[36] MCP therapists might make use of acceptance-based strategies in Session 2, which focuses on cancer and meaning. For instance, when patients describe their identities and how cancer may have affected them, acknowledgment and acceptance of difficult changes that affect their role identities (e.g., not being able to throw a football with a son or a lack of sexual intimacy) in combination with behavioral change strategies that support their identities (e.g., watching a football game with a son or cuddling with a partner) could be encouraged.

Socioeconomic Status Barriers

Among Chinese immigrants, socioeconomic status (SES) barriers present another significant challenge to the delivery of all interventions, including MCP. Many interviewees expressed concerns regarding Chinese cancer patients' level of education, cancer awareness, and immigration status, noting that the latter can deter undocumented Chinese immigrants from accessing "nonessential" care such as a psychosocial intervention.

It is noteworthy that the Chinese are the only ethnic group ever to have been excluded from the United States by federal law on the basis of race, a legal history that has contributed to the significant SES variation within the Chinese American population as well as to a greater proportion of foreign-born versus US-born Chinese Americans.[56] The Chinese Exclusion Act of 1882 barred immigration from China to the United States and denied citizenship to Chinese Americans until its repeal in 1943.[57] Following the Lyndon Johnson administration's 1965 Immigration and Nationality Act, which dismantled racial quotas and allowed skills- and family-based immigration, more prosperous and often college-educated Chinese emigrated to the United States.[57] However, Asian Americans experience a higher rate of poverty than non-Hispanic Whites, with 16.1% of Asian Americans living in poverty as opposed to 10.4% of Whites,[58] contributing to what some scholars have called the making of "two Asian Americas."[56]

Given the demographic heterogeneity among Chinese immigrants that is the legacy of the Chinese Exclusion Act, the MCP intervention would need to address a variety of needs, which might vary by SES category. One interviewee described a bimodal income distribution affecting cancer stigma and beliefs among Chinese immigrants in California: "The Chinese in the South Bay are very different from [those in] San Francisco: highly educated, with more exposure to newer information so their old stigmas[s] can be reversed." On the other hand, poorer and undocumented immigrants were described as potentially "fearing" the Immigration and Naturalization Service and therefore more reluctant to share information and participate in MCP.

Interviewees also described that immigrants' long work schedules would result in difficulty accessing care: "Their families are working 14–15 hours a day, and so [participating in MCP] is hard because people are working." Participants made a number of recommendations to address barriers to treatment among low-income Chinese patients. These included providing transportation from patients' homes to therapy, providing child care to caregivers, and having MCP sessions take place in the hospital or hospice setting to better integrate psychosocial and cancer care and to increase retention rates. Given the potential for mistrust in undocumented immigrants, some interviewees further emphasized the importance of obtaining "buy-in" from patients' oncologists, palliative care specialists, or other trusted medical health professionals who have already established relationships with Chinese immigrant patients.

Care Arrangements Within the Family

Interviewees voiced the central role of family in Chinese cancer patients' illness, including patients' fear of becoming a burden to family members, the common practice of designating a family member to make medical decisions for the cancer patient, and the desire for inclusion of family in MCP. This is consistent with prior research describing Chinese cancer patients' anxiety about becoming a burden on the family compounding their own distress[59] and presents a significant challenge in delivering a culturally sensitive psychosocial intervention in this population.

One interviewee distinguished between a "family-centered" model of care and a more Westernized, "patient-autonomy" model, explaining, "The bioethical models are different. You have to work with the family." A family-based model can present certain communication challenges around disclosure of cancer diagnoses, as another interviewee described:

> Families might want to protect patients. . . . Families don't want them to know they have cancer. If the family is blocking [disclosure of cancer diagnosis to the patient]—and we encounter this a lot—I try to establish a relationship with the family and patient and say, "Okay, let's go talk to the patient together. I'm not going to tell them [the patient] anything. But let's just ask them [the patient], 'You had all these tests, and when the test results come out, do you want the doctor to tell you what's going on, or would you rather they just talk to your family?' And if the patient says, 'I want to know,' you say to the family, 'Do I lie to [the patient], or should we work out a solution?' "

A number of service providers emphasized the importance of identifying the family member responsible for the patient's care in providing optimal care to the patient: "It's much more of a family thing . . . you have to identify who the main decision maker is in the family. If it's the patient himself, that's great. If it isn't, then you kind of have to [work with that person]."

These comments echo the literature on disclosure of diagnosis for Chinese patients, which illustrates the complexity of cultural attitudes toward truth-telling. One study of Chinese cancer patients found that cancer patients were more likely than families to believe that patients should be informed of the diagnosis and that attitudes toward such a disclosure were influenced by disease stage.[60] A Taiwanese study found that cancer patients strongly proclaimed their rights to be informed about their disease over their family before releasing information to family caregivers.[61]

In adapting MCP for this population, researchers and clinicians should be cognizant of the role of filial piety in the care arrangements for Chinese cancer patients. Mok et al.[62] found that family caregivers of terminally ill patients in Hong Kong believed their roles were important to their loved ones and led to increased meaning in both parties' lives. In another study of family caregivers of Taiwanese terminally ill cancer patients at risk of experiencing depressive distress, results indicated that family caregivers who felt confident in their knowledge of how to take care of the patient at home or were sufficiently aware of the patient's thoughts and feelings about disease experiences were less likely to suffer from depressive distress,[63] suggesting that psychosocial interventions should be developed to include family caregivers and enhance their understanding of the patient's disease experiences. Given the complex family dynamics described by interviewees and in the literature,[60–63] it will be important for MCP therapists to learn how to sensitively discuss cancer-related issues in a way that honors patient rights and, if desired by the patient, includes their families. Therapists should consider a family-centered approach in adapting MCP with Chinese immigrant patients to enhance satisfaction and alliance.[64]

Cultural Synchronicity in MCP Language and Concepts

As recommended in the EVM, culturally adapted treatments must use language that is culturally syntonic so it is received as intended.[22] In addition, treatment concepts and theory must be relevant to the client's cultural context.[22] Several interviewees described potential cultural and linguistic difficulties of translating a spiritually centered psychosocial treatment such as MCP. Specifically, interviewees expressed concern regarding the translation of the word *legacy*, which is used throughout the MCP intervention. One interviewee called it a "very strong" word indicating "a social action . . . something really extraordinary," suggesting that the word be further contextualized in translation so that *legacy* is "more tangible and related to family." Another interviewee wondered whether the concept of *creativity* would translate to a Chinese immigrant population: "I think you have to explain 'creativity' to them—that there's a lot of different achievements; it could mean a lot of different things." In one session, patients are asked to explore meaning derived from creativity and responsibility. One interviewee stated that in her experience, Chinese people are "really focused on basic needs. . . . There's not much time to focus on the creative arts." The word *creativity* may need to be reframed in the adaptation to encompass creativity not only in the arts but also in everyday life. Chinese words approximating the meaning of *resourcefulness* or *talent* may be more culturally salient. For instance, one interviewee suggested that creativity be framed experientially, in terms of Chinese immigrants' "practical surviving" or hobbies.

Another interviewee wondered whether asking about "connecting with life through love, beauty, and humor" in one of the MCP sessions might be "too abstract," recommending that therapists tie experiential sources of meaning back to the family, which would be received as more culturally syntonic. One interviewee stated that humor is not

> . . . as normalized as it is in Western culture. . . . I think people would say, "Let's just laugh about it." And find fun about some things [to make cancer] easier to deal with, but I don't know that they see the importance of humor as seriously as Western culture does.

Therapeutic Alliance

Interviewees discussed the importance of establishing trust with patients, families, and communities in order to secure "buy-in" for the MCP intervention. One interviewee stated that because Chinese patients may exhibit some "initial inhibition," establishing "trust" and "being comfortable is key" to reach "untapped distress [that is] pushed under the surface." Another interviewee also emphasized the significance of trust, "especially when discussing vulnerabilities and emotions surrounding the diagnosis." Only after trust is established, one interviewee observed, will patients "share their personal histories and experiences," especially given that such sharing may be "culturally and socially discouraged."

There is much in the literature suggesting that the therapeutic alliance, defined as the collaborative bond between therapist and patient, is a key factor in a successful treatment. Three decades of psychotherapy research have consistently identified the therapeutic alliance as the single most important factor in determining rates of attrition, premature treatment termination, and general clinical outcomes.[65,66] A meta-analysis of 79 studies showed that the therapeutic alliance has a consistent and moderate effect on psychotherapy outcomes.[67] In the cultural adaptation literature, it has been suggested that therapeutic alliance is enhanced by the therapist's awareness of his or her own cultural biases,[68] modification of the therapeutic relationship to the client's culture, development of trust and credibility, and the promotion of cultural empathy.[69] This is consistent with findings that ethnic-specific programs are associated with lower premature dropout and increased length of treatment,[70,71] underscoring the importance of cultural responsiveness and sensitivity. Practitioners delivering MCP to Chinese immigrants should be required to complete "cultural competency/responsiveness" training to gain the specific knowledge, attitudes, awareness, and clinical skills necessary for effective cross-cultural communication in the clinical setting.[33,72]

REFERENCES

1. Chen MS. Cancer prevention and control among Asian and Pacific Islander Americans. *Cancer*. 1998;83(S8):1856–1864.
2. McCracken M, Olsen M, Chen MS, et al. Cancer incidence, mortality, and associated risk factors among Asian Americans of Chinese, Filipino, Vietnamese, Korean, and Japanese ethnicities. *CA Cancer J Clin*. 2007;57(4):190–205.
3. Guidry JJ, Torrence W, Herbelin S. Closing the divide: Diverse populations and cancer survivorship. *Cancer*. 2005;104(Suppl 11):2577–2583.
4. Yu MY, Hong OS, Seetoo AD. Uncovering factors contributing to under-utilization of breast cancer screening by Chinese and Korean women living in the United States. *Ethnic Dis*. 2003;13(2):213–219.
5. Reeves TJ, Bennett CE. *We the People: Asians in the United States*. Washington, DC: United States Census Bureau; 2004.
6. MLA Language Map Data Center. Data center results; 2008.
7. Thorne SE, Hislop TG, Armstrong E, et al. Cancer care communication: The power to harm and the power to heal? *Patient Educ Couns*. 2008;71(1):34–40.
8. Surbone A. Cultural aspects of communication in cancer care. *Support Care Cancer*. 2008;16(3):235–240.
9. Green CR, Anderson KO, Baker TA, et al. The unequal burden of pain: Confronting racial and ethnic disparities in pain. *Pain Med*. 2003;4(3):277–294.
10. Lam WW, Fielding R. The evolving experience of illness for Chinese women with breast cancer: A qualitative study. *Psycho-Oncology*. 2003;12(2):127–140.
11. Lin JS, Finlay A, Tu A, et al. Understanding immigrant Chinese Americans' participation in cancer screening and clinical trials. *J Community Health*. 2005;30(6):451–466.
12. Ho RT, Chan CL, Ho SM. Emotional control in Chinese female cancer survivors. *Psycho-Oncology*. 2004;13(11):808–817.
13. Hsiao S, Gau M, Ingleton C, et al. An exploration of spiritual needs of Taiwanese patients with advanced cancer during the therapeutic processes. *J Clin Nurs*. 2011;20(7–8):950–959.
14. Lin H, Bauer-Wu SM. Psycho-spiritual well-being in patients with advanced cancer: An integrative review of the literature. *J Adv Nurs*. 2003;44(1):69–80.
15. Mok E, Wong F, Wong D. The meaning of spirituality and spiritual care among the Hong Kong Chinese terminally ill. *J Adv Nurs*. 2010;66(2):360–370.
16. Chiu L. Spiritual resources of Chinese immigrants with breast cancer in the USA. *Int J Nurs Stud*. 2001;38(2):175–184.
17. Breitbart W, Rosenfeld B, Gibson C, et al. Meaning-centered group psychotherapy for patients with advanced cancer: A pilot randomized controlled trial. *Psycho-Oncology*. 2010;19(1):21–28.
18. Breitbart W. Spirituality and meaning in supportive care: Spirituality- and meaning-centered group psychotherapy interventions in advanced cancer. *Support Care Cancer*. 2002;10(4):272–280.
19. Breitbart W, Poppito S, Rosenfeld B, et al. Pilot randomized controlled trial of individual meaning-centered psychotherapy for patients with advanced cancer. *J Clin Oncol*. 2012;30(12):1304–1309.
20. Breitbart W, Rosenfeld B, Pessin H, et al. Meaning-centered group psychotherapy: An effective intervention for improving psychological well-being in patients with advanced cancer. *J Clin Oncol*. 2015;33(7):749–754.
21. Conner NE, Eller LS. Spiritual perspectives, needs and nursing interventions of Christian African-Americans. *J Adv Nurs*. 2004;46(6):624–632.
22. Domenech-Rodriguez M, Wieling E. Developing culturally appropriate, evidence-based treatments for interventions with ethnic minority populations. In: Rastogi M, Wieling E, eds. *Voices of Color: First-Person Accounts of Ethnic Minority Therapists*. Thousand Oaks, CA: Sage; 2004.
23. Borrego J, Anhalt K, Terao SY, et al. Parent–child interaction therapy with a Spanish-speaking family. *Cognit Behav Pract*. 2006;13(2):121–133.
24. Bernal G, Sáez-Santiago E. Culturally centered psychosocial interventions. *J Community Psychol*. 2006;34(2):121.

25. Cardemil EV. Cultural adaptations to empirically supported treatments: A research agenda. *Sci Rev Mental Health Pract.* 2010;7(2):8–21.
26. McCabe KM, Yeh M, Garland AF, et al. The GANA program: A tailoring approach to adapting parent–child interaction therapy for Mexican Americans. *Educ Treatment Children.* 2005:111–129.
27. Roosa MW, Dumka LE, Gonzales NA, et al. Cultural/ethnic issues and the prevention scientist in the 21st century. *Prev Treatment.* 2002;5(1):5a.
28. Rodríguez MMD, Baumann AA, Schwartz AL. Cultural adaptation of an evidence based intervention: From theory to practice in a Latino/a community context. *Am J Community Psychol.* 2011;47(1-2):170–186.
29. Smith TB, Rodriguez MD, Bernal G. Culture. *J Clin Psychol.* 2011;67:166–175.
30. Miranda J, Bernal G, Lau A, et al. State of the science on psychosocial interventions for ethnic minorities. *Annu Rev Clin Psychol.* 2005;1:113–142.
31. Sue DW, Arredondo P, McDavis RJ. Multicultural counseling competencies and standards: A call to the profession. *J Counseling Dev.* 1992;70(4):477–486.
32. Rogers EM. *Diffusion of Innovations.* New York, NY: Simon & Schuster; 2010.
33. Kagawa-Singer M, Kassim-Lakha S. A strategy to reduce cross-cultural miscommunication and increase the likelihood of improving health outcomes. *Acad Med.* 2003;78(6):577–587.
34. Hall GC, Hong JJ, Zane NW, et al. Culturally competent treatments for Asian Americans: The relevance of mindfulness and acceptance-based psychotherapies. *Clin Psychol Sci Pract.* 2011;18(3):215–231.
35. Falb MD, Pargament KI. Relational mindfulness, spirituality, and the therapeutic bond. *Asian J Psychiatr.* 2012;5(4):351–354.
36. Masuda A, Hayes SC, Fletcher LB, et al. Impact of acceptance and commitment therapy versus education on stigma toward people with psychological disorders. *Behav Res Ther.* 2007;45(11):2764–2772.
37. Steinhauser KE, Christakis NA, Clipp EC, et al. Factors considered important at the end of life by patients, family, physicians, and other care providers. *J Am Med Assoc.* 2000;284(19):2476–2482.
38. Lin H, Bauer-Wu SM. Psycho-spiritual well-being in patients with advanced cancer: An integrative review of the literature. *J Adv Nurs.* 2003;44(1):69–80.
39. Yang K, Yin T. Defining the content domain of health-related quality of life for terminally ill cancer patients. *Nurs Res.* 1999;7:129–144.
40. Xu Y. Death and dying in the Chinese culture: Implications for health care practice. *Home Health Care Manage Pract.* 2007;19(5):412–414.
41. Markides KS, Coreil J. The health of Hispanics in the southwestern United States: An epidemiologic paradox. *Public Health Rep.* 1986;101(3):253–265.
42. Mendoza FS, Fuentes-Afflick E. Latino children's health and the family–community health promotion model. *West J Med.* 1999;170(2):85–92.
43. Smith LK, Pope C, Botha JL. Patients' help-seeking experiences and delay in cancer presentation: A qualitative synthesis. *Lancet.* 2005;366(9488):825–831.
44. Holland JC, Kelly BJ, Weinberger MI. Why psychosocial care is difficult to integrate into routine cancer care: Stigma is the elephant in the room. *J Natl Compr Canc Netw.* 2010;8(4):362–366.
45. Lambert SD, Kelly B, Boyes A, et al. Insights into preferences for psycho-oncology services among women with gynecologic cancer following distress screening. *J Natl Compr Canc Netw.* 2014;12(6):899–906.
46. Wilson K, Luker KA. At home in hospital? Interaction and stigma in people affected by cancer. *Soc Sci Med.* 2006;62(7):1616–1627.
47. Ryan H, Schofield P, Cockburn J, et al. How to recognize and manage psychological distress in cancer patients. *Eur J Cancer care.* 2005;14(1):7–15.
48. Corrigan PW, Kleinlein P. On the stigma of mental illness: Practical strategies for research and social change (pp. 11–44). Washington, DC, US: American Psychological Association, xv, 343 pp.http://dx.doi.org.ezproxy.gc.cuny.edu/10.1037/10887-001; 2005.
49. Corrigan PW, Watson AC, Miller FE. Blame, shame, and contamination: The impact of mental illness and drug dependence stigma on family members. *J Fam Psychol.* 2006;20(2):239.
50. Tsang HW, Tam PK, Chan F, et al. Stigmatizing attitudes towards individuals with mental illness in Hong Kong: Implications for their recovery. *J Community Psychol.* 2003;31(4):383–396.
51. Tsang HW, Tam PK, Chan F, et al. Sources of burdens on families of individuals with mental illness. *Int J Rehabil Res.* 2003;26(2):123–130.
52. Ku TK. Culture and stigma towards mental illness: A comparison of general and psychiatric nurses of Chinese and Anglo-Australian backgrounds. Unpublished master's thesis; 2007.
53. Yang LH, Kleinman A. "Face" and the embodiment of stigma in China: The cases of schizophrenia and AIDS. *Soc Sci Med.* 2008;67(3):398–408.
54. Hwang W, Wood JJ, Lin K, Cheung F. Cognitive-behavioral therapy with Chinese Americans: Research, theory, and clinical practice. *Cognit Behav Pract.* 2006;13(4):293–303.

55. Corrigan PW, Penn DL. Lessons from social psychology on discrediting psychiatric stigma. *Am Psychol.* 1999;54(9):765.
56. Lee E. *The Making of Asian America: A History.* New York, NY: Simon & Schuster; 2015.
57. Ngai MM. The architecture of race in American immigration law: A reexamination of the immigration act of 1924. *J Am History.* 1999;86:67–92.
58. Ramakrishnan K, Ahmad FZ. *State of Asian Americans and Pacific Islanders series: A multifaceted portrait of a growing population.* Washington, DC: Center for American Progress; 2014.
59. Lee J, Bell K. The impact of cancer on family relationships among Chinese patients. *J Transcult Nurs.* 2011;22(3):225–234.
60. Jiang Y, Liu C, Li J, et al. Different attitudes of Chinese patients and their families toward truth telling of different stages of cancer. *Psycho-Oncology.* 2007;16(10):928–936.
61. Tang ST, Liu T, Lai M, et al. Congruence of knowledge, experiences, and preferences for disclosure of diagnosis and prognosis between terminally-ill cancer patients and their family caregivers in Taiwan. *Cancer Invest.* 2006;24(4):360–366.
62. Mok E, Chan F, Chan V, et al. Family experience caring for terminally ill patients with cancer in Hong Kong. *Cancer Nurs.* 2003;26(4):267–275.
63. Tang ST, Li CY, Liao YC. Factors associated with depressive distress among Taiwanese family caregivers of cancer patients at the end of life. *Palliat Med.* 2007;21(3):249–257.
64. Hwang W. The psychotherapy adaptation and modification framework: Application to Asian Americans. *Am Psychol.* 2006;61(7):702.
65. Horvath AO, Greenberg LS. *The Working Alliance: Theory, Research, and Practice.* Vol. 173. New York, NY: Wiley; 1994.
66. Solomon P, Draine J, Delaney MA. The working alliance and consumer case management. *J Mental Health Admin.* 1995;22(2):126–134.
67. Martin DJ, Garske JP, Davis MK. Relation of the therapeutic alliance with outcome and other variables: A meta-analytic review. *J Consult Clin Psychol.* 2000;68(3):438.
68. Vasquez MJ. Cultural difference and the therapeutic alliance: An evidence-based analysis. *Am Psychol.* 2007;62(8):878.
69. Comas-Diaz L, Caldwell-Colbert A. *Applying the APA Multicultural Guidelines to Psychological Practice.* 2006. Retrieved September 24, 2006, at www.division42.org/ContEd.
70. Takeuchi DT, Sue S, Yeh M. Return rates and outcomes from ethnicity-specific mental health programs in Los Angeles. *Am J Public Health.* 1995;85(5):638–643.
71. Yeh M, Takeuchi DT, Sue S. Asian–American children treated in the mental health system: A comparison of parallel and mainstream outpatient service centers. *J Clin Child Psychol.* 1994;23(1):5–12.
72. Betancourt JR, Green AR, Carrillo JE, et al. Defining cultural competence: A practical framework for addressing racial/ethnic disparities in health and health care. *Public Health Rep.* 2003;118(4):293–302.

11

Cultural and Linguistic Adaptation of Meaning-Centered Psychotherapy for Spanish-Speaking Latino Cancer Patients

ROSARIO COSTAS-MUÑIZ, OLGA GARDUÑO-ORTEGA, CARLOS JAVIER GONZÁLEZ, XIOMARA ROCHA-CADMAN, WILLIAM BREITBART, AND FRANCESCA GANY

INTRODUCTION

Latinos are the largest, fastest growing minority group in the United States. Approximately 50,000 new cancers are diagnosed among Latinos every year.[1] Although Latinos have lower incidence rates than non-Hispanic Whites for the most common cancers, they are more likely to be diagnosed at a more advanced stage.[1] Many patients with advanced cancer suffer from psychological distress and symptoms, end-of-life despair, and hopelessness,[2,3] further complicating their illness management and recovery. This suffering may impact patients' survival and care.[4]

A recent meta-analysis comparing the psychological morbidity of ethnic minorities with cancer, across studies with varying study designs, sampling methods, stages, diagnoses, and outcome measures, demonstrated that US Latino cancer patients show significantly worse distress, depression, and overall health-related quality of life (QOL) than non-Hispanic White and other minority patients.[5] For example, Latina breast cancer patients report almost twice the rate of depressive symptoms,[6] breast cancer survivors report poorer mental health,[7] and Latinos with prostate cancer report lower health-related QOL[8] than non-Hispanic White and African American patients. Furthermore, Latinos with varied cancer diagnoses have high rates of clinically significant depression and significant rates of depression recurrence 24 months after post-depression care treatment.[9] Even though Latino cancer patients are at higher risk for poor mental health outcomes, they are less likely to receive psychological/psychiatric services and interventions.[5]

In this chapter, we describe the considerations for, and process of adapting, a psychotherapeutic intervention. We provide a brief review of the efficacy of interventions developed, adapted, or delivered to Latino cancer patients; describe the therapy concepts and applicability of these concepts to the patient population; present the conceptual frameworks, plan, process, and methods used in adapting meaning-centered psychotherapy, which is the source of the cultural adaptation; and describe the future directions of the cultural adaptation program.

PSYCHOSOCIAL INTERVENTIONS FOR LATINO CANCER PATIENTS

A meta-analysis[10] showed that interventions targeted to a specific cultural group are four times more effective than interventions provided to groups consisting of participants from a variety of cultural backgrounds, and those conducted in the participants' native language (if other than English) are twice as effective as interventions conducted in English. Another meta-analytic study[11] confirmed that culturally adapted psychotherapy is more effective than unadapted psychotherapies by an effect size of 0.32. Latino participants with low levels of acculturation appeared to benefit greatly from culturally adapted mental health interventions.[10]

Despite the fact that Latino patients and advanced cancer patients in general are at higher risk of psychological disturbance, psychosocial treatments focusing on reducing psychological symptoms and improving quality of life in Latinos are scarce.[5] Efficacy studies of psychotherapy interventions on improving psychological adjustment, well-being, and hope at the end of life[5,12–14] have not been adapted for minority groups. Few interventions have been developed to reduce psychological symptoms among Latinos diagnosed with cancer: (1) Dwight-Johnson and colleagues[15] tested the effectiveness of the Multifaceted Oncology Depression Program in low-income Latino patients; (2) Ell and colleagues[16] adapted an intervention, Alleviating Depression Among Patients with Cancer (ADAPt-C), for predominantly female Hispanic patients with cancer; (3) Penedo and colleagues[17] tested the efficacy of a group-based cognitive–behavioral stress management program for use with Hispanic men with prostate cancer; and (4) Napoles and colleagues[18] adapted a peer-based cognitive–behavioral stress management program for Spanish-speaking Latina breast cancer patients. Two of these interventions are comprehensive programs that include problem-solving psychotherapy,[15,16] whereas the other two are based on a group- and peer-based cognitive–behavioral model.[17,18] Almost all of these interventions excluded patients in palliative care, and most of the samples were composed of stage I or stage II patients. All the interventions stressed the importance of addressing the unique needs and themes experienced by Latino cancer patients, which are often neglected in unadapted approaches.

Meaning-centered psychotherapy (MCP) is among the most promising adaptations due to its underlying model, research, and intervention practices. MCP provides a good fit for addressing the needs of Spanish-speaking Latino patients with advanced cancer who want support while coping with cancer. In the next section, the themes and goals of MCP are described in conjunction with the importance of meaning and spirituality to Latino cancer patients.

SPIRITUALITY AND MEANING-MAKING IN LATINO CANCER PATIENTS

Individual meaning-centered psychotherapy (IMCP) is a manualized 7-week intervention designed to assist patients with advanced cancer in sustaining or enhancing a sense of meaning, peace, and purpose in their lives as they face limitations due to progression of disease and treatment.[13] This intervention is grounded in the writings of Frankl[19] and informed by the work of Spiegel et al.,[20,21] Yalom et al.,[22] and Kissane et al.[23] MCP uses didactics, experiential exercises, and psychotherapeutic techniques (e.g., reflection, clarification, and exploration) that promote the use of sources of meaning as resources in coping with advanced cancer.[13] Seven 1-hour sessions address specific spiritual and existential themes related to meaning, cancer and identity, legacy, hope, and the finiteness of life.[13]

For Latinos, spirituality is a fundamental component of the healing process. Spirituality serves as a source of comfort, enhanced confidence, and lessened fears. Ethnic minority women diagnosed with cancer stress the importance and significance of spirituality on their recovery and consider their faith an important source of support.[24] Furthermore, religion is deeply rooted in Hispanic culture; 94% of Hispanics in the United States report a religious affiliation.[25] Moreover, among cancer patients, Latinos report higher religious and spiritual unmet needs[26,27] and use religious coping strategies more frequently than non-Hispanic Whites.[28,29] Also, among Latinos diagnosed with cancer, spiritual beliefs are highly correlated with health-related QOL.[30]

A systematic review of spiritual, religious, and existential-related research in Latino cancer patients, conducted by our research team, found that overall study findings supported spirituality as a central component to the cancer experience of Latinos. Spirituality provided healing, strength, lessened fears regarding the diagnosis, and helped through the recovery process.[31] The belief in a transcendent being/power provided patients with the strength to fight, and accepting their illness as God's will was significant in enhancing the patients' quality of life. Furthermore, religious beliefs and religious practices, such as prayer, attending church, and reading the bible, were particularly critical in helping to provide a positive view through the course and outcome of the illness. The Functional Assessment of Chronic Illness Therapy—Spiritual Well-Being (FACIT-Sp) was the most frequently used scale to measure spiritual, religious, and existential well-being, which is composed of two subscales: Faith (religious well-being) and Peace/Meaning (existential well-being). The majority of articles focused on spiritual themes, compared with religious themes and/or spiritual coping (either religious or spiritual), and only a few studies focused on existential themes (i.e., meaning, purpose in life, etc.). The results of the present review suggest that spirituality and religiosity play an important role in Latinos' coping, whereas existential themes were less prevalent in the literature examining spiritual outcomes in Latino cancer patients.[31]

Few studies have focused on the existential needs of Latino cancer patients. Moadel and colleagues[26] found that between 50% and 65% of Latinos reported wanting help to find hope, meaning in life, spiritual resources, and wanting to talk to someone about finding peace and finding meaning in life. Of these patients, 25–51% reported unmet spiritual/existential needs, which included wanting help in overcoming fears, finding hope, talking about peace of mind, finding meaning in life and spiritual resources, and having someone to talk to about the meaning of life and death.[26]

McClain and colleagues,[3] who studied a sample of predominantly non-Latino White terminally ill patients, found significantly stronger associations with the meaning factor (measuring existential well-being) than with the faith subscale (measuring religious well-being) with respect to hopelessness, desire for hastened death, and suicidal ideation. They conclude that the ability to find or sustain meaning in one's life during terminal illness might help to deter end-of-life despair to a greater extent than spiritual well-being rooted in one's religious faith. However, this finding could potentially differ or become even stronger with patients from different ethnic backgrounds. For this reason, to meet their needs, it is important to determine the associations between existential and religious well-being and psychological coping for other minority groups, such as Latino cancer patients, to understand the differential contribution of meaning, spirituality, and faith to depression and end-of-life despair.

Cultural adaptation is the systematic modification of an intervention protocol to consider language, culture, and context in such a way that is compatible with the client's cultural patterns, meanings, and values.[32] Cultural adaptations involve a planned, organized, interactive, and collaborative process, which includes the participation of persons from the targeted population for whom the adaptation is being developed.[33] A fundamental controversy in the field of adaptations is the fidelity–adaptation dilemma, which consists of a dialectic involving arguments favoring fidelity in the delivery of an evidence-based intervention as designed versus arguments favoring the need for adaptations in the delivery to reconcile intervention–consumer mismatches in accord with the needs and preferences of a subcultural group.[34,35]

Localization and transcreation[36] are the two strategies used to adapt the intervention manual following the Ecological Validity Model (EVM). Localization refers to adjusting language to the needs of the target speech community.[36] In transcreation, the source text is rewritten in the target language to convey the concepts and achieve the aims of the source text while accounting for both language and cultural considerations.[37,38] Transcreation not only renders the text of written materials into another language but also infuses culturally relevant context and themes. In transcreated materials, the text is reconstructed to meet the literacy and culture of the target audience.[38,39]

WHY ADAPT?

Proponents of the cultural adaptation of interventions[40,41] have presented a variety of arguments to support their position, including demographics, cultural sensitivity, ecological validity, ethics, and the preponderance of evidence. Racial and ethnic minority populations are growing in the United States. Adapting interventions presumably better enables engagement and retention of linguistic, ethnic, and racial minority groups. Treatments are more likely to be sustained if they are culturally congruent and community grounded. Most interventions are conducted with non-Hispanic White, fairly educated, and middle-class patients, which makes them nongeneralizable to ethnic minorities and individuals with diverse cultural backgrounds.[34] Racial and ethnic minorities have rarely been included in samples used for validating the efficacy of evidence-based interventions.[42] In addition, clinicians have an ethical responsibility to offer the best possible treatment by taking into account the values, culture, and context of their patients.[43] Finally, there is ample scientific evidence showing that interventions that are culturally adapted are more effective with linguistic, ethnic, and racial minority groups than are unadapted interventions.

Meta-analyses have demonstrated that adapted psychotherapy interventions[10,44] are far more effective than non-bona fide treatment, bona fide treatment, and evidence-based interventions. Griner and Smith[10] found an average effect size of 0.45, indicating a moderately strong benefit of culturally adapted interventions. Interventions targeted to a specific cultural group were four times more effective than interventions provided to groups consisting of clients from a variety of cultural backgrounds. Interventions conducted in clients' native languages (if other than English) were twice as effective as interventions conducted in English. Benish and colleagues,[11] based on a meta-analysis that included published and unpublished studies and also studies with culturally adapted psychotherapy versus unadapted but bona fide (i.e., conventional) psychotherapy, confirmed that culturally adapted psychotherapy interventions are more effective than unadapted, bona fide psychotherapies by an effect size of 0.32. Psychotherapies showed improved outcomes when the illness myth was adapted in a manner consistent with client cultural worldviews. According to Benish et al.,[11] the illness myth is the client's values and beliefs surrounding etiology, symptoms, course, consequences, and acceptable treatment options, which are pivotal when considering cultural adaptations of psychotherapy, particularly when addressing incongruence between client worldviews and predominant assumptions that are implicitly and explicitly woven into conventional psychotherapeutic practice.

Several models have been proposed to guide the process of cultural adaptation or transcreation of interventions and psychotherapy, including, but not limited to, the multidimensional model for understanding culturally responsive psychotherapies,[45] ecological validity framework,[46,47] cultural accommodation model,[48,49] cultural sensitivity framework,[50] cultural adaptation process model (CAPM),[51] psychotherapy adaptation and modification framework,[40,52] and heuristic framework for the cultural adaptation of interventions.[53] However, EVM[34] and CAPM[51] were selected as conceptual models for the MCP cultural adaptation for two reasons. First, these two models are complementary models: One guides the process (CAPM), whereas the other (EVM) guides the adaptation of the content and components of the intervention. Second, these models have been used together successfully to adapt interventions for Latino individuals and families, providing attention to the needs and predominant values of the Latino culture.[54]

MEANING-CENTERED PSYCHOTHERAPY

MCP is a manualized psychotherapy intervention developed for the specific spiritual and meaning-making needs of patients with advanced disease.[13,14] The basic concepts of MCP include the following:

1. Meaning of life: Life has meaning and never ceases to have meaning even up to the last moment of life; meaning may change in this context but it never ceases to exist.
2. Will to meaning: The desire to find meaning in human existence is a primary instinct and basic motivation for human behavior.
3. Freedom of will: We have the freedom to find meaning in existence and to choose the attitude toward suffering.
4. The three main sources of meaning in life are derived from creativity (work, deeds, and dedication to causes), experience (art, nature, humor, love, relationships, and roles), and attitude (attitude one takes toward suffering and existential problems).
5. Meaning exists in a historical context: Thus, legacy (past, present, and future) is a critical element in sustaining or enhancing meaning.

Substantial research has evaluated and supports the intervention's efficacy for producing favorable outcomes for patients with advanced cancer. Randomized controlled trials using intent-to-treat analysis have been conducted with advanced cancer patients using individual and group formats. The efficacy of MCP is strong for both individual and group formats.[13,14] In both individual and group MCP, participants demonstrated significantly greater improvement compared to the control condition for the primary outcomes of quality of life and spiritual well-being, including both components of spiritual well-being—sense of meaning and faith. MCP has been carried out at a comprehensive cancer center and is in the process of being adapted for caregivers, survivors, and hospice settings and culturally adapted for Spanish-speaking and Chinese immigrant patients.

This chapter discusses the ongoing activities and plan for the cultural adaptation of MCP for Latinos diagnosed with advanced cancer. The description of this cultural adaptation process has two overarching goals: (1) to provide an example of the process of adapting a psychotherapeutic intervention for chronically ill patients for researchers and clinicians interested in culturally adapting interventions and (2) to describe a method for tailoring a psychosocial intervention to the specific needs of Latinos with a chronic disease. An additional aim is to add transparency to the process of adapting efficacious programs and contribute to the emerging field of cultural adaptation of interventions.

ADAPTATION FRAMEWORK

CAPM[51] and EVM[55] provide the framework for the IMCP adaptation.[34] CAPM is a complementary process model to EVM. It describes three phases of adaptation: the formative phase, adaptation iterations, and intervention and measurement adaptation.[51] This chapter describes the preliminary results from the formative phase of the MCP linguistic and cultural adaptation. Following the EVM, the research information-gathering process will focus on seven areas: language, context, persons, metaphors, concepts, goals, and methods.[55]

Cultural Adaptation of Meaning-Centered Psychotherapy: Formative Research Phase

Domenech-Rodriguez and colleagues[51] describe that during the formative research phase, a collaborating team is initiated that is composed of a treatment developer and the cultural adaptation team. The team assesses the following: the fit of the intervention's concepts and techniques, the relevant literature, the populations' intervention interest and needs through collaboration with key informants and community members, and possible intervention adaptations based on the reported target populations' needs.[51] This stage informs the design and content of the needed adaptations. Some of the strategies that can be used include conducting a literature review, administering quantitative surveys to assess characteristics and preferences of potential participants, and, most important, conducting qualitative research with potential participants and experts who are experienced in working with the targeted groups. During this stage, it is important to establish an advisory committee or a systematic partnership including intervention program developers, agency administrators, program staff, community members, and other staff members interested in the program adaptation.[51]

For the cultural adaptation of MCP, the cultural adaptation team had three general objectives for the formative research phase: (1) to understand the Latino cancer patients' experience of making meaning after their cancer and their understanding of the IMCP concepts (meaning of life and identity after cancer, purpose in life, legacy, and sources of meaning); (2) to assess the acceptability of the goals (enhance hope, make sense of the cancer experience, and develop a sense of legacy), metaphors, and concepts of IMCP to patients and mental health providers of Latino patients; and (3) to assess the feasibility of the therapeutic methods (didactic teaching of the philosophy of meaning, session exercises, homework, and open-ended discussion) and goals of IMCP. The cultural adaptation team, which iscomposed of experts on Latino psychology, psycho-oncology, immigrant health, linguistics, and translation, employed qualitative and quantitative research methods through the mixed methods approach (questionnaire and interview techniques) to gather information in these three areas. Hence, patients and providers were approached to conduct the formative research.

In the provider phase, providers who deliver mental health services to Latino cancer patients completed a questionnaire that explored three areas of focus: (1) psychotherapeutic needs of Latino cancer patients; (2) providers' use and the acceptability of IMCP main concepts (i.e., meaning, purpose in life, experiential sources of meaning, etc.) and the feasibility of the strategies of IMCP (i.e., reflections, assignments, etc.); and (3) barriers to the use of psychotherapeutic services. Our provider sample was evenly distributed in the United States and Latin America; half practiced in the United States, half preferred speaking English, and three-fourths were Latinos. Providers were recruited from the 72 National Cancer Institute-designated US cancer comprehensive centers, 8 oncology centers that provide psycho-oncology services in Latin America, along with 5 national and international organizations that have a high membership of Latino providers of mental health or psycho-oncology services.

In the patient phase, patients completed a mixed method approach with a quantitative and qualitative phase. First, patients completed a questionnaire composed of questions assessing acceptability and feasibility of the goals and therapeutic methods of IMCP and also including scales measuring spiritual well-being (including meaning and faith), hopelessness, quality of life, psychological symptoms, acculturation, religiosity, fatalism, and familism. Then, using purposive sampling, a select group of patients were interviewed to understand their psychotherapeutic needs, acceptability of MCP main concepts (i.e., meaning, purpose in life, experiential sources of meaning, etc.), and the feasibility of the strategies of IMCP (i.e., reflections, assignments, etc.). In the first part of the qualitative interview, patients answered questions about their experience with cancer, as well as questions about the importance or relevance of existential themes and coping after the diagnosis. In the second section of the interview, the interviewer presented the key definitions, reflections, and questions of the seven IMCP sessions and five metaphors of the intervention. Patients were asked to react to the definitions, questions, reflections, and metaphors; the interviewer used the teach-back technique and asked patients to describe what words and phrases they liked and which were more difficult to understand.

Meaning-Centered Psychotherapy: Adaptation Plan Guided by the Ecological Validity Model

Bernal et al.[46] developed a framework, the EVM, consisting of the following eight dimensions that need to be addressed to adapt interventions to be culturally sensitive: language, persons (facilitators), content, treatment concepts, treatment goals, treatment methods or strategies, metaphors, and context.[55] The following sections address the dimensions of the EVM as they pertain to our adaptation of the IMCP.

Language

Language-appropriate interventions are more than the mechanical translation of the interventions. Special efforts are directed toward ensuring the use of culturally syntonic language for certain treatments. Culturally responsive language is instrumental in ensuring that the intervention is received as intended.

The adaptation team assembled a panel of Spanish speakers who represented a diversity of broad speech communities from the Spanish-speaking world (i.e., Puerto Rico, Mexico, Colombia, Argentina, Venezuela, Uruguay, Dominican Republic, Spain, etc.). A list of all key MCP terms and concepts (i.e., identity, sources of meaning, and transcendence) was distributed to the bilingual consultants. They were asked to produce a translation for each term on their own, and they were warned to preserve the language register or style. All translations were collected, and consensus was achieved for each word based on the term that was most commonly used by all panel members. For example, meaning has two translations to Spanish, *significado* and *sentido. Sentido* was kept because it is more frequently used in the context of existential issues. Furthermore, all study materials were then directly translated. Two translators were involved in the translation and quality control process, and after consensus was accomplished, subject matter experts or bilingual mental health professionals vetted all professional jargon.

To improve the use of culturally syntonic language, the main reflections and questions of the intervention were translated into Spanish and presented to Spanish-speaking patients. Patients were presented first with the translation and were asked to react to the translation and then, if needed, were offered standardized explanations or descriptions discussed by the advisory committee. The teach-back technique (asking the patient to explain, in his or her own words, what he or she understood)[56,57] was used to identify words or phrases that were difficult to understand or for which the original meaning was not accurately conveyed in the Spanish translation. Patients showed the most difficulty understanding the meaning and use of the literal translation of words and phrases such as "sources of meaning," "legacy," "attitudinal sources of meaning," "creative sources of meaning," "transcendence," and "creative call." After providing further explanation, patients were able to offer alternative phrases and explanations to these and other words and phrases that they believed would better convey the desired meaning.

Persons

Persons refer to the similarity and differences between the client and therapist, and the relationship between these individuals. Cultural factors shape this relationship. In the Latino culture, physical proximity and nonverbal communication are essential in building and sustaining client and therapist rapport; often, Latinos prefer physical proximity and generally expect nonverbal gestures, such as a hand on the shoulder from a therapist. To ensure awareness of such factors, our cultural adaptation team is composed of experienced bilingual and bicultural investigators and interviewers, with representation from varied Latino backgrounds, including members from Puerto Rico, Mexico, Cuba, Nicaragua, Colombia, Argentina, and Spain.

Content

Content is defined as cultural knowledge, which refers to cultural values, shared understanding, practices, and traditions. In the Latino culture, these may include collectivism, familism, sympathy, personalism, gender roles, time orientation, and so on. Existing treatments should be adapted to incorporate cultural values and social norms.

Patients were asked to react to the content and language of key definitions, reflections, and questions of the seven MCP sessions. Patients often offered alternative phrases and narratives that were more consistent with their values and language. Examples and narratives illustrating collectivism, familism, and other cultural values can be integrated into the manual. Also, in this formative phase, the adaptation team examines whether cultural values, such as familism and religiosity, and acculturation moderate the relationship between meaning and existential coping with the psychological adjustment of Latino cancer patients. These might be possible factors that may also moderate the intervention efficacy.

Treatment Goals

Goals of the treatment should be congruent with the goals of the clients. It is desirable to frame goals within the values, norms, and traditions of the group in question. The goals of MCP are to help patients to enhance hope, make sense of the cancer experience, and attain a sense of legacy.

The acceptability of the goals (enhance hope, make sense of the cancer experience, and develop a sense of legacy) was explored with mental health providers and patients. All patients and 78% of the providers reported that "making sense of the cancer experience" is an important goal. Seventy-eight percent of patients and 90% of providers reported that "finding meaning in life or thinking about the purpose in life" was an important therapeutic goal. Seventy-seven percent of patients and 70% of providers reported that "understanding the purpose in life after a cancer diagnosis" was an important goal. Last, for 77% of patients and 63% of providers, "reflecting on the heritage or thinking about life contributions" is an important therapeutic goal. The concepts of hope and meaning appeared to be highly acceptable for patients and providers. The goals of finding purpose in life and developing a sense of legacy were acceptable for 63–78% of patients and providers.

Treatment Concepts

The treatment concepts refer to the constructs used within a theoretical model in which the therapy is based. The degree to which the treatment concepts are consonant with the culture and context is critical. Concepts of the intervention should be congruent with the belief system of the clients.

Key concepts of MCP include meaning, search for meaning, hope, purpose in life, connecting with life, courage, death and dying, identity, life's limitations, sources of meaning, legacy, and meaningful death. More than 50% of the providers reported that hope (80%), purpose in life (61%), meaning (59%), connecting with life (58%), and courage (57%) were important themes that they explored in psychotherapy with their patients. Themes that were less used in psychotherapy by these providers were death and dying (47%), sources of meaning (27%), legacy (26%), and meaningful death (16%).

Treatment Methods

The treatment methods are the procedures for achieving the goals defined in the treatment. Methods should consider the context and the values of the population. Integrating the family, in appropriate situations, is a compatible strategy with the Latino culture given the importance placed on the family.

We asked patients and providers questions about the acceptability and feasibility of the therapeutic methods (session exercises, homework, and open-ended discussion). Half of the patients reported that they would participate in psychotherapy, and 38% were unsure. In terms of preferences, almost half preferred psychotherapy that lasted one hour, and two-thirds preferred to meet every week. Thirteen percent of the patients preferred individual therapy, one-fourth preferred therapy with family sessions, and another one-fourth preferred group therapy. The most acceptable therapeutic strategies endorsed by patients were doing a project (i.e., photo album and crafts) for their family (40%), video recording their thoughts to share them (30%), and writing reflections (20%). Providers reported that the most acceptable therapeutic techniques were asking patients to do a project (23%), asking patients to write reflections (23%), and asking patients to record their thoughts to share them (9%).

Metaphors

Metaphors refer to the cultural expressions, imagery, and sayings that might be used in treatment or concepts shared by the population in question. The intervention should include culturally consonant ideas, images, and refrains. Sayings and idioms have been described as useful means of introducing metaphors in the therapy with Latinos. Metaphors are the cultural expressions, sayings, or stories that might be used in treatment and should be culturally consonant.

To illustrate the ideas and philosophy of MCP, the psychotherapy includes metaphorical language. These metaphors were presented to patients who were asked to react and express their understanding and opinion of them. The majority of patients understood the metaphors; some of them indicated that some of the metaphors were complex and difficult to understand, and others provided examples from their own lives. For example, patients were presented with the following story about Frankl's experience in concentrations camps:

> Frankl describes how even in the concentration camp, he and his fellow prisoners

> experienced the beauty of the mountains of Salzburg or a particularly vivid sunset more richly than before because of their circumstances. They found solace in the fact that whatever their individual fates, the beauty of nature, of which they were a part, would continue beyond them.

A 50-year-old Latino male responded to this story as follows:

> I liked that you found more beauty in things than before in things you did not notice—like it happened to me with art . . . I found more . . . enjoyment than before . . . the metaphors are a bit too hard [difficult] . . . by hard [difficult] in the sense that we should find something more down to earth—for a simpler example—in order for *Don Tribulcio* [a common folk or "Joe the Plummer"] can say: *Oh okay I get it. . . .*

This participant's reaction demonstrates the need to transcreate (the source text is rewritten to convey the concepts and achieve the aims of the source text while accounting for both language and cultural considerations) some of these metaphors to achieve localization (adjusting language to the needs of the target speech community).[36] During this phase, patients are asked to offer their own metaphors with the same underlying message of the original metaphor.

Context

Context considers aspects and processes such as acculturation, educational attainment, literacy, and migration patterns and history. For immigrants, the cancer experience can be embedded in their migration history. Many immigrants face the triple burden of adjusting to the disease and treatment, adjusting to a foreign culture, and adjusting to a new and unknown health care system. The therapy situation can also be a foreign and new experience for them, different from their usual folk practices and known ways of dealing with emotional strain.

TABLE 11.1 ADAPTATIONS TO THE INTERVENTION

Dimension	Possible Adaptations
Language	Incorporation of phrases and words used by the patients during the qualitative interviews to the manual to increase the cultural fit.
Persons	Inclusion of bilingual and bicultural interventionists and training of interventionists on the MCP theoretical and methodological model, cultural adaptation of psychotherapy, and Latino psychology.
Goals	Provide justification and relevance of the MCP goals to patients and providers, specifically the goals of finding purpose in life and developing a sense of legacy, which were less familiar and used by providers.
Content	Adapt the sessions content using patients' language when possible and to include examples that illustrate key concepts such as familism, collectivism, and migration experience.
Concepts	Provide more definitions and examples, using patients' own language, of the providers' less used concepts, such as death and dying, sources of meaning, legacy, and meaningful death.
Metaphors	Adapt or replace metaphors when necessary with metaphors provided by patients or metaphors that are more relevant to the patient experience. Incorporate Latino-specific sayings into the manual.
Context	Consider the patients' varying levels of education and literacy when translating the concepts and language used in MCP. Include teach-back techniques to ensure patients understand the language and concepts presented to them. Contextual issues (i.e., literacy and migration) will be considered when adapting the language, content, and metaphors of the MCP intervention.
Methods	Therapeutic methods: Assignments can be completed during the session to facilitate engagement and decrease difficulty related to literacy. Incorporate family members to one session if the patient is receptive. Research methods should also be culturally responsive: Incorporate research instruments that have been validated in Spanish.

FUTURE DIRECTIONS

The cultural adaptation team is in the process of analyzing and interpreting the results of the formative phase research. These findings will inform the adaptation and transcreation of the MCP protocol into Spanish. The next steps after the adaptation/transcreation of the protocol will be (1) a pilot feasibility study; (2) protocol revision and new adaptations, based on the findings of the pilot study; (3) efficacy study; and (4) replication in community and international settings. After the formative phase is completed, some possible adaptations to the intervention by the cultural adaptation team may include those shown in Table 11.1.

SUMMARY

In this chapter, the formative phase of the cultural adaptation of meaning-centered psychotherapy for Latinos with advanced cancer was illustrated. The adaptation was motivated by the high prevalence of Latinos with advanced cancer and the need for effective psychotherapeutic interventions that can assist them to cope with the diagnosis, maintain or increase a sense of meaning and purpose in life, increase spiritual well-being, and improve psychological adjustment. CAPM[51] and EVM[55] provide the framework for this adaptation.[34] This chapter described the detailed results of the formative phase of the MCP linguistic and cultural adaptation. Following the EVM, the research information-gathering process focused on seven areas: language, context, persons, metaphors, concepts, goals, and methods.[55] The cultural adaptation team combined quantitative and qualitative strategies to conduct the initial phase of the adaptation. An ongoing adaptation plan is being developed and implemented. Given the need for psychosocial interventions for Latinos diagnosed with advanced cancer, this significant contribution will address the critical lack of palliative cancer care interventions for Latino Spanish-speaking patients.

REFERENCES

1. American Cancer Society. *Cancer Facts & Figures for Hispanics/Latinos.* Atlanta, GA: American Cancer Society; 2009.
2. Smith EM, Gomm SA, Dickens CM. Assessing the independent contribution to quality of life from anxiety and depression in patients with advanced cancer. *Palliat Med.* 2003;17(6):509–513.
3. McClain CS, Rosenfeld B, Breitbart W. Effect of spiritual well-being on end-of-life despair in terminally-ill cancer patients. *Lancet.* 2003;361(9369):1603–1607.
4. Somerset W, Stout SC, Miller AH, et al. Breast cancer and depression. *Oncology.* 2004; 18(8):1021–1034.
5. Luckett T, Goldstein D, Butow PN, et al. Psychological morbidity and quality of life of ethnic minority patients with cancer: A systematic review and meta-analysis. *Lancet Oncol.* 2011;12(13):1240–1248.
6. Eversley R, Estrin D, Dibble S, et al. Post-treatment symptoms among ethnic minority breast cancer survivors. *Oncol Nurs Forum.* 2005;32(2):250–256.
7. Bowen DJ, Alfano CM, McGregor BA, et al. Possible socioeconomic and ethnic disparities in quality of life in a cohort of breast cancer survivors. *Breast Cancer Res Treat.* 2007;106(1):85–95.
8. Krupski TL, Sonn G, Kwan L, et al. Ethnic variation in health-related quality of life among low-income men with prostate cancer. *Ethnic Dis.* 2005;15(3):461–468.
9. Ell K, Xie B, Kapetanovic S, et al. One-year follow-up of collaborative depression care for low-income, predominantly Hispanic patients with cancer. *Psychiatric Services.* 2011;62(2):162–170.
10. Griner D, Smith TB. Culturally adapted mental health intervention: A meta-analytic review. *Psychotherapy Theory Res Prac Training.* 2006; 43(4):531–548.
11. Benish SG, Quintana S, Wampold BE. Culturally adapted psychotherapy and the legitimacy of myth: A direct-comparison meta-analysis. *J Counsel Psychol.* 2011;58(3):279–289.
12. Lorenz K, Lynn J, Dy S, et al. Evidence for improving palliative care at the end of life: A systematic review. *Annal Intern Med.* 2008;148(2):147–159.
13. Breitbart W, Poppito S, Rosenfeld B, et al. Pilot randomized controlled trial of individual meaning-centered psychotherapy for patients with advanced cancer. *J Clin Oncol.* 2012;30(12):1304–1309.
14. Breitbart W, Rosenfeld B, Gibson C, et al. Meaning-centered group psychotherapy for patients with advanced cancer: A pilot randomized controlled trial. *Pscyho-Oncology.* 2010;19(1):21–28.
15. Dwight-Johnson M, Ell K, Lee PJ. Can collaborative care address the needs of low-income Latinas with comorbid depression and cancer? Results from a randomized pilot study. *Psychosomatics.* 2005;46(3):224–232.
16. Ell K, Xie B, Quon B, et al. Randomized controlled trial of collaborative care management of depression among low-income patients with cancer. *J Clin Oncol* 2008;26(27):4488–4496.
17. Penedo FJ, Traeger L, Dahn J, et al. Cognitive behavioral stress management intervention improves quality of life in Spanish monolingual

Hispanic men treated for localized prostate cancer: Results of a randomized controlled trial. *Int J Behav Med.* 2007;14(3):164–172.
18. Napoles AM, Ortiz C, Santoyo-Olsson J, et al. Nuevo Amanecer: Results of a randomized controlled trial of a community-based, peer-delivered stress management intervention to improve quality of life in Latinas with breast cancer. *Am J Public Health.* 2015;105(Suppl 3):e55–e63.
19. Frankl VE. *Man's Search for Meaning.* New York, NY: Washington Square Press; 1984.
20. Spiegel D, Bloom JR, Yalom I. Group support for patients with metastatic cancer: A randomized outcome study. *Arch Gen Psychiatry.* 1981;38(5):527–533.
21. Spiegel D, Yalom ID. A support group for dying patients. *Int J Group Psychother.* 1978;28(2):233–245.
22. Yalom ID, Greaves C. Group therapy with the terminally ill. *Am J Psychiatry.* 1977;134(4):396–400.
23. Kissane DW, Bloch S, Smith GC, et al. Cognitive-existential group psychotherapy for women with primary breast cancer: A randomised controlled trial. *Psycho-Oncology.* 2003;12(6):532–546.
24. Ashing-Giwa KT, Padilla G, Tejero J, et al. Understanding the breast cancer experience of women: A qualitative study of African American, Asian American, Latina and Caucasian cancer survivors. *Psycho-Oncology.* 2004;13(6):408–428.
25. Espinosa G, Elizondo V, Miranda J. Hispanic Churches in American Public Life: Summary of findings. *Interim Rep.* Mar 2003;2:1–29.
26. Moadel A, Morgan C, Fatone A, et al. Seeking meaning and hope: Self-reported spiritual and existential needs among an ethnically-diverse cancer patient population. *Psycho-Oncology.* 1999;8(5):378–385.
27. Moadel AB, Morgan C, Dutcher J. Psychosocial needs assessment among an underserved, ethnically diverse cancer patient population. *Cancer.* 2007;109(2 Suppl):446–454.
28. Culver JL, Arena PL, Antoni MH, et al. Coping and distress among women under treatment for early stage breast cancer: Comparing African Americans, Hispanics and non-Hispanic Whites. *Psycho-Oncology.* 2002;11(6):495–504.
29. Culver JL, Arena PL, Wimberly SR, et al. Coping among African-American, Hispanic, and non-Hispanic White women recently treated for early stage breast cancer. *Psychol Health.* 2004;19(2):157–166.
30. Wan GJ, Counte MA, Cella DF, et al. The impact of socio-cultural and clinical factors on health-related quality of life reports among Hispanic and African-American cancer patients. *J Outcome Meas.* 1999;3(3):200–215.
31. Costas-Muniz R, Hunter-Hernandez M, Rodriguez M, et al. Spirituality in Latino cancer patients: A systematic review of spirituality, religiosity and existential factors in Latino cancer patients. *Psycho-Oncology.* 2014;23:385–385.
32. Bernal G, Jiménez-Chafey MI, Domenech Rodríguez MM. Cultural adaptation of evidence-based treatments for ethno-cultural youth. *Professional Psychol Res Pract.* 2009;40:361–368.
33. Castro FG, Barrera MJr, Holleran Steiker LK. Issues and challenges in the design of culturally adapted evidence-based interventions. *Annu Rev Clin Psychol.* 2010;6:213–239.
34. Bernal G, Scharrón-del-Río M. Are empirically supported treatments valid for ethnic minorities? Toward an alternative approach for treatment research. *Cultur Divers Ethnic Minor Psychol.* 2001;7:328–342.
35. Castro FG, Barrera MJr, Martinez CRJr. The cultural adaptation of prevention interventions: Resolving tensions between fidelity and fit. *Prev Sci.* 2004;5(1):41–45.
36. Gany F, Diamond LC, Meislin R., et al. Ensuring access to research for non-dominant language speakers. In: Schenker M, Castenada X, Lainz AR, eds. *Migration and Health: Research Methods Handbook.* Oakland, CA: University of California Press; 2013.
37. Macario E, Isenberg JA, Quintas I. Drugs + HIV: Learn the Link Campaign. How IQ Solutions and the National Institute on Drug Abuse (NIDA) adapted a television PSA for Hispanic teens. *Cases in Public Health Communication and Marketing*; 2007.
38. Quinn GP, Hauser K, Bell-Ellison BA, et al. Promoting pre-conceptional use of folic acid to Hispanic women: A social marketing approach. *Maternal Child Health J.* 2006;10(5):403–412.
39. Solomon FM, Eberl-Lefko AC, Michaels M, et al. Development of a linguistically and culturally appropriate booklet for Latino cancer survivors: Lessons learned. *Health Promotion Pract.* 2005;6(4):405–413.
40. Hwang W-C. The Formative Method for Adapting Psychotherapy (FMAP): A community-based developmental approach to culturally adapting therapy. *Prof Psychol Res Pract.* 2009;40(4):369–377.
41. Nicolas G, Arntz DL, Hirsch B, et al. Cultural adaptation of a group treatment for Haitian American adolescents. *Prof Psychol Res Pract.* 2009;40(4):378–384.
42. La Roche M, Christopher MS. Culture and empirically supported treatments: On the road to a collision? *Culture Psychol.* 2008;14:333–356.
43. Trimble JE, Mohatt GV. Coda: The virtuous and responsible researcher in another

culture. In: Trimble JE, Fisher CB, eds. *The Handbook of Ethical Research with Ethnocultural Populations & Communities*. Thousand Oaks, CA: Sage; 2002.

44. Huey SJJr, Polo AJ. Evidence-based psychosocial treatments for ethnic minority youth. *J Clin Child Adolesc Psychol.* 2008;37(1):262–301.
45. Koss-Chioino JD, Vargas LA. Through the cultural looking glass: A model for understanding culturally responsive psychotherapies. In: Vargas LA, Koss-Chioino JD, eds. *Working with Culture: Psychotherapeutic Interventions with Ethnic Minority Children and Adolescents*. New York, NY: Wiley; 1992:1–22.
46. Bernal G, Bonilla J, Bellido C. Ecological validity and cultural sensitivity for outcome research: Issues for the cultural adaptation and development of psychosocial treatments with Hispanics. *J Abnorm Child Psychol.* 1995;23(1):67–82.
47. Bernal G, Saez-Santiago E. Culturally centered psychosocial interventions. *J Community Psychol.* 2006;34(2):121–132.
48. Leong FTL. Toward an integrative model for cross-cultural counseling and psychotherapy. *Appl Prev Psychol.* 1996;5(4):189–209.
49. Leong FTL, Lee SH. A cultural accommodation model for cross-cultural psychotherapy: Illustrated with the case of Asian Americans. *Psychotherapy.* 2006;43(4):410–423.
50. Resnicow K, Soler R, Braithwaite RL, et al. Cultural sensitivity in substance use prevention. *J Community Psychol.* 2000;28(3):271–290.
51. Domenech-Rodrıguez M, Wieling E. Developing culturally appropriate, evidence-based treatments for interventions with ethnic minority populations. In: Rastogi M, Wieling E, eds. *Voices of Color: First-Person Accounts of Ethnic Minority Therapists*. Thousand Oaks, CA: Sage; 2004:313–333.
52. Hwang W-C. The psychotherapy adaptation and modification framework: Application to Asian Americans. *Am Psychologist.* 2006; 61(7):702–715.
53. Barrera MJr, Castro FG. A heuristic framework for the cultural adaptation of interventions. *Clin Psychol Sci Pract.* 2006;13(4):311–316.
54. Bernal G, Rodriguez MMD. *Cultural Adaptations: Tools for Evidence-Based Practice with Diverse Populations*. Washington, DC: American Psychological Association; 2012.
55. Bernal G. Intervention development and cultural adaptation research with diverse families. *Fam Process.* 2006;45(2):143–151.
56. Caplin M, Saunders T. Utilizing teach-back to reinforce patient education: A step-by-step approach. *Orthop Nurs.* 2015;34(6):369–370.
57. Farris C. The teach back method. *Home Healthcare Now.* 2015;33(6):344–345.

12

Adaptation of Meaning-Centered Group Psychotherapy in the Israeli Context

The Process of Importing an Intervention and Preliminary Results

GIL GOLDZWEIG, ILANIT HASSON-OHAYON, GALI ELINGER, ANAT LARONNE, REUT WERTHEIM, AND NOAM PIZEM

ADAPTING PSYCHOLOGICAL INTERVENTIONS TO DIVERSE CULTURAL SETTINGS

Different cultures define and construct the meaning of health and health-related issues differently.[1] Studies show that perceptions of both mental and physical illnesses as well as their implications vary across different sociocultural groups.[2,3] Implementation of psychosocial interventions and psychotherapy protocols in different settings and cultural environments should be sensitive to these divergent perceptions. With this idea as a preliminary premise, we started the challenging journey of adapting meaning-centered group psychotherapy (MCGP) to Israeli patients coping with cancer.

The setting of cancer evokes existential thoughts and feelings.[4] These thoughts and feelings constitute a challenge to the patients' and their social environments' (such as friends and relatives) sense of meaning. The need to understand and make sense of the illness seems to be universal. However, the framework of contents and constructs as well as the values that allow for the exploration of questions such as "Why me?" or "Why now?" may differ between cultures. Even values that are a cornerstone of Western medicine, such as patient autonomy, are not necessarily shared by patients/families of all cultural backgrounds.[5]

To import and transfer interventions between cultures and to supply adequate psychotherapy services within diverse cultures, it is important that professionals take the view of both "cultural competence" and "cultural humility."[6] Whereas cultural competence means that professionals should actively seek knowledge about the communities they serve, cultural humility means they should be reflective concerning their own values and cultural beliefs.[6] The importance of cultural sensitivity in both senses (competence and humility) cannot be underestimated. Regardless of the level of match between the professionals' background and culture in which they work, professionals should always be aware that the values and beliefs they carry shape the care they provide.

Nevertheless, while implementing therapies in a different setting than the one in which they were developed, one should balance the need to adhere to the original model and the need to be flexible and sensitive to the participants' cultural characteristics. Psychotherapies and medical treatments are moving toward individually tailored therapies. Individually tailored therapies are consistent with the idea of sensitivity to cultural diversity and subsequently can maximize therapy effectiveness.[7,8] However, individually tailored psychotherapies may result in difficulties in research and costly implementation.[9]

Having a clear definition of culture within the context of therapy and health behavior as a basic premise may serve as a guideline in balancing individually tailored therapies that are specific to a culture/group/individual and cost-effective therapies that offer the same treatment to larger groups.[10] For example, Pasick and D'Onofrio[11] define culture in the context of health behavior as "unique shared values, beliefs, and practices that are directly associated with a health-related behavior, indirectly associated with a behavior, or influence acceptance and adoption of the health education message." Using this or similar definitions enables practitioners to balance between individually tailored therapy and "common ground therapy" by seeking the common beliefs and values concerning health, sickness, and disease within a specific culture that influences personal health behavior.[12]

The idea of balancing between common and individual aspects of psychotherapy is strongly tied to the question of what should be retained and what may be transformed or reshaped while adapting psychotherapy. Adaptation is not a strange concept to the psychotherapy world. During the past decade, there have been adaptations of psychotherapy (even within the same theoretical approach) in various aspects, including setting (couch, chair, and Internet), time frame (number of sessions per week and short-term psychotherapy), and clients (individual, couple, and groups).[13] Although there are many existing protocols for translation and adaptation of measures and questionnaires (e.g., see Beaton et al.[14]), there are almost no protocols for intervention adaptation. This is partially due to the lack of clear statistical and methodological guidelines in the case of psychotherapy. However, interventions that include fidelity measures may be perceived as noting the critical elements of the intervention that exist across cultures (e.g., in mental health field, the fidelity outcome project of evidence-based practices[15]).

Most literature recommendations on psychotherapy adaptations derive from adaptations of intervention manuals for minorities. It is generally agreed that adaptation should consider engagement (attending the therapy) and outcome (effectiveness) as well as any known aspects of the culture that may influence attendance or outcome. For example, such aspects as differences in language, customs, traditions, stressors, and resources should be considered while adapting psychotherapy.[16] Even aspects that may be considered trivial and hence overlooked, such as the average distance between the residence of the patient and the therapy center or issues of health insurance, should be considered while adapting the psychotherapy. In accordance with Bernal's recommendations,[13] we suggest that adaptation should retain the essence of the psychotherapy by retaining the key theoretical constructs, theory of change, and basic procedures. In this chapter, we use this framework of retaining the essence of psychotherapy to describe the adaptation process of MCGP in the Israeli context.

MEANING-CENTERED GROUP PSYCHOTHERAPY

Meaning-centered psychotherapy (MCP) was developed by Breitbart and colleagues.[17,18] MCP is a manualized intervention provided in either individual or group format. It aims to help patients with advanced cancer to sustain or enhance a sense of meaning in life.[18] It utilizes psychoeducational and experiential techniques, and—inspired by the work of Frankel[19,20]—it addresses themes that are related to the impact of cancer on the sense of meaning and identity.[21] Accordingly, following Bernal's[13] focus on key theoretical constructs, theory of change, and basic procedures as essential across cultures, we aimed to keep these constructs as close as possible to the source. Accordingly, key theoretical constructs such as existential meaning and experiential exercises that promote changes in the system of meaning of one's self were retained.

The MCGP[21] is the group intervention version of MCP. The MCGP is based on eight weekly sessions. Each session addresses a specific theme related to the concepts and sources of meaning. These include Session 1: Concepts and Sources of Meaning; Session 2: Cancer and Meaning; Sessions 3 and 4: Historical Sources of Meaning; Session 5: Attitudinal Sources of Meaning; Session 6: Creative Sources of Meaning; Session 7: Experiential Sources of Meaning; and Session 8: Transitions (Reflection and Hopes for the Future).

Randomized controlled trial (RCT) studies have shown that MCP is beneficial in both its individual and its group format in improving spiritual well-being, quality of life, and sense of meaning and in reducing anxiety.[22,23] There is evidence that MCGP is feasible and eligible for RCTs,[24,25] and that it is an effective treatment in comparison to supportive group psychotherapy.[26] MCGP may also be beneficial for caregivers of persons diagnosed with cancer.[27]

SOCIOCULTURAL ASPECTS OF ISRAEL

Israel can be described as a tapestry of people from different origins, cultures, and religions living in an area of 21,643 km^2 with a density of 353.1 people/km^2.[28] In 2013, the total population of Israel was 7,984,500 people; almost half the population is concentrated in 14 large cities.

Israel is considered a Western country with family structure and cultural values that follow a more traditional and patriarchal Middle Eastern paradigm.[29] In comparison to populations of other Western countries, the Israeli population is relatively young with a relatively high number of children per family and low age at first marriage.[30]

The data presented here draw a complex picture of the Israeli society. On the one hand, according to many standard rankings, Israel is similar to developed Western countries. The standard of living in Israel is relatively high: It is 18th of 188 nations on the United Nation's Human Development Index, with high rankings in education and health and low infant mortality rates.[31] On the other hand, it is similar in many respects to traditional societies (higher rates of children per family and lower age at first marriage). As part of the traditional values, extended family members are in many cases involved in caregiving and medical decisions.

The picture becomes more complex when considering population subgroups in Israel. The Israeli Central Bureau of Statistics reports that Jews (including small percentages of non-Arab Christians and undefined groups) make up 79.4% of the Israeli population; Arabs comprise 20.6%. The Arab population is subdivided into Muslims (84.3%), Druze (8%), and Christians (7.7%). More than 3 million immigrants of Jewish origin have arrived in Israel since its establishment in 1948. Approximately one-third of these immigrants were born in Africa or Asia (approximately half were born in the former Union of Soviet Socialist Republics (USSR)), whereas two-thirds were born in Europe or America.[28]

As a result of this complex structure, issues of national history, origins, and religion are continuously debated in Israeli discourse. In addition, the ongoing violent conflict between Jews and Arabs, in addition to the fact that more than one-fourth of the Israeli population is composed of Holocaust survivors and their descendants, brings issues of terror, mortality, and military conflicts into the daily public discourse. The reality of the Holocaust is preached on an almost daily basis in Israel by both conservatives and liberals, who consider themselves as defending the very existence of Israel and Israeli citizens.[32] Thus, it is not overstated to describe a meaning-centered therapy with persons experiencing life-threatening illness as touching the heart of complex constructs in the Israeli culture.

According to the Israel National Cancer Registry,[33] the cancer incidence in Israel is higher than the mean of member countries of the Organization for Economic Co-operation and Development (OECD), whereas cancer death rates are lower than the OECD mean. Age standardized cancer incidence rates in Israel (per 100,000) are 286.11 and 316.62 for Jewish males and females, respectively, and 222.35 and 201.01 for Arab males and females, respectively. Age standardized cancer death rates in Israel (per 100,000) are 96.7 and 81.1 for Jewish males and females, respectively, and 100 and 66.2 for Arab males and females, respectively. The highest incidence rates are among the 75 years or older age group. Approximately 8% of people age 65 years or older are diagnosed with cancer, and cancer cases in this group constitute approximately 53% of the total cancer cases in Israel.[34] The majority of elderly cancer patients still live in their own homes, with care provided by close family members (because of the fairly traditional family structure in Israel). At least 40% of primary caregivers are spouses, with a majority being women (66%).[34]

THE ADAPTATION PROCESS OF MEANING-CENTERED GROUP PSYCHOTHERAPY

The adaptation process consists of four stages: Identifying the need and having the desire, translating the manual, pilot intervention, and a second pilot intervention accompanied by structured assessment.

Identifying the Need and Having the Desire

Our view is that any adaptation and/or translation of intervention must be based on a desire to do so. Desire is not only a "gut feeling" but also the combination of a clinical need for an intervention, scientific evidence for the expected outcomes, and being comfortable with conducting and assessing the intervention.

Our team includes psychologists experienced in working with cancer patients in both individual and group settings. Whereas we are all clinicians with experience in psycho-oncology, the first two authors are also researchers who have experience in psycho-oncology research. After participating in a workshop on MCP, we believed that this protocol may serve both clinicians and clients to support the existential work that is done in psycho-oncology units. Given ethical considerations and the amount of investment needed to adapt an intervention, it is important to be sure that the intervention has the potential to benefit patients. Thus, we read and discussed within our team the accumulating research evidence showing the benefits of MCP for persons with cancer as presented in this chapter.

Translating the Manual

After obtaining permission from the developers of the intervention, the manual was translated into Hebrew by a student of clinical psychology who is a native English speaker and familiar with the basic concepts of the intervention. We preferred translation by a student and not by a professional translator because we agreed that translation by someone who is familiar with the basic concepts and theories may better retain the essence of the intervention. Four experienced clinicians discussed this translation (two of them attended the MCP workshop). Final language adjustments were done based on this discussion.

Pilot Interventions

The pilot study included two group interventions. The goal of the first group intervention was to examine the working process and to "fine-tune" the translation. The second group intervention was accompanied by standardized measurements intended to obtain preliminary results concerning the outcomes of the interventions. Both group interventions were conducted in a hospital setting and were moderated by two experienced clinicians. The Helsinki Committee of each hospital approved the two group interventions.

The first group included six advanced lung cancer patients (age 65 years or older). Patients were heterogenic in terms of time since diagnosis, religiosity, and gender (one man and five women). None were born in Israel. The second group included seven women 1–4 years post-diagnosis of stage IV breast cancer.Both group interventions were conducted in public hospitals in Israel and were free of charge for the participants.

We first discuss the adaptation of the two group interventions together and then the preliminary results based on the self-report measures applied during the second group intervention. Adaptations of the MGCP can be classified as adaptations of the framework and setting and adaptations of the contents.

Contextual Adaptations

Framework adaptations included adding more sessions (up to 12 sessions) due to patterns of self-disclosure, communication, and the fact that the interventions were being implemented in Israel. Our experience with group interventions in Israel (including the MCGP pilot groups) taught us that participants tend to share a lot and show deep involvement with other participants. The participants were eager to give advice and share their own experience and homework assignments with other members of the group; they did not necessarily adhere to the time limits. We decided that additional meetings would enable more participants to be fully involved with the others in the group. This would allow them to fully express themselves and to fully share their experience and homework assignments.

In addition, group cohesion issues were addressed while taking into account cultural aspects. The nature of the Israeli culture makes it difficult to differentiate between the personal and the public and between the original goals of the MCGP and social aspects of the group. Thus, the strong need of the participants for social support and for sharing experience was reflected in the second group intervention through a "WhatsApp Group" started by the participants. "WhatsApp" is a smartphone application that allows people to exchange text messages, photos, and videos between group members. These groups are very common in Israel. An average family can have several different groups: kids only, parents only, the entire family, and so on. It was almost natural for the MCGP group to form such a group.

This WhatsApp group had a practical goal of sharing information. It also allowed group members to exchange emotional support. The creation of this group is a sign of group coherence. Although we do not recommend that moderators initiate such a group, we do recommend that they join the group if they are invited. They should leave the group at the end of the intervention to enable the participants to continue using it as an independent support group. We also decided to allow the last session to be conducted in a festive setting, such as the home of one of the participants or a café. This was considered as another sign of group coherence and a "thank-you" ceremony for the coordinators of the group.

Interestingly, women in the second pilot group kept in touch with each other after the intervention ended. When one of the participants died a few months after the end of the intervention, the group applied (as a group) to the moderators and asked for another session. The session was dedicated to meaning. It seems that this pattern is very relevant to Israeli society, which acts as a tribe or unified group after traumatic events.

Content Adaptation

Adaptations of the intervention content were based first on Frankel's book as related to personal stories of first- and second-generation Holocaust survivors. Frenkel's book is perceived in the Israeli culture as connected directly to the Holocaust, which, as previously mentioned, is apparent in the Israeli discourse. Thus, the book may bring into the discussion Holocaust issues at the expense of other issues. Also, the Hebrew translation of Frenkel's book is very old and difficult to read. Based on these reflections, reading the book was only optional and not mandatory.

Second, adaptations were based on specific life events, such as immigration and loss, that are common in Israeli society. More time was needed for exploration of these issues. Older participants may have immigrated to Israel and may have lost or been separated from close family members. It is also likely that older participants have a Holocaust background or are themselves survivors or related to Holocaust survivors. Others may have experienced losses through the Israeli wars and terrorist attacks. Thus, it is not uncommon for an Israeli family to experience multiple losses. For example, an association of one of the participants in the second group during the Legacy Project stated, "Wow where do we grow up? . . . I lost a brother in the war and was left as a 10-year-old girl with parents that are Holocaust survivors . . . the whole Jewish legacy is hiding here . . . I'm a pride to my parents. . . . Only the cancer disturbs . . . it's not related to anything." The participant spontaneously associated between the cancer and other actual and potential losses within the Israeli cultural context.

Third, adaptations were based on the relations between the ongoing conflicts and threats to Israeli society and issues of existential fears and meanings. The participants believed that the existential situation in Israel does not leave them space to discuss their illness. However, the disease sometimes does serve as a metaphor or analogy to the current existential situation in Israel.

Fourth, private names almost always have a specific meaning. Jewish–Israeli names are usually based on meaningful Hebrew words or meaningful biblical and historical figures. It is also common to name children after deceased relatives, relatives who were killed during the Holocaust, or soldiers who were killed during military combat. It is very common in traditional families to change the name of patients diagnosed with chronic illness (replace the name with another name, add a new name, or replace a letter in the name) in order to change their fate.

Other issues include the support system in the Israeli culture. The combination of a dense population under a constant threat results in feelings of shared fate and responsibility. In times of national and/or personal crisis, Israelis seek and accept support from relatives, friends, neighbors, and even strangers. Israelis easily share their positive and negative experiences, thoughts, and feelings with others.

Children play a significant role in Israeli society, and the parental role is considered very meaningful. Children and childbirth play a significant role in the Legacy Project. Interestingly, all children in the public education system have to complete a "Roots Project" during the seventh grade. The project deals with the history, roots, and legacy of the children's families. Sometimes it is mixed with the Legacy Project of the MCGP.

All these adaptations were based on the rationale that the history and sociocultural aspects of any environment are important to understanding group-based interventions because the group serves as a microcosm of the environment[35] and is reflected by it. Therefore, therapists carefully traced themes that are grounded in the Israeli culture.

Of note, Israel is a young country that was established after the Holocaust. It is also a country that copes with cultural diversity due to immigration as well as ongoing internal and external conflicts. These aspects form a unique baseline for coping with cancer in general and specifically for participation in MCGP. In his discussion of the psychological aspects of politics in Israel, Bar-Tal[36] suggests that emotions are cultural–societal reflections that can be understood beyond the individual level. Accordingly, the collective emotional orientation of fear is functional in times of conflicts and overrides hope as a cognitive orientation.[36] This phenomenon of emotional and cognitive orientation may occur when persons in Israel must cope with different existential challenges beyond politics. Accordingly, special therapeutic attention should be given to the fear default. Attention should also be given to attempts to explore meaning and hope.

Patterns of familial support and organization may also differ between Israel and other societies. Israel's cultural climate includes modern as well as traditional aspects.[37] These may influence the patterns of familial and social support while coping with stressors.[38] Israel's cultural climate can also influence parental aspects of caring for children while coping with cancer.[39,40] Accordingly, due to tied familial and communal relationships, the adaptation seems to be needed when addressing the relational meaning that stems from the familial context. For example, a single religious woman who had difficulties with the Legacy Project said, "What do I leave after me if I have no children?" She continued,

> Why did I come to this world? . . . To be a mother? Is this my destiny in this world? There are many mothers in the world, so what makes me so special? Maybe the fact that I grew up in a traditional-religious home. . . . In the religion they say that after a person fulfilled his mission in this world he has to go. . . . I got cancer and if my goal and mission is to be a mother I still didn't fulfill it. . . . Maybe I need to look for other missions in other places maybe I haven't found it and still looking.

This woman died a few months after the end of the group but not before she made a detailed will that specified who would raise her dog and who would get her car. She also left a detailed notebook with letters and pictures for her relatives and friends.

Standardized Evaluation of the Second Group

Addressing the meaning and identity and enhancing a comprehensive, integrative, and coherent sense of self and meaning are critical to coping with advanced cancer. Having cancer—especially in advanced stages—challenges one's sense of self and may alter it due to implications of illness and treatment.[41,42] Thus, central to the understanding of the experience of the self in coping with cancer is the concept of self-clarity. This refers to the level of clarity, consistency, and confidence one has with regard to his or her beliefs about the self.[43,44] Having a clear sense of self is related to the sense of meaning in life,[45] which in turn is related to positive strategies employed while coping with cancer.[46]

Accordingly, we chose standardized evaluation instruments concerned with both meaning and identity issues (sense of meaning and sense of self-clarity) as well as with symptoms of anxiety and depression that are common among cancer patients. All of the chosen instruments are available in Hebrew and have satisfactory psychometric properties. Instruments were administered before the intervention started, four times during the intervention (after meetings 3, 6, 9, and 12), and 2 months after the intervention.

Instruments

The Life Regard Index (LRI) was used to assess the sense of meaning in life.[47] The LRI has two subscales—Fulfillment (FU) and Framework (FR). These refer to the fulfillment of life goals and to having and progressing toward personal goals and having a framework or perspective from which life goals can be derived and viewed. The questionnaire includes 28 items rated on a Likert scale ranging from 1 (highly disagree) to 5 (highly agree). Half of the items are phrased in negation. The authors of the questionnaire[47] reported high retest reliability (r = 0.94). Others have reported high internal consistency reliability (Index = 0.8, FR = 0.79, FU = 0.87).[48]

The Self-Concept Clarity Scale (SCCS)[43] was used to examine the extent of clarity, consistency, and stability in one's self-beliefs. The SCCS has 12 items rated on a 5-point Likert scale ranging from 1 (highly disagree) to 5 (highly agree). High scores indicate high clarity. The authors of the SCCS reported a Cronbach's alpha of 0.86, indicating high internal consistency reliability. The retest reliability was 0.79 and 0.70 over a period of 4 and 5 months, respectively.[43]

The Hospital Anxiety and Depression Scale (HADS)[35] was used to assess anxiety and depression. HADS consists of 14 items. Each item was rated from 0 to 3 according to severity of anxiety and depression. Eight items require reverse scoring. After this, depression and anxiety subscale totals can be summed. Each subscale score can range from 0 to 21. The reliability of the scale in both the original English version and the Hebrew version is satisfactory and ranged from 0.83 to 0.92.

Results

We had complete data for only six participants (one of the participants did not complete all of the questionnaires). Unfortunately, we could not perform significance tests with only six participants, and thus we present the descriptive data for each of the six participants (Figures 12.1–12.5). To simplify the data, we present only three of the six time points (the first measure before the group started, the fifth measure taken after the last meeting, and the sixth measure taken 2 months after the last session). Depression (Figure 12.1) metrics decreased for four of the six participants (and did not change for one participant) after the end of the last session. We identified a relapse in the depression measures 2 months after the intervention. The mean depression measures decreased after the last session (from a mean of 13.05 before the intervention to a mean of 10.33 after the last session) and relapsed 2 months after

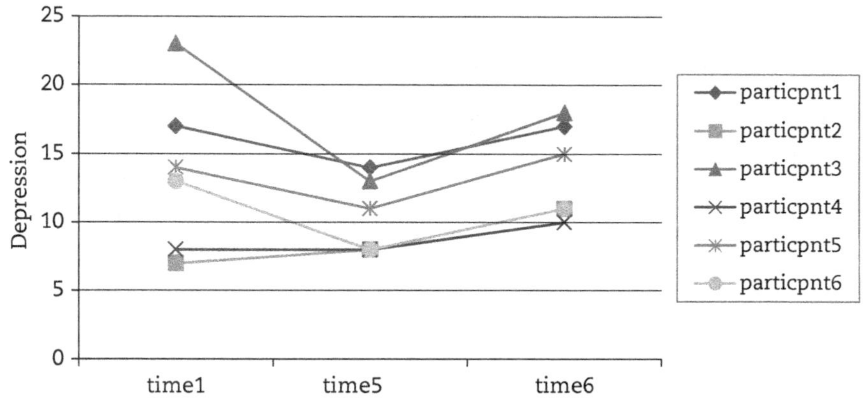

FIGURE 12.1 Depression levels of the six participants by time.

the intervention (mean = 13.67). Anxiety levels (Figure 12.2) decreased between the first session and last measure for four of the six participants (and did not change for one participant). The mean anxiety scores decreased from a mean of 16.14 before the first session to 14.00 after the last session, with a small relapse 2 months after the intervention. The results for the self-clarity measures (Figure 12.3) were mixed: Three participants reported higher levels of self-clarity after the end of the intervention, one reported almost no change, and two reported negative change. The FR metric (Figure 12.4) increased for some of the participants and decreased for others, but whereas decreases ranged between 1 and 4 points, increases were at least 10 points. The FU metric (Figure 12.5) increased for five of the participants (2–12 points) and decreased for one participant (only by 1 point). The means for both FR and FU metrics increased when comparing the measures before the intervention to the measures 2 months after the intervention (FR from a mean of 50.72 to a mean of 52.50; FU from a mean of 52.14 to a mean of 54.67).

CONCLUSIONS

Our conclusions are limited because we conducted only two pilot studies with a small number of participants and no control groups. The data are both quantitative and qualitative and indicate that MCGP was beneficial to most of the patients in terms of depression, anxiety, and meaning fulfillment. Adaptations made to the content and framework seem to be appropriate.

There are also indications of depression and anxiety relapses after completion of the intervention. Therefore, we recommend "booster sessions"—that is, periodic additional therapy sessions that will reinforce the initial progress. The individual data also seem to indicate higher variability within the participants after concluding the intervention compared to the beginning of the

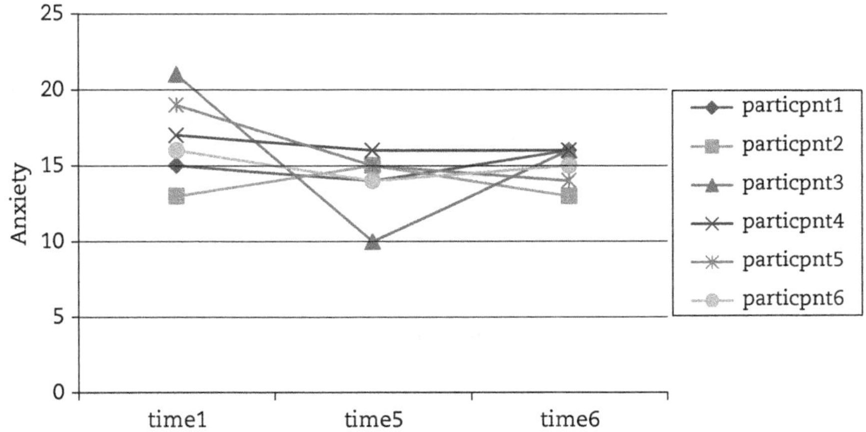

FIGURE 12.2 Anxiety levels of the six participants by time.

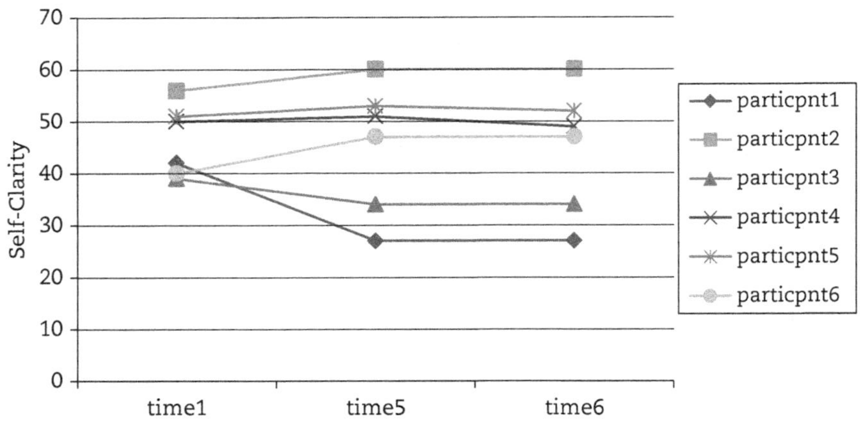

FIGURE 12.3 Self-clarity levels of the six participants by time.

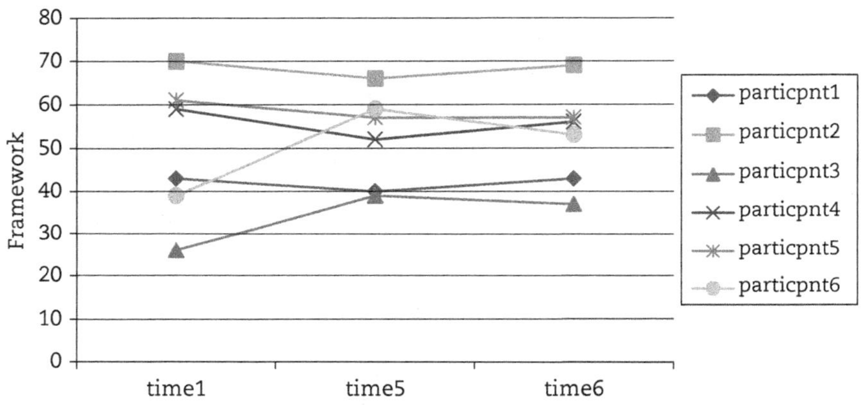

FIGURE 12.4 Framework levels of the six participants by time.

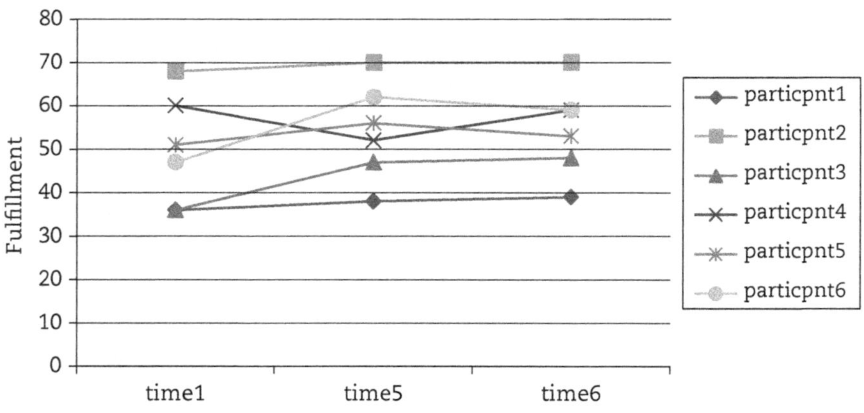

FIGURE 12.5 Fulfillment levels of the six participants by time.

intervention (in all measures except self-clarity). This finding implies that different people may utilize the MCGP differently. The next step should be a large-scale study in several cancer centers to validate our preliminary results. In addition, more research is needed to target the profiles of patients who can benefit more from the intervention and target patients who may need a different form of intervention.

Notably, the pilot study described here included Israeli Jews. In Israel, there are two ethno-national groups characterized by different cultures, traditions, and customs: Jews and Arabs.[49–51] Despite each group's religious-based differences, these groups do share a heritage, language, customs, and ethnic ancestry.[52] The majority of Israeli Arabs have been described as having traditional collectivistic tendencies, whereas most Israeli Jews have been described as having more modern and individualistic tendencies.[53–55] These differences are expressed in both formal service utilization and social support utilization. A study based on an analysis of national hospitalization records found that Israeli Arabs significantly underutilize mental health services compared to Israeli Jews.[56] Another study on patterns of social support showed that Israeli Arabs tend to use familial support, whereas Israeli Jews tend to use support provided from spouses, friends, and professionals.[57] Accordingly, efforts to adapt this protocol and implement it and assess its effectiveness among different ethno-cultural groups in Israel are needed.

Case Example

To demonstrate some of the issues discussed in this chapter, we present excerpts from two group sessions of our second MCGP interventions. Participants were seven women diagnosed with stage IV breast cancer, 1–4 years after diagnosis. We have changed identifying information such as age and place of birth. Cultural issues in these meetings included the Jewish heritage and legacy, the meaning of names in the Israeli culture, and the place of war and the Holocaust in the Israeli discourse. We have minimized our interpretations (text in brackets) in order to let readers judge and evaluate the excerpts for themselves.

> The fifth meeting started as all other meetings with a "check in" round. L brought book dealing with healing from cancer which she decided to give as present to somebody else in the group. L says the she gets free sessions of acupuncture and she wants to pass over the "giving." [The concept of giving is a central issue in the Jewish religion and heritage.] A express her thanks to the group for not letting her leave the group as she intended in the last meeting and she said she needs the group in order to be able to discuss not only her strengths but also her weaknesses. After a short discussion the coordinators move towards reviewing the homework assignments. A few minutes are given to participants who didn't complete the assignments at home to complete it onsite. O mentions that the legacy project enabled her to share feelings with her own family. L asked to be the first to talk. She describes her childhood with two Holocaust survivor parents and a big brother that was killed in one of the Israeli wars. She talks about how she always had to be the strongest person in the family. She has three names: Two of them are names of grandmothers that were killed during the Holocaust. Her third name is an Israeli name given to her by her late brother. She talks about the way the whole Jewish heritage is concealed in her privet life and how she tries to find the meaning of her cancer diagnosis within this complex heritage. [L's familial situation brings into discussion the complex issue of the Jewish heritage, Holocaust, and Israeli war. She brings to attention the extent to which the past legacy is connected to the present and the extent to which private meaning is connected to the public. She also bring into discussion the deep meaning of names in the Jewish and Israeli traditions.] E says that her own name comes also from her grandmother. After she was diagnosed a rabbi she trusts suggested adding another private name with a meaning that is connected to healing. She said she is confused and don't know what name she should use. Her original name is very important to her since it symbolizes the legacy and tradition that are very important to her and that she wants to transfer to her children. Another participant tells that she's called upon her great grandmother and she tells the group about the difficulties that her father had in fighting to let the family immigrate to Israel. She tells the group how important is the religion in her family and that her believe in God helps her to cope [As mentioned previously, family support and family involvement are "built" into the Israeli culture.]

In the next meeting, while discussing the rest of the homework assignments one of the participants tells the other about the country her family immigrated to Israel from. She said she comes from an individualistic culture and she's jealous about the family support the other participants get. The group discusses the things that they want or don't want to take and keep from their families and their mothers. They discuss the idea that each person has a role in life and that one can't die before he or she have fulfilled this role. Another participant tells the group how her family immigrated to Israel when she was 9 years old but she's still part of the culture in her original birthplace. Her Israeli husband has even learned the language of that country in order to be more connected to her cultural roots. She tells the group that her name has meaning both in Hebrew (in Israel) and in her mother tongue. She talks about the feeling of being different when she came to Israel and didn't know the language and customs. She says that her experience in being different helps to cope. She says, "I take with me the idea that I'm different and this helps me to cope and to make progress."

REFERENCES

1. Helman CG. *Culture, Health and Illness.* Boca Raton, FL: CRC Press; 2007.
2. Kirmayer LJ, Bhugra D. Culture and mental illness: Social context and explanatory models. In: Salloum IM, Mezzich JE, eds. *Psychiatric Diagnosis: Patterns and Prospects.* New York, NY: Wiley; 2009:29–37.
3. Angel RJ, Williams K. Cultural models of health and illness. In: Cuéllar I, Paniagua FA, eds. *Handbook of Multicultural Mental Health: Assessment and Treatment of Diverse Populations.* New York, NY: Elsevier; 2000:25–44.
4. Kim Y, Schulz R, Carver CS. Benefit-finding in the cancer caregiving experience. *Psychosom Med.* 2007;69(3):283–291.
5. Deiss R. Ethics and multiculturalism in the patient–physician encounter. *The Virtual Mentor.* 2007;9(8):523–526.
6. Tervalon M, Murray-Garcia J. Cultural humility versus cultural competence: A critical distinction in defining physician training outcomes in multicultural education. *J Health Care Poor Underserved.* 1998;9(2):117–125.
7. Kohn-Wood LP, Hooper LM. Cultural competency, culturally tailored care, and the primary care setting: Possible solutions to reduce racial/ethnic disparities in mental health care. *J Mental Health Counsel.* 2014;36(2):173–188.
8. Ross S, Anand SS, Joseph P, et al. Promises and challenges of pharmacogenetics: An overview of study design, methodological and statistical issues. *JRSM Cardiovasc Dis.* 2012;1(12).
9. Garland AF, Hawley KM, Brookman-Frazee L, et al. Identifying common elements of evidence-based psychosocial treatments for children's disruptive behavior problems. *J Am Acad Child Adolesc Psychiatry.* 2008;47(5):505–514.
10. Egede LE. Race, ethnicity, culture, and disparities in health care. *J Gen Intern Med.* 2006;21(6):667–669.
11. Pasick RJ, D'Onofrio CN, Otero-Sabogal R. Similarities and differences across cultures: Questions to inform a third generation for health promotion research. *Health Educ Q.* 1996;23(Suppl):S142–S161.
12. Baider L, Goldzweig G. The magic of dreams: Conflicts and quandaries within multicultural societies in transition. In: Silbermann M, ed. *Cancer Care in Countries and Societies in Transition.* New York, NY: Springer; 2016:47–64.
13. Bernal G, Domenech Rodríguez MM. Advances in Latino family research: Cultural adaptations of evidence-based interventions. *Family Process.* 2009;48(2):169–178.
14. Beaton DE, Bombardier C, Guillemin F, et al. Guidelines for the process of cross-cultural adaptation of self-report measures. *Spine.* 2000;25(24):3186–3191.
15. McHugo GJ, Drake RE, Whitley R, et al. Fidelity outcomes in the national implementing evidence-based practices project. *Psychiatr Serv.* 2007;58(10):1279–1284.
16. Lau AS. Making the case for selective and directed cultural adaptations of evidence-based treatments: Examples from parent training. *Clin Psychol Sci Pract.* 2006;13(4):295–310.
17. Greenstein M, Breitbart W. Cancer and the experience of meaning: A group psychotherapy program for people with cancer. *Am J Psychother.* 2000;54(4):486.
18. Thomas LPM, Meier EA, Irwin SA. Meaning-centered psychotherapy: A form of psychotherapy for patients with cancer. *Curr Psychiatry Rep.* 2014;16(10):1–6.
19. Frankel VE. *The Unheard Cry for Meaning.* New York, NY: Simon & Schuster; 1978.
20. Frankel V. *Man's Search for Meaning.* New York, NY: Washington Square Press; 1963.

21. Breitbart W, Poppito SR. *Meaning-Centered Group Psychotherapy for Patients with Advanced Cancer: A Treatment Manual.* New York, NY: Oxford University Press; 2014.
22. Breitbart W, Poppito S, Rosenfeld B, et al. Pilot randomized controlled trial of individual meaning-centered psychotherapy for patients with advanced cancer. *J Clin Oncol.* 2012; 30(12):1304–1309.
23. Breitbart W, Rosenfeld B, Gibson C, et al. Meaning-centered group psychotherapy for patients with advanced cancer: A pilot randomized controlled trial. *Psycho-Oncology.* 2010;19(1):21–28.
24. Spek N, Uden-Kraan CF, Vos J, et al. Meaning-centered group psychotherapy in cancer survivors: A feasibility study. *Psycho-Oncology.* 2014;23(7):827–831.
25. van der Spek N, Vos J, van Uden-Kraan CF, et al. Effectiveness and cost-effectiveness of meaning-centered group psychotherapy in cancer survivors: Protocol of a randomized controlled trial. *BMC Psychiatry.* 2014;14(1):1.
26. Breitbart W, Rosenfeld B, Pessin H, et al. Meaning-centered group psychotherapy: An effective intervention for improving psychological well-being in patients with advanced cancer. *J Clin Oncol.* 2015;33(7):749–754.
27. Applebaum AJ, Kulikowski JR, Breitbart W. Meaning-centered psychotherapy for cancer caregivers (MCP-C): Rationale and overview. *Palliat Support Care.* 2015;13(06):1631–1641.
28. Statistics TCBo. *Statistical Abstract of Israel 2015.* http://www.cbs.gov.il/reader/shnatonenew_site.htm; accessed February 2016.
29. Goldzweig G, Abramovitch A, Brenner B, et al. Expectations and level of satisfaction of patients and their physicians: Concordance and discrepancies. *Psychosomatics.* 2015;56(5):521–529.
30. McNicoll G; United Nations Department of Economic and Social Affairs, Population Division: Population, resources, environment and development database, Version 4.0. *Population Dev Rev.* 2006;32(4):790–791.
31. *Human Development Reports 2015.* http://hdr.undp.org/en/2015-report; accessed February 2016.
32. Bar-On D. Israeli society between the culture of death and the culture of life. *Israel Stud.* 2005;2(2):88–112.
33. State of Israel Ministry of Health. *National Cancer Registry.* http://www.health.gov.il/ENGLISH/MINISTRYUNITS/HEALTHDIVISION/ICDC/ICR/Pages/default.aspx; accessed February 2016.
34. Goldzweig G, Merims S, Ganon R, et al. Coping and distress among spouse caregivers to older patients with cancer: An intricate path. *J Geriatr Oncol.* 2012;3(4):376–385.
35. Zigmond AS, Snaith RP. The Hospital Anxiety and Depression Scale. *Acta Psychiatr Scand.* 1983;67(6):361–370.
36. Bar-Tal D. Why does fear override hope in societies engulfed by intractable conflict, as it does in the Israeli society? *Political Psychol.* 2001;22(3):601–627.
37. Lavee Y, Katz R. The family in Israel: Between tradition and modernity. *Marriage Fam Rev.* 2003;35(1-2):193–217.
38. Goldzweig G, Hubert A, Walach N, et al. Gender and psychological distress among middle- and older-aged colorectal cancer patients and their spouses: An unexpected outcome. *Crit Rev Oncol Hematol.* 2009;70(1):71–82.
39. Hasson-Ohayon I, Braun M. Being a parent and coping with cancer: Intervention development. *Palliat Support Care.* 2011;9(2):149–152.
40. Braun M, Hasson-Ohayon I, Perry S, et al. Motivation for giving birth after breast cancer. *Psycho-Oncology.* 2005;14(4):282–296.
41. Park CL, Zlateva I, Blank TO. Self-identity after cancer: "Survivor," "victim," "patient," and "person with cancer." *J Gen Intern Med.* 2009;24(2):430–435.
42. Wong JC, Payne AY, Mah K, et al. Negative cancer stereotypes and disease-specific self-concept in head and neck cancer. *Psycho-Oncology.* 2013;22(5):1055–1063.
43. Campbell JD, Trapnell PD, Heine SJ, et al. Self-concept clarity: Measurement, personality correlates, and cultural boundaries. *J Pers Soc Psychol.* 1996;70(1):141.
44. Bigler M, Neimeyer GJ, Brown E. The divided self revisited: Effects of self-concept clarity and self-concept differentiation on psychological adjustment. *J Soc Clin Psychol.* 2001;20(3):396–415.
45. Błażek M, Besta T. Self-concept clarity and religious orientations: Prediction of purpose in life and self-esteem. *J Religion Health.* 2012;51(3):947–960.
46. Jim HS, Richardson SA, Golden-Kreutz DM, et al. Strategies used in coping with a cancer diagnosis predict meaning in life for survivors. *Health Psychol.* 2006;25(6):753.
47. Battista J, Almond R. The development of meaning in life. *Psychiatry.* 1973;36(4):409–427.
48. Debats DL. The Life Regard Index: Reliability and validity. *Psychol Rep.* 1990;67(1):27–34.
49. Al-Haj M. The status of the Palestinians in Israel: A double periphery in an ethnonational state. In: Dowty A, ed. *Critical Issues in Israeli Society.* Westport, CT: Praeger; 2004:109–126.

50. Kupermintz H, Salomon G. Lessons to be learned from research on peace education in the context of intractable conflict. *Theory Pract.* 2005; 44(4):293–302.
51. Suleiman R. Planned encounters between Jewish and Palestinian Israelis: A social-psychological perspective. *J Soc Issues.* 2004;60(2):323–337.
52. Muller JZ. Us and them. *Foreign Affairs.* 2008; 87(2):18.
53. Al-Krenawi A, Graham JR. Culturally sensitive social work practice with Arab clients in mental health settings. *Health Soc Work.* 2000; 25(1):9–22.
54. Mikulincer M, Florian V, Weller A. Attachment styles, coping strategies, and posttraumatic psychological distress: The impact of the Gulf War in Israel. *J Pers Soc Psychol.* 1993;64(5):817.
55. Haj-Yahia MM, Sadan E. Issues in intervention with battered women in collectivist societies. *J Marital Fam Ther.* 2008;34(1):1–13.
56. Al-Krenawi A. Mental health service utilization among the Arabs in Israel. *Soc Work Health Care.* 2002;35(1–2):577–589.
57. Pines AM, Zaidman N. Israeli Jews and Arabs: Similarities and differences in the utilization of social support. *J Cross-Cult Psychol.* 2003;34(4):465–480.

13

Replication Study of Meaning-Centered Group Psychotherapy in Spain

Cultural and Linguistic Challenges

FRANCISCO GIL, CLARA FRAGUELL, AND JOAQUÍN T. LIMONERO

Don't you worry about being important in your life, others will give meaning to your life.

FILM: *A Pastisserie in Tokyo*

DIRECTOR: NAOMI KAWASE

INTRODUCTION

Patients diagnosed with advanced cancer (stage IV) present a greater degree of complexity regarding physical and psychological symptom management.[1–3] For this reason, patients with advanced illness require an intervention model tailored to their specific needs. One such model, meaning-centered group psychotherapy (MCGP), aims to maintain or promote meaning in life, improve quality of life, diminish psychological distress and symptom burden distress, and enhance emotional and spiritual well-being in patients with advanced cancer.[4–9] As Gilbert[10] notes, the body of literature maintains that one of the most important components of well-being is the ability to love and be loved, to care for and be cared for. To care and to be cared for is one of the most important components in psychotherapy group models, and MCGP is no exception.

BACKGROUND

Receiving a cancer diagnosis can trigger feelings of threat and uncertainty for both patients and their families. In stages III and IV of diseases such as cancer, the therapeutic objective is to maintain quality of life and increase survival time for the patient. The literature shows that sustaining a sense of meaning is important for patients with cancer and can enhance psychological and physical well-being through the following examples: (1) Enhancing a sense of meaning improves emotional adjustment to illness; (2) in addition to the high prevalence of emotional distress observed, sustaining meaning allows patients to endorse good quality of life despite physical symptoms attributable to disease or cancer treatments; and (3) patients who experience that their life has meaning have a better emotional adjustment to illness, and their quality of life and physical comfort level are higher. Until recently, there have been no psychological interventions demonstrated to enhance meaning in patients with advanced cancer. Breitbart and colleagues[4,5] developed MCGP for patients with advanced cancer (stages III and IV). This model of psychotherapy aims to encourage patients in their search for meaning through experiences, choosing one's attitude, life reflections, and connection to and development of one's legacy. MCGP sessions consist of didactics, experiential exercises, and discussion in the group setting.

OBJECTIVES, PROCESS, AND TECHNIQUES

The objectives of MCGP are to help patients with advanced cancer live life to the fullest, to maintain and expand meaning in life, and to live peacefully and with a purpose in life. Specifically, the objectives of MCGP are as follows:

- To encourage cancer patients to seek and create meaning in life, despite uncertainties and limitations of their disease
  - To find meaning in past experiences
  - To discover new sources of meaning in life

- To seek ways of overcoming practical limitations
- To discover new ways to reconnect with life transcend
- To learn how to distinguish between the limitations one can change or overcome and to accept those that cannot be changed
- To integrate a diagnosis of cancer into one's life history
- To express feelings and emotions
- To improve one's psychological adaptation by attributing meaning to life

Each session addresses a specific topic: introduction to the concept of meaning, cancer and meaning, sources of meaning, and closing.

Clinical Vignette: Group Session 1

As an illustration of the group process, the following is the transcript of Session 1 of the first group—concepts and sources of meaning. The patients are J, C, M, and T The therapists are Paco and Maribel.

Paco: For this first session, we have given you a sheet. We will have eight sessions over the course of 2 months. We will talk about the meaning and the purpose of life. There are difficult moments, there are moments of difficulty making meaning to our lives or maintaining the meaning of our life or, sometimes, the disease gives us an experience of personal growth. We will start the first session talking about Víctor Frankl. . . . I'll start by giving you a prompt: Remember one or two experiences [or moments] in which life has been especially significant for you, regardless if that experience seems extraordinary or trivial. It could be, for example, something that helped you overcome one difficult day or, on the other hand, a moment in which you felt very alive. Tell it to the group.

T: When I married, the day after getting up, I felt a sense of freedom because I was not allowed out of my old house. I now had my own house, it was like a bird that opens the cage and flies, and I felt in those moments free, and that newly married experience, in my house, my husband, was extraordinary. The other experience that has marked me very much was my mother's death 6 years ago. She was diagnosed with cancer, we were told that it was terminal, and I have not passed yet, so this is one thing that has marked me.

Paco: Thanks, and those experiences you had, what meaning did that have in your life?

T: They were positives, positives, I have missed my mother, but it has been positive, it has given me more strength to life.

Paco: To grow?

T: To grow, yes, because my mother was a negative person, everything was so bad, everything made her scared, or if she was not going with her husband to shop, she could not go shopping alone. It has given me more strength, because I've seen the effect on my mother, and I do not want to be like her.

Paco: Thanks T. J?

J: Things that reinforce my meaning of life? When I travel, day to day is very repetitive, then, when the holidays arrive and you can go to a specific place that you like.

Paco: And something that was significant to you?

J: A moment that affects me a lot is when I am with my family and friends, their support.

Paco: Is friendship something that moves and gives you strength, meaning, in these times of diagnosis?

J: Yes.

Paco: Thanks. C?

C: For me, the lifestyle before, moments full of meaning were those related to work, because it was the priority and also when I am learning things, also traveling. I liked these very much, and I am very curious with everything, seeing things, observing, and work. For me, these are very meaningful.

Paco: And any negative experiences?

C: Negative, 1 year ago my father died. He spent several weeks in a coma, and the situation was irreversible and that was very hard. For me, it was the most difficult experience.

Paco: And what source of meaning do you attribute to these experiences?

C: According to this classification, it would be creative and experiential.

Paco: For you, J?

J: Experiential, too.

Paco: And for you T, it would be also experiential? As legacy?

T: Yes, my mother, is what has given me direction.

Paco: M, talk to us about one or two experiences.

M: Positive, meetings with my daughters. . . . Before the illness I worked, and I was out on the street, I was working in commercial Pharmacy and now . . . [Crying]

Paco: Do you feel OK?

M: Yes, you are sad, you don't give what you have to give. . . .

C: I appreciate it now, I did not appreciate it before, I thought it was just my job, and now I am missing not being able to work.

M: Yes, and it's a shame, does life have meaning? If you don't do anything?

Paco: But, you said that your daughters were the ones who give you meaning in this life.

M: Yes, but I can't be on the top of my daughters, my daughters have their life, I don't want to overwhelm them. I can't tell to my daughters help me, I have to help them. The only goal I have is to reach 28 of May, which is when my daughter gets married. Nobody tells you if you're going to die, nobody tells you how long you'll live with this disease. I was a very active person, was all day working, and now I don't do anything. I laughed before, jumping, dancing, singing, and now nothing, all the expression from my face has gone. Nothing has meaning, I don't want to die, I don't want to suffer, but I think that maybe, I don't know, if there were something more positive, I don't tolerate the chemo [chemotherapy]. I had patience, but every day you wake up, every day it's the same, before I paid attention to my image, my hair was blonde, and now I don't dye it blonde . . . [silence]

Paco: For me, I see much value in what you're doing.

M: No, I don't know, if my daughters tell me something, I change the face. In reality it is difficult . . . I was at the table, and I was absent, and someone could think the next year I will not be here, they don't value it . . . I don't see future. Nobody tells you if you will live 1, 2, or 3 years.

Paco: When you heard J, C, and T, what feelings did you have when they talked about their sources of meaning?

M: So, now that I don't have much meaning, much strength, I would like to change, and I think I have it, but it comes, and nothing happens.

Paco: What do you need?

M: I think that I need to have more contacts with people who have the same experience and who know how to help me, through the experience of others, and also try to help them.

Paco: This is the reason why we are all here together. You have testified important experiences with meaning. I have to say a couple of things: First, that I am committed, together with Maribel [co-therapist] to be here together with all of you, and I ask your commitment to attend group sessions. There will be sessions that can contribute to you and others not as much. Coming and sharing is what helps most. For this reason, I ask the commitment that you come to group sessions. And the second, is that I will send a book by mail, Víctor Frankl's book, "Man's Search for Meaning," that you begin to read, and discuss it at the next meeting. Before finishing, I don't know if you want to comment something or any questions. . . . We will see in the next session. Thank you for coming.

QUALITATIVE ANALYSIS OF RESULTS: CONSTRUCTED AND EMERGENT THEMES

In this section, experiences of participants from the three groups included in our pilot study are presented, and the issues or themes from these experiences are reflected in the MCGP (Table 13.1). Both were proposed (constructed themes) or emerged from the analysis of the transcription (emergent themes) (Table 13.2). We present the constructed and emergent themes along with some quotations.

Constructed Themes

Attitudinal Sources of Meaning: Encountering Life's Limitations

Attitudinal sources of meaning are derived from Frankl's core theme that our last vestige of human freedom is to choose our attitude toward suffering and life's limitations. In order to understand this source of meaning—how to transform personal tragedy into a triumph or how one has succeeded despite adversity—we present the following themes found in the transcriptions:

- Coping, fighting spirit

> I want to live, I want to fight. I don't think "I want to die tomorrow." They must fight, everything is possible. There are sometimes very bad, very bad moments, but then you have to be strong. I trust the doctors and treatments that they are giving me.

- Avoidance

> I looked at TAC and came out a phrase of "tumor" and put another phrase that came out of "metastases" . . . and have not already returned to look at anything else.

- Acceptance

> I will have to live with this tumor all my life; they have already told me and I am mentally prepared.

- Limitations

> I live now mentored, as if they had tied my hands, they take care of me very well. I'm doing well, but I think that someday, I have to return to my life as before, this is a nightmare, I mean, I don't control the situation, I am still in shock.

TABLE 13.1 DEFINITIONS OF THE PRESENTED TOPICS

Topic	Definition
Coping	Strategies used to cope with any situation, such as avoidance, negotiation, and projection
Limitations	Obstacles that are derived from the disease, such as physical or intellectual side effects due to chemotherapy
Personal growth	Process of thinking and learning about the events that happen in one's life
Acceptance	Feeling by which a person admits that his or her situation will not change but, rather, the new circumstance is incorporated into his or her life
Search for meaning	Thoughts on the meaning of life, both past and present
Anger because of the disease	Reaction of anger or rage against the disease for its negative consequences
Crisis of knowledge	Commotion at the time one becomes aware of the disease or its level of severity
Resilience	A person's ability to resist and overcome ongoing assaults
Death	Permanent end of the biological functions of a living being; in this case, due to oncological disease
Personal relationships	Bond linking two or more individuals and that is the basis of life in society; may be with family members, friends, coworkers, etc.
Incomprehension	Feeling misunderstood by others
Need to share	Need to explain and live the experiences of the disease to others
Connection with nature	Individual connection with the elements of nature
Connection with beauty	Individual connection with beautiful elements
Pleasurable activities	Activities that produce pleasure
Outstanding things	Situations and/or activities that have yet to be accomplished before dying
Illusions	Hope something happens
Legacy	What remains when somebody dies
Family history	History of one's own family
Past times	Narration of the past
Threat	Feelings of danger caused by the disease
Benefit of group therapy	Personal perception of the effectiveness (or ineffectiveness) of group therapy
Sadness/apathy	Inability to feel emotion and motivation; state indifference or sadness
Uncertainty	Doubt, lack of knowledge about what will happen
Loss of social role	Loss of social role that unfolds with the diagnosis of disease
Current routine	Everyday life while patients are participating in group therapy

- Personal growth

    Since it happened to me, I have no appreciation for money, what I want is to be able to live, to live long.

- Search for meaning

    Now, I will have to fight to see a grandchild! I have this objective ...

- Anger

    When I think more about it is when I am alone in my bed. I think: "Why do I have this, my God! We were so happy before."

- Knowledge crisis

    When you detect cancer with a CAT [computerized axial tomography], and tell you that there is nothing to do ... everything stops.

- Resilience

    Sometimes, you can't move, by pain, or by the side effects of the chemo : You lose weight, weakness ... but you can tolerate it.

- Death

    Once I was so sick, it was a headache ... I said "God, take me, hopefully right now mom, I die ... come to me, do not make me suffer so ..." I wished with all my heart, and I felt peace when I thought that everything was going to end.

TABLE 13.2 FREQUENCY TABLE OF BUILT AND EMERGING TOPICS

Topic		Group 1 ($n = 7$)	Group 2 ($n = 5$)	Group 3 ($n = 10$)	
		No. (%)	No. (%)	No. (%)	P
Attitudinal sources of meaning	Coping	40 (14.4)	22 (9.9)	20 (8.8)	
	Limitations	24 (8.7)	6 (2.7)	12 (5.3)	
	Personal growth	17 (6.1)	4 (1.8)	6 (2.7)	
	Acceptance	11 (4)	10 (4.5)	2 (0.9)	**
	Search for meaning	8 (2.9)	3 (1.3)	1 (0.4)	**
	Anger due to the disease	5 (1.8)	8 (3.6)	3 (1.3)	*
	Crisis of knowledge	4 (1.4)	4 (1.8)	9 (4)	
	Resilience	3 (1.1)	0 (0)	1 (0.4)	
	Death	0 (0)	4 (1.8)	5 (2.2)	
	Subtotal	112 (40.4)	61 (27.4)	59 (26.1)	
Experiential sources of meaning	Personal relationships	18 (6.5)	27 (12.1)	9 (4)	*
	Incomprehension	7 (2.5)	1 (0.4)	2 (0.9)	
	Need to share	4 (1.4)	3 (1.3)	7 (2.6)	*
	Connection with nature	2 (0.7)	2 (0.9)	0 (0)	
	Connection with beauty	1 (0.4)	0 (0)	0 (0)	
	Subtotal	32 (11.6)	33 (14.8)	18 (8)	
Creative sources of meaning	Pleasurable activities	17 (6.1)	1 (0.4)	9 (4)	**
	Outstanding things	5 (1.8)	4 (1.8)	2 (0.9)	
	Illusions	5 (1.8)	11 (4.9)	3 (1.3)	*
	Subtotal	27 (9.7)	16 (7.2)	14 (6.2)	
Historical sources of meaning	Legacy	16 (5.8)	6 (2.7)	5 (2.2)	**
	Family history	5 (1.8)	14 (6.3)	12 (5.3)	
	Past times	0 (0)	15 (6.7)	6 (2.7)	*
	Subtotal	21 (7.6)	35 (15.7)	23 (10.2)	
Emerging topics	Threat	53 (19.1)	25 (11.2)	48 (21.2)	**
	Benefit of group therapy	10 (3.6)	19 (8.5)	23 (10.2)	
	Sadness/apathy	9 (3.2)	5 (2.2)	4 (1.8)	*
	Uncertainty	7 (2.5)	10 (4.5)	11 (4.9)	**
	Loss of social role	4 (1.4)	6 (2.7)	1 (0.4)	
	Current routine	2 (0.7)	13 (5.6)	25 (11.1)	**
	Subtotal	85 (30.7)	78 (35)	112 (49.6)	
	Total	277	223	226	

$^{*}p < 0.05$; $^{**}p < 0.001$.

Experiential Sources of Meaning: Connecting with Life Through Love, Beauty, and Humor

These are essentially sources of meaning that are derived from our "experience" of life, connecting with life through love, beauty, and humor. To exemplify this source, we present the following themes found in the transcriptions:

- Personal relationships

  It gives me meaning to go to my town, see my brothers and nephews . . . all this for me is very important and, if they are not here, I can go to see them. . . .

- Misunderstanding

  My husband says to me : "I don't know if you are aware that there are some moments that you are wrong, I see that some moments you are active and there are moments that you are not active; I do not know if you do this because of the disease or because you want to abuse of me." Then, I start to cry. During long time, I have had problems with some persons caused by the disease . . . "Why do I have to suffer?"

- Need to share

> I'm talking about everything with my wife, the disease at home is something normal. My daughters ask, I explain what I have to do, the tests . . . it is not taboo, I don't have to make sacrifices. Before, when I was worse, I didn't explain anything, I didn't want to worry my wife, I didn't want to see my daughters suffering . . . but that is why I am here, because I need to talk about it and express it.

- Connecting with life (nature and beauty)

> Now, you see things that before you didn't see, and I didn't consider it. Now, you breathe, and see trees.
>
> The beauty, I really like to travel, I feel most connected with beauty when I visit monuments or museums . . .

Creative Sources of Meaning: Creativity, Courage, and Responsibility

Through creative endeavors, we are afforded the capacity to transcend our given bounds by actively infusing something of ourselves into the world. To exemplify this source, we present the following themes found in the transcriptions:

- Pleasant activities

> It has given meaning to my life and my job, it has always been very important to me and, later, the things that I liked to do, now I can't do, like traveling, reading, my tastes . . .

- Opportunity to recover what one had always wanted to do

> I have stopped painting during these years, because I went to work and I didn't have much time. And now, I'll return to painting on Tuesdays.

- Issues to do

> You have to enjoy. I say to my daughter . . . now we are only my wife and myself, then, less opportunity to enjoy. Although, now I can still enjoy . . .

- The illusions

> The only goal I have is to reach May 28, when my daughter gets married. . . . My daughter's wedding will be her happiest day, and from there, what God wants.

Historical Sources of Meaning: Life as a Legacy That Has Been Given

The patients are witness of their living legacy as a cohesive whole, by integrating past memories, with present accomplishments, toward future contributions. To exemplify this source, we present the following themes found in the transcriptions:

- The legacy

> I thought to write a diary, write letters to the people you love. . . . Perhaps, there are things that you can't tell them, because at this time you do not know how to explain it . . . and so many things that you have inside, and you would like that they had present.
>
> I would like to let them know that I've been always a cheerful person, a person who liked to laugh and to live. Now, I'm not this kind of person, but before, I was so. I always liked to do things . . . I want to think that I was a person who desired to give everything, to make people happy . . . many things!

- Issues past and present

> I have not been able to be the same person as him, I do not have what he had [father] . . . I have had very difficult work. I have always been on the road, I have not been with them [children], as I wanted to be. Now, I am more with them than ever before. Now, I'm happy with what I have. . . . My life has been happy, my mother also had to work hard, lived for us, I would like to be as she was for me.
>
> I think that now the relations between parents and children are much more sincere, more sincere than they were before.

Other Emerging Themes in Spanish Adaptation

In the qualitative analysis, along with the themes constructed by Dr. William Breitbart from his meaning-centered psychotherapy model, arise the following emerging issues:

- Threat

> Now everyone, 90% die of cancer!

Yes, but ... also I think that it depends on how you are. ... For example, now I know that my cancer is stopped, it has not affected the spinal column, and I think that I am more positive for this. If it was progressing, and I was affected by several sites, I don't know how I would be. I think I would be much more down. It would be difficult to find positive things.

- Benefit from attending to the group

I have to say one thing about the first day that I walked out of here ... well today I am also very touched by the girl [a participant in the group], and I can't stop thinking about her ... she touched me, but I think it was good for me. Even last week, I had a visit with my psychiatrist and I told him "I am not able to go to the group. ... I am very touched, but I think that I should wait.

- Sadness

At the end of the year, I was not interested in anyone. We were 30, and on Christmas day, we were having dinner. I went to take my pills and I thought of not returning, I did not care if I was happy or not.

- Uncertainty

I had to be operated on in a month. And, they tell me that I have to wait 3 months. ... I always feel the fear of waiting.

- Loss of the social role

They brought me my grandchildren at seven in the morning until seven in the evening, and for some reason, they have removed me from them, and this hurts.

- Current routines of patients

The next Monday, I can't attend the group because I am going to the doctor. And on Thursday, they will tell me if I'm going to the operating room or not, if the treatment has affected me ... I have the visit with the doctors, and they will decide.

Table 13.2 presents frequencies of occurrence of constructed and emerging themes in each of the groups and compares these between the groups. From Table 13.2, it can be seen that threat is an emerging theme, not proposed by William Breitbart and colleagues in the English version of MCGP. This topic occurs most frequently in the first (19.1%) and third group (21.2%), and it is the second most common theme in the second group (11.2%). Coping is another prevalent theme: It is the second and third most frequent theme in the first (14.4%) and the second group (9.9%), respectively. Other frequent themes are limitations (third most frequent theme in the first group (8.7%)); personal relationships (most frequent theme in the second group (12.1%)); and current routine and the benefit of group therapy as the second (11.1%) and third (10.2%) most frequent themes in the third group, respectively.

To determine if there were differences between groups with respect to the constructed and emerging themes, we performed a chi-square analysis. In this analysis, we observed that there are statistical differences between groups for approximately half of these themes.

CHANGES IN SPIRITUAL WELL-BEING AND PSYCHOLOGICAL FUNCTIONING AFTER MCGP

The results of the three pilot groups of MCGP show a reduction of anxious and depressive symptoms and hopelessness and increased spiritual well-being and meaning, similar to the results of Breitbart et al.'s study (Table 13.3 and 13.4). Also in support of Breitbart et al.'s findings,[4] both meaning and feelings of peace increased for participants after the intervention (Figure 13.1).

TABLE 13.3 CHANGES IN SPIRITUAL WELL-BEING AND PSYCHOLOGICAL FUNCTIONING AFTER MCGP RESULTS PRE- AND POST-INTERVENTION (N = 37)

Pre-intervention	Post-intervention	p
Hopelessness = 6.76	5.81	0.07
Depression = 14.73	15.35	0.09
Anxiety = 2.29	2.16	0.1
Meaning/peace = 2.28	2.79	0
FACIT (meaning/peace/faith) = 2.06	2.53	0

Source: Adapted from from Breitbart W, Rosenfeld B, Gibson C, et al. Meaning-centered group psychotherapy for patients with advanced cancer: A pilot randomized controlled trial. *Psycho-Oncology*. 2010;19:21–28.

TABLE 13.4 CHANGES IN SPIRITUAL WELL-BEING AND PSYCHOLOGICAL FUNCTIONING AFTER MCGP RESULTS PRE- AND POST-INTERVENTION (N = 13)

Pre-intervention	Post-intervention	p
Hopelessness = 5.54	4.69	0.306
Depression = 8.31	6.54	0.061
Anxiety = 10.85	8.62	0.105
Meaning/peace = 2.56	2.83	0.243
FACIT (meaning/ peace/faith) = 2.29	2.44	0.388

CONSIDERATIONS FOR THE APPLICATION OF MCGP IN SPANISH CANCER PATIENTS

Based on the results of the three pilot groups of MCGP for Spanish patients with cancer, we will consider the following adaptations for future studies:

- Increase the number of patients to 10–12 because we estimate a loss of 4 or 5 patients during group sessions.
- Extend the estimated survival time requirement of participating patients to avoid withdrawals for progress of aggravation disease
- Include cancer patients with stage III or stage IV cancer.

These MCGP trials have prompted plans for a future validation study in which we will compare the MCGP model with the compassion/meaning-centered group psychotherapy (CMCGP) model.[11]

DISCUSSION

In the qualitative analysis, we identified six emerging themes not covered by the foundational MCGP for English-speaking participants: threat, benefits of group therapy, sadness, uncertainty, loss of social role, and the importance of a patient's current routine. Furthermore, we discovered that for half of all the themes found (constructed and emerging themes), there were no statistically significant differences between the groups.

Our results indicate that some of the most widespread feelings verbalized by patients were feelings of threat, which coincides with results reported by Van der Spek et al.[12] Van der Spek et al. conducted MCGP with Dutch patients and found that the "threat to identity" was one of the main subjects related to meaning. In our study, some participants also mentioned having a loss of meaning in their lives. These were mainly losses related to physical limitations due to their treatment or the disease itself.

However, many patients reported experiences of personal growth as of result of their disease process; they reported greater awareness of their own life and even an increase in the connection that they had with nature or with beauty. Van der Spek et al.[12] also found an increase in patients

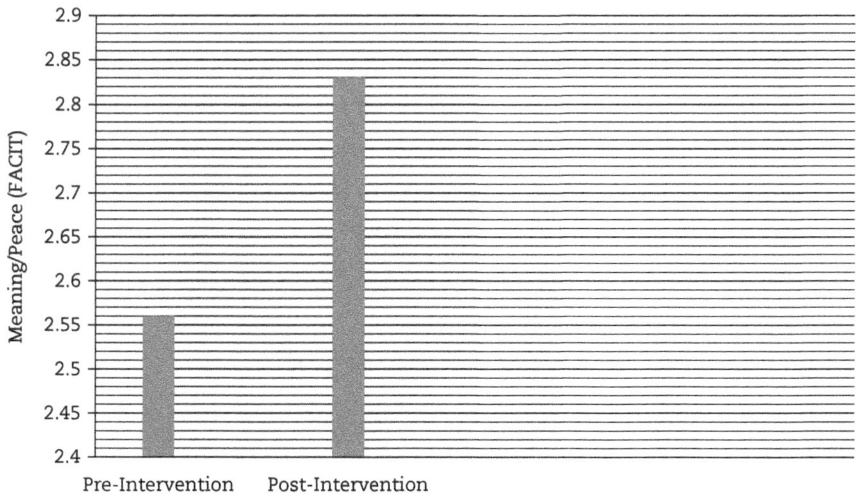

FIGURE 13.1 Patient-reported changes in meaning and feelings of peace before and after intervention.

experiencing life more fully and truly valuing the small things in life—both themes that we have considered as personal growth.

Another common theme among patients was acceptance of both their diagnosis and their prognosis, despite the sense of crisis that often accompanies knowledge of a poor diagnosis/prognosis. Many patients described an acute awareness of the severity of their situation, but many were able to reach acceptance regarding this difficult information.

Loneliness, misunderstanding, and isolation are themes that also arise. Having strong relationships can play an important role for patients and, thus, it is mentioned as one of the most important sources of meaning. Not surprisingly, this theme is strongly related to both feelings that one is misunderstood and the need to share.[13] This ambivalence for patients is usual in these circumstances, such that patients may often experience the need to feel close to others while simultaneously distancing themselves from friends and family.

According to prior research[12,14–16] and in accordance with the results of our study, it is possible for patients living with cancer to experience the disease in an adaptive way by drawing meaning from the experience and transforming it into a source of personal growth. Ryff and Singer[17] observed that psychological well-being consists of two dimensions: living life with purpose and the quality of connections with others. Therefore, it is important to know the barriers associated with difficulty finding meaning in order to promote the creation and adaptation of meaning-based interventions for patients with advanced illness.

Not only do the results of this study validate the themes proposed by Breitbart et al.'s foundational MCGP but also other themes emerge. This finding is important in the context of the adaptation of MCGP for Spanish patients. It would be interesting to determine if these results are similar for Latin American patients, who have similar sociocultural aspects as Spanish patients, and whether these similarities in culture could play an important role in the construction of personal meaning. On the other hand, it would also be helpful to add any new themes that may emerge in order to discuss issues that patients consider to be important.

Although significant differences in themes were found between the MCGP groups, this may be considered normal or even expected because the participants within each group had varied sources of meaning.

FUTURE DIRECTIONS

Three factors are known to have major psychological benefits: maintaining a compassionate attitude toward others, accepting the help of others, and developing a self-compassionate attitude (be sensitive to one's own vulnerability).[10,18–21] In addition, maintaining or promoting a sense of meaning in life improves quality of life and emotional and spiritual well-being in patients with advanced cancer.[4–8] As Guilbert[10] notes, science still shows that one of the most important components of well-being is the ability to love and be loved, to care for and be cared for.

At the molecular level, increased activity of telomerase and the length of the telomeres are related to an increase in survival, lower recurrence, and lower cancer progression. Also, it has been observed that a reduction in anxiety symptoms (intrusive thoughts) is associated with an increase in the activity of telomerase.[22,23] The contemplative techniques (compassionate meditation) reduce anxiety symptoms and increase the activity of telomerase.[24]

Our next project will compare the benefits of two psychological interventions—MCGP and CMCGP—in patients with advanced cancer. The aim of CMCGP is to reduce the emotional distress of patients with advanced cancer by maintaining or increasing their capacity for compassion, self-compassion, meaning, and mindfulness.

Paul Gilbert[10,25] developed compassion focused therapy (CFT), which is a process of development of compassion toward oneself and others; this intervention aims to increase well-being and quality of life. The approach to CFT, although it takes elements borrowed from Buddhist teachings, has a neuroscientist, evolutionary, and psychosocial approach, linked to the psychology of the care. Three variables—feeling safe, caring, and sharing a sense of belonging—are not only associated with a lower tendency for depression, anxiety, and stress but also related to a neurohormonal profile that corresponds with high levels of endorphins and oxytocin.[26,27] In addition, research has shown that the same brain processes operate in compassion and self-compassion, and the brain systems are the same. For this reason, Gilbert[25] proposed that psychotherapists should focus on searching for a mode of stimulating the ability to experience positive emotions associated with feelings of security and well-being in their patients; this is achieved through developing compassion toward oneself and others and increasing sensitivity to perceive and accept compassion of others. This requires access to an implicit emotional system, proposed by the CFT. CFT evolved with the care system of mammals and humans, or system of affection (a neuropsychological-specific structure), that gives rise to our feelings of security. From a psychotherapeutic perspective, Gilbert[25] proposes "the development of inner warmth" that favors working with emotions in a compassionate and kind way. This feeling of caring for others and self-care (compassion and self-compassion), in addition to sharing the same identity or sense of belonging to a group, are two of the goals that we intend to achieve through CMCGP.

Many psychological schools include compassion within their therapeutic approach. Also, for thousands of years, practicing Buddhists have promoted the development of compassion for oneself and for others in order to achieve improvement of one's personal well-being.[25]

In response to the need for interventions focused on enhancing spiritual well-being, we developed CMCGP using the constructs of compassion, self-compassion, meaning, and mindfulness. The first steps of evaluation are compassion, self-compassion, meaning, mindfulness, and spiritual well-being; the second evaluation measures are personal growth, emotional well-being, and quality of life. CMCGP is an eight-session manualized psychotherapy intervention influenced by the work of Paul Gilbert,[10] Kristin Nef,[19–21] Christoffer K. Germer,[18] and William Breitbart.[4–6] It utilizes didactics, discussion, reading, and experiential exercises that focus on themes related to compassion, meaning, and advanced cancer. Also, the intervention focuses on helping patients with advanced cancer develop or increase a sense of compassion and mindfulness in their lives through the use of compassion meditation with visualization techniques. Each session addresses specific themes related to an exploration of the concepts of compassion and self-compassion, the sources of meaning, and the relationship and impact of cancer on one's sense of meaning and identity. For example, in Session 3 ("promoting my self-compassion"), to promote self-compassion, patients are asked about what self-compassion is for them, and during the session they practice a self-compassion meditation for 15 minutes. After each session, patients are given specific activities to practice as homework, including meditation techniques and other exercises. The focus of each session is on issues of compassion, meaning, and purpose in life in the face of advanced cancer. The elements of support and expression of emotion are limited by the focus on experiential exercises, didactics, and discussion related to themes focusing on compassion and meaning (Table 13.5).

TABLE 13.5 WEEKLY SESSIONS COVERED IN CMCGP

Session No.	CMCGP Session Topic
1	Concepts of compassion
2	Concepts and sources of meaning
3	Promoting self-compassion
4	Cancer and meaning
5	Giving and accepting compassion
6	Historical sources of meaning (legacy: past, present, and future)
7	Encountering life's limitations
8	Termination: Awakening of compassion and meaning

In the future, we will evaluate the changes made at the level of spiritual and emotional well-being, quality of life, and survival. We will perform a study on peripheral blood telomerase activity to determine the possible relationship between emotional and spiritual well-being, quality of life, survival, and any increase in the activity of this telomerase enzyme in both interventions (MCGP and CMCGP).

We are also considering the development of new studies comparing online versus in-person CMCGP in advanced cancer patients in order to reduce the attrition effects observed in a previous study.[28]

SUMMARY

The efficacy of MCGP provides us with a beneficial intervention to address emotional and spiritual suffering in patients with advanced cancer. We need to consider alternative approaches (e.g., telemedicine) for patients who might benefit from group interventions but are too ill to travel.

REFERENCES

1. Gil F, Costa G, Pérez X, et al. Adaptación psicológica y prevalencia de trastornos mentales en cáncer. *Med Clín*. 2008;130(3):90–92.
2. Gil F, Costa G, Pérez J. Does chemotherapy reduce stress? *Palliat Support Care*. 2010;8(4):455–460.
3. Gil F, Costa G, Hilker I, et al. First anxiety, afterwards depression: Psychological distress in cancer patients at the diagnosis and after the medical treatment. *Stress Health*. 2012;28(5):362–367.

4. Breitbart W., Rosenfeld B., Gibson C., et al. Meaning-centered group psychotherapy for patients with advanced cancer: A pilot randomized controlled trial. Psycho-Oncology. 2010;19:21–28.
5. Breitbart W, Poppito S, Rosenfeld B, et al. Pilot randomized controlled trial of individual meaning-centered psychotherapy for patients with advanced cancer. *J Clin Oncol.* 2012;30(12):1304–1309.
6. Breitbart W, Rosenfeld B, Pessin H, et al. Meaning-centered group psychotherapy: An effective intervention for improving psychological well-being in patients with advanced cancer. *J Clin Oncol.* 2015;33(7):749–754.
7. Gil F, Breitbart W. Psicoterapia centrada en el sentido: "Vivir con sentido." Estudio piloto. *Psicooncología.* 2013;10(2–3):233–245.
8. Gil F, Breitbart W. Psicoterapia de grupo centrada en el sentido: Vivir con sentido. In: Gil F, ed. *Counseling y Psicoterapia en Cáncer*. Barcelona, Spain: Elsevier; 2014:305–312.
9. Park N, Peterson C, Seligman MEP. Strengths of character and well-being. *J Soc Clin Psychol.* 2004;23(5):603–619.
10. Gilbert P. *Terapia Centrada en la Compasión.* Bilbao, Spain: Desclée de Brouwer; 2014.
11. Gil F. Model of Compassion/Meaning-Centered Group Psychotherapy (CMCGP). In elaboration 2015.
12. Van der Spek N, Vos J, van Uden-Kraan CF, et al. Meaning making in cancer survivors: A focus group study. *PLoS One.* 2013;8(9):e76089.
13. Ettema EJ, Derksen LD, van Leeuwen E. Existential loneliness and end of life care: A systematic review. *Theor Med Bioeth.* 2010;31(2):141–169.
14. Thorton AA. Perceiving benefits in the cancer experience. *J Clin Psychol Med Settings.* 2002;9(2):153–165.
15. Tedeschi RG, Calhoun LG. Posttraumatic growth: Conceptual foundations and empirical evidence. *Psychological Inquiry.* 2004;15(1):1–18.
16. Henoch I, Danielson E. Existencial concerns among patients with cancer and interventions to meet them: An integrative literature preview. *Psycho-Oncology.* 2009;18:225–236.
17. Ryff CD, Singer BH. Contours of positive human health. *Psychological Inquiry.* 1998;9(1):1–28.
18. Germer CK. *The Mindful Path to Self-Compassion. Freeing Yourself from Destructive Thoughts and Emotions.* New York, NY: Guilford; 2009.
19. Neff KD. Self-compassion: An alternative conceptualization of a healthy attitude towards oneself. *Self Identity.* 2003a;2:85–101.
20. Neff KD. Development and validation of a scale to measure self-compassion. *Self Identity.* 2003b;2:223–250.
21. Neff K. *Self-Compassion: Stop Beating Yourself Up and Leave Insecurity Behind.* New York, NY: Morrow; 2011.
22. Ornish D, Lin J, Daubenmier J, et al. Increased telomerase activity and comprehensive lifestyle changes: A pilot study. *Lancet.* 2008;9:1048–1057.
23. Ornish D, Lin J, McChan J, et al. Effects of comprehensive lifestyle changes on telomerase activity and telomere length in men with biopsy-proven low-risk prostate cancer: 5-Years follow-up of a descriptive pilot study. *Lancet.* 2013;17:1–9.
24. Schutte NS, Malouff JM. A meta-analytic review of the effects of mindfulness meditation on telomerase activity. *Psychoneuroendocrinology.* 2014;42:45–48.
25. Gilbert P, Choden. *Mindful Compassion.* Oakland, CA: New Harbinger;2014.
26. Carter CS. Neuroendocrine perspective on social attachment and love. *Psychoneuroendocrinology.* 1998;23:77–818.
27. Panksepp J. *Affective Neuroscience.* New York, NY: Oxford University Press; 1998.
28. Applebaum AJ, Lichtenthal WG, Pessin HA, et al. Factors associated with attrition from a randomized controlled trial of meaning-centered group psychotherapy for patients with advanced cancer. *Psycho-Oncology.* 2012;21:1195–1204.

14

Enhancing Meaning at Work and Preventing Burnout

The Meaning-Centered Intervention for Palliative Care Clinicians

LISE FILLION, MÉLANIE VACHON, AND PIERRE GAGNON

INTRODUCTION

Working in palliative care (PC) can be challenging, distressing, and rewarding. PC involves several types of stressors, such as organizational, professional, and emotional. The cumulative impact of all types is particularly demanding. This chapter focuses mainly on emotional stressors. By the very nature of their work, health care providers or caregivers practicing in PC settings encounter emotional demands and ethical challenges. They have to deal with repeated deaths, distress of patients and family, ethical concerns, and their own personal suffering, all in a work environment that is nowdays less supportive and more demanding. This chapter provides a reflection of and suggestions for dealing with these caregivers' particular challenges. It describes the development and evaluation of an intervention, the purpose of which is to create a framework and strategies for preventing burnout, clarify caregiving intentions, reconnect with mindful choices, and reinforce actions and work engagement. The chapter first provides an understanding of workplace stress, stressors specific to PC, psychosocial risks factors that may lead to burnout or engagement at work, and key ingredients retained for intervention. It then describes the elaboration and validation of the meaning-centered intervention (MCI) for enhancing meaning at work in PC practice. Next, the chapter briefly depicts the MCI. Finally, it summarizes quantitative and qualitative evaluations conducted with PC nurses, and future directions are discussed.

PALLIATIVE CARE AND WORK STRESS

The European Agency for Safety and Health at Work states that "there is increasing consensus around defining work-related stress in terms of the 'interactions' between employees and their work environment."[1] Within this model, stress can be said to be experienced when the demands from the work environment exceed the employee's ability to cope with them. Stress at work contributes to negative outcomes at both organizational and individual levels. For the organization, work-related stress is notably associated with high rates of absenteeism.[2]

Palliative care consists of providing comfort and support and improving quality of life for patients living with fatal diseases such as cancer.[3] Palliative care practice research repeatedly suggests that professionals providing PC could be particularly at risk of experiencing workplace stress. Although they are confronted with the same professional and organizational challenges as all practicing nurses or clinicians, those working with the dying have to cope with specific emotional demands.[3] When PC is provided in acute care settings, emotional stressors specific to the care of terminally ill patients and ethical concerns may become particularly challenging (for discussion, see Fillion et al.[4]).

At the individual level, stress experienced at work is related to a high incidence of health problems, compassion fatigue, burnout, and job dissatisfaction (for review, see Vachon and Fillion[5]). Stress can be observed at the physiological, psychological, and behavioral levels of analysis. It is an ongoing process affected by both individual and environmental factors. The individual is constantly responding to and interacting with the environment; whether the stress is a benefit or harm depends greatly on the individual's cognitive appraisal of the stressor and subsequent coping process.[6]

Stress, Burnout, and Engagement

Maslach and colleagues define *burnout* as a psychological syndrome in response to chronic interpersonal stressors on the job, and they reported three key dimensions: overwhelming exhaustion, feelings of cynicism and detachment from the job, and a sense of ineffectiveness and lack of accomplishment.[7]

In contrast, the same group of researchers conceptualizes work engagement as being the opposite of burnout.[8] They define *work engagement* as a persistent, positive affective–motivational state of fulfillment in employees that is characterized by vigor, dedication, and absorption. Work engagement entails energy and involvement. It encompasses the individual's relationship with work. It also includes sustainable workload, feelings of choice and control, appropriate recognition and reward, supportive work community, fairness and justice, meaningful work, and high levels of activation and pleasure.

Interestingly, the following questions can be asked: Are burnout and work engagement interrelated? Are the same factors involved in both long-term outcomes?

Occupational Stress, Psychosocial Risk Factors, and Mismatch Theory

The French Ministry and a group of international experts[9] suggested defining occupational stress as psychosocial risk factors that could be classified along six axes: intensity of work, social climate, emotional demand, autonomy, values, and safety issues. Each factor suggests some conditions of the working environment, but each also has some individual component characteristics. Inspired by the Maslach focus on the person–environment fit model[10] to explain either the burnout process or work engagement, we recently proposed to define occupational stress as psychosocial risk factors, whereas burnout would be defined as the result of a chronic mismatch between work environment and the person.[5]

Burnout may arise from chronic mismatches between people and their work settings in some or all of the previously mentioned six axes. Alternatively, people may vary in the extent to which each of the six axes or areas are important to them. Some people may place a higher weight on autonomy than on values, whereas others may be prepared to tolerate a mismatch regarding workload if they receive praise, good pay, have good relationships with colleagues, and find their work meaningful.

To prevent burnout and promote work engagement, we recently discussed interventions combining both organizational and individual components to decrease psychosocial risk factors.[4,5] Without neglecting the organizational importance, the intervention presented in this chapter targets the individual level (increasing individual resilience to the psychosocial risk factors), delivered in a group format. While taking into consideration the necessity and complexity of integrating organizational and individual interventions, we have developed a strong individual component that can be easily implemented in a work environment format. Before presenting the intervention, we first discuss the main ingredients of the intervention according to four psychosocial risk factors faced by PC care providers: social climate, emotional demands, autonomy, and values. The presentation of a conceptual framework to integrate these ingredients and to suggest intervention strategies follows.

Social Climate, or the Importance of Human Connections

Social climate corresponds, on the one hand, to the relationships between workers and, on the other hand, to the relationship between the worker and the employing organization. Social climate must be considered in connection with the concepts of integration (in the sociological sense) and recognition.[9]

Mismatch may arise when people lose a sense of personal connection with others in the workplace.[5] Social support from people with whom one shares praise, comfort, happiness, and humor affirms membership in a group with a shared sense of values.[11] Team communication problems have long been identified as an issue in PC, as in other specialties. Payne[12] found that conflict with staff contributed to both emotional exhaustion and depersonalization subscales of the Maslach Burnout Inventory.

The capacity to communicate and connect deeply with other human beings (e.g., patients, family, colleagues, and superiors), to interact with compassion and a sense of values, and to be able to mobilize social support from colleagues appears to be part of a first ingredient for the choice of intervention. The group format was notably selected for this reason.

Emotional Demands, or the Capacity to Find Meaning with Suffering

The emotional demands are related to the need to regulate, control, and shape one's emotions at work. Having to control or hide emotions is demanding.[9]

Palliative care has been recognized as being associated with emotional demands. The mismatch may particularly appear when requirements to display or suppress emotions on the job are challenging and when the therapeutic relationship, human connections, or empathy could be compromised.[5]

Although the literature has been somewhat divided as to whether or not the care of the dying is a major stressor in hospice PC settings, our PC research in acute care settings clearly demonstrated the link between having to cope with high patient and family distress and showing higher distress and lower job satisfaction.[13] Similarly, research in the burnout area has focused explicitly on emotion–work variables and has found that these emotional factors account for additional variance in burnout scores over and above job stressors.[8]

In contrast, "being with the dying" is also described by caregivers as one of the most rewarding aspects of their work. Caregivers working in specialized PC units often report less emotional burden and better work satisfaction than care providers from other care settings.[14] A survey of 464 palliative care staff in New Zealand[15] did not identify "death and dying" issues as a major contributor to creating a stressful work environment. Participants reported that these issues were manageable as long as there were sufficient and appropriate organizational support practices, such as acknowledgment of the deaths, the use of rituals, and the availability of debriefing, if required. In fact, under humane conditions, working with death and dying, finitude, and facing suffering could even be described as a source of meaning.[16]

In an in-depth qualitative study of palliative care nurses (N = 11), we found that the connections that nurses make with their patients in confronting death can involve both suffering and meaning.[17] We described three patterns of nurses' experience of death confrontation: integrating death, fighting death, and suffering death. Whereas some nurses reported feeling frustrated (discordance) or powerless (consonance), others sometimes experienced feeling nourished from their contacts with dying patients (empathic resonance). We also observed an oscillation process from one mode of confronting death to another in relation to contextual changes.

Some situations are particularly difficult and may sometimes be considered traumatic exposures, also known as secondary or vicarious traumatization or compassion fatigue.[18] Emotional demands and compassion fatigue may lead to burnout.[5] In contrast, when caregivers have developed a capacity to accept, face, and cope with suffering, they may experience compassion satisfaction.[5]

How to deal with emotional demands and suffering was a second ingredient retained for the choice of intervention.

Autonomy and Control, or Capacity to Make Mindful Choices

Autonomy at work involves the worker being an active participant in the production of wealth and in the driving of his or her professional life. It refers to flexibility in the work situation, participation in decision-making, and opportunities to use and develop skills and competencies. The notion of autonomy includes the idea of professional development and achievement and also the ability to take some pleasure in one's achievement.[9]

The mismatch occurs when there is no recognition, insufficient control or resources to properly do the work, and lack of personal reward at work. The issue of control is related to lack of efficacy or reduced personal accomplishment. Mismatches often indicate that individuals have insufficient control over the resources necessary to do their work or insufficient authority to pursue the work in what they believe is the most effective manner.[5] Caregivers consistently report having difficulty performing their tasks because of a lack of organizational resources.[19] At the individual level, how can autonomy and reward be activated?

One of our previous qualitative studies described how the perception of being able to make a difference for a person and a family at the end of life was a personal reward for nurses providing PC.[20] In a subsequent quantitative study involving a sample of 209 PC nurses, we also demonstrated the importance of autonomy and acknowledgment. Among the best predictors of job satisfaction and distress were autonomy and reward.[13] With a larger and more representative sample (N = 751), we replicated these findings and explained even more satisfaction and distress.[4]

Finding ways to increasing a sense of autonomy and a capacity to make meaningful choices at work was a third ingredient retained for the choice of intervention.

Values and Coherence, or Being Aware of What Really Matters

People who are asked to act in conflict with professional, social, or personal values experience ethical suffering or moral distress. The conflict of values may be associated with incoherence between workers' beliefs and the aim of the work or its side effects, or it may be associated with a pressure to act in opposition to their conscience. People may feel constrained by their job setting to do something unethical and not in accord with their own values.[9]

Alternatively, there may be a mismatch between people's personal career goals and the values of the organization. People can also be caught in conflicting values of the organization, such as when there is a discrepancy between a cost-efficacy culture and high-quality service or when the values of the organization and those of the worker are in conflict. A variety of organizational pressures can lead to people not being able to do their jobs properly, a decrease in quality patient care, and an increase in moral distress.

A report that presented strategies to reduce burnout among oncologists found that optimization of career fit (a balance between personal and professional values) led to increased job satisfaction.[21] When there is a misfit between the values of an individual and those of an organization, moral distress may result. Moral distress in the workplace occurs when there is incoherence between one's beliefs and one's actions and possibly also outcomes.

How does one make sense and deal with moral distress? We propose that awareness of values is a first step. Being aware of what constitutes one's core values and deep intention at work was a fourth ingredient retained for the choice of intervention.

Enhancing capacity to pay attention to human connections, fragility in the context of stress, facing suffering, making meaningful choices at work, and being aware of what constitutes one's core values and intentions all correspond to existential issues particularly vivid and directly linked to finitude and human conditions.

DEVELOPMENT OF A MEANING-CENTERED INTERVENTION

Although existential dimensions are crucial in end-of-life caregiving, they are rarely addressed in supportive or individual interventions for PC caregivers. Similarly, awareness of rewards and benefits associated with aiding end-of-life patients, an experience frequently reported by nurses as satisfying in our preliminary work, is not integrated in the therapeutic process. The positive workplace elements (i.e., rewards and benefits) could stimulate providers to find meaning in their work and, consequently, enhance their well-being and job satisfaction.[4]

Existentialism, Meaning, and Logotherapy

Given the existential issues raised in palliative care practice, Frankl's[22] existential approach, *logotherapy*, appears to be a relevant tool for caregivers and palliative care stress. This approach holds three cardinal assumptions: (1) Humans have the freedom and the ability to find meaning as long as they are conscious, (2) humans have a basic will to find such meaning, and (3) humans carry within themselves the knowledge that life has meaning. *Freedom of will* does not mean being free from determinants (biological, psychological, environmental, and sociological) but, rather, refers to the human capacity to choose an attitude toward conditions of life. Even in stressful situations, there are only three choices: flight, fight, or transcend. *The will to meaning* refers to Frankl's principle that humans are motivated to find meaning. Those who experience an "existential vacuum"—that is, those who do not find meaning in their lives and cannot be guided by it—can experience severe emotional distress. Logotherapy proposes three ways or basic avenues to explore meaning through experiential, attitudinal, and creative values.

Experiential Values

A first avenue could be through *experiential values*, the openness and capacity to pay attention to what is happening. Meaning can emerge from simple experiences through the beauty of art, nature, and love. The natural beauty of flowers, the works of artists, as well as the nurturing human relationships of a compassionate caregiver can help people find meaning. Whereas life and PC practice offer intense moments of human connections that may bring meaning to people's lives, lack of consciousness and sensitivity may keep people from appreciating beauty and its intense moments of human connections. This requires the capacity to shift attention to bring meaning through experiential values in general and at work. The construct of experiential values seems similar to *mindfulness*, often described as "paying attention in a particular way: on purpose, in the present moment, and nonjudgmentally."[23]

Attitudinal Values

A second avenue is through *attitudinal values* or acceptance of what is, allowing things to be just as they are, in order to see more clearly how best to respond or become response-able. According to Frankl, meaning can take place in accepting what cannot be changed, instead of resisting it and creating even more tension. Situations that bring extreme physical or emotional suffering can serve as a springboard to meaning. Otherwise, without meaning, suffering may turn into despair and self-destruction. Frankl notes that "suffering guards us against apathy."[24] Humans grow and mature through suffering. Although a caregiver may feel powerless toward inescapable suffering, his or her attitude toward it—for instance, in being present—may make a difference in creating space, safety, and courage to allow and integrate suffering. Acceptance is not resignation. Acceptance means actively responding to emotion. It constitutes a key therapeutic ingredient in many cognitive therapies—part of what is often called the third-wave generation in cognitive–behavioral therapy, notably acceptance and commitment therapy.[25]

Creative Values

A third avenue, *creative values*, corresponds to the sense of engagement in concrete actions, closely related to our deep intention as human beings and according to our personal intuition of how to be in the flow of the present experience. Many health care providers are drawn to their profession by the wish to help people. Creative values represent what we give to the world, what we add to life, and what we contribute to. Caregivers rarely take the time to evaluate and recognize their actions on a daily basis. If they were to do so, however, they might benefit from such perspective. Although caring is part of caregivers' daily tasks, becoming conscious of their actions and their consequences on patients' well-being and aware of the profound intention to serve others could add meaning and satisfaction to PC practice. In fact, this is a core element of compassion, which includes not only empathy toward suffering but also a profound intention to help alleviate suffering.[26]

We suggest that logotherapy, "therapy through meaning" (or meaning-centered therapy), with the three avenues and related therapeutic processes, can help enhance meaning at work, increase satisfaction, and prevent burnout by decreasing the four risk factors of occupational stress. Next, we summarize how the exploration of these three sources of meaning via logotherapy, as proposed by Frankl, can be associated with a decrease in psychosocial risk factors in PC settings. Figure 14.1 illustrates these relationships.

First, exploring experiential values can lead to a better capacity to pay attention to what is good and nourishing at work. It can reconnect the caregiver with pleasure, joy, and humans connections, and it can directly contribute to improving social climate. Second, exploring attitudinal values can help cultivate a different relationship with life finiteness and suffering experiences at work, in facilitating acceptance of emotion instead of trying to control or suppress it. The nature of PC

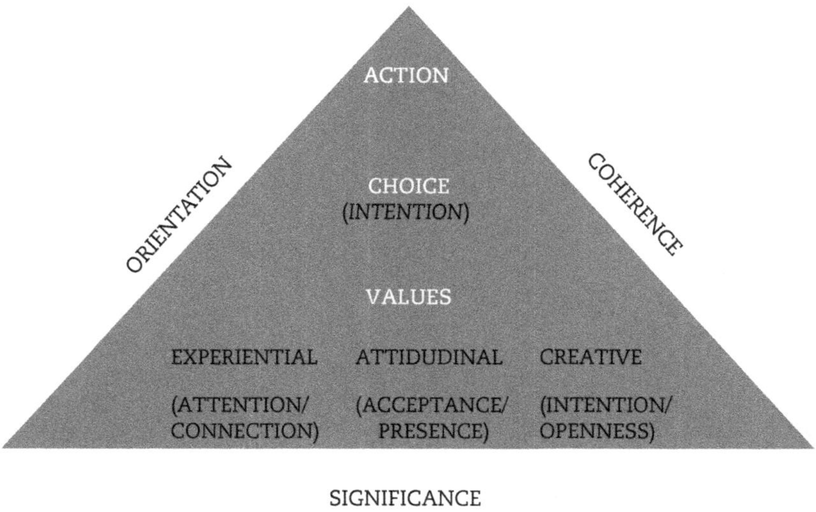

FIGURE 14.1 Therapeutic ingredients and process of the meaning-centered intervention at work with palliative-care/end-of-life caregivers.

forces caregivers to confront life's finiteness and suffering. A greater capacity to acknowledge and integrate suffering experiences can help decrease emotional demands. Third, exploring creative values can clarify the profound intention of being a caregiver and bring awareness of the availability of choices and possibilities of increasing coherence between actions, intention, and values. This could help increase the sense of autonomy and control. Finally, exploration of all avenues or sources of meaning could result in a better awareness of values, more coherence between values and actions, and the capacity to act when faced with incoherence.

Logotherapy may provide concrete ways to help find meaning at work, leading to more satisfaction at work. Meaning at work can be defined according to three dimensions: significance, orientation, and coherence. Significance refers to "the value of work in the subject's view and his definition or representation of it." Orientation corresponds to "what the subject is seeking in work and the purposes that guide his actions." Coherence is "the effect between the subject and the work he performs, between his expectations, his values and the actions he performs daily in the work environment."[27] From Frankl's perspective, meaning at work is also a contribution to society. Moreover, he states "that the job at which one works is not what counts, but rather the manner in which one does the work."[25]

The goal of the intervention for PC caregivers is to enhance meaning at work in coherently linking values and intention with choices and actions. In exploring experiential, attitudinal, and creative values, it aims to increase the capacity to pay attention to what is meaningful at work. Consciousness is the vehicle. Paying attention helps one to be more present, less unconsciously reactive to stressful situations, more able to accept what is, and more response-able. Being response-able in this situation involves the capacity to recall one's deep intention, make mindful choices, perform coherent actions, increase the match between work environment and the person, and therefore promote work engagement and meaning at work.

Development of the Meaning-Centered Intervention for Palliative Care Caregivers

Based on logotherapy, Breitbart and colleagues[28] developed the MCI for cancer patients with advanced disease. We used their first 8-week program as the foundation for the development of the MCI for PC caregivers (MCI-PC). The original MCI has eight weekly sessions and aims to help cancer patients maintain meaning in their lives, despite the life-threatening nature of their illness. Each session lasts 1½ hours and focuses on one of the logotherapy themes.[29] Sessions comprise a mix of didactic presentations, discussions, experiential exercises, and home exercises. To better serve our first targeted group of caregivers, namely PC nurses, we adapted the original format and content.

Elaboration Process

The eight-session format was reformulated into four sessions lasting between 2 and 2½ hours each. If we add the time dedicated to home exercises, this could represent the equivalent of half a day of work, and it could be managed more practically for organization. It was assumed that active work and home lives reduce nurses' availability for participating in the intervention. The original didactics, discussions, and exercises were all revised and adapted to cover topics relevant to nurses and caregiving at the end of life.

For instance, adjustments were made to the sequence of activities in each session. A single, uniform, and logical structure was retained and applied for each session. All sessions start with a centration practice in order to focus the attention of the participants and create space for exploration. Then, a group discussion or a sensitization activity follows, preceded by an associated didactics. Most exercises were tailored to fit the experience of clinicians in palliative care. For example, in dealing with the topic of suffering, emphasis was placed on distinguishing patients' and clinicians' experiences of suffering. Clinicians' experience of suffering and emotional stressors were addressed directly and discussed in terms of existential distress, powerlessness, and multiple losses. We discussed most decisions with Breitbart and colleagues. Then, we conducted content validation with experts and wrote a first draft manual for participants. We developed a training program for facilitators and pilot tested this adapted intervention with a sample of PC nurses (for details, see Fillion et al.).[30]

CONTENT AND FORMAT OF THE MEANING-CENTERED INTERVENTION

The intervention briefly presented in Table 14.1 was designed to cover five themes of logotherapy: (1) characteristics of meaning; (2) sources of meaning; (3) creative values in terms of personal

TABLE 14.1 MEANING-CENTERED INTERVENTION, OBJECTIVES, CONTENT, AND ACTIVITIES

Session	Objectives/Topics	Content	Activities
I	Introduction	Presentation of facilitators/ participants	
		Clarification of MCI objectives and participants expectations/rules	
	Meaning	Open questions about themes of the book and meaning	Group discussion
	Ways to discover meaning	Exploration of meaningful experiences in life and at work	Small group + large group discussion
	Didactic	Meaning/existential vacuum	Mapping and mini-lecture
II	Exploration of intention and creative values	Historical perspective exploration of accomplishments; clarification of intention to be caregiver	Reflect on their career from three perspectives: past, present, and future
		Responsibilities in general and at work	Personal reflection/small and large discussion
		Differences/similarities	
		Response-able and meaning	Mini-lecture
		Hope, goals, wishes	Make a wishful list before end of life
III	Suffering, coping strategies (acceptation, staying present) and attitudinal values	Create a link between suffering and meaning, and establish that which the participants do personally to avoid or respond to suffering at work and elsewhere	Discussion on "good death" and "good end-of-life accompaniment"
		Attitudes one can adopt when facing one's and others' suffering	Mini-lecture
		Own attitude toward suffering and develop strategies to face it, starting with acceptance	Narration, small group exchange
		Contamination of suffering, emotional demands, transformation of suffering, and opportunity to grow	Mini-lecture
		Experience of the finiteness of life	Goals exchange/time-limit instructions
		Establishing priorities (intention/ attention/choices/actions)	Mini-lecture
IV	Emotional experiences, humor, and experiential values	Explore how emotion-filled experiences and "being mode" can be a source of meaning	The three meaningful experiences/pictures matching
		Love, nature, art, and meaning	Mini-lecture
		Humor and meaning	Narrative stories
		Active coping strategies reinforcement	Matching stressors and coping strategies
		Integration of three ways to find meaning at work	Personal reflection
		Action plan	Group discussion
		Group processes exploration/ conclusion/home exercise (action plan)	

exploration of intention as a nurse and a sense of accomplishment at work; (4) attitudinal values through suffering experiences at work, and; (5) experiential avenues explored with emotion-filled experiences, presence, and sense of humor.

The material used for the intervention includes a participants' handbook. The material is provided to participants on a weekly basis, and the format retained was a customized binder. It contains the information introduced in the didactics, as well as the handouts for activities and home exercises. In addition, each participant receives the book *Tuesdays with Morrie*.[31] This book relates the true story of a retired university professor who is dying of a rare degenerative disease. The reader witnesses his physical degeneration and emotional connection with those around him through the eyes of an older student. This text was selected for three reasons: Its focus on end-of-life accompaniment, Morrie's existential attitude toward his illness, and the student's personal and spiritual journey throughout his professor's death process. All meetings last approximately 2½ hours and follow the same structure. Next, the content of each session is briefly described (see Table 14.1).

Session 1: Search for and Sources of Meaning

The goal of the first session is to explore the concept and characteristics of "meaning" as well as three ways to become aware of personal "sources of meaning"—that is, what gives meaning to their lives and, specifically, to their PC work. A significant portion of the first session is spent on introduction and group functioning. The session includes two activities and one didactic.

The first activity consists of a reflection around the selected book. The purpose is twofold: to set the tone for the entire intervention and to allow participants to ponder and structure their thoughts about meaning, life, death, and dying. A didactic presentation on the characteristics of meaning and the consequences of experiencing the absence of meaning (called an existential vacuum), such as depression and burnout, follows. The second activity seeks to identify moments and experiences that bring meaning to the participants' lives and work. Participants are invited to write on paper, in the shape of a green leaf, examples of meaningful situations. Following a short didactic on the three ways of finding meaning, illustrated by a poster of a tree with three strong branches, the facilitator invites participants to pin their paper leaves under the appropriate branches as a way of mapping sources of meaning.

This task of focusing on creative, attitudinal, and experiential values through examples generating and mapping is repeated at the end of each session.

Session 2: Historical Perspective, Intention, and Creative Values

The goal of the second session is to explore the source of meaning in relation to creative values. Participants are invited to adopt a historical perspective on their lives and to recall or reconstruct their profound intention to become a caregiver; explore the sense of accomplishment at work or elsewhere; and/or explore goals, hopes, and wishes. It comprises three activities and two didactics.

The first activity aims to bring to mind the manner in which the choice and practice of PC impact the caregivers' lives and how PC has influenced their personal life trajectory and their sense of identity and continuity. The participants are invited to identify the values that guide their work and restate their profound intention of being a caregiver. Specifically, they are asked to reflect on their career from three perspectives: past, present, and future. They discuss their choice of being a nurse or a PC clinician, recall their intention at that time and now, articulate that which they feel they have accomplished professionally, and reflect on what they have learned from their PC practice. Finally, they are asked to share future projects they would like to achieve, as well as identify what they would like to transmit to other caregivers or be remembered for.

The second activity aims to define what it means, for each participant, to be responsible by identifying each person's responsibilities, for whom and for what each person is responsible, and who imposes those responsibilities. Furthermore, participants are asked to reflect on differences and similarities between home- and work-related responsibilities. A didactic on responsibility and response-abilities follows.

The last activity focuses on future hopes and goals with the purpose of bringing consciousness to and integrating the session's themes. Participants are invited to list five things (hopes, wishes, and goals) they would like to realize in their lives. They then indicate whether they believe they have control over each one and describe concrete actions they are currently taking to reach their goals.

Session 3: The Meaning of Suffering and Attitudinal Values

The purpose of the third session is to explore the experience of patients and caregivers with regard to palliative care, create a link between suffering and meaning, and establish that which the participants do personally to avoid or respond to suffering at work and elsewhere. It includes three activities and the same number of didactics.

A discussion revolving around the previous week's home exercise opens the session's activities. Participants are asked to discuss the concept of "good death" and reflect on what a "good" end-of-life accompaniment would look like. They are invited to elaborate on how a caregiver could contribute to a patient's "good death" and whether they would feel at ease accompanying a dying patient in that manner. The facilitator's role is to detect and explore the participants' potential anxiety and emotions about death, such as powerlessness, guilt, a sense of failure, and uncertainty, while emphasizing the positive aspects of PC work. The didactic focuses on attitudes that one can adopt when facing one's and others' suffering.

The second activity is intended to help the participants become conscious of their own attitude toward suffering and develop strategies to deal with it. The participants are asked to relate and narrate one critical workplace situation in which they experienced suffering. Caregivers' strengths and abilities to acknowledge, accept, hold, and contribute to the integration experience of the suffering are highlighted. The didactic elaborates on the increased complexity that clinicians face (emotional demands), how they sometime believe that they must ignore or put on hold their own suffering in order to care for their patients, and how the way they handle patient suffering can impact their own suffering. Three strategies are explored: (1) trying to view things differently—that is, through an attitudinal change of creating a space for what is (openness and acceptance) instead of reacting to; (2) transforming a dramatic situation into an invitation to be response-able—that is, through the creative avenue (intention/choice/action); and (3) transcending suffering—that is, through the experiential avenue and the present moment (being with/presence).

The purpose of the third activity is to explore the finiteness of life. It stimulates a reflection on how to support dying patients to identify what is important and precious to them and also on how hope can be marshaled until the very end of life. Participants are invited to share the content of their lists' priorities of five things in small groups. The facilitator interrupts the group and invites its members to review their lists, imagining they have no more than 1 year to live, and discuss whether the content and priorities of the lists remain the same. The facilitator then invites the participants to pursue their discussion, knowing that they have only 1 month to live, and then 1 week. The facilitator invites them to transform concrete goals (doing) into "being with" and "connecting" ones, which is expected to lead to specific actions and greater hope.

Session 4: Emotional Experiences, Humor, and Experiential Values

The main purpose of the fourth and final session is to explore how the being mode, particularly emotion-filled experiences, can be a source of meaning and how humor can help ground oneself and distance oneself from extreme suffering, often exacerbated by thoughts and reactions. Both the being mode and humor are aspects of experiential values. This section contains three activities and two didactics.

The purpose of the first activity is to provide the participants with an experience in which intense and positive emotion is central and explore its value and meaning. Participants are asked to remember three moments that they identify as wonderful or magnificent. With these in mind, they are asked to choose from a selection of pictures the one that makes them feel particularly alive. One by one, participants are encouraged to share their experience. The facilitator can explore how beauty and experiential avenues connect people to a broader and more solid aspect of themselves (i.e., the existential self). Other themes can also be explored: What moments were particularly important for someone? Do people feel as if they were part of something greater than themselves? Have these emotion-filled experiences changed since the beginning of their PC work? Did some participants not find pictures that represented something beautiful? Why? This is followed by a didactic on "being mode" and the capacity to fully appreciate the richness of emotion-filled experiences.

The second activity aims at highlighting the role of humor as a source of meaning. Participants share a joke, an anecdote, or an event that took place at work and that they found amusing. The facilitator holds the space for all participants to take part in the benefits of humor and laughter and then explores the way caregivers make or do not make space for humor at work. Finally, the didactic defines humor and its functions.

The purpose of the third activity is to identify organizational or individual strategies to help deal with emotional stressors in the workplace. First, the facilitator recalls the different active coping strategies discussed during the four sessions—for example, finding meaning in a sense of accomplishment (actions related to intention), changing one's attitude under dire circumstances (openness, acceptance, and space), and using humor and nourishing social connections. The participants are invited to list at least three sources of work-related stress and then develop strategies, individual and organizational in nature, that would help them transform otherwise difficult situations. Participants are invited to focus on strategies that can be implemented in their work environment (action plan).

Intervention Closing

Participants are reminded that they contributed to their own growth and the growth of others, including that of the facilitators. The facilitators ask all participants to talk about their growth process in the group. The facilitators express gratitude for participation and active engagement in the group.

EVALUATION OF THE INTERVENTION

After adapting, validating the content, and test piloting the intervention with a group of PC nurses, we conducted two studies with PC nurses to document the capacity of MCI to increase work satisfaction and quality of life of PC caregivers.

Study 1: Enhancing Meaning in Palliative Care Practice—A Randomized Controlled Trial

This study was a randomized waiting-list group design. The objective was to test its efficiency to improve job satisfaction and quality of life in PC nurses.

Design, Variables, and Participants

The MCI-PC intervention represented the independent variable. Job satisfaction and quality of life were selected as outcomes and were measured at pre-test, post-test, and 3-month follow-up. Job satisfaction outcome included two measures—general job satisfaction (General Satisfaction subscale of the Job Diagnostic Survey) and perceived benefits related to PC work (Benefit-Finding instrument). The quality-of-life outcome also included two measures—the spiritual (Spirituality subscale of the Functional Assessment of Chronic Illness Therapy) and emotional aspects (Vigour subscale of the Shortened Profile of Mood States). Confounding variables of participants' sociodemographics, work-related dimensions (organizational and professional stress), and distress were statistically controlled for (see Fillion et al.[32]).

The sample was voluntarily recruited from the PC nurse population of three regional districts of the province of Quebec, Canada. Inclusion criteria were nurses fluent in French, working within the selected districts, able to claim that 20% of their caseload involved PC, and able to commit to the four-session schedule. The final sample used for data analyses included 109 participants comprising an intervention group ($n = 56$) and a waiting-list group ($n = 53$).

Results

Analyses of covariance for repeated measures were used to verify the effect of intervention on both outcome variables. The intervention had no impact on general job satisfaction. No group effect or interaction was detected. It was proposed that our selected instrument is limited in measuring general job satisfaction. This measure focused mainly on nurses' intention to remain at work. A measure of satisfaction related to nursing aspects such as quality of care and quality of the relationship with the dying patient, or a measure of meaning at work, could be more sensitive to the MCI content and the PC context.

The intervention shows, however, an effect on specific satisfaction toward PC. Perceived benefits of working in PC were significantly higher after the intervention and at the follow-up for the experimental group. The intervention thus improved the participants' perception of benefits of working in PC.

The intervention had no impact on the spiritual and emotional quality of life. No group effect or interaction was detected. The sample's scores on those outcomes were already relatively high at baseline. The probability of increasing the participants' spiritual and emotional quality of life after any event was decreased because they had already scored high at the beginning. The results for these outcomes could be understood through the "healthy worker" prism[33] and suggest a selection bias as an alternative explanation. Recruiting on a voluntary basis has limitations. We discussed suggestions to facilitate enrolment, notably facilitating participation during working hours.

In summary, the PC nurses in the experimental group reported more perceived benefits of working in PC after the intervention and at follow-up. However, spiritual and emotional quality of life remained unaffected by the intervention. To explain null findings, theoretical and methodological challenges related to existential interventions, such as choice of outcomes, and selection bias (participants recruited were healthy workers) were discussed.

Study 2: An Awakening Experience—An Interpretative Phenomenological Analysis of the Effects of an MCI Shared Among Palliative Care Nurses

The purpose of the second study was to explore palliative care nurses' existential experience of an MCI and to describe the qualitative effects of the MCI from the nurses' point of view.

Method and Results

Ten palliative care nurses were interviewed before and after participating in a group intervention. Data were analyzed using interpretative phenomenological analysis.

Two essential themes emerged from the analysis and are briefly presented here (for more details, see Vachon et al.[34]). First, the MCI expanded nurses' existential awareness in four ways: (1) by increasing their awareness of life's finiteness, (2) by opening them up to new meanings and purposes of suffering, (3) by having them become more aware of sources of meaning and purpose in life, and (4) by giving them access to a state of mindfulness.

Awareness of Life's Finiteness

The majority of participants recalled having experienced a particularly powerful moment in the intervention. In the activity on life's finiteness (Session III), most nurses reported that, for the first time, they really became aware of their own life's finiteness. One nurse mentioned that even while working with dying patients, she had not thought of her own life's finiteness before. She experienced that new reality as a shock that also triggered her urgency to be fully alive:

> I knew I was going to die one day, but I never thought of myself dying. You know? So . . . it was . . . at the moment, it was a real shock . . . a reality shock. . . . If it would happen to me now, I just . . . I would fight it. . . . That's the way I am. I would react the same as I always do . . . I am not ready. I have so many things I need to do in my life. . . . I was angry. Not now! I said: I am alive and I want to be alive! When I got back to my car, I turned on the music . . . I needed to feel alive . . . so much. (Participant 9)

Meanings and Purposes of Suffering

Nurses were invited to explore the meaning and purpose of suffering. Participants reported that this exploration encouraged them to change their attitude about suffering, to accept that it is also part of life, and to become open to its meaning and purpose:

> We were brought to realize that suffering can give purpose. . . . It made me feel almost good . . . and it hit me hard at the same time, it made me see how difficult it was for me to accept suffering. Difficult to accept that it is there. So, I manage to escape it. . . . And instead, I can embrace it more and trust that . . . it is there for a reason, that I will learn from it, that it will reveal things about me. (Participant 5)

Sources of Meaning and Purpose in Life

Many nurses mentioned becoming aware of their own way of achieving meaningful living. Many realized how their work of accompanying patients at the end of life was a way to achieve their own life's purpose.

> I realized how important it was to remember the deep values that brought me here . . . especially when I am overwhelmed and tired. I am here to complete a personal and a professional journey. I really want to keep in touch with that on a daily basis with my patients. (Participant 1)

Mindfulness

Participants reported having developed a new capability of being more fully aware on a daily basis, especially when life was moving too fast. They talked of the MCI as a way of "taking a pause" and increasing their awareness:

> It was a pause in time, to restart on a good footing. . . . I felt calmer. I am often asked to respond quickly at work and at home. Now I am able to say stop, to breathe . . . one thing at a time. I hope it will continue like this. (Participant 8)

The second essential theme was the group's containing function for nurses. The group process allowed nurses to (1) develop a shared language to talk about their spiritual and existential experience and (2) experience validation through sharing their experience with peers. The MCI seemed to provide a safe space where nurses could express freely their personal experience, explore it, and create meaning out of it.

Essentially, nurses identified the group as having positive effects by allowing them to develop a shared language:

> To put words, to put these words on the experience . . . I think that it gives tools, in effect, somewhat personal tools to deal with . . . a difficult work, but with life in general, I think. But . . . the way I see it, for sure . . . you know, these four meetings, but it could have lasted . . . it could have been eight meetings, four meetings, we are now equipped, but I think it is also useful at times, once in a while, you know, to make sure to revisit these values. (Participant 6)

Nurses reported that they hardly had time, in either their personal or their professional lives, to express their experience and to witness others' experience. It seemed to help nurses to feel recognized and validated through sharing experience:

> Well, it reassured me . . . I am not alone with this. . . . Now, when I entered a patient's room, I feel more confident. I think I can be good for them. (Participant 2)

DISCUSSION

The qualitative study was useful to support our first assumption that the MCI-PC can enhance meaning in linking coherently values and intention, choices and actions. In exploring experiential, attitudinal, and creative values, participants seem to increase their capacity to pay attention to what is meaningful at work. A second assumption also received some support: Consciousness or awareness could be the vehicle for linking it. Allowing nurses to expand their existential awareness may also have been an awakening experience, allowing them to be more aware of their lives' sources of meaning and intention and calling them to live an authentic life according to their values. However, we do not know what the long-term impact of this intervention will be.

FUTURE DIRECTIONS

In addition to the study discussed in this chapter, we also conducted a second qualitative study to explore how the MCI-PC could be relevant for nurses working in very challenging situations, notably nurses working in bone marrow transplant units.[35] The results supported the usefulness of the MCI-PC to increase existential awareness and concrete benefits, but they also documented the difficulty of some nurses to self-regulate their emotional reaction in empathic situations. Furthermore, participation in this intervention was associated with some awareness of a need to improve self-care strategies not only to regulate participants' emotion but also to increase their stress resilience in general.

We therefore incorporated a more structured component of mindfulness (experiential values) into our four-session MCI-PC intervention. Specifically, we adapted some mindfulness-based stress reduction practices and integrated them according to a 4-week format suggested in the literature.[36] In addition, we included an organizational component. Prior to the 4-week intervention, a 1-day workshop was offered to all members of a PC unit. Using the appreciative inquiry approach, one goal was to clarify shared values among the PC team. We suggested an original way to combine organizational and individual interventions. We are currently documenting this new adaptation in the context of a broader research project. The next step is to pre-test its efficacy in selecting a mixed-method approach (quantitative and qualitative methodology) to document and explore in-depth how this MCI with a mindfulness-based component contributes to improving meaning at work, well-being, work engagement, and preventing burnout.

SUMMARY

Meaning, as an overarching concept, brings light to both the stress and the benefit of working in palliative care. It also links the individual to his or her own system of values, relationships, the organization to which he or she belongs, and his or her more global environment. With the help of existential psychology, group dynamics, new psychotherapeutic techniques, and work psychology, we can achieve a better grasp of the concept of meaning in palliative care and design adapted, pragmatic, and feasible interventions to enhance it.

Despite these advancements, more research is needed to document original ways to better integrate individual and organizational components in order to optimize the fit between the environment characteristics and the caregiver's sources of meaning.

REFERENCES

1. Cox T, Griffiths A, Rial-Gonzalez E. *Research on work-related stress.* Luxembourg: European Agency for Safety and Health at Work, Office for Official Publications for the European Communities; 2000.
2. Verhaeghe R, Mak R, Van-Maele G, et al. Job stress among middle-aged health care workers and its relation to sickness absence. *Stress Health.* 2004;19(5):265–274.
3. Ferris FD, Balfour HM, Bowen K, et al. *Modèle de guide des soins palliatifs.* Ottawa, Ontario, Canada: Association Canadienne des Soins Palliatifs; 2002.
4. Fillion L, Truchon M, L'Heureux M, et al. *Impact of work environment on nurses' job satisfaction and well-being: Improving end-of-life care and services.* Final report. Montreal: IRSST; November 6, 2014. Available at http://www.irsst.qc.ca/publications-et-outils/publication/i/100782/n/work-environment-on-nurses-job-r-846; accessed November 2015.
5. Vachon MLS, Fillion L. Stress and burnout in palliative care. In: Bruera E, Higginson I, von Gunten CF, et al., eds. *Textbook of Palliative Medicine and Supportive Care.* 2nd ed. Boca Raton, FL: CRC Press; 2015.
6. Lazarus RS, Folkman S., eds. *Stress, Appraisal and Coping.* New York, NY: Springer; 1984.
7. Maslach C, Schaufeli WB, Leiter MP. Job burnout. *Annu Rev Psychol.* 2001;52:397–422.
8. Maslach C. Engagement research: Some thoughts from a burnout perspective. *Eur J Work Organ Psychol.* 2011;20:47–52.
9. Collège d'expertise sur le suivi des risques psychosociaux au travail. *Mesurer les facteurs psychosociaux de risque au travail pour les maîtriser*; 2011. Available at http://www.college-risquespsychosociaux-travail.fr; accessed November 2015.
10. French JRP, Rodgers W, Cobb S. Adjustment as person–environment fit. In: Coelho GV, Hamburg DA, Adams E, eds. *Coping and Adaptation.* New York, NY: Basic Books; 1974:316–333.
11. Vachon MLS. Four decades of selected research in hospice/palliative care: Have the stressors changed? In: Renzenbrink I, ed. *Caregiver Stress and Staff Support in Illness, Dying, and Bereavement.* Oxford, UK: Oxford University Press; 2011:1–24.
12. Payne N. Occupational stressors and coping as determinants of burnout in female hospice nurses. *J Adv Nurs.* 2001;33:396–405.
13. Fillion L, Tremblay I, Truchon M, et al. Job satisfaction and emotional distress among nurses providing palliative care: Empirical evidence for an integrative occupational stress-model. *Int J Stress Manag.* 2007;14:1–25.
14. Fillion L, Desbiens JF, Truchon M, et al. Le stress au travail chez les infirmières en soins palliatifs de fin de vie selon le milieu de pratique. *Psycho-Oncologie.* 2011;5(2):127–136.
15. Huggard J. *A national survey of the support needs of interprofessional hospice staff in Aotearoa/New Zealand.* Unpublished master's thesis, University of Auckland, Auckland, New Zealand, 2008.
16. Fillion L, Saint-Laurent L. Les conditions favorables liees a la pratique infirmiere en soins palliatifs: les points de vue des infirmières. *Les Cahiers de Soins Palliatifs.* 2003;4(2):5–42.
17. Vachon M, Fillion L, Achille M. Death confrontation, spiritual–existential experience and caring attitudes in palliative care nurses: An interpretative phenomenological analysis. *Qual Res Psychol.* 2012;9(2):151–172.
18. Figley CR, ed. *Treating Compassion Fatigue.* New York, NY: Brunner-Routledge; 2002.
19. Fillion L, Saint-Laurent L, Rousseau, N. Les stresseurs liés à la pratique infirmière en soins palliatifs: les points de vue des infirmières. *Les cahiers de soins palliatifs.* 2003;4(1):5–40.
20. Fillion L, Saint-Laurent, L. Les conditions favorables liées à la pratique infirmière en soins palliatifs: les points de vue des infirmières. *Les cahiers de soins palliatifs.* 2003;4(2):5–42.
21. Shanafelt T, Chung H, White H, et al. Shaping your career to maximize personal satisfaction in the practice of oncology. *J Clin Oncol.* 2006;24:4020–4026.
22. Frankl VE. *The Doctor and the Soul: An Introduction to Logotherapy.* Oxford, UK: Knopf; 1955.
23. Kabat-Zinn J. *Wherever You Go, There You Are: Mindfulness Meditation in Everyday Life.* New York, NY: Hyperion; 1994:4.
24. Frankl VE. Logotherapy. *Isr Annal Psychiatry Relat Discipl.* 1967;5(2):142–155.
25. Hayes SC, Strosahl KD, Wilson KG. *Acceptance and Commitment Therapy: The Process and Practice of Mindful Change.* 2nd ed. New York, NY: Guilford; 2011.
26. Rushton C, Kaszniak AW, Halifax JA. Framework for understanding moral distress among palliative care clinicians. *J Palliat Med.* 2013; 16(9):1074–1079.
27. Morin E. *The meaning of work, mental health and organizationalcommitment.* Montréal:IRSST;2008. Available at http://www.irsst.qc.ca/ publications-et-outils/publication/i/100415/n/sens-du-travail-sante-mentale-et-engagement-organisationnel-r-585; accessed November 2015.

28. Greenstein M, Breitbart W. Cancer and the experience of meaning: A group psychotherapy program for people with cancer. *Am J Psychother.* 2000;54(4):486–500.
29. Frankl VE. Logotherapy and the challenge of suffering. *Rev Existent Psychol Psychiatry.* 1987;20:1–3.
30. Fillion L, Dupuis R, Tremblay I, et al. Enhancing meaning in palliative care practice: A meaning-centered intervention to promote job satisfaction. *Palliat Support Care.* 2006;4:333–344.
31. Albom M. *Tuesdays with Morrie: A Young Man, an Old Man, and Life's Greatest Lesson.* New York, NY: Bantam Doubleday Dell; 1997.
32. Fillion L, Duval S, Dumont S, et al. Impact of a meaning-centered intervention on job satisfaction and on quality of life among palliative care nurses. *Psycho-Oncology.* 2009;18(12): 1300–1310.
33. Tummers GER, Landeweerd JA, van Merode GG. Work organisation, work characteristics, and their psychological effects on nurses in the Netherlands. *Int J Stress Manag.* 2002;9:183–206.
34. Vachon M, Fillion L, Achille M, et al. An awakening experience: An interpretative phenomenological analysis of the effects of a meaning-centered intervention shared amongst palliative care nurses. *Qual Res Psychol.* 2011;8(1):66–80.
35. Leung D, Fillion L, Duval S, et al. Meaning in bone marrow transplant nurses' work: Experiences before and after a "meaning-centered" intervention. *Cancer Nurs.* 2012;35(5):374–381.
36. Mackenzie CS, Poulin PA, Seidman-Carlson R. A brief mindfulness-based stress reduction intervention for nurses and nurse aides. *Appl Nurs Res.* 2006;19:105–109.

APPENDIX 1

Transcripts of a Full Course of an Eight-Session Meaning-Centered Group Psychotherapy Intervention with an Exemplar Group Conducted as Part of a Randomized Clinical Trial

NOTE TO READERS

The following transcripts were derived from audio recordings conducted of an entire eight-session intervention in an exemplar meaning-centered group psychotherapy (MCGP) group during a randomized controlled trial. Institutional review board permission was granted to publish these de-identified transcripts for educational and training purposes. The therapists/group facilitators conducting this group were Drs. William Breitbart and Allison Applebaum (two of the authors of the MCGP chapter in this textbook that this appendix is intended to supplement; see Chapter 2). Patients are identified only by a letter, not related to their names or any other characteristics. Professions, places, and other potential identifiers were changed to help preserve patient anonymity. We have also kept the language intact, including erroneous use of language, in order to keep it genuine and authentic.

SESSION 1: CONCEPTS AND SOURCES OF MEANING—INTRODUCTIONS AND MEANING

Therapist 1: Thank you all for coming here today. This is the first session of meaning-centered group psychotherapy, and I appreciate you coming because it's hot out there, not everyone feels great all the time, and some people probably have to travel a bit of a distance as well to get here. So I want to thank you for being here.

Today I want to accomplish a few things. My mother taught me that when you meet someone new, you should introduce yourself. So let's start with that. I'm Dr. William Breitbart and I'm Chief of the Psychiatry Service.

Therapist 2: I'm Dr. Allison Applebaum, and I'm a clinical psychologist and have worked in cancer centers for the past few years and am excited to meet all of you today.

Therapist 1: Now if you could each maybe share just a bit about yourself, starting with you, S, just tell us who you are and maybe one of two things about yourself that are important to you.

S: Ok, I'm S, I don't live in the city, I live about two hours away. And so the fact ... coming in for chemo ... which I just started, is emotionally and physically hard on me. That might some it up.

P: I'm P, I live on Long Island, I used to be a lawyer. I'm ... I'm a lawyer with cancer now. ... I never thought I'd say that.

Therapist 1: You're a lawyer with cancer. ... You'll see one of the things we'll be doing in here, is talking about how cancer has affected our identity.

L: My name is L, I'm from Brooklyn. I'm a retired registered nurse, health administrator. I was diagnosed with liver cancer in November.

Therapist 1: Ok, thanks for being here.

C: My name is C, I'm not retired yet, I'm jealous of those who are. I run a rehab and detox. I'm clean and sober for almost 30 yrs. And I can't figure out how I ended up having cancer. I thought this was a great idea to do this group. I need it. So I'm excited about it. Cause I run groups, that's what I do. I do what you do. I just don't have a "Drs. thing" behind my name. My education is in the streets. . . .

Therapist 1: C brings up an interesting point that I want to talk a little bit about. That is, what we're going to do together, and what this is, and how this might be different from other types of support groups. We're really involved in a research study. We're comparing two different kinds of support interventions and when we recruit people like yourselves to be in the study, we randomize to a standard support where people talk about their feelings and what it's like to deal with cancer and the doctors and family and side effects of medication, etc., or they get randomized to what you got, which is meaning-centered group psychotherapy. This is slightly different than standard support therapy in that what we're all going to do together for once a week for next the 8 weeks is go through a learning experience together. It's a bit more structured than freewheeling kind of, "let's talk about what's on our minds today" therapy. Each session is going to be made up of a little bit of info about the importance of meaning in life, especially when living with cancer. It's going to focus on connecting with and learning about the various sources of meaning, and trying to connect with those, trying to be flexible and moving from one source of meaning to another. So these groups will be partly didactic, very briefly, nothing too difficult, not like college level coursework, but just a little discussion of information. And then we're going to have an experiential exercise, basically we're going to ask you a question to respond to, we'll have you write down your answers to them and discuss them with the group. And these exercises are a way of learning something through doing that exercise, to reinforce the learning. So the goal of our meeting together for 8 weeks is really to teach you something about the importance of meaning and the sources of meaning. We're all human beings. As creatures, we *create* things. We create values, and we create meaning in our lives. And I think to be fully alive and live fully, involves creating a life that has meaning, that has identity, that has direction. Another word for direction might be hope, purpose, you know? And that's always important, those kinds of ideas are important in living life fully when you're healthy and even more important in living life fully when you're living with cancer. So that's the overall goal that we're trying to accomplish.

Now, Dr. Applebaum and I . . . you can call us Bill and Allison, by the way . . . we're here to facilitate the group and the discussion. So on some level, we're also teachers, but the fact that this is also a group and the fact that you all are people that have had more or less degree life experience, you've accumulated wisdom on your own. And so I totally expect that we're going to learn something from you. And so in doing the group together, while Allison and I are going to be the official facilitators and lead you along the path of what needs to be done each week, feel free to stop, interrupt, make a comment, point out something, say something about what you believe, question something that someone else has said.

Now this is not a regular support group. But the fact of the matter is that we'll meet weekly for the next 8 weeks and share experiences and grow to care about each other and there will be some support that occurs. We can't prevent it . . . we don't want to discourage it either . . . but it will happen, but the main focus is really to learn some of these lessons about meaning. We want to ensure you that this is safe and confidential environment. Anything you say is confidential for a number of reasons. One, this is a clinical, psychotherapy setting but also, it's a research setting. I don't know if you recall the informed consent you signed, but because it's research, it's doubly protected and everything that you say and do, answer you give on those forms, it's all very private information. The only people who see that are me and those who are involved in analyzing the data and they've all gone through rigorous training in maintaining privacy and there aren't too many of those people.

The other thing you should know, we want to keep it a safe place, not only in terms of confidentiality, but also, where nobody gets hurt. So, there are going to be stimulus questions that may ask about your cancer experience, in fact today we're going to begin by asking one of these questions. We'd like you to share what you're comfortable sharing, we don't want you to share anything that makes you uncomfortable, we want you to share as little or as much as you feel you'd like to share. If you have something to say about what someone else has said, let's say you disagree or it rubs you the wrong way, make an effort to say it in a way that is not hurtful, and we'll do our best to help you with this, and Allison and I will do the same.

You can get a lot out of the group if you don't say a lot. You can listen and participate in that way. But obviously everyone will get more if you participate fully. You have control over what you say, reveal.

Therapist 2: Yes, and to add to that, we have 8 weeks together, our time is short, an hour and half each week, and we do want to encourage you to come as much as possible and participate as much as you can. We recognize that things may come up in terms of health and how you're feeling but we want to emphasize that what you put in will really help what comes out of this therapy for you.

Therapist 1: Right. There are a number of reasons for you to come. It's important, because it's a research study and we need to get comprehensive information in order for us to make statements about how effective this therapy is. But the other thing is that you're going to get a lot out of it and you all will have a much richer experience the more you attend. The fewer sessions you attend, the fewer people there are, the less sharing there is, and so on. So try as much as you can to attend the meetings and let us know in advance if you can't make it.

Therapist 2: So, you have a form in your binder about guidelines. We're not going to read through that right now, but do take a look over the next week. You may have noticed that there are video cameras and audiotapes. The purpose of these is twofold. The first is to make sure that Bill and I are doing our jobs right and really adhering to a manual because this is research. The second reason, and maybe the more important reason, is to help us to understand how you are making meaning of your experience, to help us learn more about meaning-making. Again, these tapes are shared only within our team, within a small group of people.

Also, you all are welcome to share your contact info with each other and form that type of support, but it's not something that we'll do in here or facilitate, necessarily.

Therapist 1: Since this is research, it's a little like if you were participating in a chemotherapy trial, so we collect data like the video and audio so that one of the team members can listen and make sure that we're following the treatment manual. This is a manualized treatment that follows a specific course. It's meant to assure/check that we're doing it according to the manual. We may occasionally use the video to train other therapists, but main purpose is to make sure that we're doing it right.

You have in front of you a couple of items. This basically is your handbook for the whole therapy. And we're going to go through it bit by bit, starting with today. The other thing you have in front of you is *Man's Search for Meaning* by Victor Frankl, and that's something for you to read at your leisure. You might find it helpful. When we developed meaning-centered psychotherapy a few years ago, it was inspired by the work of this particular psychiatrist, Dr. Victor Frankl, and his ideas about the importance of meaning in human life. And he's someone who survived the concentration camps and then wrote down his ideas about importance of meaning. This is a book about his story, and some of the concepts we'll be talking about are drawn from it. He didn't design this therapy with cancer patients in mind, but what we did is adapt his work to the unique experience of patients with cancer.

So we've done a bit of an overview and ground rules, and in a moment we'll go over the content of the first session. But at this time it might be a good idea to go around the room and ask people to talk this time a little bit more about their cancer experience, if you feel comfortable.

S: Ok, um, I originally got breast cancer in 2004, and, I'm a librarian working with young adults, and I was getting a biopsy, I had had a liver transplant, and because of many complications with that got a delayed diagnosis. I certainly didn't have cancer in mind when the breast doctor called me. It was a Monday night at 9 pm at work, and I was devastated and shocked, to hear something like this. I don't think of things too much scarier than cancer to get. I had a lot of complications because of my transplant. Because my liver was not very good, I couldn't have the chemotherapy that would have been suggested, and there was no plan B had my liver failed, and regular chemo wasn't an option, so I had radiation, so I went on Arimidex, that kept me in good shape until this past October. And prior to that my cancer markers went up and I had a second liver transplant. So I had a new lease on life. Where I was barely there, kept alive with transfusions, I then had a great will to live, and I do have an optimism, and as soon as I got my liver transplant, I was now living back in Technicolor, everything meant so much to me, for the first time in my life, I wanted attention, I wanted to show off how good things could be in medicine, I gained 30 lbs of good weight back. So I was pretty upset when I found out in October that it had metastasized to the left lung. At least I have a liver that is good enough to withstand the chemo. But what I'm having a hard time with is that this chemo is not necessarily for a finite amount of time, but for the rest of my life, to contain the cancer. So, I'm frightened. And, I hate needles, so whereas actually the pills I'm on for my liver are for life, I'm ok with that. But I really have a very hard time with needles, you'd think after all of this, it would be ok, but the IV is an experience I dread every 2 weeks out of 3. And just recently, I have hope that I'll survive, that the drugs will work, but I all of a sudden am finding myself more anxious and wondering about meaning. I had to retire from the library, I'm working there part time, 4–6 hours a week. It's therapy to get involved in something else entirely, and I love my relationship with my niece, but when I have too much free time, I feel like I don't have time and need to be productive. I need to have fun or accomplish something. So I have a newfound need to find meaning and purpose in life. . . .

P: I don't know when it started but I had some problems with food going down. It was minor, intermittent . . . but in January I told my doctor that I had problem swallowing. I got an endoscopy in February, and the doctor saw inflammation throughout my esophagus and saw a mass and did a bunch of biopsies and sent off to a lab and they all came back negative and he didn't believe it, and wanted to re-do it. The 2nd pathology report . . . came back . . . and I have cancer. It's hard. It's not usually so hard. I have cancer of the esophagus, its metastasized to the liver, and doctors tell me that I have to take, similar to you S, a pill daily, and another medication, and I will take it until the neuropathy gets so bad that I have to stop it, in which case he will put me on something else, and then he'll put me on something else as long as I will live. It's hard to accept the fact that I'm 49 years old, I was always the caretaker for my family, I have a wife, three children, my little guy is 4 years old, and if the statistics are true, then there's a 90% chance that I won't be here for him next year . . . and as he grows up, he'll know me more as a concept than as a person, and I don't like that at all. Most of the time I don't think about it, most of the time I think about taking care of things at the house. I have my own practice with a partner. I'm a trial lawyer and I can't do it anymore. My anxiety is just too great right now, I just can't try cases anymore. I'm in the process of giving away all of my cases to a couple of other attorneys. Trying to keep busy, doing some other things, there's a social aspect to going into court that I like, but it's mostly now to adjourn things, minor things. Mostly, I'm ok.

Therapist 1: Thanks, P.

Therapist 2: Thank you for sharing.

Therapist 1: S and P brought up important issues which reminded me of something I didn't say when I was trying to talk about goals of this treatment. One of the things that's most difficult in the face of cancer and these kinds of threats is to be able to still have courage and the will to live, even though you have cancer and these potential limitations, the courage to still love deeply, even though there's the risk that you might lose people you might love. And the courage to be able to still care about things in the world and to take care of yourself. And one element of being able to have this courage, and to overcome these obstacles, has to do with legacy. And you'll see, as we go through our work together, that one of our sessions really has to do with overcoming these limitations, the scary limitations in some cases. One element that has to do with that is legacy, and how you're remembered and what you leave behind. And now is perhaps . . . of all the moments of your life that are important, now, dealing with cancer is an extremely important time in your life, in terms of how you live it, with courage, with hope, because it's going to teach a lesson to all the people in your life. We're all watched all the time, by our kids, our relatives . . . and we teach by example.

L: That's another large responsibility.

Therapist 1: It is. Maybe even . . . even a benefit?

P: Nurse is getting nursed.

Therapist 1: What was that?

P: The benefit, that the nurse is finally getting nursed.

Therapist 1: Exactly.

Ok, go ahead L.

L: Well in 1984 I had colon surgery, and I had a couple of transfusions. At any rate, somewhere around 89 or so, they diagnosed me with hepatitis C. I went for treatment, transfusions, in 1992, which was not really that successful. For some reason, a lot of African Americans don't respond well to the treatment and I was on interferon for about a year and lost about 20 to 30 pounds and decided that I wasn't going to go that route unless I had to. I was asymptomatic for the most part, my energy levels were good. I retired about 13 yrs ago, I had a stressful high powered job and I knew that that would have killed me, and so I backed out. I decided, last year, that I needed to deal with this hepatitis C and I stated going back to . . . GI docs, and the doctor that I spoke to told me that as long as it wasn't bothering me, we'd do sonograms every 6 months. But, on one of those they saw the tumor. Because of its size, I wasn't a candidate for transplant, and because of the damage of 25 yrs of hepatitis C, a resection was not something they could do. The procedure was an embolization, which I had in January. I get CT scans every three months, and had one on July 2. The tumor I had was 5 by 5 and it apparently has liquefied and is shrinking, but they see two new growths. Since a lot of this was happening in the winter and I was feeling blue, I realized when the weather got better and I was still feeling that way, that I needed to get some help, some counseling, and talk about it. So, that's where I am. My reaction to the whole thing, I wasn't really surprised when I got the diagnosis, but I was hoping that it wouldn't happen. I have a 40 year old son and 2 grandchildren who live in Georgia, and I have property there and had planned to move, but that's been put on hold. That said, the treatment I have been getting here, I'm pleased with. I worked with an organization that monitored hospitals in the city, and so I have a lot of feelings about healthcare and how patients are treated, but this has been a good experience for me, how I've been treated here. But . . . how I've responded is by retreating, becoming a couch potato, isolated, I don't talk on the phone. I was a woman of faith, but there's a lot of confusion in terms of what meaning my life has, and where do I go from here. And sometimes it's just hard to rise to the occasion. And the comment you made about people looking up to you, I try to put up a good face most times. I just don't know how hopeful I am.

Therapist 2: Thank you so much for sharing.

Therapist 1: I think this experience will help . . .

L: Hopefully.

Therapist 1: You brought up a couple of words that we're going to really spend some time thinking about. Responsibility . . . and all of that business. I don't want to get too ahead of myself, so we'll get back to that later today. . . . C? You've been listening to everyone very intently.

C: I do this, so it's . . . being in a group is what I do. My word is denial, and I already have a bunch of medical issues. Hypertension, diabetes, I had pulmonary edema in 1990, couple of heart attacks. So what happened for me is that I was trying to cross the street, and I couldn't get across the street. I was too tired to get across. So I go to my doc who saved my life in 1990. He takes my blood, he calls me back, and says, "I need you to go to the ER because you're anemic and your blood count is 7.3. How do you feel?" I say, "I'm fine, just tired, why? Doc, calm down, I'm ok. I just need to get across the street." Next thing I know, I needed to get blood tests and colonoscopy. I knew something was up when the doc said "We need to talk." I mean, I'm the guy who delivers the news, that's my job, so I said to the doc, "You can tell me, tell it to me straight." They told me I had cancer. Yeah, right. Said I had colon cancer and I needed to have surgery. I changed my diet, started eating liver, spinach, for iron, Popeye was my hero! Next thing I know, I go in and have the operation, I'm ok, ready to go, they say, "Mr. X, you need to start chemo, and then they hit me with . . . you have stage 3 cancer." Because I was in denial. I didn't want to believe that . . . see, I'm that guy who's blessed, because I grew up when it was ok to smoke, to drink, I'm from CA, it's where I got my tan. And I was in the heat! So I smoked and had a great time! I was that guy who was free love. . . . I saw Jimmie Hendrix and all these amazing artists back in the day . . .

So I'm ok. I appreciate all of your courage in here.

I knew I was in trouble last week (very tearful). I had a full head of braids. And then, all of my braids, they just broke. My hands on the outside now are as black on the inside from the chemo.

Therapist 1: So you saw a lot of changes.

C: And I had a staff member be disrespectful in a meeting this week, and I'm normally ok to work with, and normally can handle things like that ok. But I lost it on him. I just lost it. So, I'm in trouble. But, during my last chemo session this wonderful lady came in. She said, "We're going to be doing an experimental therapy group. What do you think?" I said thank you, I could not wait to get here. I'm scared, so scared, so I can appreciate. . . . So here I am.

Therapist 1: Glad you're here, C, glad you're here.

S: Can I just say something?

Therapist 1: Sure.

S: I used to be called the Queen of D'Nile (denial). (Everyone laughs.) And I think there's something about cancer . . . where denial only works up to a point, and at that point, I need other coping skills.

Therapist 2: And I think that's what you're going to get here.

C: Can I share one more thing?

Therapist 1: Of course.

C: I sit on the 3rd floor to get my chemo every other week, and what's interesting, is in this room, I have all of these different people, different races, nationalities, religions. And I say, "Damn!" What got me here, what got me this, is that cancer is the only thing that's not prejudice! It's just not prejudice. You know what I mean?

P: I also find it funny that at least every other person is really sick, but most of us, we're looking ok! I sorta wouldn't think twice that any of you were sick!

Therapist 1: The comment I want to make . . . it seems like all of you have a lot in common. And it's clear already that you've begun the process of sharing with each other and supporting. And you all have in common that you look great, but on the inside there's this suffering and whenever we human beings encounter an obstacle, a limitation, when we're living our lives fully and then anticipate fully having to give up our work, seeing changes that indicate that our bodies have physical limitations, we suffer. That's what causes suffering, coming up against life's limitations.

I think one of the things we want to do today is an experiential exercise to give you an idea of what we mean by meaning. So if you open up your books to the first tab, you'll see there a picture of Viktor Frankl, and it's from his work that we developed this therapy. There are three principles that he espoused that are really important for us to introduce today.

The first is that as human beings, we have a will, a need, basic primary need to find meaning in our lives. We're meaning-making creatures. It's one of the things that we're driven to do, to find meaning in our lives. He believed that life had meaning/has meaning, from the very first moment of life to the very last. And if we ever feel that our life doesn't have meaning, it's not because we don't have meaning, but because we've become disconnected from that meaning.

When you talk about having a void, L, Frankl would have called that an existential vacuum. No meaning, where did it go? It's not that there is no meaning, it's just that you've just become disconnected from it. That's the second principal, that, if we feel that there isn't any meaning, we've become disconnected from the meaning.

The third is that we have the freedom to choose our attitude towards anything that limits us, anything that causes suffering. The freedom to choose our attitude towards anything in life. There may be something that limits us physically, limits our idea of how long we might live, but there's nothing that can limit our attitude, how we think about the problem, we have the choice to do this, the possibility of taking something that is potentially a tragedy and overcoming it and making it into a personal triumph.

Frankl talked about his experience in the concentration camps. They took everything away, they controlled his life, but they could not control the attitude he had.

Ok. The next page is two definitions of meaning, but I want to ask if people would be interested in reading them. P, will you take a stab at reading?

P: Definition of meaning. Number one. Having a sense that one's life has meaning involves the conviction that one is fulfilling a unique role and purpose in life that is a gift. A life that comes with the responsibility to live to one's full potential as a human and in so doing, achieving a sense of peace, contentment, and transcendence through connecting to something greater than oneself.

Therapist 1: This is Frankl's definition. What this definition is basically saying is that meaning is the result of living a life that is full, living a life that you intend, that is unique to you, living a life that you direct, writing your own life story, and so, if you're living a life in which you're fulfilling your unique role and purpose, then you'll be living a life of meaning. He talks about this life being a gift, I don't know if everyone agrees that life is a gift, certainly, when I was born and aware of being alive, I didn't ask to be. But, if people are religious, you might think of it as a gift from god, but even if you're not religious, when you're given something precious like life, it's reasonable to think that you should treat it like something precious, like a gift, you shouldn't mistreat it, you should take care of it.

He used the word responsibility, and that's the word that you used L, when I mentioned that our children observe us, and we're teachers. One of the basic ideas of Frankl and other existential philosophers is that we have a responsibility to live our life to the fullest. And one way that I like to think about this word responsibility is what *is your ability to respond to being alive*? How are you going to respond to being alive? What are you going to create? The other way of thinking, is that we're responsible for everything in our lives. Are we responsible for having cancer? Not to that extent. But we're responsible for how we respond to it. The real question is how do we respond . . .

If you're able to live this way, transcend your own individual concerns and connect to something greater than yourselves, your family, your friends, your community, your race, your ethnic group, fellow NYers, Americans, able to connect to something greater than yourself, you can achieve a sense of transcending these physical limitations. So that's one definition of meaning.

How does that strike you guys?

P: I'd rather not have to deal with it, but yeah . . .

Therapist 1: Which part would you rather not deal with?

P: Before I had cancer, my life had a meaning, but I really didn't think about it. I was a husband and a father and I had my job and those things just worked. And I just worried about money and my relationship with my kids and if my wife was interested in sex, but now, every day I get to worry about those things again, it's a gift.

Therapist 2: We're going to be spending some time in this group talking about how your identity may have changed pre and post cancer.

Therapist 1: Meaning, identity, hope, they're all very much related. Do you have some thought about that, L?

L: No, what I was thinking, this philosophy applies to life in general. So if you come with baggage, you have a double amount of baggage. One of the reasons I'm here is not because I've been having so much trouble with cancer, but because I have baggage. I want to free myself . . .

Therapist 1: Does the baggage relate to not being able to live life fully and fulfill a unique purpose?

L: To some extent, yeah.

Therapist 1: What do you think, C?

C: I think I'm in recovery again. You know? Last time I had real drink, real drug, was 1982, sep 2nd, at noon. Only thing I do now is eat! So, I have to now . . . I'm in recovery again, I have another title, I have to say, I'm a cancer survivor. . . . This gentleman, Frankl, he was in a concentration camp. I grew up being . . . I was that guy, black was beautiful. It's all about the degree of blackness. I'm darker than most black people, other than people in Africa. And so I always had to fight. The fight is not new, it's just an added fight. I can respect where Frankl is coming from, because I've been in a concentration camp in my own culture.

Therapist 1: Thanks for sharing that, C.

For some people, having cancer wakes them up to a reality of how precious and how short life is, and an enhanced sense of meaning in life. You were saying P that every day you can worry about the mundane is a gift.

P: Correct.

Therapist 1: The next page is very important. Frankl spoke about there being some very predictable and very common sources of meaning in life. The first one is through experiential sources of meaning, the meaning you get through your relationships, through love, your connectedness with nature, art, beauty. You can think about the experiential sources of meaning as anything you encounter in this world through your senses, touch, smell, taste, sight. And just think about someone you love, your four year old, P, and what it's like to experience him. The meaning you derive from experiencing life and all the sensations of your body.

The second is through creative sources of meaning, through your work. So that is being a counselor, or a librarian, nurse, or lawyer. A lot of people derive meaning from their work, but also through their dedication to things they care about in the world, like peace.

Things that people connect to, and care about in the world.

Fourth, meaning occurs in a historical context. The meaning in our lives is influenced enormously by our legacy, our family, the legacy we create and the legacy we leave behind.

And finally, we can derive meaning through suffering, the attitude we take towards suffering. We can derive meaning from the attitude we take.

L, do you want to read that second definition of meaning?

L: Sure. Meaningfulness refers to moments that make life worth living. When you feel needed or alive. Things from the past, when you look back on them you still find to be very important.

Therapist 1: If you remember, one of the things I was talking about, to be fully alive means to be creating meaning in your life, identity, direction, hope, love, relationships, and it makes sense that if you are feeling alive, it's those moments that you create meaning that make you feel most alive. And that's the subject of our experiential exercise for today.

Therapist 2: Would someone like to read the experiential exercise on the next page?

S: Sure. But, first, can I share some of my reactions to what you just said?

Therapist 1: Of course.

S: They're pretty heavy. Certainly, there have been times when I've really connected. I used to work with teenagers, the group I really love. The subtext was that you can really make a difference in life. The fulfillment I found in doing that is really missing from my life right now. You don't know when it's going to take root. And now, my students, they're 28, and they reach out and tell me how I've impacted them. And that's meaningful, and that's missing right now. The other thing you said was about connecting to the world, but for me, I've actually tried to disconnect from the world, I've stopped watching the news, I find the news so taxing, so horrible, and I feel that justice doesn't exist, and my plate is too full, and so I have built up defenses, not just about cancer, but about the global problems as well! I just don't want to hear about it . . . and you're talking about being connected to the world, and I'm trying to make an effort not to be connected!

Therapist 1: I'm glad you shared this, S. Let me address those points quickly, and then we'll go into the exercise, which I think is going to provoke a lot of reactions and really feed into this discussion. By connectedness, I'm really referring to . . . not necessarily to Fox news or CNN, but the things in life that give your life a sense of meaning. Connectedness to something greater than yourself. God, nature. So I would assume there are things greater than, more transcendent than, the news. And so really, the important thing is being connected to things that bring meaning, like your work with kids, S.

S: Can I just say one other thing?

Therapist 1: Sure.

S: I was thinking, I used to be the most unassertive person in the world. But it was only when I got my liver transplant, I had a life to protect, that I started saying "no," that doesn't work for me, because I was so protective of my liver, of me. So my sweetness of life was right there, and I wanted to protect it. I became so intense. I realized that I don't feel that with the cancer. I feel angry, not protective. I feel angry that I have the cancer!

Therapist 1: We'll get back to anger in a little bit, anger is important. Anger results any time . . . we all have a trajectory of a life that we anticipate. Any time that trajectory is interrupted, we can fall. And so you can have a couple of reactions. One is to get really down and depressed and a experience a feeling of loss of meaning. The other, is to get angry.

So . . . let's quickly do this exercise . . . and basically, what I'd like you to do is write down one or two experiences when life felt particularly meaningful to you, or a moment when you felt really alive, and take a few moments and right down your thoughts, and then we'll share it.

Therapist 2 (after 5 minutes of writing) : Ok, so maybe in the interest of time we'll get started, as I'm noticing that our session is moving quickly towards the end. Would anyone like to volunteer to go first?

L: I'll go first. I've been told by friends and family that I have the "gift of helps." I guess because of my nursing background I help folks. So I had a group of seniors. My dad is 98, my mom lived to 92. I have a group of seniors in my community. I help them navigate the healthcare system. I feel like a highlight for me has been helping them to navigate the healthcare system, getting them services, helping them to get the help they need to stay healthy.

Therapist 1: So you have provided help. Compassion.

L: Yes, compassion.

Therapist 1: When you've been compassionate, how did that make you feel?

L: Useful, that I'm using a talent I have, using knowledge I have.

Therapist 1: Using your talents, living to your full potential . . .

L: Thank you.

Therapist 1: It's interesting, you're giving, not taking.

L: Yes, I have difficulty taking.

Therapist 1: Thanks, L. P?

P: The birth of each of my three children. I remember each time. The sense of elation I felt was unparalleled to anything else, but also, the sense of dread. The first one, how do I diaper the baby? How do I take care of it? I guess maybe the middle one, not so much. My kids are 18, 16, and 4. So, clearly we had a "whoopsy" baby, which was unbelievable, since I was a parent of teenagers, and that just, what doesn't kill you makes you stronger. On one hand we couldn't go to sleep because the teenager was out, or we were up because the baby was up. Anyway, so that's the first, personal thing that I'm most happy about.

Professionally, it's a client I had. He was a 30 something man who was retarded and lived with his parents, on Staten Island, and he was their boy. He fell down the steps in their home and he went to the ER, and he had 3 different surgeries on his neck due to previous issues with his spine, and when the doctor in the ER took an x-ray that showed a problem, the doctor just sent him home. Unbelievable. Anyway, he's quadriplegic now, and I represented him, and we sued the hospital and I met this guy several times and he was actually . . . he should be a model for everyone. He's one of the happiest men I've ever met. I got him enough money that they would be able to make it accessible for him, and enough money to have a caretaker. So he can come home and be with his parents.

Therapist 1: Let me make a quick comment, and people feel free to step in. L, you were talking about compassion, but it's also an example of love. And so, really, your story, your example of a meaningful moment was really a source of meaning that we would identify as experiential, love, connectedness with people you care about. You had several sources of meaning, P, love of your children and wife. Very often, important life events are profoundly meaningful, because they have such an impact on so many aspects of our lives, like having children. You became a father. It's very important to your identity, and all this love came into your life. And then you talk about work, and how meaningful work is. And an example of work that is, a case that is, so meaningful. What was so remarkable about him was that despite the fact that he was quadriplegic, he was happy. He controlled the attitude towards his suffering experience. Your life is made up of all these moments when we have choices. . . . This guy chose to have hope, he chose to have a life despite suffering. Hope, this was a choice.

C, you want to go?

C: I didn't have a connection to my children because of my drug history. But, a number of years ago my daughter sent me a note, saying that I'm the greatest dad in the world. That was the happiest moment I can remember, other than the time that I first picked her up. And I looked at her and it scared the crap out of me, and now, I finally got her back. And now, every Wednesday, no matter what happens, we talk, and about everything. I've been alive ever since. It's given me a sense of purpose. And the other thing, I don't have a formal college education. I don't have a paper like you guys have on your walls, I'd love to have that. I don't have something on the wall that says I graduated from . . . but I did pass an exam to become a certified counselor. But, the doctor I work for now came into my office and told me to come in and run the detox group, and I said I don't have any formal training, and she said, "C, you have 20 years of experience of working with people and I believe in you." And that's . . . now I have doctors calling me and asking me what I think!

P: My job, I know an awful lot of lawyers, and I've sued an awful lot of doctors, and none of them are really smarter than you are. I mean, they have degrees on their walls, and some are just brilliant academically, but in terms of being life smart? No, no they're not smarter than you.

C: But you can understand of the importance of my passing that test, for my certification? I can't wait to go to work each day . . .

P: Of course.

Therapist 1: You know, people think that you only get meaning in life from happy things, like the birth of children or winning some prize, but it also comes out of suffering experiences, experiences that you might think were shameful, or you might be insecure about, failings, C, your story, your meaningful moment comes out of overcoming limitations, not having an education, not being . . . not believing in yourself, but there it was, you had done enough, you experienced redemption, right? And it didn't just come to you out of the blue, you did something to deserve these doctors believing in you, you did something right with your daughter, that led her to write that letter and re-establish that relationship.

S, you want to go?

S: Yeah, one of the sweetest moments . . . I couldn't have children of my own due to my liver problems. My niece, who's 7, means the world to me. One of the happiest moments was being able to swim with her, and be her playmate, and have her run into my arms and hug me, and at that time last summer, I had enough substance not to be knocked over by her, and to feel the weight of her and her energy and her love and her enthusiasm and her positivity. . . . I was enfolded in it. And at the same time, getting so much pleasure, drinking in nature, nature is so spiritual for me, so meaningful. So being outdoors, and connecting with her, and with nature, it's just been such a gift.

And then, because I had a pretty good attitude when I went back after my liver transplant, I went on rounds with the doctors and saw the patients because I could talk to them one way, in a different way than the doctors. I didn't have that piece of paper, but having been through it, I was on the other side, and we all have bumps in a serious operation, there were certain things I was able to say to them about the bumpy road . . . just specific things I said due to my experience . . . about the healing process, and it was really good. I hadn't been a nurse or a doctor, but now, when I got to see my doctor, I usually try to take an afternoon and see patients who are having problems pre or post transplant.

Therapist 1: Thank you S. Which sources of meaning do you think your two stories tap into?

S: Love, absolutely.

Therapist 1: And what else?

S: Well, experiential, all the senses. And compassion . . .

Therapist 1: And creativity. . . . It was almost like a job, it was a cause, that you were dedicated to, and you were doing something valuable with your life, seeing these patients. It was unpaid work, but took dedication. A really great example of the creative source of meaning.

Therapist 2: You know, S, you began by saying I'm not sure if what I've written down is as meaningful as what others in the group have shared, and I just want to note that, what we each find meaningful is very intimate, is very unique to us all, and personal and different, what might be meaningful to one of us, may not be to others.

Therapist 1: Exactly. The other thing is that, no one else can give you meaning, only you can. The purpose of this group is not for us to give you meaning, but for us to help you find and reconnect with meaning. What you've done today is the beginning of that process of discovering these different sources of meaning in your life. And over the next seven sessions, what we're going to be doing is speaking specifically about each of these different sources of meaning and how they each can be resources for you. Next week we'll be speaking about how cancer has impacted your identity, but after that, each session will be focused on each of these different sources of meaning, and then we'll have a review session at the end.

The other thing is, I'd like to suggest you begin to read this book in front of you, *Man's Search for Meaning*. Read as much as you'd like. Also, feel free to look at the session two material before we meet next week so that you can prepare for what we'll be discussion.

P: So there's homework?

Therapist 1: It's just a suggestion. The book is a quick read, you don't need to read the whole thing. But some people really enjoy it and find it a good, "food for thought," so to speak.

Therapist 2: Any other questions?

Therapist 1: Ok, we look forward to seeing you all next week.

SESSION 2: CANCER AND MEANING—IDENTITY BEFORE AND AFTER CANCER DIAGNOSIS

Therapist 1: I'm going to try to keep us on time so let's get started. Welcome back, this is the 2nd session of meaning-centered group psychotherapy. Glad that people are back today. And, we have a new group member, T, who wasn't here last week because of a problem with pain. We're thrilled that you're here.

T: I was in the hospital.

Therapist 2: We're so glad that you're out and feeling better.

Therapist 1: What we did in the first session is we all introduced ourselves to each other and so maybe we should do that to catch you up to speed, and then quickly review what we did in the first session before getting to the material for today's session, which is that we're going to focus on the issue of identity, how meaning and our identity relate to one another. A lot of us get our sense of meaning from various roles we play in life, who we are, being a wife, a teacher, a daughter, a son, parent, so we're going to be talking about identity and meaning. But to get started, let's do intro again.

Therapist 1: I'm Dr. Breitbart, please call me Bill. I'm a psychiatrist, and actually this intervention, this counseling, called meaning-centered psychotherapy is something that I developed.

Therapist 2: I'm Dr. Allison Applebaum, you and I actually talked on the phone last week. I'm happy to see you here today. Please call me Allison.

Therapist 1: So if you all could introduce yourselves, if you can just talk a little bit about your cancer experience, the short version . . .

P: My name is P, I have esophageal cancer, with mets to liver. It's stage 4, inoperable. I'm married, have three kids, and I'm 49 years old. My parents recently came up from FL to help take care of me.

L: My name is L, I have liver cancer, and I was recently diagnosed. I'm not a candidate for a transplant or resection. I have no symptoms and am feeling fine at least right now, although had ups and downs.

C: Hi, I'm C. I have colon cancer. Found out about it because I was feeling just so damn tired. I run a rehab/detox unit and I've made good friends in groups before. So this is a good place.

S: My name is S, I have breast cancer, with mets to left lung, which has really reduced my capacity. I have no wind, and I've had a chronic problem even before that where I needed 2 liver transplants. So I've been ill for a long time. And I'm a reference librarian in a public library.

T: I'm T, I have breast cancer and now it's in the lining of my lung, and I recently had chest tubes put in. I'm on oxygen because of that. But, it has metastasized, not in major organs, but it is in my spine and neck.

Therapist 1: And that's why you had pain?

T: Yes, lower back pain.

Therapist 1: Tell us about your home and work life?

T: Well I don't work, I was going to school, studying landscape design but I can't make it up there anymore. I'm not married, I don't have children. But I have brothers and sisters who come up. I'm from the Bahamas . . .

Therapist 1: Well we're really glad to have you here . . . and we hope everyone's health holds out so all can be here for the remaining groups. Does anyone have any thoughts or comments about our first session?

P: We were talking outside about how someone should do a sitcom about this group, if you wanted to put together four more disparate people together you couldn't. . . . Was this random?

Therapist 1: Totally random, for the purpose of research.

L: I don't know, I don't think we're really that different. Maybe culturally . . . but otherwise, not so much. . . .

Therapist 2: Well these are all things that are going to come up today when we talk about identity . . .

Therapist 1: What I hope you got from the first session is while people may appear on the surface to be different, we all share an awful lot as humans, our mortality, which everyone is confronting, but what also seems to be universal is this need to find/search for meaning, to create a life of meaning, direction, and identity. And identity is the focus of today's session.

Just as a review, T, what we did last week is we focused on the importance of meaning in human experience, that we're meaning-seeking creatures, that as humans, we create. We create meaning and when we confront obstacles, limitations, that cause us to suffer, like illness or pain, or the fear of death, that we suffer and part of the suffering experience is losing connection and contact to the things in our lives that give our lives meaning. Last week we talked about two different definitions of meaning . . . do you remember them? Which one made most sense to you?

Therapist 2: You can take a look back in your binder . . . this isn't a test!

Therapist 1: The first definition of meaning: having a sense that one's life has meaning involves the conviction that one is fulfilling a unique role and purpose in life that is a gift. A life that comes with the responsibility to live to one's full potential as a human and in so doing, achieving a sense of peace, contentment, and transcendence through connecting to something greater than oneself.

The other definition had to do with moments in life when you felt most alive, because of the meaning associated with relationships with people.

Then we talked about predictable sources of meaning. First was the experiential source of meaning. We're human beings, we have senses, we derive meaning through experiencing life, through love, our love relationships, romantic, filial, love of children, connection to things that are beautiful about life, like sea air, being in nature, good food, all sorts of things. . . .

Therapist 2: Like the meaning you all derived from connecting as a group before we started today.

Therapist 1: The second source is through creativity, the things we do that engage us in life, our dedication to values, causes. The third is the more difficult one to understand . . . and we're going to have an exercise about that, it's finding meaning through the attitude we take towards experiences that cause us to suffer, understanding that we have the freedom to choose our attitude. . . . You can choose your attitude, how you respond, to suffering. Humans have control over the attitude that you take, towards the predicament that you're in, and it's through that attitude that you can derive meaning, by taking something that's potentially an adversity and making it into a triumph. And the fourth source of meaning is through our legacy. The legacy we inherit, the legacy we create, and the one we leave behind. So meaning occurs in a historical context.

So the focus of today is on the connection between meaning and identity.

Therapist 2: Before we jump right in, I know we had a suggested some home reading, to read the first part of *Man's Search for Meaning*, and so I just wanted to touch base and see if you have any thoughts about the reading, questions, etc. . . .

Therapist 1: Did anyone read it?

P: Actually, I read more than half, the first part was compelling . . . the fact that anyone survived just astounds me . . . but the fact that he got something out of it and didn't want to come out and kill every German . . . was just . . . amazing. But, it just makes sense. If you're just living to satisfy needs, you might as well be a rat in a maze. So that part makes sense. But I still have a hard time getting over the randomness of cancer . . . to good to bad people, and to be able to derive meaning from that, I'm just not there yet, to be able to make meaning out of any of us having cancer.

Therapist 1: Thanks P. When we're talking about meaning, we're talking about your ability to continue to feel that you're living a life of meaning and value and purpose, an inner sense of "my life has meaning, even though certain things have been taken from me due to the cancer . . ." . . . that you're still in touch with the things that give life a sense of purpose and value and . . . as opposed to sitting around and trying to figure out "what does it mean" . . . that's not what we're trying to figure out. This group is not about figuring out "Why did I get cancer?" but, instead, how can you maintain meaning in the face of cancer. There may be a little connection for some people, perhaps cancer opens you eyes to new things, but that's not what we're saying here.

T: I actually think I already read that, maybe even in HS or college . . . but I'm guessing I was in a very different mindset at that time. Hopefully I'll have a more mature view about it now . . .

Therapist 2: The main reason VF wrote it was the crystallize his ideas about being in situations where you can control hardly anything, but ultimately you can control your attitude . . . and I think he may have gone so far as to say that the people who were able to maintain a sense of meaning, those were the ones who got through. I don't necessarily agree, I think luck had a lot to do with it as well . . .

Therapist 1: Luck was a major factor for sure. He was saying that the ones who were lucky enough to not be killed managed to survive better—not longer—but with more hope, if they had the attitude that there was something to survive for.

So we have two exercises today about identity. If you turn the page in your book to the second tab. . . . There are really 2 questions here. One is for you to describe "who are you." And the other is to write down how that answer is affected by cancer. What I'd like is for you to start with the first, and then we'll have a discussion, and then get to the second. I'd like you to answer the first question by thinking about your perspective before you had your cancer diagnosis so we can make the contrast to how cancer has changed those answers. . . .

L: I am a daughter, a mother, a grandmother, a sister, a friend, and a neighbor. I attempt to respect all people in their views, which sometimes can be difficult. I represent myself honestly and frankly without being offensive, at least I try. And my philosophy is to do unto others as they would have done unto you. I'm somebody who can be very private and not always share all my needs and concerns. It's questionable as to whether I am not worthy. I also have been working on accepting love and affection and other gifts from other people. I'm more of a caregiver than someone who gets care from others, I don't like to receive care, but I'm beginning to, . . . actually . . . this is may be the one thing that my illness has caused me to kinda mull over. That I'm more accepting of people wanting to do things.

Therapist 1: Thank you. That's really interesting. I want to make some comments, but first let's hear from someone else.

P: I'm very terse because what I wrote down, they're more speaking points. I am a father, I . . . that's probably the foremost thing I think of when I think of who I am. I'm the guy that my kids come to for . . . for the four year old, the answer is candy, the 18 and 16 year olds, when they really want to know something, they ask me, and rely on me to drive them around. I'm a husband, married 26 years in 2 weeks, my wife . . .it's been P and A as long as I've been an adult. . . . I'm comfortable with that, I like that, I love my wife. The third one is, I am a lawyer, that's clearly a part of my identity, at cocktail parties people have questions for me. . . . I like the fact that people come to me for advice, and I like the fact that sometimes I can help people, and I like that what I do is interesting. Also, I'm a son/brother, I'm a member of a family. I have three brothers and a mother, stepfather, and father, far away in CA, haven't spoken to him very much. My stepfather is my father.

Since cancer, my parents have come up and have taken over caretaking roles that I used to do. While I wouldn't have identified as son/brother pre-cancer, it's all come back.

Therapist 2: Thank you.

Therapist 1: T, you want to take a stab?

T: I am a family member, first and foremost. I'm a member of my immediate family. A sister and daughter. I'm a horticulturist and garden designer, avid reader, my dog's best friend, someone who was active, walking, and a baker and dessert maker.

Therapist 1: C you want to go?

C: It's funny. I don't have anything about family, I've been alone for so long. I put down that I'm a teacher and a student of my culture. I am a true friend, loyal as a puppy. I'm like . . . I guess I'm like a big dog that would sit in someone's life. And . . . I say this with a smile on my face, I'm a good lover. I take my time. I'm patient. I've never had a relationship that lasted for more than 12 years, so P, I congratulate you for getting to 26 years. And, I'm a good learner, and . . . I'm in recovery. This is interesting because I knew about recovery, but I'm in denial of this cancer, and so I'm struggling with that. Because I act like I'm ok and cool and I already know what it is to be struggling, to be in a Holocaust, just from my culture.

Therapist 1: Thanks C. S, do you want to go?

S: Well in terms of pre-cancer, I'm my niece's loving aunty who she currently adores . . . she's 7, I'm not sure how long that will last, but right now, that's really important to me, and it's brought my brother and me closer. I'm active and am always ready for an adventure. All my friends knew I was a "yes let's do it person," enthusiastic, open. I'm a young adult librarian, with a real connection to the teens. I really loved working with them, especially on the advisory council, I really just loved it, and oftentimes would stay very late with them, into the night. I was just, really . . . connected. . . . I ran around a lot and I was rarely home before 11pm. . . . My friends always asked why I wasn't home more. It wasn't that I didn't like home, it's just that I wanted to be out, experiencing life. I also love concerts, music concerts, and I danced. And I dated; I was the essence of positive, a very good friend, I'm really proud of that, and proud that I was capable of more intimate relationships despite two ex-husbands. . . .

Therapist 1: Thanks guys. Do you have any questions for each other about the things that you said? Were there any commonalities that you noticed?

L: I guess the commonality, that most of us spoke about, except for C, is being a member of a unique group, family, and for most of us, that was in the top position. That was most important.

S: I have a comment but I don't know if it's what you're asking for. L was talking about being a giver, but that it's basically hard for her to receive. I've had friends who are like that and it's frustrating to want to give to a person like you, but you also don't want to take people's wishes lightly . . . I know I'm probably speaking out of turn for all of your friends, L, who want to be generous back to you.

L: Most of them have been, ok . . . because they, you know, sit me down and do what they want to do. I guess most of my good friends are very strong willed people like me and they listen and do for the most part what they want. And I don't get offended for the most part.

Therapist 1: It was actually quite striking . . . that there were many similarities in what you shared about your identities pre-cancer. For many people, the first, the most important source of your identify, had to do with your love relationships, family relationships, your role in a family, being a daughter, father, an aunt, being a member of immediate family. So it's from these connections that we derive meaning in life, through our connectedness with people we love. And often they are members of our family. And, often, these are our sources of identify, as a member of a family, as a father, an aunt . . .

L: These roles are also source of pain.

Therapist 1: Yes, but also a source of meaning. And do you remember which source of meaning? It's the experiential source of meaning. Through love, connectedness with people. Someone made a comment that C didn't mention this source of meaning. C, you said something interesting. You said you've been alone too long. But you also said that you're a good lover, and a loyal friend, loyal as a puppy. So for you, love, experiential sources of meaning through love, is very relevant for you too. You derive a sense of meaning through love, . . . friendship and romantic love. Those are all similar, all love, right? But let me ask you something, C, did you leave out being a son, or a family member, for a specific reason?

C: Well, I was never . . . I never knew my dad. I didn't really know my mother until I was older. And I have a brother and a sister, and I was thinking about that, I have a younger brother, we've never been close. Not close man. And I have a sister who did something that offended to me and I haven't spoken to her in years. So, in a way, my job became more of my family, the people I worked with, people in recovery, were my family. Because I became more connected to them. But outside of that, no . . . no real family. So in a sense, family has been a disappointment, pain. So everyone talks about family reunions, I'm not there. I don't have that. That's not a part of my life.

Therapist 1: So again this idea that the things that give us meaning are the sources of pain comes up. The other thing I heard that was common for other people, besides love, connectedness to people, . . . is connectedness to other kinds of experiences in life, like dancing, and T, you were talking about baking, cooking . . . so it's not just relationships, it's relationships to the world, and being in nature, and engaging in pleasurable things, like dancing and eating. And in addition to that, several people talked about their identify coming from what they did for work, being a nurse, a lawyer, a librarian, being in recovery and being a counselor is very linked for you, C, and so that, that's a creative source of meaning. We derive meaning through things we create, the work we do in our lives. And you added something interesting, L . . . that had to do with . . . I think I used the word compassion. . . . It had to do with caring for other people.

L: Well, you know, you talked about our profession, but I didn't actually talk today about my professional life, I didn't say anything about being a nurse or a health care provider, but I talked about being caretaker. A caretaker in general, to the people in my life.

Therapist 1: Exactly. So this creative source of meaning doesn't just come from a job you get paid to do, but from the person you create in the world. So you, L, you've created a person who is a loving, giving, caring person. And so you've created a virtue, a value, . . . that compassion is important, caring for others is important, so it's not just job you do, but the kind of person you become and create in the world, and what values that represents. Being a loyal friend, friendship is important. And being a teacher. And you may not get paid to be a teacher, C, but you're a teacher nonetheless.

C: In my profession I need to teach what it is to be in recovery. I need to help people understand how to stay in recovery. And I teach because I've done it myself and I'm lucky enough to be with people willing to share their experiences, and I soak that up. I was speaking to friend in recovery who said he had never been in school, but I asked him how long he had been getting high, and he said 20s years . . . and so I told him, "Boy, you have a doctorate in getting high!" And so do I! I have life experience that makes me an expert that allows me then to teach others.

And now, I'm sitting here trying to figure out where you're trying to go with this, and

I gotta be honest, its stirring up a lot of feelings for me, to be sitting here and talking about my cancer.

Therapist 1: We'll get a real good opportunity to talk about this in the next exercise. ... But also, I don't want to forget about the comment made that the things that give us meaning also can give us pain.

This exercise is really an effort to take the important roles we play and to help you realize how they're connected to various sources of meaning ... we talked about creativity, love, work, our dedication to deeds, the kinds of people we've made ourselves into ... and also legacy and history. C, I think you mentioned being a student of history, and how your legacy has impact this role. C, could you talk a little more about that?

C: Just as this gentleman who wrote this book here that I haven't read yet, I think it's important, I got a chance to grow up in a very important time in my culture. I was that guy who couldn't walk on the sidewalk, a man actually pushed me and mom off of a sidewalk, my mom immediately moved us from Columbus to California where it wasn't so profound. But I appreciate my culture and I like teaching about it, but I'm not one of those people who is going to wave a flag and want to kill, but help others understand that there's a rich history. History is important, and there can always be change, and that's why I teach. I'm not an activist or anything, but at the same time, I do find the value of teaching history. I think people take a lot for granted. And my people didn't.

Therapist 2: So history is important to who you are and how you now lead your life.

C: Very. And ... I'm proud of L ... she's an administrator! She's a beautiful black woman, a sister, who is an administrator, in a high position!

Therapist 1: So pride and your history are related. And P, you didn't say it overtly, but history is important to you, particularly your role as a father and the legacy you're creating.

P: That's the word that got me upset last time. With my four year old I don't know what I'm going to leave. My older ones know who I am, and I'm happy about that. But I am concerned, I do want to leave a legacy. Part of my identity is my being a lawyer, what I found out post cancer is that I'm really well respected, and not because I'm the best lawyer around, but because I treat everyone with respect. I'm respectful, I'm assertive. There is no one in my industry who has anything bad to say about me.

Therapist 1: So that's a good transition to the second question of how cancer has impacted your answers. P, would you mind going first?

P: It's ... on the one hand, I get a little ... my kids continue to mature and ... perhaps they never finish maturing. But the thing is, in terms of my being a father, that aspect of my legacy, it's really about my little guy. ... My older ones ... they're in denial. They know I have cancer, they know it's serious, but no one really talks about it. And, they're in many ways Jewish American Princesses who have a lot of growing up to do, they are selfish in a bunch of ways that I wish they weren't. And as much as I love my wife she has some shortcomings and has difficulty seeing that. But I'm afraid that I'm not going to be able to show them that the world doesn't revolve around them. I want to be there to guide them. As far as my wife, we used to be equal breadwinners, and clearly we're not now. My wife is the primary breadwinner. She got a brand new job as an executive director soon before I had my diagnosis. And, so ... there's a whole bunch of things. I'm sad that she has all this stuff, we've always been confidants, and always told each other things that aren't going right, and now, I think she holds back to try not to hurt me.

The lawyer thing I told you, I've accomplished something great. I did ok. And the people seem to respect me and I appreciate that.

Therapist 1: So having cancer hasn't changed the answers to who you are, in terms of your identity, or the sources of meaning that are so much related to your identity, but they've actually made those things more important, brought in an urgency. Your legacy, your role as a father is more important to you than ever. Connecting with your brother is more important. And having an appreciation of who you were as a professional and how people saw you, cancer was an opportunity to hear about what people thought about you that you may not have had the opportunity to hear otherwise ...

L, want to go next?

L: I'm having difficulty with this, in terms of being able to crystallize my thoughts and speak about them.... Let everyone else go and come back to me.

S: Um, I feel I'm much more genuine since I have cancer. I just try to say what I really mean. And I like that. That's actually the one positive. Instead of feeling the need to please everyone, I seem to be a little more comfortable with just stating the case.

I have friends that have offered to help over the years and I always said no, I didn't want to test the friendships, didn't want to find out they didn't want to do what I might have needed. I just wanted status quo. But I've had so many situations now where I've needed to ask for help and was relieved that they were actually just very compassionate and really are there for me. I didn't want to find out they wouldn't be, and I also . . . take pride in being strong, and it's scary to admit you're weak, and the silver lining has been finding out that they're genuine too.

I used to be able to live in denial. I may have had a liver problem and breast cancer but believe it or not it didn't really impact my life. But now, with my difficulty breathing, I can't dance anymore. I can't do things I used to do, I get so winded that my being able to not let this disease impact me is . . . everything I do is impacted by the fact that I'm breathless. And I'm jealous in a way of my friends who can do all these things that are fully taking advantage of summer. Now, it's a little more distant. . . . I miss fully engaging in summer.

That leads into . . . I find myself feeling very anxious and frantic inside, this free-floating anxiety that undoes me. . . .

Therapist 1: I want to make a few comments about what S said. Lots of similarities with what P shared in a sense. Cancer has resulted in things that are not all negative. And what I think this cancer experience has done for you S is that you realize that you're free . . . you have freedom. To just be. You can be yourself. The problem is that when you discover that you're free, that's a little scary. To be free and responsible to do and choose attitude, that's scary.

The anxiety you describe, and the jealousy, that's very interesting. That indicates to me that you wouldn't be jealous unless there wasn't a part of you that very much wanted to live life fully, right? You guys still want to live life fully, even in the face of the threats of cancer, you still have the courage to want things.

P: You're equating jealousy with courage?

Therapist 1: Yes, you still want stuff. As long as there's that desire, there's a way to get some of it. The other thing I want to say, you were talking about care. L brought up care before. Caregiving. And you brought up this interesting thing. Cancer gave you permission to take care of yourself. It's actually one of the very common things that happens when you have cancer. Suddenly you realize, if I don't take care of myself, I can't take care of anyone else. So I need to do everything I can to take care of myself in order to take care of others, otherwise I won't be able to. Sometimes that means allowing others to help take care of you. Sometimes it's a gift you give other people to allow other people to take care of you.

L: I agree. Well. . . .

I guess something that S said. I've always had a reputation for being "no-nonsense," cutting to the chase, telling it like it is. I still feel the freedom to do that, but I now make the effort to couch it in a more positive manner, and I'm kinder and more diplomatic in my delivery. I've also found that I'm trying to secure—I have a son who has a family, he's 40—I'm trying to secure his financial well-being in ways that I don't know if I should. That's my need to do that. That has very dramatically changed over the past 6–8 months.

Therapist 1: So that's part of your legacy.

We're all humans, we're mortal, we have to die. The hardest thing you can do is face death. Most people can't do that easily. I'm not going to sit here and say that you need to accept eventual death lightly, but the task is to be able to turn around and look at the life that you lived and accept that and say that there are some things that I didn't do, some things that I did, achieve some redemption, reconciliation, tie up the loose ends, etc.

C, you want to go?

C: Ok. I was just thinking. I think I've become more open, not so guarded. I have some fears. I've been worried about the death part of this process, I'm like, I'm on borrowed time already, at this point. I feel like I have the grim reaper on my shoulder. My mother was very spiritual, Pentecostal, always praying. Everyone else in the church became a member, but I would just sit, not get into it. But now, I pray every morning, and I'm rocking, I'm not just sitting. So I've become a little more open to this process. And I have a history of being direct.

Therapist 1: C, do you think the experience you're having praying, do you think that's because you're developing a close relationship to God or does it remind you of your mom? Makes you feel closer to her?

C: I think a bit of both. I was made to go to church, but now, it's a choice. I'm really just appreciative to be alive, sit here with all of you, every new experience.

Therapist 1: And we haven't had a lot of examples of attitude, but in this part, we have heard a lot. The choice you make in how to see things, being more open, spiritual, more honest.

Therapist 2: More direct with your desires.

Therapist 1: These all have to do with attitude. Thanks C. T?

T: Um, well, I'm the youngest sibling. And now they all seem to be gathering around me.

Therapist 2: So you've been embraced more deeply?

T: Yes, absolutely. I find myself not being as closed off as I used to be. I don't really have any secrets, but I'm more of an open book than I ever was. What's changed most is I can't continue my studies in garden design. So now I've shaped them around what I can do. When I couldn't do the garden, I did the window boxes, or did the design inside the church. And I've started painting planters, as opposed to being on the ground itself planting. But I've had to change what I can do to be creative. And my dog . . . well, I'm no longer able to be his active best friend. So I can't really interact with him in the same way and he no longer lives with me.

Therapist 1: So let me make some comments. The whole purpose of this exercise was to talk about the relationship between meaning and our identity, and how cancer has affected it. You can see from the discussion today that there are these predictable sources of meaning, so interconnected with who we are and our identities, and even cancer doesn't eliminate these sources but sometimes cancer poses challenges, limitations . . . like once doing landscaping and now painting at home . . . but what's really important is that when cancer exerts a physical or other type of limitation, you can find a way to do a part of what was meaningful and also remember that there are a bunch of sources of meaning and you can move from one to another when you feel that sense of loss. So you need the flexibility to move from one to another.

We're out of time, so next week we'll meet again and begin talking about legacy. The next two sessions will focus on historical sources of meaning, the first part is the legacy that we inherited from our families and our experiences, so if you want to jot down a few notes before next week, that would be great. And if you haven't read any of *Man's Search for Meaning*, do that.

Any other issues?

Therapist 2: No I think you covered it all

SESSION 3: HISTORICAL SOURCES OF MEANING—LIFE AS A LEGACY THAT HAS BEEN GIVEN

Therapist 2: Welcome everyone to our 3rd session, it's great to see everyone. Today we're going to be talking about historical sources of meaning. But before we get into today's material, I'd like to start by reflecting for a moment on what it's been like for me to sit here for the past two sessions and listen to you and those things that have really stood out to me. Last week you each spoke about how your identities have shifted in some way since your cancer diagnosis and what struck me is not so much how your identities have changed, but how the diagnosis has highlighted or brought to light aspects of your personalities or lives that are meaningful to you.

L, I'm going to start with you. Last week you spoke about many relationships, being a mother, grandmother, friend, caretaker, both in the context of work and outside of work, and you spoke about the struggle you have in letting others take care of you. You used the word worthy, you said "I don't know if I'm worthy of this care." Worthy is an important word, one we should listen for and think about as we talk about meaning.

P, you also spoke about relationships last week and your role as a father and particularly the strong sense you feel about creating a legacy for your children and especially your youngest child and what that legacy is going to be. You also spoke about your renewed sense as a brother and a son, with your stepfather and youngest brother who've come back into your life to take care of you. . . . And, I notice that you're all dressed up today, I'm guessing for work?

L : Well, actually for you, but . . . yes, for work.

Therapist 2: I appreciate the suit! So you spoke about how people have told you how much they respect you in your profession of law . . . and I imagine that will play a big part in your legacy.

S, you spoke about your relationship with your niece in the first session and how important she is. You described so vividly a desire to live your life in "Technicolor," and I'm guessing no one would disagree with me when I say that it sounds like you've completely been living your life in Technicolor. You also said last week that you've become more genuine, taking more time, thinking more about "what does S want" and as a group we acknowledged that we do have a choice, that we're authors of our lives, that we can choose what we want to do tonight, this year, in this life. At the same time, though, we had noted that having that choice is scary because it also means that we're responsible for our lives . . .

L, P, and S, you didn't explicitly say these words or identify these specific sources of meaning but in all of your stories, it was clear to me that creative and experiential sources of meaning have played a large role in your identities.

T, what really stood out to me is your love for design and gardening and how, even in the face of the limitations you're facing, you haven't given up on any of that, you've adapted your approach, scaled down, you're doing window boxes, painting planters, instead of working on your hands and knees in the garden. This attitude you've taken towards the situation is really significant.

C, last week what really struck me about you is when you started speaking you said, "I'm not like everyone else in this room, I'm not going to be able to talk about family relationships, but then you went into talking about how you've been a teacher and a counselor and a leader in your community, and I was sitting there thinking, "Wow, that's about connectedness! That's about what relationships are about!" And I was also struck that you've already found that connectedness here in this group, and you've already had some nice moments that you've shared in here with P.

And this is really a nice segue into today's topic which is historical sources of meaning. C, you spoke really eloquently about your history and how important your lineage is to you, and teaching and sharing has been a big part of who you are. That is a big part of what we're going to talk about today.

Therapist 1: Thanks Therapist 2. You know I'm hearing this for the first time too and I have a few thoughts about what you said. You know, this whole 8-week journey we're taking together is focused on meaning. But, we derive meaning from a number of sources, which we've been talking about. But meaning exists in a person's life, it's not some abstract thing, it's within your life. So what's really critical is to live a life, to create a life, that has some meaning, a life that has some direction, a life that in which you create an identity. When Therapist 2 was talking about L and highlighting the word *worthy* and talking about fulfilling a role as father for P and fulfilling those responsibilities, and S living a genuine life, what we're really talking about is creating that life that you want to live. Sometimes what happens is that we run into obstacles to creating that life. Sometimes those obstacles occur during our lifetime, like developing cancer. Sometimes the obstacles have to do with what we've inherited, our genes, resources of our families, things like that, things we carry from our past that introduce a set of limitations as well. And so the real task is to be able to encounter these limitations, either things that come up or things that are inherited and get over them, transcend them, and that's the real task, transcending through the attitude you take—positive, negative, not being defined by history. Also, you can transcend by connecting with something greater than yourself. And that connectedness is a source of meaning. If there's one thing that you leave this 8-week intervention with, I hope, it is the notion that meaning comes from being connected, to people, the world, your past, nature . . . meaning is all about being connected, and so I think the session that we're focusing on today in terms of the historical context of meaning and the legacy we've inherited is going to confront us with some of these things in the past that perhaps have shaped us in a way, perhaps positives, perhaps neg, perhaps things we've had to overcome, or things that have given us a foot up. And sometimes what happens if you don't live a life that you didn't really want, you can feel guilty, that you haven't fully lived authentically . . .

Therapist 2: Maybe we can open this up for some reflection on what Therapist 1 and I just shared?

T: Well what you said about me is accurate, I can't do design for a large resort, I have to scale everything I do, down.

Therapist 2: So similar to what S said last week, you've made a choice to continue, but just in an attenuated form.

T: Right, I'm always busy. I am still cooking, making sorbet, ice cream, all those things.

L: I think she was on target. I don't remember saying the word "worthy" but I guess it's something I would say . . .

Therapist 1: But it rings a bell?

L: Yeah, it rings true.

Therapist 2: Other thoughts?

Ok, then what we can do is segue into the experiential exercise for today, on legacy and historical sources of meaning. I'm wondering if before jumping into the questions, if we can discuss together what this work legacy means to you?

L: To me it means, what you're leaving behind, what you stand for, how you would like to be perceived by those persons who are important to you, there are those people who want to be important to everyone, but that's not my thing. Just to be important to the few people in my life who are really important to me.

Therapist 1: So you think about it in terms of how to be remembered?

L: Yes.

Therapist 1: That's the focus of next week's session. Today we're going to be talking about the legacy we've inherited, in our families, from generations and generations.

S: With reference to what you're saying, not the legacy I'd leave, but the one I received, I think legacy is what I've gotten certainly from my parents, expectations, and examples that they've left. I think I was pretty lucky ... I wouldn't be who I am ... without what my parents taught me. We didn't spend a lot of time on illness, didn't milk illness, if something was wrong, we took care of it, and moved on. I was constantly moving on, and not weighing self down.

Therapist 1: So it's lessons learned from your parents, like the attitude you take towards illness?

S: Exactly. And they both had a sense of adventure which I clearly got.

Therapist 1: Anyone else? In terms of what legacy means?

P: I agree with what both of you said. You know, it really ... is what comes to you and what you leave. I'm not sure that I've thought much about the legacy that's come to me.

Therapist 1: C?

C: I have two comments. Thanks, Therapist 2, because you did your homework and you talked. I wasn't sure what your role was, and it was good to hear you. Co-facilitators sometimes just lay back, and I was wondering when you were going to come forward, for you.

For me, my legacy is a little different. The legacy that was given to me was negative, because my mom and dad's relationship changed and he left. And I guess I reminded my mom about my dad, in the way I was, the way I walked and talked, and I got beat for that.

Therapist 1: So you're talking about legacy as lessons you were taught, sometimes lessons were positive, sometimes negative.

C: I certainly understand that, but that was the legacy given to me.

Therapist 1: Gotcha.

Therapist 2: T, anything to add?

T: I don't know so much about the legacy, but when I think about the word, I think about what people would think or say about me, what type of person I convey to the world.

Therapist 1: What I'm hearing is the term legacy, you think of it as what you leave behind. So this idea, this legacy that you inherited is novel, new, you haven't thought about it in this way much or appreciated this other way of thinking about it. And one of the things about meaning, is that meaning occurs in a historical context ...

So this idea of legacy that you've inherited from the past and how it influences who you are as a person and meaning in life and who you are is something you haven't really thought about, and that's what we're going to focus on today. We want you to appreciate that meaning exists in that historical context, is partly shaped, by our past legacy, what we inherited.

T: Your inherited legacy, that means from birth?

Therapist 1: Yes, where your parents are from, your lineage.

T: Everything you're related to that came before.

Therapist 1: Yes, even your genetic makeup. So a lot of what you've inherited in the past you can't go back and change, but what you can change is what you do when you move forward with the life that you create, and I think that's part of what we want to explore today.

Therapist 2: Ok, so maybe we can go into the exercise. Why don't you take a few minutes to review the questions—for those who have already completed—or complete now for the first time for those who didn't, and then we'll go around and listen and discuss your answers.

T, can we start with you today?

T: Ok. So, when I look back on my life and upbringing ... my family offers me the most significant memories. One being, I'm much younger than my brother and two sisters, so at one point I felt like an only child, they're three years apart each, and then there's a six-year gap, and then me. So in some ways I felt like an only child. And I do remember the recurring theme that I was "too young," too young to go bike riding, to go to the movies, not old enough to join them . . . so I felt excluded.

And then I wrote down about my name. I know how I got my name. My father didn't want an Irish name, like my siblings . . . so he chose T. Although ironically it actually is Irish, but he didn't know. I have read about the meaning of my name a long time ago, and if I remember correctly, it has something to do with harvesting crops, or something like that.

And events that touched my life? The major events I'd say, the first was going away to boarding school at age 13, and then the second was when I was 16 I just sort of, I contracted a very rare circulation disorder that came out when I was at boarding school that almost killed me. I was taken to the children's hospital of Philadelphia and they thought I wouldn't survive and I was the first person to survive that in the US.

Therapist 1: Thank you, T. I'm going to wait to comment until a few more people have gone. L?

L: I considered myself to be a cross breed, a product of an African American woman and Afro-Caribbean man. They married in 1939, very unusual for those cultures to be together, but it was a very proud black household. I was raised in an extended family type situation. My grandmother raised 6 children on her own. We all lived together in a 4-story brownstone, where my dad still lives. At times there were 13 of us there. My cousins were more like brothers and sisters to me.

As the oldest girl child in my generation, I got a lot of opportunities that most African American children didn't get. At age 9 I spent the summer in Europe and got to visit 10–13 countries. My uncle was in the service and could bring his family there. So that started my wanderlust for travel.

I was very close to my family, my father. As an adult, they were also my best friends, very supportive. Education very important to them, my dad is 101. Still a doctor. One of the oldest living black doctors. Which is rare. Productivity, responsibility, both were very important to them. So, yeah, I think that's it.

Therapist 1: That's very rich. Can I say a few things? That's really interesting that T and L, your stories, they almost represented the opposite ends of a certain spectrum. From the perspective of the kinds of things that I think about when I think about sources of meaning and how meaning in your life form. T, you talked about being the only child, felt like the only child, and the more powerful events in your life were about being sent away, being on your own, and so I got the sense that being disconnected from everyone else, those moments were moments of meaning. And for L, your moments were all about family and connecters, and family being supportive and resources for each other. You, T, you talked about being the youngest, and you L, the oldest, roles which have different sets of expectations. What you talked about L was being the oldest child in a family with high standards and expectations, and you T were talking about being "too young," not being able to do very much. "You aren't even baked yet!" That was the message you got. The ingredients were raw.

So you wonder how those two sets of expectations affected how you both went about creating a life. Would you say they did?

L: Oh yes, burdensome at times, even, such high expectations. I was supposed to be a mentor, supposed to be a teacher, someone the younger children looked up to, not an easy rode necessarily.

Therapist 1: And T how'd that feel?

T: Lonely. I was left alone.

Therapist 1: Were you burdened by that?

T: I don't think so . . .

Therapist 1: So the issue of having this family history, experiences you had as a child, for you, sometimes they're burdensome, and sometimes, not, they can be gifts.

L: Yes, I see the general experience as a gift, I had many gifts, I was very blessed, but at the same time a lot was expected of me, I *could not* fail.

Therapist 1: So do you think being alone was a burden, T?

T: Yes and no. I learned how to entertain myself, so I didn't get bored. And I don't now.

Therapist 1: So you developed that ability to be on your own. Sometimes good things become burdensome, sometimes negative things become gifts, right? They encourage you to grow in other ways.

C, do you want to take a swing?

C: A couple of things. I was raised in . . . I didn't know I was raised in a broken home. My dad left, my mom took care of us. Significant things happened. I took my brother and sister at age 9 across country, from Columbus, Ohio, to Fresno, CA, on the Greyhound bus. And now

I look back and wonder how these three little kids survived across country. So I've always been the guy who took care of the family.

I didn't know we were poor. I had a track coach. I ran, I was good enough to almost go to the Olympics. But during my first track meet that we went out of town, we stayed in a hotel, and it was the first time I had gotten into a bed that had a top sheet and a bottom sheet, and I never knew you were supposed to have a top sheet and bottom sheet. And when I got home, I went out and bought sheets for me and my siblings.

So the people in my family, they made the difference. We were all raised with respect. Yes Ma'am, no Ma'am, that's how we spoke. My mom was raised down south and that was how I was raised.

My last name is an English name that was given to slaves, many generations ago, and my first name, that's my dad's name. And that's pretty much it. I'm a survivor, so, I hope I ended up like my dad, as my mom always said I would.

Therapist 1: Can you talk a little bit more about being a survivor? In relation to what you just told us about your family?

C: I listen to the news these days and I'm trying to figure out how a nine year old got his siblings across the country.

Therapist 1: Did you do that for a specific reason?

C: My mom had moved from Columbus to California to be a cook in a restaurant and we had to go live with her and that was the only way to get there. And I was told to take care of my siblings, and I did that, and I've always done that. Always. I've always been a caretaker. Always figured out how to do what I need to do. Always would take the brunt, to make sure they were ok.

And I still do that now. When I found out I was an addicted person, when I found out I had cancer, I survived those things, and still am.

And I've learned to say, the most important thing for me, so that I don't use or drink, is to say that my feelings got hurt, because if I don't, I'll use. If I keep it in, it will be destructive.

Therapist 1: One of the quotes in front of you, from Nietzsche, is, "He who has a why to live for can bear with almost any how." It sounds like you found a How to survive, right? The question I'm wondering about, is the why? What was the why that you had?

C: I wish I knew.

Therapist 1: You mentioned a higher power?

C: Yes, that's part of it. Absolutely. I believe in a higher power.

Therapist 1: It sounds like you overcame a lot of limitations, all these things, and being connected to something greater than yourself, that might be part of what allowed you to transcend?

C: Yes.

And there are other people for whom religion is really important.

L: Yes . . .

Therapist 2: Would you mind sharing a little bit about that?

L: I was raised in an evangelical setting and church was a basic activity. And, um, I guess what they say, the apple doesn't fall very far from the tree. My grandmother was very . . . very spiritual. No smoking in the household. The denomination I grew up in was particular ascetic, no jewelry, women wore skirts, not pants, but it was also very inspiring, these were people who came here through Ellis Island, bought property, and made sure their children got an education.

Therapist 1: Thank you. S?

S: My father, who was English, was very religious, Jewish, and had been orthodox in England, and became a little less religious at one point, Conservative, but truly believed, loved being in Temple, and really had a relationship with a rabbi. And my mother wasn't religion. I personally hated Hebrew school with a passion. And I actually skipped it at one point and didn't know what to do with myself and had said to my father at one point at 12, I said to him, "I just can't do it." I said, "Believe me, dad, God does not hang out at Temple Israel." And I remember him asking me where I thought God was, and I wasn't prepared for the question, and it took me a while and I was looking around at the trees, it totally resonates with the rest of my life, and I said, nature. So I think maybe the term is that I'm spiritual, but when it comes to organized religion, I'm not comfortable, I really find nature is the extension to me of God and things that are bigger than ourselves and meaning in life. So that's in terms of religion.

On the other hand, even though I didn't really like Passover and the other holidays, after he died, I've been the one who puts together these holidays, in his honor, because it was so important to him. I feel something is wrong if the holiday goes by without observing it.

I had been very lucky, with my father being English, we went to England and other countries a lot, and while my parents weren't into spending money on clothes, they were really into culture and travel and education, and when I was 15 I was really into French because my parents would speak French at the dinner table when they wouldn't want us to understand what they were saying, so when I was 15 or 16 I went to France and studied French and I got 9 weeks around Normandy and the University of Grenoble and then went to the Sorbonne the next summer.

My parents on paper were perfectly suited to each other, loved travel and adventure, but didn't get along at all and I was in the middle of this triangle. They were both used to being the star, but they wouldn't give each other the star power. My father was really compelling, and my mother, so beautiful, and so the two egos that didn't get along, and my brother was young, and my mom would use me as a shield, and my dad would look towards me to save him. It was really a painful situation.

My mother really believed education was important, I was a math major. My mother had to convince my father that I needed to go to college, he was convinced I was going to waste the education and just get married. So a strange combo of things to come from, but it was, and somewhere down the line, I got in over my head with math and changed majors to something that I always found solace in, which was books. I was a tomboy when I was younger, and I really escaped through books. When other girls were mean to me, I would find myself go and escape through reading.

Ok, I think that's a lot, that's it.

Therapist 1: You said so much that was meaningful, thanks for sharing all of that. All of you have shared so much. One of the interesting things about families and growing up in religious traditions and how they've influenced us, and for some of us the religion we grew up in continues to sustain us. S, you describe becoming somewhat alienated from religious tradition, but what was really poignant was that as an adult you've taken up the Passover tradition, and it's very meaningful, so I'm wondering what about it is so meaningful?

S: One year I thought about it as our Thanksgiving. Thanking God that we survived. A real thanksgiving, continuation of tradition, of a people, and maybe this is what you're getting at, there's been so much adversity in our lives, all of us in this room are here because of adversity, but we overcame, and Passover is about that, overcoming . . .

Therapist 1: So the actual content of the Passover story was meaningful to you in terms of survival and freedom and things like that, right? I wondered whether when you do celebrate Passover, that that is a way that you feel more connected to your family, childhood, times that you did this with your family when you were younger?

S: I'm glad you said that, because when I hear the songs I used to hear in Hebrew school, that was my favorite part, those songs bring back my childhood, they're a "shortcut" to my childhood.

Therapist 1: So no matter good, bad, mixed, it feels meaningful to touch base with your childhood, your heritage, periodically.

S: Yes, and I feel very connected to my father at that time.

Therapist 1: And safe maybe?

S: Yeah, because I'm with my family too.

Therapist 1: Thank you. P?

P: Ok, so each of you here . . . when everyone else spoke, a bell went off for me. C, you spoke about divorced parents. For me, when I grew up, my dad left, I was the only one I knew of all of my friends who didn't have a dad, and for a long time, that was the defining thing. My mother never said that I was like him, which I guess is a really good thing.

And L, when you spoke, you spoke about devoted family. My mom is incredible. When my dad left, we were stuck in suburbia with no car, no phone, nothing. And she had four kids, I was the oldest, and she went and got us, and had a master's degree in education, no job because of the new baby, and she took a civil service test, and with an M.A. in education the only thing she could do was be a parole officer, and that's what she did to take care of us. She raised 4 boys by herself. 5 years later she remarried, and I eventually realized that her new husband was a good man. So my mom raised us, but like you, L, there was never a question about education or college, it was, "You're going to college, you're going to school after college." There was no thought that I or my siblings weren't going to go on, because education was so, so important.

And then the next thing I wrote down was being Jewish. The difference there was that I don't remember having any discussions about whether God exists. Jewish is a culture thing that I am glad I am a part of but defines me and also separated me growing up in Suffolk County, where at the time it was only 10% Hewish. So the fact that I didn't have this understanding of what Jesus was separated me from my friends, or at least I felt that.

And the last thing I wrote down was being the oldest brother. And C I thought about you. When my mom went to work I learned to cook and took care of everyone every night at a very young age. I learned how to cook basic things. I think that what that . . . coming from divorced parents and having a father who did some bad things . . . so it . . . well, being a good father is just so important to me. It's only recently that I've spoken to my father and forgiven him.

Therapist 1: How did that happen?

P: It's a complicated story. My brothers. . . . Each of us reached out to him at separate times. It's a crazy story but a friend of mine had interviewed with him, for a job, about 20 years ago. And put it together that this guy—this architect—was my dad. My last name is so uncommon that it was clear that it was he, living in CA. And soon after that I called him up, and he was very nice, and happy to hear from me, and flew me there . . . and then . . . I guess I upset his wife, and upset his life, and then he told me that he didn't want more contact with me. This was a while ago. But what happened was that my youngest brother has always been the peace-maker, the conciliator, and interestingly he formed the strongest relationship with my father, maybe because he was in diapers when he left, but anyway, he re-established ties with him and my father was going to visit him and I was going on a trip and I saw my father and it was interesting, because I always remembered him as a big burly guy, he had had two back surgeries, was hunched over, a little man. He looked like a little man. And I was sorta distant, and he was very deferential, was happy to meet his grandchildren, which is hurtful that he considers them his grandchildren because they don't consider him their grandfather.

Anyway, that was about 10 year ago, and since then . . . there have been small steps to repairing. Bringing back religion, I'm not religious at all. I think that what you said about nature. I think it's all about energy. If you believe that everything is energy and energy is God then you believe in God.

Getting back to the Jewish thing, I was sitting in temple on high holy days with my children. I want them to have an identity at this point, so we're sitting in temple and the rabbi was talking about forgiveness on Yom Kippur and he starts talking about how when you don't forgive, it eats up you, it's not necessarily about the person who did something wrong, but it's for you, it eats away at you. And that coincided with my wanting to really reach out and forgive my father, I didn't confront him, but forgave him, just for me.

Therapist 1: Thank you P. We're running out of time but I want to comment on the two things about what you said that were striking. How your past and your family made being a good father so important to you, and then, this notion of forgiveness. I'm just wondering if forgiveness comes up for others? When you think about families and backgrounds?

S: Well I forgive my parents for the pressure they put on me. My mother came first, and I was to her just a barrier to my father. But I've forgiven her for that, to move on. I think being actively angry at someone is to say that that person is living rent free in your head. I think that's the best saying ever.

Therapist 1: And forgiving others is also connected to forgiving ourselves, right?

L: Yes, yes. I have very high expectations, and when others don't meet it, I sometimes get very angry. And it does more damage making me feel badly than them. So forgiveness is good in terms of cleansing and encouraging, and yeah, proceeding.

C: Like you, religion, forgiveness, that was big for me. I was made to go to church; I was made to be observant. I don't think I really forgave my mom for thinking that I was like my dad, and for the last 5 years of her life I didn't talk to her. I have a sister who tricked me into talking her. I just know that I speak my peace, so that I take care of me, you're absolutely correct, that's freeing. I try not to put my energy on someone else, so I really work hard at not doing that.

Therapist 1: Thanks C.

Therapist 2: So moving forward, today was focused on the past. And next week we're going to focus on the present and the future, the legacy that we're living, and the one we hope to leave in the future. The legacy you live and will give.

Therapist 1: It's a little more like what you guys were talking about in terms of your definitions earlier today about legacy.

Therapist 2: Ok, are there any questions before we finish?

Therapist 1: Ok, we'll see you all next week then.

SESSION 4: HISTORICAL SOURCES OF MEANING—LIFE AS A LEGACY THAT ONE LIVES AND WILL GIVE

Therapist 2: Welcome to our fourth session of meaning-centered psychotherapy. It's really wonderful to see you all here today.

Therapist 1: We just want to let you know that C couldn't make it today but he's looking forward to re-joining us next week.

Therapist 2: And we have S joining us by phone today. S, can you hear us?

S: I'm here. Hi everyone!

Group: Hi S!

Therapist 2: Wonderful. Ok. So today, we're going to pick up where we left off last week discussion legacy. Last week the focus was on the legacy that we're given, those things that we didn't choose. Our families, our cultures, our histories, where we were born, our names even.

Therapist 1: Yes, and our discussion was really rich and highlighted how this given legacy can be positive or negative, that for some of us, we've had an advantage, so to speak, because of what we were given, while for others, we were at a disadvantage, or had challenges or obstacles to overcome as a result.

Therapist 2: Today the focus is really on the present and future—the legacy that you live and will give, the one you are actively creating now, and the one that you will leave for others.

Therapist 1: So today, yes, it's really about ... when we asked you all last session to define "legacy" for us, many of you, most of you shared thoughts that really had to do with this notion of legacy. The second part, what you hope to leave for others when you are no longer here. Which, I know, is a difficult thought. So, we started a bit late today and for time sake, I want to jump right in to the experiential exercise, which is really focused on the ways in which you are actively, currently, creating your legacies, and those things which you hope to pass on to others.

Therapist 2: Were you all able to take a look at the exercise in the interim?

P: Yeah, I took a lot.

S: So did I.

Therapist 2: L, T?

L: Yeah, I didn't right anything down, but I have a sense of my answers.

T: Yeah, I'm sorry I also didn't do any writing this week. So I'd prefer to not go first today.

Therapist 2: S, since you're on vacation and calling in—which, by the way, we are so, so happy about!—would you like to go first?

S: Sure. In 1975, 30 years ago, when I found out that I was sick with a very serious liver problem, despite the fact that I didn't drink or anything. They were already wondering about my life span, if I should work, and I already knew that I couldn't have children. My greatest accomplishment? I've lived my life despite being ill, I've held a career, had two marriages, close relationships, been self-sufficient, and was really into sports and dance. Despite what the doctors were saying, I contained that someplace and did everything I wanted to do, and maybe even more, because life was already precious.

And in terms of my career, I really loved my career, and in terms of a legacy that I might leave, it's the message to the teens that I work with that they can really make a difference. I've never thought of myself as creative in the artistic sense, and I've always rationalized it by saying that everyone needs an audience, but in my career, I was incredibly creative, thinking out of the box so often.

Another key aspect of my legacy is my perseverance. I persevered when I got divorced the first time, I realized that I couldn't just keep my house by the work I did as a librarian, and so I took out a loan and bought my husband out of the house, and that took a lot of time and energy, to get the money together, but I did, so that I could have some stability in my life. More importantly, in terms of perseverance, is seeking what I desperately need. Of course that's been getting a very good doctor at MSKCC, and so in terms of legacy and medicine, I would say, teaching others to not always accept what one doctor says to you. It took me a long time to learn to defend myself and seek info elsewhere. And of course, being an active part of my niece's life, is a key aspect of my legacy, and I hope those things that I deem important, she will too.

Therapist 1: I hope that you'll still have something to say about the 2nd part of the exercise, S., but what's interesting about what you're saying, P and L were talking about family and creative sources of meaning in terms of work, and experiential sources of meaning in terms of love, and you spoke about creative sources of meaning as well in the less traditional ways, but also, what you spoke about is the importance of the attitude that you took towards the circumstances you were in, in the face of suffering and limitations—with the house, for example—that attitude was something that you're quite proud of in terms of how you've lived your life. Is that correct?

S: Yeah, you've put it in a nutshell.

Therapist 1: Are you aware of times when you had to make a choice? Were you conscious of this?

S: When I was sick at the other hospital, I made some potentially risky decisions in terms of my health, but they were choices that felt right for me, not necessarily the doctors, and they turned out ok.

Therapist 1: So there were moments when you had to choose, to wonder whether you were going to give up, move forward . . .

S: Definitely. I was actually in a coma in March, 2008, I thought I was paralyzed, because I couldn't move anything, and I remember thinking, did I flatline? But I was just determined to live, determined to get out of there. But I remember hearing the nurse say to my brother, "She's a fighter, she'll survive."

Therapist 1: I know L and P you talked about what you're most proud of, but this notion of making certain choices in your life and being conscious that you have to make a choice to move forward and fight for something or not, the attitude you took, that was relevant for you guys too, right?

L: Yes, the situation with my job was that. The CEO gave me such a hard time when I put my resignation in, they fought it, but I stuck with my decision to go back to school. I wanted to go back to school, I had started a master's program a long time ago, but I wanted to set an example of education for my son. But, you know, I wanted to set an example and it worked out beautifully for me, liberated me.

Therapist 1: You, P?

P: I'm sort of processing something S said about not accepting the first opinion. My current doctor's opinion has been his opinion since the beginning. He told me that I have a death sentence and that the chemotherapy is the means of "execution," but we just don't know for how long. I'm just, I'm mulling over whether or not to accept that opinion, or go for 2nd, 3rd, or 4th opinions like S. My conversation with the doctor after this morning, I need to think about it more.

Therapist 1: What about that notion—not about statistics—when someone says to you that you have a death sentence, you picked up on an attitude that he was conveying, that . . .

P: That my cancer has a 2% chance of being cured, that 90% of patients with my cancer die within two years.

Therapist 1: So what you heard from your doctors is, "You're on death row, resign yourself."

P: Yes.

Therapist 1: And so the question is now about your attitude. Do you resign yourself? Or do you try to take the attitude that you're still alive, that you can live fully as long as you're alive, you can live a meaningful life drawing on these sources of meaning that you can use as resources of meaning.

P: It is an attitude . . . it's a way part of me feels. I've always prided myself in being rational, in facing the truth. I'm a statistician for God sakes! I know what statistics mean.

Therapist 1: And is being rational inconsistent with maintaining an attitude that as long as I'm alive I'm going to live fully?

P: No, not at all. The other part of me, I know I have a lot to live for. But I take it one goal at a time. This summer I wanted to teach my daughter to drive. And she got her license two weeks ago.

Therapist 2: Congratulations!

P: Thank you. It's good. She now gets to pick me and her mom up at the train station. And I wanted to be around for her birthday. And for my anniversary, and my next son's birthday, and you know. I want to be there for them.

Therapist 1: I don't want to leave this particular subject without opening it up for discussion, if this resonates with others in the room.

T: To not be discouraged?

Therapist 1: Yes, in the attitude that P is taking.

T: My oncologist keeps telling me it's a matter of when, not if, I'm going to be going back into the hospital. But, you know, I don't really plan on going back in there! And that's really my attitude. I don't like to think about the when, I like the "if." Things like that comment, I don't think that's helpful, it's coming from a negative place.

Therapist 1: And you have a choice to come from the negative or positive place.

L: But a lot of times, we can be exposed to so much that we can become desensitized. And I think the physicians really need to work on that . . . being sensitive and understanding how to speak to patients.

P: I agree. He provided info he knew to be true, medically and statistically.

Therapist 1: The fact of the matter is that you're going to journey through this cancer trip here, and be bombarded by all sorts of info and attitudes about what your attitude should be, but the only thing that is consistent is you and your responsibility, and choosing your attitude.

L: That's a very good point. It is what it is. People have attitudes, they're human and it's what you do with that.

T: Yeah, you know when my lung collapsed, I had been walking around with a gallon of fluid in my lung, and no one thought it was a problem that I was having trouble breathing. I went to see my doctor and he told me that I needed surgery, but my surgeon at that time had just left the hospital. And the doctor said to me, "Your surgeon dumped you!" And I was like, "Um, actually, my surgeon dumped this hospital!"

Therapist 1: That's the attitude. T, we didn't get to your answers yet, but can we get to those?

T: Well, my first is keeping my family's legacy alive. My parents are still alive, and when I was little so were my grandparents and great grandparents. And what my grandma used to say is that we should use the good china, the good crystal. Why save it? What's the point of having it behind glass, to prevent it from breaking? If you do that, you'll never use it. If you have nice things—whatever those things are—use them. I think it's a good metaphor. So that's what was passed on to me.

And then, for me, I guess my creativity has to do with my ability to design outdoor spaces, gardens, and perennials and annuals. Those gardens can go on long after I'm no longer around. The design will always be there, even if the plants die.

And, one of my greatest accomplishments was surviving that rare disease when I was 16. I was in a lot of pain, and the doctors were sure that it would kill me because my organs were shutting down, but, somehow, I managed to get through that, to get cured for that. And given what I went through, the hospital now has a protocol about how to cure it. So that's definitely my legacy.

I have a great love for animals. I've taken care of many dogs and cats, and birds in the Bahamas. My respect for nature and animals is huge.

And among my friends, I've always been the voice of reason, the moral grounding. People always ask me if I think "Is this ok?" People are always asking me for advice. And I'm a loyal friend, a very good friend.

Therapist 1: So you're a bit of a philosopher as well? You advise your friends on the moral way to live?

T: I guess so, I didn't think about it like that so much. But yeah.

Therapist 1: And you got that from who?

T: My mother. She may have been a bit aggressive in sharing what she thought was wrong and right, but it was clear to us.

Therapist 1: So with T, we're hearing a lot of the same things in terms of sources of meaning. A lot more of the historical legacy and how the values and wisdom you've inherited allows you to be a teacher and a friend and do good in the world. And you've contributed in a profound way to decreasing suffering in the world, in terms of your illness and being the first to live.

T: Exactly. Not too long after I left the hospital then, a boy in Boston had the same thing and they were able to cure him, treat him much faster. They hadn't seen this since WWII, and then me! They still don't know what causes it.

Therapist 1: You said something about using the good china even though it may get broken, and please remind me of this because I want to come back to it after then second part of the exercise.

The second part of the exercise focuses on the future, on life lessons you've learned that you want to pass on to others, kids, family, the people you love, people you're close to? The general public, the animals . . .

Therapist 2: L do you want to get started again?

L: Ok. I guess the thing is that I'm a type A personality. I always speak what I feel. But it's important to know that you can't control the attitudes of other people, that you need to "let go, and let God." It's a saying we have in

Church. Because when you are constantly hating, it does more to destroy you than the other person. And so I hope that others recognize that it's important to let go.

Therapist 1: So you can't control others' attitudes?

L: You can try, but really, you can't control them.

Therapist 1: And this is related to forgiveness what we had talked about last week?

L: Yes.

That's the main one. The other has to do with . . . I've always been very responsible. Especially in taking care of my child. I would never buy things for me unless he was fully taken care of. I've never been a person that's liked having bills. I like putting my head on the pillow and not think about the rent or my next bill. I've always been practical. When I turned 61, I bought the car of my dreams!

Therapist 1: Which car?

L: A Lexus, 350. A sedan.

Therapist 2: Nice!

T: All the bells and whistles?

L: Yes, I did it for me. I mean, I complain about how expensive the gas is, but, I wanted to do it, that was for me. I rewarded me.

Therapist 1: So the idea that you want to pass along to your son is?

L: It's important to do for you, do things that take care of you. If you can't take care of you, no one will. That we're worthy of care.

Therapist 2: There it is again! Worthy!

L: Ha! You know, at first I didn't remember saying that, but now . . . now I get it. Yes, that's definitely something I would have said.

Therapist 1: So it's ok to take care of ourselves but not when compromising ourselves, either.

L: Right, like, that was my one splurge. But I wouldn't feel comfortable buying a pair of $400 shoes, or, what's that deli down on Houston street? Famous for their pastrami?

Therapist 1: Katz's deli.

L: Yes. It's $15 for a sandwich! Can you believe it? I remember when it was $5! I wouldn't do that. That's unnecessary.

Therapist 1: Thank you. P?

P: I don't know. The future? Lessons to pass on? Um, I think, . . . I don't always act this way, but I try. I think it's important to be patient, it takes time for things to happen. If you're patient and persistent, and you know you're right, people will come around, or it will get to the point where it doesn't matter. So I think it's important for my kids to learn patience, learn to take their time in waiting for things to happen.

The other thing is a little different. I've always thought I've been accepting of people's differences. My partner, she's a very bright woman, I respect her in a thousand diff ways. One of the things I don't respect is that she looks at things as black and white. There is always one right way. And one of the things she would think you're wrong about is $400 shoes. She has signed Manolo Blahniks! I didn't know what those were before her! But she thinks that that's the right thing to do. Get the best stuff, it lasts the longest. To me, a Coach bag will last just as long as Louis Vuitton! But I think that this is important. In terms of people, just this group, we are all so different, there are many who don't accept other people's differences. Maybe the shoes weren't a good example, I'm not sure, but it's about acceptance.

Therapist 1: And acceptance takes patience.

P: Yes, so I really hope that my kids become patient and accept other people's differences.

Therapist 1: So it's interesting. L, you talked about attitudes and caring for ourselves, and being forgiving and loving and caring and open, open to life's experiences. We can't really have experiential sources of meaning—love—unless you're open to it. But you said something that was really striking, P, that builds a little bit on the discussion we had before, which is that you wanted your kids to be patient, and you wanted them to learn to take their time, to wait, so it had a lot to do with time.

P: Yeah.

Therapist 1: That's been on your mind a lot. How you look at the time that you got.

P: Yeah . . .

Therapist 1: You must be having trouble being patient and waiting . . .

P: No, I mean, I've been keeping myself busy, and I don't have the stamina that I used to, but it's more of wanting to use the time I have to the fullest. I mean the thing is, in comparison to you, T, with your lung collapsing and your being sick as a child and you, S, with your being so sick and the surgeries, I haven't been sick. I've lived my entire life without any real health issues, thank God. Which is part of the incongruity of the situation, everyone who sees me says, "Boy, you look great!" I wish I didn't look so good because I lost 10 lbs because I can't eat. I don't know, it's hard to find meaning in the disease, you know.

Therapist 1: What about meaning in the time?

P: The time? What I'm doing is setting little goals for myself. I want to be alive for my daughter's birthday. And then the anniversary. And then my son's birthday. And so on and so forth. I want to be alive for my birthday, too! I want to be alive when I'm 50.

S: Can I say something?

Therapist 2: Please, yes.

S: When I had my transplant, I was seeing a therapist to help me through the transplant as well as my recent divorce, and then she asked me about the birthday coming up and how I was feeling about it and I hadn't really thought about it, but at that time, I felt so differently about that birthday because I didn't know that I would be alive at that birthday, but then it was a true celebration, to be alive at that day. And you, P, probably feel that way, with all these milestones. . . . They mark that you've lived, you're alive, you've made it and are still functioning.

P: Yes, exactly. It's funny, I've always downplayed my birthday. Never really celebrated. But this year, I think I want to have a party. I want to really, really celebrate!!

Therapist 1: Well you know the comment you made about the Coach versus the Louis Vuitton bag? I'm going to bring in the using the good china comment now. T talked about an attitude in her family that you should use the good china, don't keep it in the breakfront behind the glass, use it every day, even though it might break.

T: And it does!

Therapist 2: And that relates a little bit to what we're talking about now. Do you live life fully, do you love and take the chance and live fully and love deeply every day in the setting of this illness, knowing that it could end, that the time could end, that you could risk losing people that you love?

Therapist 1: Exactly. Do you have the courage to live and love fully even though there are risks involved in that?

L: I can try.

T: It takes knowing how to. It takes effort. You have to sort of train yourself, learn how to live like that to a certain degree.

Therapist 1: What do you think S?

S: I think it's a matter of choice. No doubt, courage is involved, to take a big bite out of life, but we don't know what our time limits are, and of course you can say that no one does but for us, it's much more tangible. But for us, it's just so much clearer. Once you're told about the endgame, it's scary and certain part so your close down to be on guard against more bad news, but also, coming down to always making the choice, and choosing life, and if you choose life, choose it big, choose it juicy, choose what's meaningful to you. This really goes into my legacy and being proactive.

Therapist 1: P, what do you think about what S just said?

P: I know that I try to do that, I'm trying to do the things that I like, you know, there's pauses periodically, but I'm trying to spend time with the friends that I like, opposed to those who you see out of obligation. I don't have time for that. I do reflect, and I know, at 49 years old, I still have so much. I have a wife and kids who can take care of me, a family who can, I'm lucky in a lot of ways. I just want to keep being lucky.

S: I wish you a lot of luck.

Therapist 1: Do you think we ever make our own luck?

S: To a certain extent.

L: I think we do.

T: Sometimes it's there, we just need to recognize it. Maybe it's just a way of looking at a certain situation.

L: It's looking at your life with openness, not closeness.

Therapist 1: That's true, and does this relate to what was S was talking about?

L: Yeah, I can relate to a lot of what she said. There were many times that I didn't live life to the fullest before cancer and after, and you can't just change immediately who you are, you have a history.

Therapist 2: Exactly, and that's what we were covering last week, about our histories and the legacies that we were given.

Therapist 1: And today is about how you live now. Do you guys think how you live now is going to be important in terms of lessons for your kids and family and friends, how you face this struggle? What do you think the lessons are that others will learn?

L: Well, for me, it's to try to be as realistic as possible. I don't want to paint too rosy a picture. I want to be able to talk to my son and his wife about what is happening and some of the fears I have without myself or them really freaking out. And so far this has gone well. At the same time, a lot of people I thought would be very supportive have surprised me by their silence. Perhaps they just don't know what to say, it's like when someone dies, people don't know what to say.

Therapist 2: Anyone else?

T: I want people to remember that I don't sweat the small stuff, I don't spend all my energy, I don't get fully consumed with this stuff.

S: Yeah, keep your perspective about what's important, and we do, we all get caught up, so much energy is spent unnecessarily on things that are not that significant. And I can't change that for everything, but certainly, I don't have time for the type of group dynamics where you have catty people or office politics. I don't have patience for that, it's a waste of my time. And also certainly, I want others to know that I'm not passive, not losing hope, and that there are many ways to look at a situation.

Therapist 2: It sounds like many of you are saying that you've learned important lessons that you want to pass on to others, but that the experience of having cancer has been an important source of lessons learned about life that perhaps you may not have learned otherwise, especially the idea about how precious every moment of life is, and living life fully.

Therapist 1: Is that fair to say?

S: I would say so.

L: Yes, and it's like the car I bought.

Therapist 2: How so?

L: I would never have done that before. But now, why wait? What's the point?

Therapist 1: I'm going to ask a question that is a little difficult, no, not a little, very. Cancer has opened your eyes to living fully and that's something you learned that you want to pass on to others. I'm wondering whether through this cancer illness you think that there's any sort of important lesson to pass on to your kids and others about mortality, the fact that we're all mortal, and whether you think it's maybe important to teach your kids and family not to fear death? Maybe that's something?

T: I don't know if it's for me to teach them. I know they're afraid of it enough, independent of me, and they don't want to talk about it.

Therapist 1: I was thinking in terms of teaching others not to fear death.

T: Yeah, but they don't want to hear that from me.

P: I don't know how you can teach that other than to live every day with enough courage to live to the next day. When I first told my daughters about my diagnosis, it was difficult, and they said "No daddy, you're not like that, you're stronger," and I want to teach them, not that that's not true, that I'm not strong, but that I'm human.

Therapist 1: Do you think that the way that you go through this, to teach your kids how you live through this every day, the attitude you take towards this, you'd like to teach them not to be afraid of death through that?

P: I'm still afraid of death, so I don't know how to teach them.

S: That's what I was going to say. I'm afraid of death. It's hard for me to teach what I haven't taught myself yet.

P: Well, I mean, I' afraid of not being alive, not necessarily death. I'm afraid of the people I'm going to leave behind, I'm afraid it's going to hurt them too much.

Therapist 1: So you're afraid of their sadness, their loss?

P: Yeah, day to day I worry. I mean, I'm starting to have difficulty swallowing, eating. I'm throwing up all the time. This is the first tangible change. And the way that I am emotionally is very much tied to how I feel physically. Like today, it was hard to come, but I was ok enough to come.

Therapist 2: We're so grateful that you came here today, P.

P: So just to finish the thought. I mean, the cancer . . . it's getting worse. The effects, they are tangible. And I don't know if I'll be more afraid when it gets worse.

L: I have sorta mixed emotions. My first reaction when I go the diagnosis was, you know, I was raised to talk about death. Talk about illness and reality. When my grandmother died, I touched her body and all that. And being a nurse, I don't have a fear of death, per se. But I also, when I was diagnosed, didn't really have a zest for life, just withdrew a bit. The processing of the whole thing. So while I say I'm not fearful about death, I'm not sure about the unknown and how this disease entity is going to take over. Right now I live alone. I don't plan to move in with my children, I don't want to be a bother or burden to my children.

Therapist 1: Anyone else want to say something about my particularly uplifting question?

S: I think I'm more afraid of the pain or losing my lung functioning, or being afraid of not being able to catch my breath. I think I'm more afraid of a painful death than death itself.

Therapist 1: I may have mentioned before, whether we officially have the role or not, we're teachers, to our kids, our loved ones, relatives, friends, family, and people who are looking at us and how we live, learn from us, so the way that you face this beast in front of you, that itself will teach. It's reasonable to assume that how you go through this, the attitude you take, is going to teach important lessons. And maybe, that will help you in some way to deal with the fear, to be able to help others. Maybe you can draw courage from that. I know that I certainly draw courage that way.

P: I was just thinking, I was watching this interview with this CNN guy, who has the same cancer as I have. And he was saying, he hopes he finds God before he dies. And I was thinking, how is that going to happen? How does that happen?

Therapist 1: Well, you know, what we're doing in here is not necessarily about finding God, although if that is your way to meaning, then . . . in some ways, we are doing that. But I think what's more important is not necessarily that you find meaning, but that you are actively searching for it. Frank's book, it's "Man's Search for Meaning," not "Man's Got Meaning," right? It's the goal that you set, right? You may not reach the goal, and as a result could feel you've fallen short, but you'll surely feel you've fallen even more behind if you don't even search.

P: True. Yeah.

Therapist 1: So I know that we're out of time. Therapist 2, could you remind people what we're going to be doing next week?

Therapist 2: Sure. So, a lot of what we've talked about today has touched upon attitude. The topic of next week is your attitude as a source of meaning. How the choices you make, the approach you take to suffering—of any kind—may serve as a resource for you. And so if you can take a look at those questions for thee experiential exercise before next week, that would be wonderful.

Also, we have a suggested assignment, to be completed at any point, which is to share your story. Would someone mind volunteering to read this out loud? The assignment is on the last page of the fourth session materials in your binder.

T: I'll go. Ok.

"Share your legacy and tell your story. Tell your story to loved ones in your life in any manner that is comfortable to you. The key is to highlight experiences that have been a source of pride and meaning for you, and things that you'd like to accomplish but have yet to do. As you share your story, become aware of how it feels to have your words witnessed, validated and heard by those who love you most."

Therapist 1: That's a suggested homework. It's optional, but can be very helpful. Any questions?

Therapist 2: Ok, great. We looked forward to seeing you all next week.

SESSION 5: ATTITUDINAL SOURCES OF MEANING—ENCOUNTERING LIFE'S LIMITATIONS

Therapist 2: Welcome back everyone! It looks like we've established our seating in here! Everyone has the same seats!

T: Yeah, it would feel funny to sit anywhere else.

Therapist 2: Not a problem. We have a tendency to get comfortable where we are.

Therapist 1: Welcome back everyone to session five of meaning-centered group psychotherapy.

Therapist 2: We're going to jump right back into the work here. In our last few sessions we've been discussing legacy, the one you were given, the one you are currently creating, and the one you hope to leave behind. And at the end of last session we had mentioned the exercise—the suggested homework—of sharing your legacy with your loved ones, and so I just wanted to check in and see how that exercise went for you. Did any of you begin this? Maybe we can spend a few minutes or so chatting about what this experience was like?

Therapist 1: Did anyone do it?

S: I actually had a hard time doing it.

L: I found it difficult also. I wrote down a lot of stuff but I didn't talk to anyone about it, the opportunity didn't come. But it was even hard just putting the material together.

Therapist 2: T, did you do the exercise?

T: Well, I wrote down that "my life story is still unfolding . . . I'm just 38, I've accomplished a lot of things that I've wanted to, but there are still so many things that I have yet to do." There are other things, though, like using my design skills to create a design architect firm.

Therapist 1: I guess the exercise was really a suggestion for the possibility to share the legacy you shared in here with loved ones in your life, but it sounds like there may not have been opportunities for this?

S: I don't know. I sorta feel like it's easier to think about passing my parents' legacy on to my niece than mine, since those were people she didn't know.

Therapist 1: And L, you said it was difficult?

L: It was difficult altogether. I mean, I'm a person who is brutally frank and sometimes it can be very cutting. And I started thinking about some experiences in the past where I guess I had been rude, not intentionally. And ... thinking back on these experiences in a way was mortifying, so it was hard to really want to think more about them.

Therapist 1: Well today then I think is going to be really interesting. We're going to introduce the idea of some kind of a legacy project, which is also optional. We'll talk about that later. But it's related in some ways to what you all are bringing up right now.

S: What I find my concern is in terms of talking to a 7-year-old is that I find that I'm so protective of her that I'm hiding things from her, I don't want her to know how sick I am, I don't want her to be scared for me, if I go swimming and run out of breath, I don't want her to know the reasons why. So sharing this legacy with her is hard for me.

Therapist 1: Right, of course, it's much different to share your story with a 7-year-old than with someone who is a peer so to speak.

Today, we're going to move forward with our discussing the various sources of meaning. And just as a review, these sources of meaning are through experiences, through experiences of love, and beauty, and humor, what we experience in the world, through creativity, what we put ourselves into, and through attitude, which today's session is going to focus on. We have sessions coming up focusing on these various sources of meaning, in terms of creativity, next week, and then experiential sources of meaning, in our seventh session.

Today's focus is on what we call the attitudinal source of meaning, which really refers to the situations in our lives where we've encountered some kind of limitation and as human beings, we're often driven to create a life and a trajectory or direction, forward, up, and so when you encounter limitations that prevents this movement, it can cause us to stress or suffer. There are all sorts of limitations—the ones that you all are experiencing now in terms of cancer and your physical capabilities, fatigue, stamina, pain—and for all of us, the ultimate limitation is the finiteness of life, the fact of death. And so what this attitudinal source of meaning is about is, no matter what situation you find yourself in, your sense of control and loss, what is it that you do still have the ability to control? And this boils down to the attitude that you take towards your situation. The idea is that you're trying to transcend or overcome the limitations, live fully within the limitations.

Sometimes it's a difficult concept to really grasp, but through the experiential exercise I think we'll be able to flesh this all out. We're all confronted by the same limitations of the finiteness of life, and this is made all the more real with cancer. So that's the focus of today's exercise.

Therapist 2: Ok, did you all have an opportunity to take a look at the exercise? If not, why don't you take a few minutes now to do so and then we can go through the questions together.

Would someone like to volunteer to go first? There are really three exercises to do today, and we'll try to get through them all. The first has to do with losses, limitations or obstacles you faced in the past, how you dealt with them, coped with them in the past, what did you do? How did you overcome them?

Therapist 1: P, you seem ready, you want to start?

P: I guess so. Life's limitations. When I first looked that question, the current situation is so much bigger than any past trauma I've had to think about. It just is. But, looking back, I guess, the first major limitation I encountered was when I was a teenager my parents split up. When I look back now, it's decades ago ...

Therapist 1: And you had shared that you've begun to reconcile with your dad ...

P: But you know, at the time, divorce I guess was coming into fashion, but as a kid I was the only one I knew who had parents who were getting divorced and so I felt in that way like an outsider. The way I dealt with it was in some degree, I rebelled. I know I hung out with kids who my mother definitely didn't approve of, I smoked and drank and did a lot of stereotypical things that teenagers do, and ultimately, it took going to college and putting some distance between myself and my family situation to start feeling better. And I dealt with the anger, and I got over it.

The second limitation was about a year before my cancer diagnosis, I was not getting along with my wife. I just, and, um, I'm not a particularly vocal person about my feelings, I felt like she would criticize me when I shared feelings and so I stopped, I just became passive aggressive. It lasted for 6 months. And I went to her eventually and I told her that I didn't feel anything anymore. And once I said it, I realized that that wasn't the case. I guess what I learned was that I have to say things before I internalize them so much that I end up saying things that are just blatant lies. So, yeah, those are the two major ones.

Therapist 1: So P, one was about your family of origin and a lot of emotion, and the second was about feeling an absence of emotion. And so both situations were challenges that involved losses, the loss of your family, and your parents splitting up, and the other was a sense of loss that you were feeling with your wife, loss of connection. When you said the way you dealt with your anger, it sounds like you had to think about the feelings you were having in order to really believe them? To accept them as true?

P: Yes, I did. With my wife, you know, I'm not perfect, neither is she. And there are certain things about her. She's not the most observant, of, things, which may be part of the reason why I ended up repressing things and doing what I did. But it's not for lack of caring, but it's just a capability that she doesn't have. And either you accept it or you don't.

Therapist 2: So it's about change or acceptance?

P: Well, did she change? It was a change in my attitude.

Therapist 1: Exactly. Did that change your marriage at all?

P: It did.

Therapist 1: For the worse? For better?

P: For the better, completely. We transformed as a couple. It went from my being monosyllabic to being a couple again.

Therapist 1: So what began as a really terrible event in some way improved you marriage?

P: Yeah, it did. But then this cancer diagnosis happened.

Therapist 1: Right. Thank you for sharing your answer to this first question, P. S, would you like to go?

S: I was going to say that my first divorce made me much more independent. I was married right after grad school and I put my husband on a pedestal. I felt surprisingly light and free when we divorced, I could build horizontally and have so many supports, and not put someone on a pedestal and be more important to me than I am. But in this relationship, he was the angry one and I had to be happy. But being out of it, out of our characteristic roles, I learned to express my anger. I realized we were playing these roles, and that my role of being happy had really prevented me from expressing my true feelings.

And then my second divorce was to a horrible man and I well . . . it accelerated the need for a transplant. I was going through pre-transplant with doctors at the time who really cared about me and had a transplant and then a divorce that he wanted to make it as horrible as possible. . . . Surprisingly, the transplant was the easier of the two things to go through. The doctors were the total antithesis to the divorce. He was so horrible. So one of the things I learned was that with some people, trying to explain yourself, trying to have logic, it doesn't matter. Sometimes you just need to give up, and I don't think that I've ever give up before, but this time . . . I realized that there are certain people that I just can't have a relationship with. It was big learning. To learn that, well, we just can't change people, we can't always impact others, that all we can do is impact ourselves, really.

And then just having a chronic disease, with my liver, I felt badly, but more so when cancer came. When we talk about terrorism . . . my body is my terrorist. I can't rely on it, I never really drank, I never did anything, I had such a clean life, and it doesn't matter. And C had said there's no prejudice when it comes to cancer, I believe it. But, I didn't realize until after that I was in a battle with my liver disease that I wasn't going to let it win, at some point of course it's my own body, it has its own say, but I have my own battle with it, I was so determined to live every moment to its fullest, not be defined by my disease.

Therapist 2: Thank you S. We're going to hold off on too many comments until everyone has gotten a chance to share. But what images you have in there, of you body as a terrorist, and how you've chosen to live life in spite, despite, all of this, and to focus on life, not illness.

S: Exactly.

Therapist 1: Your story was similar to P in terms of your ultimately thinking differently. Your attitude about a lot of things shifted. What you could expect from men, from relationships, from your body and to life. You chose to not be defeated by the divorces, and by the illnesses. So you really have the freedom to make choices.

S: Yeah, and to choose not to get married again!

Therapist 2: Ha!

OK, L, would you like to go next?

L: At a very early age I started having medical problems, gynecological problems, and I realized early that I wouldn't be able to have my own child, and I decided to adopt a child. I had a partner at that time and so I didn't see myself as a single parent, but he began to vacillate and it upset me but it made me determined to raise this child and do what I needed to do to take care of him. I ended up going into therapy in order to work out this different family structure, but I also found that I became very distrustful. I had had other relationships that hadn't worked out, and found that I was becoming very isolated. And so, yeah. That was clearly a challenging time for me.

Therapist 1: So this is the same son you speak about so proudly, he's the crowning achievement of your life?

L: Yes he is.

Therapist 1: And yet he—the circumstances of his existence in your world—were very painful and difficult at first, is that correct? What I'm struck by, is what started out as limitations, not being able to have a child, what some people would be defeated by, you pushed forward and adopted, and then when your partner didn't support it, you pushed forward even more.

L: Yeah. And the other thing is that I raised him to be very independent. I taught him that he can do anything that a woman can do, he can cook and clean and take care, in addition to being a man. And he has the sensitivity of both a man and a woman. I've raised him well.

Therapist 1: So a person could look at the beginnings of this as a tragedy, but what came out of this was a beautiful child, a son you're so proud of who brings you so much love and meaning in your life, and it all had to do with the attitude that you took in face of these obstacles. You chose to go forward. You chose to not look back.

L: Exactly.

Therapist 1: Thanks, L.
T?

T: Yes, well, first I started writing this down wrong, in terms of thinking before cancer. But I can answer it. I think the thing that happened to me, maybe two or three years before I moved to New York, I felt like everything was against me or caving in on me. During a short period of time, I broke up with my bf of five years, and I was fired, it was a magazine I was working at and they lost money and they couldn't afford me anymore, but it was a complete shock to me, so I was unemployed, and alone, and then I had found out that weekend that my landlord was evicting me, because her son and daughter in law wanted to move in. I think this was all within weeks of each other, maybe days. It was all at once. It was horrendous. I was feeling like something was pushing me away or towards, or . . . I was dealing with different forms of hurt and anger and unfairness, and I couldn't change any of it, I could find a new job, apartment or boyfriend I guess, but I couldn't change what had happened and when. I ended up moving in with my parents, which started me on the road to where I am now, in terms of plants. I was doing food shopping for my parents, I was in the grocery store and I saw all these packets of herbs, bought them, and began planting, and so I began doing that, and eventually it led to my coming to New York.

Therapist 2: So all of these catastrophes led to your coming to New York, which was a good thing you said.

T: Yes, coming here and studying was good, but then I got diagnosed with cancer. But I guess I was in a better position to be helped here medically than I was there, so I guess in that way too things worked out.

Therapist 1: That's an incredibly story, T. All these terrible things happened, and then some really good things came out of it. This exercise is about attitude, and choice, and the description you've given, all of these things that happened, they gave you a purpose, they gave you reasons to choose. Is there a certain attitude that you took that enabled you to survive all of this?

T: I don't know, I just knew that I had to move forward. I became introverted I guess, I withdrew from things socially, avoided my ex. And I focused my attention on gardening.

Therapist 1: So you protected yourself and invested yourself in this interest, that in many respects, just, blossomed?

T: Yeah, exactly. I wanted to do something that I was proud of too. Working at the magazine was ok, but I wasn't proud of that work, that didn't fully fulfill me, not in the way that gardening does.

Therapist 2: Thanks everyone, that was really interesting. All such wonderful examples of your attitudes in situations that were challenging, moments of suffering.

Let's move on to the second exercise now, which focuses on limitations and losses that you've faced since your cancer diagnosis, and equally, if not more, importantly, are you starting to find meaning in your daily life despite the fact that you're maybe a little bit more aware of the finiteness of life, of the limitations you have?

Therapist 1: It's a hard question, I know. Take a moment.

Therapist 2: S, want to get started?

S: Well, when I got cancer, I lost my left breast, and I lost my body image, and fear of, you know, not appearing attractive, and this is a very big thing, huge thing. I lost a lot of my independence, in that in that period between the operation and finding an oncologist, I needed help with everything, I wasn't supposed to drive, I was very happy that friends came up to help, I had a friend from a book group who did a lot of legal work in dealing with hospitals and malpractice, and she really came to my aid, became such an ally and a friendship ensured. She was married and had two grown children. She was the silver lining in my illness, because it brought me here, and our friendship has continued to this date, and she's taught me that there are always additional questions to ask doctors. So that was definitely a plus, it brought me hope, a terrific thing to come of something so bad.

But, um, I'm tied to MSKCC, I really hate the fact that I have to come to the city all the time, tied to chemo, for the rest of my life, and of course I hope that's for a long time, but you know, it's hard. So how did I cope? I changed my attitude as much as I could, and I regard cancer as my new job, this is what I do. My fear over getting IV needles? I've been working with another psychiatrist here on this and even working on my attitude about waiting for the PET scans, I'm getting better. So, my attitude is changed, I know what my capabilities are, I envy what others can do, because I'm very limited, but those are my new parameters.

Therapist 1: Thanks, S. L?

L: Since my diagnosis, I guess I've had a loss of motivation and drive. Now this was depression I had before the diagnosis, so it's kinda hard to differentiate what it's due to. There are some projects I had going on, like fixing the house in Georgia, but right now, I just don't. Travel? Now it's just a hassle. For people who aren't depressed, its pleasurable, but for me, I've just closed the door on many aspects of life. I stay in my house a lot, don't do too much interacting.

I've always considered myself to be a woman of faith; I was raised in the church, I've always gotten solace there, or I did in the past. I left the church that my family and parents belonged to and was going across the street, to something that my niece and nephew were a part of, and when I did, I was so emotionally overcome, and I haven't been back to church since, and I'm afraid of just losing it if I go.

Therapist 1: These were tears of?

L: Well, my father is the oldest living deacon, my mom, was so involved, I used to sing in the choir. Our lives were centered around the church, and I had taken a hiatus, and going back, it was just too much for me.

Therapist 1: Were they tears of sorrow? Nostalgia? Joy?

L: It's hard for me to explain. Well, I felt good being there, after it was all over, but it was just very draining. I felt like someone had been boxing with me.

Therapist 2: Was it cathartic?

L: I guess so, maybe. I guess I'm still just working a lot of stuff through. My emotions have never been clear cut, so I guess I'm still figuring out what it was that I was feeling.

Therapist 2: L, how did you handle the depression before? You said that this was not new to you, it was there long before cancer?

L: I, um, I never took any medication. I would never do that. I tried to keep as busy as possible, a lot of the projects I was a part of were to keep me busy. I did wonder whether I needed to go back to work, but I had had it at that point with being on the clock.

Therapist 1: I think what Therapist 2 is trying to introduce or make more accessible to you guys in the importance of being able to continue to live life fully and full of meaning and that there are these sources of meaning that are resources for you, and when you find that your legacy has meaning—for example in church—that you can draw on that for meaning. And we just want to start in here today to get a sense of how in the past, what it was in the past that you drew on in the past and what you are drawing on now in terms of sources of meaning that can be resources for you.

P, you want to go?

P: I think I talked about this before. My biggest loss was the loss of my practice, giving up my practice. My partner has been terrific, she's one of my closest friends in the world, but she's got a lot on her plate, she can't afford to retire, she has to continue to do a lot, giving away our cases that was hard, I had 60 or so cases that I had to give away, and that was very, very hard to do. My cases, my clients, they were my family, it's like cutting of your family, or cutting off an appendage, to give those files away. It was really, very hard for me. I guess the other part of the difficulty of all of this, aside from the diagnosis, the most recent difficulty is the increased problems I have swallowing. I was running late getting here today, I really need to allot about 45 minutes to eat, and I didn't today and as a result, I was throwing up for 10 minutes. I love eating, I love eating a big steak, but I can't right now. It will take me an hour to eat it. I don't like being afraid of eating. You know, it's sorta a new problem so it's, I can't tell you how I cope with it because I haven't just yet. The other thing, as far as coping with the being a lawyer part, I still go to the office, my name is still on the door. So I guess I cope by pretending I'm still involved a little bit.

The other question, about finding meaning in my daily life? My meaning has always been my family, that hasn't changed. I just told you before, I love my wife, whatever difficulties we've had, I love my kids, perhaps too unconditionally, I love my brothers, and I love my friends. As far as dealing with people, I have found that there are some people who have really stepped up to the plate, and many people who haven't. And I guess if I had thought about it more I would be distressed, but I was kinda right about some of the people who didn't, and mostly right about those who did, but not entirely.

Therapist 1: So many people have told me that it was not until they had cancer that they really understood or appreciated how much they were loved.

P: Absolutely. It kinda brings me back to why I'm expressing this, which can be sad sometimes. But still, it's a good point.

Therapist 2: You agree, S?

S: Very much so. When I was 23 I was working with a librarian who was a college age and she was in a car accident and died and since then, I've made a point of telling people how highly I regard them, I tell them now.

Therapist 1: Words count.

S: Yeah, and it's more so now.

Therapist 2: We haven't gotten to your end T . . .

T: Physical limitations are huge. I didn't have any before, and now I have so many that prevent me from doing all that I used to do. I can't go to school anymore, can't deal with getting all the way up to the Bronx, and I'm not sure if I have the stamina to actually do the work of the class and the homework. And I don't know if I'd enjoy doing all the work, because of my left lung and my energy, there's and the lung is scarred from the chest tube and catheter, so I'll never be back to full capacity, but people live with one lung, so I'll be ok. I may never get off the oxygen completely, but slowly and surely I'll get back.

Therapist 2: So a lot of us derive a lot of meaning from the work that we do, and your work, T, it's very physical as well, so how do you derive meaning given these limitations?

T: Well, I've started giving directions to other people, telling people where to place things.

Therapist 1: So you've adapted. You're still a landscape artist, you can still do the work, just differently?

T: Exactly. I'm just not the one down on my hands and knees, but I'm still in charge in a way. I'm still the artist. I just go smaller now, I do window boxes and painting planters, and doing things on smaller scales.

Therapist 2: You've made a choice not to give up this passion, just do it in an attenuated fashion.

T: Yeah, and I'm trying to sell them. I'm trying to adapt, still do things that I like to do, but it's hard to do a lot, and I can't do what I specifically want.

Therapist 1: But you can approximate?

T: Yes, similar things. And I'd like to go home to the Bahamas for a visit, I haven't been there since April, and I think by the end of September I should be able to go for about 10 days, and labor day weekend I'm going to our lake house in Pennsylvania.

Therapist 1: So even though there are physical limitations, there are still things you can do?

T: Yeah. I mean, I still have to drag around the oxygen but . . .

Therapist 1: Well you don't need to climb Mount Everest to live a meaningful life, right?

P, do you ever feel with all the treatments and everything else that you're no longer able to do all the things you used to do with your kids?

P: Absolutely. I mean, with my little guy, especially, yeah. The older ones, they're teenagers, we communicate, but it's not like we go power sailing or anything, I just pick them up from the train and take them around.

Therapist 1: One if the things I think is helpful, we're trying to teach you that these various sources of meaning can be resources to sustain meaning in your life. We want you to understand that when one source of meaning becomes blocked, like work, another, like family, can come into play. You can move from things that you do to derive meaning to ways of being—from doing—throwing a ball—to ways of being—being a father without doing so many activities, I mean you can be a father by doing so many little things, sitting down and talking, watching a game . . .

P: I won't ever be able to be a soccer coach, I can be at the game but not participate. . . .

Therapist 1: Right, but does that make you less of a dad? To be there as opposed to be in it?

P: No, it's just that my older ones, they had me do that for them, and my little one, J, he's 5 now, he'll never have that.

Therapist 1: Ok, but you're still being a dad to him at those moments?

P: I am.

Therapist 2: Ok. Before we run out of time, let's try to tackle this third question here. This one's a hard one, I'm not going to pretend it's not. But, I, you know, another limitation, the ultimate limitation, is death. Everyone always is aware of that, even before cancer, but with cancer, we all become more aware of it. So the last question is really asking you to think a little about what would be a—if you had to die—what would be the ideal way, the best way, what would be the circumstances, how would you want to be remembered. I know this is hard, but let's see if we can get through this last one.

L, do you want to start?

L: Um, I hope I'll be remembered lovingly as a good role model and as a person who had values and standards that were clear for others to see. That it is known that I cared and gave to others, helped when I could. And that, you know, my attempt was to steer the young people in a positive direction, talk about things that were meaningful, give them standards that were important for them to achieve. With education being important, meaningful work, doing the right thing.

Therapist 1: In terms of the other part of the question, in terms of a good or meaningful death?

L: A good or meaningful death? I don't know how to answer that. One without too much pain, hopefully! I don't fear dying, per se. I believe in an afterlife. But I do fear the process. The discomfort, pain, whatever. If that gets to be a part of the process, I won't have control but that's what I fear.

Therapist 1: T?

T: Um, I wrote, dying with dignity and on my own terms, no matter where I may be. But ideally, at home, as opposed to the sterile hospital or hospice. And I want to be remembered for the person I am, nothing glorified, nothing more. I don't want people to say about me things they wouldn't say to me now. So nothing more or less, that I'm a good person, a friend, a family member. I know they all realize this. I want them to say these things to me now, just like they will then. I mean, they already say them so I know them to be true.

So basically, I just want to have a little bit of control. Dying with dignity, and on my own terms. That's what's important to me.

Therapist 2: Thanks, T. S?

S: In terms of a good death, the dying part of it, I would very much like it to be painless, and I've already arranged with long term care to try to die at home, not at the hospital, and not have extraordinary measures be taken. A good death would be if I achieved something by dying. If I could save someone's life in the process of dying, that would be a good death.

Therapist 1: A heroic death?

S: Yeah. One of the things I was thinking was maybe I should do something really adventurous and daring, where I could potentially die, like hang-gliding, but someone said to me when I suggested that, that I could just break every bone and be in pain, so I revised that, but if I knew I could just die, I would be scared, but would be great to do something really daring, really take a risk.

So, that was about dying.

I actually think it's good that I've given this thought, in terms of a living will, I want to be near a window near the air, I'm so afraid of being in an airless room, a tank, and that was even before I had trouble breathing. I really just want to be by fresh air, I want to be by nature until the end. And I certainly agree with L, I'd like to leave with integrity and standards and have people think that I've done the right thing.

Therapist 1: So these virtues are important to you, passing those on?

S: Yes, for them to remember everything that I've added to their lives, in terms of laughter and fun and adventure.

Therapist 1: So with your niece, the 7 year old, even though you don't want to frighten her, you want to pass these important things on to her?

S: Yeah, I want to encourage her by example, have her see me in this illness journey, focusing on what's real, and what's good.

Therapist 1: What do you mean by that, what's real and what's good?

S: Well, I'm not ready to talk directly about cancer with her, but I do eventually want her to know what goes on, I don't like pretense, I like to be genuine, and I want her to get that in me and to be that in her. And want her to know that I'm present for her.

Therapist 1: So related to what we've been talking about, it's not so much about doing stuff, but being present, being with her.

S: And after that I have down being silly, and being able to laugh at myself, to make fun of myself.

Therapist 2: Thanks, S. P, do you want to go?

P: I couldn't answer the first question, about a good or meaningful death. L talked about no pain. I don't want pain either, but I don't think pain or no pain adds or takes away from the meaning of the death. If I could save a person's life, or a family member's life in my death, that would be good, but I don't think that's really likely at this point though.

I don't know if I mentioned that my partner's father died of esophageal cancer at 92, at home, with all of his children around him, he told everyone that he was about to go, and he did, and he spoke to each of his kids. And I'd like to be able to do that.

Therapist 1: Would that be too painful for them?

P: Well, they're not all old enough, I'm not sure if they're all ready. Especially the little guy.

Therapist 1: How old are they?

P: 16 and 19. They understand, but ... yeah, I guess they're old enough.

This question, this is really hard. I used to think right after I got diagnosed, what would people say at my funeral? And I thought about all the good that they would say. But then I stopped thinking, because it got too hard, because I don't want to think about my death just yet. I'm not there.

T: Yeah, I'm not either.

P: If I get to the point where I'm home bound, can't drive, then I'll think about it then. But right now, it's ... yeah.

Therapist 1: I mean in the hypothetical sense.

P: Well, I'm having a hard time with that. I think I'll be remembered as a caring husband and father and son, and professional. And a good friend. Think I'll be remembered as loving to my wife and my kinds and my family, and as far as professionally, I hope that I'm remembered as someone who at the very least was competent and more likely as an intelligent and thoughtful lawyer, because sometimes I was. And I took pride, and still do, in that.

In terms of lasting impressions ...

I was talking to my 16 year old. She was talking about this time when she had to get five shots before going to kindergarten, but then I took her to a toy store, to get her a gift for getting through the shot. I have a recollection of taking her there, but I have no recollection that it was after shots, so I really don't know what's going to stick out in their minds. But I hope that they are happy that I was their father.

Therapist 2: From what you've shared, P, about your children and how you've been a father to them, I'm sure this is going to be the case.

P: Thanks.

Therapist 1: Does anyone have any thoughts they want to say to other group members?

S: L, it sounds as though, in terms of depression and hiding from life, it sounds like going to church was so much more intense than anything you've experienced in the last couple of years, and it frightened you, but it sounds like real life.

L: That's interesting.

Therapist 2: Anyone else? Anything else resonate?

L: I think most of it resonated. I think most of us in the room are sorta on the same wavelength. I don't think our value systems are that different.

Therapist 1: You all kinda want the same things, all want to be remembered for similar things. It's interesting, when we talked about being remembered, there are important people we want to remember us, like kids and spouses and parents and relatives, but you all have been witnessed by Therapist 2 and I, what you've been sharing, the highs and the lows, the challenges and losses and the fears and I don't want to let today go by and I think I'll speak on behalf of Therapist 2 as well, without acknowledging that what I've seen over the past 5 weeks and especially today with this last and very difficult exercise is that I feel very privileged that you've allowed us to share with you some very intimate thoughts and feelings and what I've been feeling and seeing is four people who have been going through the cancer experience with enormous dignity and bravery, with incredible values and incredible courage to share all of this with us. And all you've shared illustrates that. And I just want to say that I will never forget the stories you've shared and I'll never forget all of you in the room.

L: That's really nice.

T: Thanks.

L: I feel kinda guilty. Out of the group, I'm the person with the least amount of symptoms and pain and invasive treatment, and I should be living life, it's not that I don't do stuff, but I've just loss the connection to really feel enthused about a lot of stuff. I really would like to get it back, I just don't know what it's going to take.

Therapist 1: Well these may be symptoms of depression. And I'm hoping that in a few more sessions perhaps getting in touch with all of the various sources of meaning, it may give you some resources to cope with these feelings as well.

Therapist 2: I probably can't say what Therapist 1 said as eloquently, but I do want to echo that sentiment, it is a privilege to sit here and listen and observe and all of the values that each of you have shared I'm surely going to remember. We're all in this moment together, and it is an honor to sit with you and listen. Over the past 5 weeks I've seen you come to this place already in finding meaning, in the language you're using, just by virtue of it, your vocabulary as changed, the language has changed. You're all becoming your own meaning-centered therapists, in a way.

I know that in the interest of time we have to wrap up for today, so I just want to quickly reference the legacy project. Again, this is something optional, but something that many group members have found meaningful in the past. We hope that you'll take some time to integrate some of the ideas of identity and purpose and creativity and meaning into a project of some sort. It does not necessarily have to be an art project, although we've had some artists in our groups before who did things like that.

But to do something, or experience something, that combines the ideas we've talked about. So for some that might mean a collage of meaningful photos, or music that's meaningful, or perhaps something that has to do with gardening or plants. Anything that is meaningful to you, that is part of your legacy. And we can talk more about that in future week. Traditionally, in the last session, we've taken some time to share these projects with each other.

T: So this doesn't need to be completed by next week?

Therapist 2: Oh, no. No, just start thinking about it, and please feel free to ask questions if they come up.

Therapist 1: Yes, it's just a suggestion and something to think about and we would love you to bring it in. But also, we've definitely had patients who have said, "My life is a legacy project, the way I live is a project." And that's perfectly ok too.

Therapist 2: So please don't feel too much pressure. It's just an idea.

And finally, over the next week, please do try to take a look at the next session, and the exercise no creativity, courage and responsibility. Ok, we'll leave you with that and see you next week.

Therapist 1: Ok, have a good week, guys, thanks so much for all that you shared today.

SESSION 6: CREATIVE SOURCES OF MEANING—ENGAGING IN LIFE: CREATIVITY, COURAGE, AND RESPONSIBILITY

Therapist 1: Ok, so we're starting a bit late today, so let's see if we can get through Session 6 today.

Therapist 2: So last week we spoke about attitudinal sources of meaning. The attitude we have in the face of suffering and both of your stories were so poignant to me. S, you spoke about these divorces . . .

S: I'm so glad you reminded me!

Therapist 2: Haha. And you spoke about how you had become so independent afterwards, and then when you became ill, you lost that independence and you needed help and you spoke about these friends who stepped up, and one person, A, in particular, who stepped up. So even though you had built up and treasured independence, you had found this new source of meaning in being connected.

And T, you spoke about this triple whammy in terms of the relationship ending, the job ending, and getting evicted, all that occurred around the same time, and then you ended up making this transition into moving into a new life, you made a decision . . .

T: I was forced.

Therapist 2: In a sense, maybe, you were forced out of those roles, but you had a choice in terms of how you could have responded, and you chose to respond in a certain way, to move forward, to create, and to begin again and begin your life here.

And so for both of you, in negative situations, you really were able to make some gains in some very beautiful ways. Today and next week more fully we're going to be speaking about ways in which you're creative, although not necessarily artistic, but more in terms of what you're doing and putting into the world, in terms of creating.

But before we go into this, I wanted to see if there were any thoughts about last week, any lingering points you had wanted to make but didn't get a chance to? And also, I know we rushed at the end last week when we presented the legacy project, so this would be a good opportunity to see if you have any questions about it.

T: This is the scrapbook?

Therapist 2: Well it doesn't need to be. We gave that as one of many examples of things that you can do. It could be something artistic like that, or it could be baking, or writing letters to people, or mending a broken relationship, anything really.

Therapist 1: Really there are no boundaries about this.

S: Actually the whole idea of writing a letter, I think, might be my way in, especially with all that you mentioned, it might be the least intimidating. At least when I was younger, there were times when I felt like people would be defensive, I felt like it would be easier to write things down. I haven't done that in a while, it might be a little bit easier for me.

T: I was thinking, I take a lot of photographs, so I may bring in a few photographs or something like that.

Therapist 2: Absolutely, that's a great idea.

S: I think I'd be better helping someone else do this project than doing it myself.

Therapist 1: Really? It sounds like you're completely on track, S.

You know, the term legacy, we had these two sessions on it. It's related to the word *legend*. So, actually, really when you think about this project, think about the legend of S, the legend of T, it represents you, how we're going to keep talking about you, and thinking about you, for a long time.

In terms of today, we introduced the idea that meaning is so important in being able to cope with cancer illness and facing all the challenges you're facing right now. If you're able to enhance or sustain a sense of meaning, you're able to keep going, and keep coping, and moving, and you can still stay in touch with things in life that make you feel alive, then you are living a life of meaning. So we talked about meaning coming from historical sources, like our legacy, what we've inherited, meaning coming from the attitude that you take towards suffering, and two of the more common sources of meaning are through the way that we experience the world, through our sensations and experiences, through our eyes and ears and touch and taste, and that's what we're going to discuss in Session 7 next week. But today, we're going to focus on creativity, our engagement in the world. So, basically our job is, when we're born, the question is, how do you respond to this fact that you're alive? And you grow up in a family, maybe, or you find yourself alive, and hat you find the world calling to you to pursue something. And that is part of what we mean by creating a life. So in simplistic terms, it's meaning that comes from your life's work, although it could be other commitments in your life, could be a cause you're dedicated to, a value that's so important to you. What's really interesting is that this notion of having to create your life, if you're religious, you might say God created and determined this for you, but if you're not, the responsibility for creating your life lies on you. So this issue of responsibility and creativity are very much linked, the idea that how you respond to being alive, by creating a life that's unique to you, and trying to live that life to its fullest potential, and that's your responsibility.

I like to play on the word responsibility. Responsibility is really your ability to respond to life, to being alive. So I find the notion of responsibility interesting, as it relates to this exercise.

So there are four questions today, the first two have to do with ways in which you've been creative, ways in which you've engaged in life fully, and as you can probably tell, it takes a little bit of courage . . .

S: To live?

Therapist 1: Yes, to live. To live with adversity, with cancer, and threat of cancer and all that it can do to you. It takes courage to keep wanting to live, to keep loving people you might lose. So I thought maybe we'd first select one question from the first group, and one then from the second group of questions. How does that sound?

S: That works.

T: Yeah, that's fine.

Therapist 1: How would you feel about doing the courage one? Living life and being creative requires courage and commitment. Can you think of times in your life when you've been courageous, taken ownership of your life, and made a meaningful commitment to something of value to you?

S: Something that you said, about the word despite, despite the absolute of cancer, and the limitations that cancer has. When first getting cancer, and other blows from cancer, like the mets, I'm not good for a while. I don't seem courageous, I'm dissolving in a puddle of tears, or I'm frantic, or I'm wondering how I'd ever cope, and then it's eventually getting used to the idea, getting to the new normal. People ask me how I cope and I don't cope at all, really. I completely drown in fear, thinking about how much worse it could get, it's the opposite of what you're talking about, I feel like I have no courage. It's eventually getting to the point of responding, eventually learning to pick myself up. So, there's no continuum here, there are peaks and valleys, I mean I don't know if that's been your experience, T, that there's been a process of pulling together to cope, T, but I know that I'm just going through that right now, knowing that one of my cancer markers skyrocketed. I don't feel courageous at all right now.

T: I'm just hoping that the progress is slow. People keep saying to me "Well, once you get better . . ." . . .

And I keep saying, "I hope," but I don't have that much control, I only have a certain amount of control, I certainly think lifestyle and diet contribute, and I'm doing my best to eat well, healthfully, and do alternative therapies and drinking all these different types of tea that are supposed to cut off oxygen to tumors.

Therapist 1: So on one level, courage is incredibly important when coping with cancer, and like S, do you feel like you have moments when you can sum up some courage and others when you're very frightened?

T: Yeah, definitely. I remember when I first learned of the recurrence, every test was coming back with more and more bad news, and it was crushing me, I felt like I couldn't take all of it. And then I started psych meds, the psych team started showing up in my room.

Therapist 1: It's always a bad sign when that happens!

T: Exactly! But yeah, you can't control it.

Therapist 1: So what it raises for me is what exactly is courage and how do we define it. But before we get into that, it might be interesting to think about if there were there times in your life before your illness when you actually felt courageous and took ownership of your life? Maybe we could learn something about the definition of courage from something that may have happened earlier in your life.

T: Trying to control bad situations?

Therapist 1: Yeah.

S: Um, I have a couple of things. After, I guess it was courageous of me to get divorced in general, to being a librarian, that was never meant to support me fully, the salary, that had ramifications for me. So I was living in a house that my ex father-in-law built, and I just knew there was no way as a librarian that I could have my own house, and I was creative and courageous just to say, what can I do to keep this house? I took in house mates, and my father-in-law lent me money interest free for a few years. And everything I did was to figure out how I could creatively keep this house. Nobody thought I could do it, and I thought, even if I couldn't, at least it bought me three more years in the house, and I just used whatever qualities I could, it didn't hurt that someone I was going out with was in the stock market, because I was earning so little at the time, so that really dominated me, really took all my resources to become victorious over it. And I still think it's one of the best things I've ever done for myself. And my father used to say that he hated seeing me live like that, he thought that I was ruining my life. But I didn't see it that way. It was a victory. And in fact, it was almost a letdown to have the goal met, I was still in gear, so to speak. It was really a terrific experience of being independent and setting a goal and achieving it. There's nothing like doing something that you're proud of to give you a sense of self-esteem and accomplishment.

Therapist 1: I have a few comments but I'll hold off to hear your thoughts T, so that we can comment on both.

T: To the first question?

Therapist 1: Yeah.

T: Well, with my earlier illness when I was 15, I never once entertained the thought that it would kill me, I don't know if it was the arrogance of being young, I just never once thought about that. I just didn't let those thoughts cross my mind. There was nothing wrong with me before it happened, and I just didn't entertain those thoughts. And that period taught me how to be sick, how to cope with illness, because the first whole week in the hospital I was by myself, no one was there, I was sick at boarding school, and went to the hospital by myself. So I was basically on my own for a whole week and they were doing all sorts of stuff. It was incredibly scary. I was in a lot of pain. And I was doing this all alone. Of course there were doctors and nurses, but I was really on my own the whole week. They didn't know what was wrong with me, it was really, very scary. So I learned to look after myself, to take care of myself. And I learned not to take what my doctors say verbatim. I question a lot, I don't blindly follow. So that would be the number one.

Therapist 1: So very interesting. One of the things we're hoping you're going to realize from the group is that while we present the sources meaning as separate groups, they very much overlap and are interchangeable, one feeds into the other as well. So for instance, here we are talking about taking responsibility for yourself, being courageous, saving your life, one of the things that helped you do that, to be courageous, was the attitude that you took, right? You decided, what kept you going, you said in the beginning, was your attitude. You never entertained he thought that there would be any other outcome. The other thing I hear in both of your comments was that at some point for you both, you reached out to her for help. So this notion of being connected to others, those were resources for you. You used the word resource. And what we're hoping is that through these sessions, you'll see these sources of meaning as resources for coping. You reached out to family and friends, to your parents, and ... in order to preserve your lives, you asked for help, you reached out, you swam, you treaded water on your own, taking care of yourself, but also, you called out for a life line in a sense. Because together both are needed to do the job.

And I had some thoughts about what courage meant based on what you guys are talking about. Courage doesn't necessarily mean you have to do it alone, but there are times when you do and times when you don't. Courage doesn't mean that you constantly need to be moving forward and being courageous, it can involve setbacks and moments of weakness, right?

T: Yeah.

Therapist 1: And I think it was you, S, who said that you were going through this whole process to achieve this goal, and once you did, it was almost like a letdown?

S: Yeah, it was.

Therapist 1: What it speaks to is that the process of going through it was so exhilarating, and let you feel so alive, that it was that part of the journey, was even more important than the destination in a sense, and I really think that takes courage. It's a process. You don't need to be courageous all the time, but finding your way out of the hole, to be courageous, may be more courageous than actually finished things, feeling like you've "achieved courage."

That makes sense to you?

S: Yeah, it does. I think, certainly life right now we've learned is a process, it's how you're living your life. You can be a really successful person, and I feel that what you were saying and what I agree with, my interpretation, is embarking on this, and figuring out how to continue on this journey, takes courage, but in itself, gives you a goal and a reason to live. That's what I got form what you were saying. The process gives real meaning to your life. Without the process, it's not as vital.

Therapist 1: Right, it's almost like life is the struggle. Life is what you're doing, while you're on the way to the goal.

T: Right, it is happening, life is happening all around, no matter what you're feeling, no matter whether you're sitting around or not, life is still going to go on. It's about how you look at life, how you participate in it.

Therapist 1: One of the things that was really interesting for me to realize when we developed this intervention, in reading *Man's Search for Meaning*, that book we gave you, Frankl used the word "Search," and I don't think that was accidental.

S: The way he is, I don't think anything is accidental.

Therapist 1: As long as you keep moving towards meaning, searching for it, that's the key. It's a continuous process, it's more important to be on the search, than finding it. Or as important.

T: What happens when you do find it?

Therapist 1: What has happened to you when that's happened?

T: I don't know if I've found it. Or maybe, I've had realizations of meaning. I guess I find meaning in some situations, but not all across the board.

Therapist 1: Right, so in life, there are a lot of things happening, everything is changing, and there are always new challenges, always new opportunities to find meaning. And as you grow from a young person to an adult, in each stage of life, you're challenged to find new meaning in each stage of life.

T: Society can also put pressure on you.

Therapist 2: How so?

T: Well, in terms of what you're supposed to have done at different life stages. They've put certain goals, accomplishments, on our shoulders, things that you should have done. But who's to say that I've not had meaning because I'm not married with five kids?

Therapist 1: Well one of the things that's related to this idea of being responsible to create your own life involves the notion that you create a life that is unique to you and which you live to your own and full potential. So some people actually term that the authentic life, when you're truly living the life that you want to be living. Living "my" life, not the life my parents wanted me to live, or society expects me to live, and when you're living authentically, you're living on your own expectations, and are the most fulfilled and have the most meaning. And you were talking about having the pressures of society's expectation on you, you were supposed to be married, but you're not?

T: Yes, and I'm ok with that, it's better to be alone than to have been married to who I would have been married to. Yeah, this is my way, it's right for me.

Therapist 1: So you could say that you've been living your authentic life?

T: Not just doing something because it's just that time. Yeah.

Therapist 1: Exactly.

S: There was this T-shirt I saw, with a woman's face looking so over-dramatic with tears flowing down her face, and the caption read "I CAN'T BELIEVE I FORGOT TO HAVE CHILDREN!"

Group: Hahahaha.

S: See? Totally makes sense to me. Bio clocks usually dominate most woman, but in the end, it's about being authentic.

Therapist 1: And you didn't have children, right?

S: Right

Therapist 1: Because?

S: I didn't have them, and now I regret it. For a couple of reasons, the first being medical. By the time I was 25, I had liver disease and I was on prednisone and my liver doctor said that it was better that I didn't get pregnant in terms of my body and the fetus handling it.

So that was my medical reason. But emotionally, I was married to someone, we had a very good relationship, we were really tight, and I didn't want to rock the boat, because in my childhood, I was in a triangle. And in my imagination, my parents were happy until I came along.

Therapist 1: Because they fought a lot?

S: Because my father favored me, it seemed. I felt like I messed things up for her, my mom. So I was thinking, why would I mess up a good marriage with a child? Am I going to be jealous of my daughter or son?

Therapist 1: So you were fearful of repeating what happened with your parents.

S: Yeah, so anyway, that would be the emotional reason. But I didn't know how much I would really love children, I would joke and say "I really don't like babies," but clearly that's not the case. I love them. So this was something I wasn't in touch with back then, and so back then, it didn't seem like such a sacrifice not to have them, but now that I didn't, I do realize now that it's too late and I missed out. So those are two major reasons.

Therapist 1: I think one of the questions later is about unfinished business. Do you feel like this is related?

S: I feel there's something else I should be doing right now. I don't know what that is. We're talking about projects, and being connected, and doing all sorts of things, but right now, I'm only working part-time, and I'm doing what I want to do, in between coming to MSK for treatment, and I really don't have a goal and a project, I mean, obviously, to stay alive is important, but I'm talking about something bigger than myself, and of course I love seeing D, my niece, but one thing that has come up to me is that I need, I want something more. I'm not feeling that connected, because I don't really have something that I've set a new goal for. So there is some unfinished business, but I don't know yet what it is.

T: In terms of unfinished business, I guess it's about creating a family of my own, if that makes sense.

Therapist 2: Of course it does.

T: I have a niece and I didn't know I would want children either, S, but now, I love, looove seeing her and she loves seeing me. So I guess that would be my unfinished business.

Therapist 2: What interesting to me about both of these stories, and one of the bigger themes of today is about creating, and both of you have shared that you didn't have children of your own, and now there's this feeling of wanting them, wishing you had had them, knowing you like them, one thing where this may be helpful to you, is to think about it and be more flexible . . . maybe there's other ways in which that desire or need can be fulfilled by these other relationships. S, up until today I heard a whole lot about this niece of yours and T, I hadn't hear anything about your niece at all, but maybe in these roles as aunts, some of that desire and some of those needs can be fulfilled.

Therapist 1: Absolutely.

T: Yeah, I think you're right.

Therapist 1: So actually, I think one more exercise fits in nicely with what we're been talking about. The third question is about responsibilities. What are your responsibilities? Who are you responsible to and for?

T: I wrote down that I'm just responsible for myself, right now. It's a relatively easy answer for me. Honestly, I'm just responsible for me.

Therapist 2: That's living authentically, that's your life right now. Just like when you were 16 you took care of yourself, and now, you're doing the same.

T: And I'm doing an ok job.

Therapist 2: It sounds like you're doing more than an ok job, T.

S: I was also going to say that I'm mostly responsible to myself. And I guess my brother and sister-in-law and my niece as well, but I think they could all live without me. I mean, my niece is very attached to me and would be devastated without me, but they would all live just fine, I think.

Therapist 1: So you both, number one on your list is being responsible to yourselves. But what does that actually mean to you guys?

T: I'm responsible for feeding, clothing, getting medical, having a roof over my head, taking care of all things, which is not easy, and you know with even all these things that I do for myself, I still need help sometimes, I can't really work and do very much outside of taking care of the cancer. And I'm in a lot of pain. And so, yeah.

S: For me to be responsible for me, to take care of myself, I've been responsible for myself for many decades now.

Therapist 1: So you would have answered the question in the same way 10–15 years ago?

S: No, things were different then. I felt there was more potential then, I had more potential.

Therapist 1: Meaning?

S: I wasn't as sick, my illness didn't prescribe limiting so much of what I did. I mean, now, I delight doing better than what the doctors would think. My whole life I've always tried to do beyond what on paper I was supposed to do. But now I'm feeling more of the restrictions.

Therapist 1: So would have said you're responsible for other people?

S: Yeah, an entire department at work, and now I just cover one desk. I was someone who was taking care of others, close friends and cousins. I didn't need as much help as I do now.

Therapist 1: When we were first developing this, I used to do the exercise with the patients, and so when it came to this exercise, I wrote down my own answer, and I would right down everyone in my world, but not myself, not me, I left that off. So it's really amazing that both of you have come to this place of knowing that you're responsible to yourselves. One after the other, my patients had themselves on their list, but I didn't. So at first, I said to myself, this must be some selfish thing that you're all putting that down . . .

T: No, it's unselfish.

Therapist 1: Right, a patient said to me, Dr. B, that's unselfish for you to take care of yourself. If you don't take care of yourself, you can't take care of others. They said, cancer teachers you that right away. And it will burden those who take care of you, if you don't also take care. You said it's unselfish, what does that mean?

T: If I take responsibility and have my needs met, then I'm not burdening others.

Therapist 1: So being a burden is a concern?

T: I mean, I am a bit of a burden, and I do feel badly that they have to come here since I can't travel down to the Bahamas to see them, but just so that I don't have to increase their burden, it's a big thing. I don't want anyone to have to pay for anything, that's the biggest thing, that my medical costs are taken care of.

S: Yes, that's a big thing.

Therapist 2: Why does that resonate?

S: My parents died 10 years or so ago. If I don't take care of me, other people will have to take care of me on the whole. I do agree, I could become too much of a burden. I used to pride myself on being low maintenance, but I realize, that I'm very high maintenance right now. There's no other way to live with cancer, it's very high maintenance. I mean, for someone to take that on, it's a huge thing, for me, and for someone else, huge. I mean, maybe my parents would have been able to help, I don't know. It's a very big thing that you be able to take care of yourself. And even then, you can't do it all entirely, you do need some help. It's really a revelation to recognize that you're high maintenance with cancer.

Therapist 1: Being able to take care of yourself is a critical part of caring about being alive. It's the critical part of taking responsibility for creating your life, right?

T: Yeah.

Therapist 1: What you're saying, it's really, saying if I don't take care of me, who will? If I don't fulfill that responsibility myself, who will? Is that what you're thinking of?

S: Yeah, I mean, it's that cheesy analogy of being on the airplane, if the oxygen mask falls, put it on you first, and then young children.

T: Right, you can't save others if you don't save yourself.

Therapist 1: Therapist 2, did you want to make a comment?

Therapist 2: I think we're pretty much out of time, but one thing that's striking to me, S, you said that you felt like there's something more, you're not sure about what it is. And then you said, you can't take a job. But you've been doing this cancer job so well, you've been taking care so well in the high maintenance way that you need, and maybe I'm wondering if it's about the way in which you take care that can be part of the *why* for you?

S: Yeah, maybe. I mean, I'm in some ways very compliant, and to be compliant, it can really be a full-time job.

Therapist 1: What strikes me about today, most of the time when we talk about this source of meaning that comes from the work we do, my job, etc, it's interesting that there is so much creativity that comes from creating a life and caring for yourselves and being responsible for yourselves. Your life has become the job.

S: I guess I haven't really thought about things that way. But yeah, now, my goal is just staying alive and feeling well enough, keeping my health.

Therapist 1: And you sometimes wonder whether that's sufficient?

S: Right.

Therapist 1: What do you think?

S: Well, right now I think, yes. I mean, I've already been in the position of saying goodbye to life, before my second transplant. I've done this multiple time. But, recently I've begun to think more about being alive, I told you about that year in Technicolor, I'm not ready to let it go just yet.

Therapist 1: Right. Exactly.

Ok, I think we're now over our time. Thank you for coming in the rain. I'm happy that we were here together, even though it was a short and small group.

Therapist 2: Yes, thank you so much. We're really glad that we were able to meet, even just the four of us. Have a great week, and we'll see you next time.

SESSION 7: EXPERIENTIAL SOURCES OF MEANING—CONNECTING WITH LIFE THROUGH LOVE, BEAUTY, AND HUMOR

Therapist 1: So last week we held Session 6, and had T and S here, and we were thinking that we had wanted to go through all of those exercises again with all of you. We probably don't have time to do that, but let's start by quickly reflecting on the trajectory we've been on, and we'll give you guys an opportunity to discuss at least one of the questions from our last session.

In Session 1 we introduced you to this idea of meaning, and in Session 2 about how cancer has impacted this meaning. In Sessions 3 and 4 we discussed the historical context of this meaning, the legacy we were given, the one we live, and the one we hope to leave behind, and then we had a session on attitudinal sources of meaning. And in Session 6 and today's Session 7, we're going to discuss two other sources of meaning. One is through creative sources of meaning, what we covered last week in Session 6, the meaning that is derived from your work, your roles in life, things you dedicate yourself to in the world, and the things you do in the world, the things that you are in the world, and Session 7 is about experiential sources of meaning, the way that you experiences life, through your sensations, touch, sight, and smell and ears and feelings, emotions, love, connection with nature and art and beauty, how those make life so meaningful. And that's what today's session is really about.

So last week the focus was really more about doing, the active stuff you do in your life that gives you a sense of meaning, and this week's session is more about absorbing the experience of living, of being in life, listening to music, having your kids snuggle with you and tell you that they love you.

So, last week, S, you participated and we did two of the exercises, one of them had to do with times when we had courage, right? Because it takes courage to go out into the world and do and be things in the world and create a life when you're struggling with cancer.

And the second exercise was about who you're responsible to and for. And so we thought with you P and L we'd do that second question. But first, any reflections on last week?

S: Well, I can only remember what I said, I mean because what I see here in terms of courage and taking ownership of your life, of the several things I had written, the main thing that I had gone over, was after my divorce, I had a house and couldn't afford to keep it just by working as a librarian. I wouldn't have been able to get a mortgage, and I was thinking about how resourceful I was, I set a goal and I stuck to it, I did everything I could to retain the house, I did everything I needed to keep it. And I actually did manage to hold on to my house. I did have help, my father-in-law helped and I took in roommates, but it all worked out. And it was scary, but I had faith that I would be able to pull this off. And I did it.

Therapist 1: L, P, any thoughts about this notion of courage to go out there and live a life?

L: You need courage just to get up in the morning and put one step in front of the other. I guess I remember, it was probably, I guess about during the early 90s, and that was my first episode of depression, that I could put my finger on, and it was a horrible winter and I was digging out my car and driving very far, it was the year I was on interferon for hepatitis C, and I patted myself on the back that I got up every day to go to work, and if it wasn't for the staff that I had, I don't think that I would have been able to get up every day and do it. I never would have been able to make it through that winter.

Therapist 1: One of the things we talked about last time is that yes, we need courage, but we also need the help of good people. Courage doesn't mean that you don't need people or are completely fearless . . .

So that's so profoundly meaningful to you that those folks helped you, what did they do?

L: They watched my back. They did what was needed to do in order for things to keep running while I wasn't functioning at full capacity.

Therapist 1: A lot of us don't like to be in positions where we have to depend on others, but sometimes in those positions we learn that people love us so much.

P, did that happen to you?

P: In terms of what?

Therapist 1: People coming out of the woodwork, perhaps people you didn't know really loved you that much.

P: Yeah, I mean, a few did after the cancer diagnosis. There were, I guess I'm used to it now because it's become a lifetime it seems, even though it's only been five months, but feels like a lifetime. My partner has been terrific, she's a very strong woman, so I wasn't surprised. She's keeping the practice going, and she really does and she's been very selfless in terms of, not that there's that much money, not giving me a hard time about sharing it. She actually feels guilty that she's doing things that I'm not a part of and she's worried that she's not splitting it 50/50 anymore.

And a good friend of mine, a neighbor, and he's always been a friend of mine, we've spoken periodically. His wife died of breast cancer about 15 years ago and so he knows better than many what this is like, he knows how people behave after cancer comes up. He told me that you really don't know who is going to be supportive until after it happens, and, well, he's been very, very supportive. He calls, he makes sure to check in periodically, offers to get together for meals, and just cares.

Therapist 1: And what about this issues of courage?

P: I don't feel courageous at all.

Therapist 1: You're not courageous?

P: Well I jumped out of an airplane when I was 17, I went skydiving, was supposed to be 18, but I lied. So I guess that took courage. It was one of the most exhilarating experiences of my life. When you first jump out, there's like a kickback, there's a lot of pressure, you go flailing. But then, it's just quiet, it's peaceful, one of the most amazing moments of my entire life. You look around, you don't hear anything, and it's just so eerily peaceful.

Therapist 1: And you got pushed out of the plane?

P: Yeah, they push you. Once you get to a certain place in line, they push you out, you have no choice.

Therapist 1: So this sounds a lot like having cancer!

Group: Hahaha.

Therapist 1: I mean, in terms of jumping, having a leap of faith, and having chaos and then other moments of quiet. And is it all taking a tremendous amount of courage?

P: So yeah, I mean, I guess some of it was like cancer. But now? Courage? No. I don't feel courageous.

L: Well my experience I related doesn't have anything to do with cancer. Because I was going to say that I haven't felt particularly courageous since I got the diagnosis. Except for the fact that I'm not afraid to tell people and giving people the opportunity to talk about it if they need.

Therapist 1: So should we do this responsibility exercise for P and L quickly before getting into the one for today?

Therapist 2: Yes, let's take a look at the question that asks about who and what you are responsible for . . .

Therapist 1: We'll see if your number one answers are the same and T and S.

S: I still don't feel courageous about cancer. As I had mentioned last week, my cancer markers went up, I felt like there was nothing anyone could say or do to help me, and I felt like there was nothing I could say or do to help me. I was feeling the opposite of courage.

Therapist 1: Well as we mentioned last week, courage doesn't have to be constant. You can have moments of weakness, moments when you can fall apart. P, you want to take a stab at this question?

P: Who am I responsible for? I just left a four year old at home, and a 16 year old. I've always felt responsible for my kids. And one of the things that makes me feel good is being able to fulfill those responsibilities. I took my daughter to Wisconsin this weekend, put together her dorm at college, and I did it. I set her up at college. I flew there and drove and dreaded the traveling and doing chemo the next day, but I did it. I felt great because I was able to do all the things that needed to be done. So that part, that's probably the most meaningful part of what I'm doing these days. There are other things I can't do, I can't keep up with my four year old. It's just too hard for me to take him outside. I don't feel that he's getting enough stimulation from me, but I try.

Therapist 1: Anyone or anything else you're responsible to for?

P: My wife, but she's pretty self-sufficient, there's not so much I need to do for her. I feel a little responsible towards my parents, mostly, my mother is so single-minded about exploring options for me, she just, she'll always keep asking questions, she won't accept what one doctor will say. She is so single-minded, that I feel bad that . . . I know why she's doing it, she's afraid, she's going to lose her son. So I try to put her mind to ease, and tell her I'm open to second and third opinions, even though I know what the statistics are. So in a way I'm taking care of her by allowing her to take care of me.

Therapist 1: L?

L: I'm responsible to my family and community. Caring for my dad, overseeing that my son and his family are financially ok, and I function as a captain on my floor, we have a lot of, my building is almost 50 years old, so a lot of old tenants, so if anything goes wrong, I watch out for them and am in charge. I've been managing to do all that.

Therapist 1: Well this is interesting because S and T had a different number one on their list.

L: Well I have another. To the Creator, to God. To be faithful to my beliefs. It's important to me that I'm not just giving lip service so to speak to a higher power, but that I'm truly connected.

Therapist 1: This connection, do you always feel it? Are there things that make it more real?

L: Prayer makes it feel more real.

Therapist 2: Anything else?

L: No that was it.

Therapist 2: Well S and T, they had a different number one . . .

T: To myself. I'm responsible to myself.

Therapist 1: And S?

S: I mean, yeah, I feel responsible, if I were to think after that, I'm definitely responsible to myself. I gave the analogy of when you take a flight and they show you the video about the oxygen mask, about taking care of yourself so you can take care of others.

Therapist 1: What do you guys feel about that? P?

P: I don't know. I mean, I have a very full house. At any one time there's a wife and two kids and now my parents, and so it's, there's a lot more going on than just me.

L: To me, I kinda make the assumption that it's understood that I'm number one. Unless I take care of myself, it will be hard for others to, and I won't be able to take care of others.

T: No it does make sense. If you're taking care of yourself, then you're not leaving that responsibility to other people.

L: I'd love to leave it to other people.

T: Sure, I would too, but it's good that I can take care of some things. They don't need to do everything.

Therapist 1: I think what P and L, what you have on your list, your list identifies the roles you play in life, things you care about, things that you feel fully engaged in, as a father, husband, son, mother, having a relationship with God, being engaged in the world, these are some things that give meaning to your life.

And I think today's session on experiential sources of meaning also is about connecting with something greater than yourself, having moments of transcending, not being aware of time and space, when you're in love, when you're holding your child, when you're listening to incredible music, those are moments of transcendence, when life has peak meaning. The exercise today is really focused on beauty and nature and humor. We added humor because we thought it was important to relate to the fact that it's important to laugh, and that we can be transported through laughter.

S: Laughter is a great medicine, it really is!

Therapist 2: So if you guys can take a look at the exercise for today, take a few moments to write a few answers down to the question about how you connect to life and feel alive through the experience of love, beauty, and humor. . . .

T, would you like to go first?

T: Sometimes I just sit back, with my brothers and sisters and family, and sit back and listen to them, whatever they're doing, whether they're fighting or having a good time. I'm just content with having them around me, just receiving, just being in the moment.

Therapist 1: You said something really beautiful S to me outside of group that I'd like to repeat if that's ok. You were walking on the grounds of XYZ hospital and you saw this building, and it was silver and stood out to you, the architecture stood out to you, its beauty, and you felt, I think the word you used was, exhilarated?

S: I was just really excited by the prospect of seeing such an interesting and different and beautiful buildings, it was Frank Gehry architecture. I was in awe. Finding it was amazing

Therapist 1: And in that moment, did you lose a sense of the present? Of why you were at that hospital?

S: Yes, everything else just dissipated . . . time, space, everything.

Therapist 1: You were connected to everything.

S: I was pretty thrilled.

Therapist 1: Did you write down anything else?

S: In terms of love, I of course put my niece D, and I haven't really mentioned my brother, but I know he loves me even though he's not demonstrative of it, and my cousins in England, and my friends. And then I put water and great music. There are times when I hear a note of music and I can almost just start to cry. It takes you beyond your situation. I forget everything else when that happens.

Therapist 1: Do you have a favorite piece of music?

S: I don't know. It can be anything. The other day I was really struck by an opera piece, and I'm not really into opera, but I heard one aria and I couldn't believe how beautiful it was and I was so transported, so taken away by it. Really an extra, out-of-body experience. Really, really nice. More than nice. It was the tone, the sound that connects you to the universe.

Therapist 1: And what about humor?

S: Definitely. My friends at the library usually go out about once a month, we went out a few weeks ago and were laughing the entire night, before we even got to the table. We had our own jokes and had such a good time. Just such good moments.

And I also seek out TV shows that have humor in them, because they also transport me. Sometimes when I feel upset I'll just go to YouTube and try to find something funny to watch to try to put me right.

Therapist 1: L?

L: Love, of my children and grandchildren, nieces and nephews. Their sense of awe, they look at me as if I know everything, or at least did when they were little. But yes, there is great love there. Museums and concerts. And I have a love of worship, I love liturgical music. There's nothing more beautiful than hearing the songs of the Church.

In terms of beauty, I feel calm and peace near a body of water. I love the sound of the waves, it's just the calmest. I always thought of myself as a New Yorker, I would never move anywhere if it was far from water. But when I think about vacations, it's always about water.

Therapist 1: Do you have a favorite place?

L: I guess it is Barbados. I mean, there's the cultural connection.

And I see beauty in the faces of children of different cultures. I love looking at books or TV documentaries where you see children of different ethnic groups.

I also love flowers and plants, although I'm not talented like T in that respect. I'm not a farmer or gardener, but I do admire them. I love fresh flowers.

In terms of humor, years ago when I was feeling down I would always put on the movie, *Tu Wong Foo*? Or something like that? They're all dressed in drag there? It always made me laugh, always made me feel better. And then, I hope this is not misunderstood, coming from a Caribbean culture, I grew up in a community where most of my friends were Barbadian Americans, so we would have fun mocking the speech patterns, the nuances of the natives. One of the funniest experiences was going to court in Barbados and seeing all these black folk dressed up as the English, with white wigs.

T: They take it very seriously!

L: I know!

S: And that's even funnier!

Therapist 1: And P, I bet that's one thing about being a lawyer in the US I bet you don't mind not having to do.

P: That's true, I don't have a powdered wig.

Therapist 1: The children from different cultures and all that. That's very powerful.

L: Yes. I have a friend of a friend, a Nigerian doctor, a radiologist, he did a book on children of Africa and it was one of the most beautiful things I had ever seen. He was sick of seeing ads for kids who were starving and so raised money for them in this way.

Therapist 1: T, you want to go?

T: Love, I love playing with my niece and nephew, they just came back from England, I love being with them. He's 11 months old and she's three years old. They're really entertaining. Playing with them. And also I find love in gardening and my neighbors are away right now, and I'm taking care of their window boxes right now and its very cathartic. I really find love in it. Growing things, growing herbs, that makes me really happy. I find in doing that there's love.

Therapist 1: Are there certain herbs that you love to grow more than others?

T: There are some that are easier than others, but I love growing them all.

Therapist 1: So you just don't love people, but you love plants.

T: Yes. And the last thing is my dogs. I love playing with my dogs, snuggling up with them, playing with them. I used to have four dogs and slowly they passed, but even now, I just love it so much. I miss having my dog with me all the time. He was such a source of love for me.

And as for beauty, of course the garden, I appreciate the beauty of all plants, wildflowers and weeds a lot, and I feed the squirrels outside my window, to me that's beautiful.

And of course, the beauty of the island. The blue skies, the waters, the vivid colors. Everything is bright, the houses, the plants, the color of paint is different. We don't live in just white houses, its aqua and pink and orange. And the water. And sand.

Therapist 2: That sounds amazing, T. Did you have anything written down for humor?

T: Yes, laughing with my family. We all have a very dry sense of humor. And we can make fun of each other, or other people who aren't there. And one of my old girlfriends pointed out that we all like to recite shows or movies we saw, the funny lines, the parts of the movies that were good. We all do that, and find ourselves laughing. And also, watching something that is funny. These days, I don't need sad. I don't need something that makes me feel worse than I feel anyway. I'd rather watch something that's going to make me laugh. I go for comedy. And lastly, I put down laughing with my niece who is three, she likes to tell fairy tales that make no sense, and it's just so funny. I love it. And when I laugh, she laughs, and when she laughs, I laugh, so it's all very good.

Therapist 1: Thanks T.

Therapist 2: You know I just want to point out, T, that not only what you shared was wonderful, but in these groups, you've really brought a lot of humor into the room, I know I've often found myself laughing when you tell stories and when I look around the room I see others laughing as well. Just experiencing you, I feel connected in that way, receiving that humor.

Group: Yeah, agreed.

T: Thanks.

Therapist 2: P, would you like to go?

P: Well the first thing I thought of, in terms of connecting, last night I was laying on my bed, I was really tired, was just zonked. My daughter comes in and lays over sideways on my recliner in my bedroom and then my little one, he comes in and he climbs up onto her lap. And he apparently asked her to imitate him. So she would say what he said, instantaneously, and this went on for about five minutes, and they had a good time, and the two of them together, just having fun with each other, it gave me such a great feeling, it didn't matter that I was tired.

Therapist 1: What was the feeling?

P: Oh it was love. To see my two kids loving each other in that way.

T: Pride?

P: I guess. I didn't put a word on it, it just felt really, really good.

Therapist 1: I think every parent's dream or desire is that their kids be close.

P: Well I don't expect that they'll be close forever, there are 11 years between them. But the fact that they were just there, they were just silly and it was just so funny. I loved it.

The other thing, it's similar, going on family vacations, a few years ago we went to this place called Smuggler's Watch, it was another—rare—time I remember everyone being happy together for more than a few hours at a time. That doesn't happen all that too often in life.

And the last thing I wrote for love is getting away with my wife for an evening or a night. We can just sit in silence and just be, that's fine, that's enough, that's comfort, that's love. I'm very happy with that.

As far as beauty, I don't know, I haven't done it so much since my diagnosis, but before that I was trying to get into photography. I got myself a fancy camera with ten different lenses and I would go out and try to take pictures of everything. Once I was in Palm Springs and there was this river that had all these palm trees growing around it, but it was also surrounded by desert and I went out and thought I was following the map but was so busy taking pictures of rock formations and the juxtaposition of the lush palms and the vegetation that went out about 10 feet from the water that I got completely lost. Meanwhile, I'm taking all these pictures, and had so many beautiful ones.

Therapist 1: Because you were lost?

P: Well, some were because I got lost.

Therapist 1: So getting lost brought you to a place you wouldn't have gotten to otherwise?

P: I don't know. But anyway, that was beauty for me, but I don't do that anymore.

As far as humor, I'm the kinda guy, in conversations where I'm not asked to speak, most of the time I listen, but every now and then I throw in zingers. That's what I do, and most people laugh at them. They're usually self-deprecating.

The other thing I wrote down for humor, I went to pay a Shiva call to a good friend after my diagnosis, and I told him about my diagnosis at the time, and I felt weird for doing that because his father had just died, but before I left his home, he gave me all five CDs of the 2000 Year Old Man, and I played them in the car on the way home from Jersey and I just started laughing.

S: That's got to be one of the funniest things ever.

P: I guess what was especially poignant is that he was going through a tragedy and I was beginning my ongoing tragedy. And it was probably the best medicine that anyone—even the doctors—ever gave me. I listened for 5–6 hours and I may go home and listen to them again tonight. It's just hysterical.

Therapist 1: I want to ask a question. You guys all described moments of love, beauty, humor, that transcend you. Are you still able to have these experiences with cancer?

P: Yes. I mean, watching my kids was last night. It's harder, but I can.

L: Harder to appreciate?

P: Harder to get myself into the places where it can happen.

T: I'm limited more physically, so in many ways I can't do the things like gardening that were connecting me in the past. But I still can do some things.

Therapist 1: Like the things that don't require exertion, like the window boxes, that's something you still connect with.

Therapist 2: That's really the idea behind these different sources of meaning. The idea that we can receive things, we don't need to do or create in order to have meaning. We can see the colors even if we can't water the garden, we can receive these things.

I'm very struck, P, by your sharing what you experienced last night, and just connecting it to what you shared about being responsible to your children and that you had said that you're not sure that you can do that as much, but with the example last night, with you sitting there and watching your children, I imagine you're no less of a dad sitting there and enjoying that moment than at other times when you're more active.

P: But there's things, like my 16 year old wanted me to take her driving. There are other things that I can't do. I felt badly today, I couldn't take her driving today. I didn't have time, because I needed the time to eat. It takes me a while to eat and I'm losing weight and so I need to make sure that I eat. And my little guy, I mean, being with him takes a lot of energy, he's a ball of energy and I just can't keep up.

Therapist 1: Thanks, P. Thanks guys for sharing all you shared. I just want to say I think today was really beautiful session. It was beautiful and funny and filled with love.

Therapist 2: Agreed. Absolutely.

Before we go, though, let's just spend a few minutes talking about a few things. A reminder that next session is our last session. And also, I just wanted to remind you all about the legacy project. We've suggested a lot of exercises in here, and traditionally what we've done, if people have chosen to do a legacy project, we ask that you share it, or bring it in, in our Session 8. Again, this can be anything, something you've thought about as a result of these groups, something that connects some of what we've talked about in here, that's connected the sessions for you. It's wide open. Just like everyone's definition of meaning is different and personal and unique, so are these projects. So we invite you to share with us in Session 8 if you're doing one, or plan to do one, or just idea about what you might do.

Therapist 1: And if you don't do one, please don't *not* come because of that!

Therapist 2: And also in our last session we're going to spend some time thinking about what this time has been like, reflecting on this journey together. And as usual, we have some food for thought questions to go through. We'll take some time to discuss what this journey has been like for all of you and to see if anything has changed for you in terms of how you're thinking about meaning.

Are there any questions?

Group: No . . .

Therapist 2: Ok, well then we'll see each other next time for what has quickly crept up to us, our 8th session.

Therapist 1: Thanks guys. We really appreciate your being here and look forward to seeing you next time!

SESSION 8: TRANSITIONS—FINAL REFLECTIONS AND HOPES FOR THE FUTURE

Therapist 1: Hi everyone!

Therapist 2: So good to see you!

L: I brought treats?

Group: Oh, thank you!

L: Chocolate croissants!

Group: Thanks so much, L!

Therapist 2: So, welcome everyone. All of a sudden we're here at Session 8, or at least it seems like all of a sudden, and there's a lot to reflect on today and talk about today. And I had spoken to a few of you in the interim about the legacy projects, so we will want to take some time to see if anyone came in with projects this week. I know T, you had mentioned to me that you were going to bring something in, would you like to go first?

T: Sure. Well, I just brought in a series of pictures, and all of them except for one, I took of myself by myself of me. The first is me and my dog in Cape Frances . . .

Group: He's so cute!

Therapist 2: Great picture!

S: And you look great!

T: Thanks guys. I love him so much, and I'm excited because I just booked my ticket to go home in two weeks to see him, and my family. So I'll have to get some treats and other things for him. And then the other picture is just this last weekend, this is me and my college roommate, she and I went to the Walk for the Cure, I didn't walk but I registered and we went and just watched. And the third, that's me and C, my niece. Last Christmas, so she's important.

Therapist 1: So you took all of them? They're very centered!

T: Yes, I know I'm getting good at that! Thanks!

Therapist 1: So what do these pictures represent?

T: They all represent important things to me . . . people, places, time. I love my niece and my college roommate. All of them are recent, maybe all except for the dog.

Therapist 1: And the race?

T: Yeah, and last year I was chosen to be somewhat of a spokesperson, my picture is all over those adds. That meant a lot. And clearly friends are important. I have a lot of good friends who help and support me.

Therapist 2: Thanks for sharing these meaningful pictures.

Therapist 1: Are you going to share them with anyone else?

T: I showed them to my mother, many people have seen them, just not necessarily all together at once.

Therapist 1: That's a beautiful set of pictures, and what I think is beautiful, aside from having you in them, is that they represent all the people that you love and your passions in life.

T: My brothers and sisters are missing, but clearly I love them too.

Therapist 1: So they represent experiential and creative sources of meaning . . . so it's a meaningful legacy project.

Therapist 2: Thank you for bringing those in, T.

L, aside from the chocolates, did you bring anything else today in terms of the legacy project? Or should we assume that that's your legacy project?

Group: Hahaha.

L: No, no, that's not my project. We started doing family reunions back in the early 80s; we went on cruises and to the Barbados. And it always came up that I was going to get a cookbook together of family recipes, and I never did, but I would like to, because the way that my dad's generation cooked, it's different. I can do a little but the generation after me doesn't have a clue. So that's going to be my project.

Therapist 1: So there are certain foods some generations aren't cooking?

L: Yeah, certain fish, and different methods of preparation. So that's the goal. I haven't started it yet, but I will.

Therapist 1: So that's connected to legacy. Keeping your heritage going?

L: Exactly.

Therapist 2: Thanks L.

Therapist 1: Did you bring in anything S, think of a project to do?

S: I, uh, was racking my brain, nothing was coming up. My brain wasn't working.

Therapist 1: Well you had a rough week or two.

S: Yeah, I did. All of my levels, my liver functioning, everything was sky high. So it's been a rough few weeks. Luckily my ultrasounds of my kidneys came out all clear, but that said, it's been rough. My insides are very complicated, very complicated to manage!

Therapist 1: Sorry it's been rough, S.

S: Yeah, I've just been really tearful. So anyway, I wasn't really thinking so much about doing this project.

Therapist 1: So you didn't think of bringing your liver in for your project?

S: Hahaha, no!

Therapist 2: That would have been a first!

S: No, I didn't. I guess I was just feeling these past few weeks like you had been feeling, L. So I haven't been really thinking. That said, I want to do a cookbook like L, at this point in my life the man I go out with is such a damn good cook, I just know he'd really appreciate that. And he comes from such a competitive family and there's a little bit of cooking competitions between us, and would be good to maybe put them all together.

Therapist 1: So what are some of the dishes?

S: I have never bragged, but I keep hearing that I make the lightest, most delicious matzo balls and really strong, great broth.

Therapist 2: That sounds amazing.

S: So yeah, I'd really like to put a cookbook together. That's definitely one thing to do. I also want to pass down my mom's recipes. She had great recipes for the holidays.

Therapist 1: And in addition to the cookbook? Is there anything else?

S: A girlfriend actually said to me the other day, "Why don't you write?" She suggested that I write down my story, so to speak. She said that everyone finds my story really fascinating, of my liver transplant, and then of cancer . . .

Therapist 1: It's a story of survival.

S: Exactly, people love that story. Even some of my doctors have told me to write a book! So maybe I will. I actually like the idea of writing an article as opposed to a book, and I may just start writing and see what happens.

Therapist 1: Just so you know, I'm an editor of a journal, and I publish essays and stories and some nonscientific stuff, and often I publish things that patients have written.

S: That's good to know!

T: And my sister's a book agent!

Therapist 1: So there you go!

S: And then, I just jotted down a few photographs that I'm sorry I didn't bring. Just my brother and sister-in-law and my cousin and me, windblown at Montauk. It's just so full of energy. And another picture of us at a farm stand, just so colorful, so rich.

Therapist 1: So the pictures are full of life and wind and food!

S: Lush.

Therapist 1: Yes, filled with experiential sources of meaning.

S: Yes, and I was also going to bring a picture from my cousin in England that was taken at D's fifth birthday party. It's just so cute, the look on her face is just so adorable, it captures her youth and innocence, and then in the corner, there's me, and I'm so skeletal and yellow, clearly so sick, and so it really shows how far I've come. It's not the kind of photo I like to look at, but D looks so funny, and me, it just shows how far I've come. I look so, so sick in the picture. And then, after that, I have a picture that was taken this year at my birthday, where I look so healthy, and the sun was about to set, and the water is reflecting, and everyone just looks so, so great! And there's a picture of me with everyone. I look so much better in that one.

Therapist 2: That sounds wonderful.

S: Yeah, so I have a few ideas.

Therapist 1: Thank you ladies for sharing those. They're all wonderful remembrances and things to pass on to others and share.

Therapist 2 mentioned that this is our last session, so we want to talk just a little bit what it was like to go through these eight weeks together. So if you could all turn in your binders to the questions for Section 8, the group reflections and thoughts for the future, we can take some time to go through these, and use these questions as a template to talk about a few things.

So, I guess when we started and I said this was meaning-centered psychotherapy, and you said "Huh?" But what's it been like for you guys to go through this experience over the past 8 weeks and has it changed how you view your lives or you cancer experience or anything like that? What's it been like? What did you take away from it?

S: Well, I hadn't realized, I hadn't been thinking in terms of finding meaning as being a choice. That was a big thing.

Therapist 2: Yes, that's huge.

S: Also, you mentioned a transcendent experience, and as much as I had shared a lot of experiences that I've had, I hadn't really seen them as having the same meaning as having children, or something big like that. And it's comforting to know that those peak experiences where you're pulled out of yourself, that they allow you to feel at one with yourself.

Therapist 1: As fundamental as having children and things like that, right?

S: Yeah. I mean, I've been sad that I didn't, so it's good for me to think about these alternative experiences.

Therapist 1: Can you speak a little more about these transcendent experiences? What did it do to your sense of self?

S: It actually took me out of my sense of self. But, in terms of my sense of, my sense of self . . .

Therapist 1: It took you out of yourself . . . and did it teach you anything about who you are?

S: Just the obvious, that I respond to these things. And that I want to do these things, do them now, currently, and make a point to do these. But in terms of myself, well, that I have the capability of feeling very deeply, even now when I'm feeling really closed off, because even though I have friends I can crumble with, on the whole, I really don't do that, and it's probably an effort, it's something that comes naturally to me, it's about being on, rather than off. One of the things I like about being on is that you rise to the occasion and you feel better doing it, than staying home and feeling exhausted. Because even being here, it certainly makes me feel more alive to interact and hear what's going on. So it's revived me.

Therapist 1: Revival, that's a good word.

S: Yeah, revival.

Therapist 1: As opposed to survival? You talked about writing a story about survival.

S: Yeah . . .

Therapist 1: What did you like about the word revival?

S: I don't think I used it, it's not something I use really.

Therapist 1: Survival is getting through, but revive probably means something slightly different, right?

S: I mean, you can barely survive, but revival is bringing back to life.

Therapist 1: So when you're focused on things that are meaningful in life, you're bringing yourself back to life?

S: Yeah, I guess.

L: That's a very good thought, though. I guess that's how I'd have to explain it. I was surviving, I was getting up and doing what I had to do, taking care of things, but not really focusing on myself and what my needs were, and coming to these sessions and having to focus on certain things and having to think and write and focus, I feel more energized, and I guess, it has been a revival of sorts. It's definitely, it's hard to concretely say what these sessions have done, but I've certainly felt a lot better coming here weekly and interacting. Even the challenge of going on the subway is an accomplishment. So that's been really good for me.

Therapist 1: What about the session where we talked about death and all of that. Was that a downer?

T: It's reality.

L: Not for me, it wasn't.

Therapist 1: Say a little more.

L: I guess the environment and family I came up in, we talked about death a lot. My father has always talked about things he would like done when he does pass, and we were always going to funerals and I can remember family members being laid out in the house. So death wasn't hidden, it was always something that was there. And when I got my diagnosis, I said I was not afraid of dying, I just don't know what to expect and don't want to be in a lot of pain, but the idea of not being here is not frightening to me, to the point that it is to a lot of other people.

Therapist 1: I guess there's always revival after death. Were you going to say something about that, S?

S: No, no I wasn't. I think I had said at the time I would like it to be as painless as possible. I'm afraid of extreme pain and of not being able to communicate what I want, what I need, that frightens me so much, to not be able to express how I'm feeling. But more than anything, it's just the nightmare of being in extreme pain before letting go.

Therapist 1: So it makes sense to talk about this with people who might be in a place of making decisions for you if you're at a place where you can't, right?

S: Yeah. The trouble is having been unconscious, and over other things, I don't feel comforted by the fact that I might be unconscious, because I remember, and it only happened once, I was so relieved to wake up, I was going through such a nightmare and felt so dry and I kept having this nightmare and feeling totally stuck in it. And so I don't find any comfort in the idea that I would be unconscious. You can be going through something really bad when you're unconscious, too. So I wish, I don't know, had that hadn't happened in the past, I might feel more at ease about just letting myself go.

Therapist 1: Had you ever been unconscious when you were sick, T?

T: I guess so, maybe. A form of it, due to all the meds that I was given, I was coming in and out of consciousness. I was delirious.

Therapist 1: How'd you answer the first question?

T: I wrote, it's been a positive experience to find meaning for me, it makes my life feel lighter.

Therapist 2: It makes you feel lighter?

T: It's a joyful experience, not a sorrowful one. It's not like you're doing it all the time. And I guess I've realized that if you look for it, it's always there. All you need to do is look. If you look, you'll find it. Just my looking at the squirrels out my window, I can find meaning in that. So before I might not have said that, and I guess now I realize that my life really does have a lot of meaning. If you say there is no meaning, then you're really just not looking, it's like you're blocking it.

Therapist 1: So there's a choice to find meaning, to see it?

T: Yeah, totally.

Therapist 1: It's a little like what S said, about choosing to find it, to look for it, it's always there.

T: I mean, I never thought my life was meaningless, but I never sat down and looked for specific meanings, either. So I've found this a positive experience that's made me feel lighter, because there's an awful lot of stress and strain when you're sick, and it changes from week to week and day to day and so it's nice to be able to figure out what's meaningful to you, and what you give meaning, to, because you can then have that with you no matter what type of week or day you're having.

Therapist 1: What do you guys think about what T just shared?

L: I think it makes a lot of sense. And what I hear her saying, and I guess for me, meaning translates into a connectedness. Whether it's with people, or nature, or animals, or whatever, the things that you enjoy doing, that you get pleasure and comfort out of, I think it can be very simple, like the last few weeks, I was really just communicating with nature, just watching the lake, and being outside. Just simple, a little bit of nothing, but looking at God's love, let go of the stress or feel connected through my belly, on a gut level, is usually for me in nature, watching the sunset, or the water, it's always different. So I think it's interesting to find that that connectedness is life, you know, it's life at its best. And what you're saying is that you may have cancer, but, you can still connect, and still find meaning. And I think that's the point of this intervention you call this.

S : Yeah, I think T said it very well. And I think that the times that I felt that I've let go of the stress or feel connected through my belly, on a gut level, is usually for me in nature, watching the sunset, or the water, it's always different. So I think it's interesting to find that that connectedness is life, you know, it's life at its best. And what you're saying is that you may have cancer, but, you can still connect, and still find meaning. And I think that's the point of this intervention you call this.

Therapist 1: That's so well said! I hope we're recording this, Therapist 2.

Therapist 2: We are . . .

Therapist 1: This is really, this is exactly what we had hoped you guys would have come away with from this intervention.

The second question has to do with whether you have a better understanding of these different sources of meaning and if you're better able to put them to work in your life. And I think you've all already addressed some of this, begun to talk about this. I would imagine in the beginning when we talked about meaning, it was a very abstract concept, right?

T: It was. At first, I was searching to come up with something, but now, it's just right there. Once I thought about it, it was easier, it was right there.

Therapist 2: You know, the language that you're using, that's changed as well. It's really very striking.

S : You should actually be sending us these tapes! So that we have a record of this! We maybe could continue to learn from them, learn phrases we didn't fully get at first.

Therapist 1: Do you guys want to add anything to your answers? Did you get a notion from the eight weeks that we wanted you to understand that there were very available and understandable sources of meaning in life, and all you have to do is recognize that they're there, and know that a lot of it has to do with connectedness, to people, causes, work, history, values, and also, overcoming and choosing your attitude towards your suffering? And did you also get the idea that it was helpful to know these different sources of meaning so that you could move around from one to another if you had to?

Group: Yes, yes.

Therapist 1: You talked a little about missing out on something by not having children, S, but you've realized that there are these other sources that are important.

S: Right, right. I mean, I think the bigger revelation has been—I mean, I was 12 when my dad asked where God is—and I said nature, is that I've been most connected to life in that way. And every fall I go enjoy the foliage. So I've found different things than children . . . like, it was a bit of a revelation to me how animated I became when I discovered that *fantastical* building, and how much pleasure I got in that moment. That was big for me. That excitement, I can re-live it in re-telling it, it's another source of meaning, another moment that is meaningful to me . . .

Therapist 1: Thanks, S. T, anything to add to that second item? You all have taken it up so well so I understand if you don't have anything to add . . .

T: Yeah, I sorta answered that one. If meaning seems like it's not there, I guess you're not looking. For me, the meaning will always be there. And I'd like to continue to fill my life with meaningful things, and this will help me identify what those things are. It's made it more concrete, more specific for me. It's helped me to find meaning and I do have a better understanding, to answer your question directly.

Therapist 1: Anything to add, L?

L: Um, I guess the one thing I tried to do in terms of meaning, especially having been very down, is attempt to look at the glass half full, to try and see the world in a more positive way. That I'm more consciously doing.

Therapist 1: You're choosing the attitude you're taking.

L: Yeah.

Therapist 1: Someone said meaning is a choice and you're saying hope is a choice?

L: I guess I am. I like that! Hope is a choice.

Therapist 1: Which brings us to the last exercise. If you guys can take a few minutes and write down some thoughts about your hopes for the future. . . .

T, would you like to go first?

T: Well my hopes for the future are to get better and live life to the fullest physically, given all that cancer has limited for me. I've been limited physically much more so than mentally. But they're, the symptoms, they're getting better. So I'm hoping they'll get so better that I don't have them anymore. And also, to make as much as I can with what limitations I'm feeling. Not let the physical stuff consume me, and not wallow in self pity. It's ok to do that once in a while, but to stay there is not good. So to do the best that I can, given whatever is going on, on a given day. And to keep my mind in a positive place. To choose to be hopeful, not hopeless. I don't want to choose hopelessness. What's the point of going on if you're hopeless?

So, to be as light as I can to fill each day, is what I hope to gain.

Therapist 1: A lightness.

T: Yes. To have my mind as free of anxiety and worry as possible. I'll be able to enjoy more that way.

Therapist 1: Thanks T. That was really beautiful. You've really become a meaning-centered therapist. L, you want to go?

L: Ok. I guess, uh, I guess, again, my hope is to try to stay in some kind of good shape for as long as I can and take advantage of the fact that I feel pretty ok most of the time. I also want to work on being less intimidating, and be easier to get along with. And there are people who I've offended, and so I want to make some amends.

Therapist 1: Amend friendships.

L: Yes. And to be more open to people's imperfections. No, that's not the right word.

Therapist 1: Forgiving?

L: To be more tolerant. And not always have to be jumping in and doing things on my own. And also, to accept offers and love from others without feeling like I'm being a burden. And I want to share my family experiences with my grandchildren.

Therapist 2: So your legacy is important to pass on.

Therapist 1: And all those things are particularly meaningful given all that you said the first week. Those things were all so hard for you.

L: Yeah. They were. I hadn't come here as the most open person.

Therapist 1: Are those tears of sadness, L? Joy? Mixture?

L: They're just . . . emotions.

Therapist 1: Emotions. Ok. Thank you, that was beautiful, L.

S?

S: Um. Well. I said that my hope is that I can keep active and feel well enough to function and be actively participating in life. It's like my first goal, and then my second one is to set goals, because I feel that I'm more on track when I have something to work towards. Um, and I want to peruse my interests and find some new ones as well. I think it's time for new ones. And, I really liked what you said about choosing to be hopeful, T. And I certainly hope to be a part of D's life. I really do. I had also written that at home, to live life to the fullest, and I have to say to hurry up and fit everything in. For example, there's a concert I want to see, why should I wait to see if someone has extra tickets, I'm going to go ahead and just buy them. And I have a whole list of things that are meaningful and that make me content, that I want to do. And then of course I had mentioned writing an article about my life and what it's been like to deal with all this illness and have it filled with hopefulness. And I want to include the heroes I've met along the way, who've been so helpful, other patients, the doctors, people who have been heroes to me and the small joys that carry me through. Small can be very meaningful. It gives you the light to go on. That is what I wrote down.

Therapist 2: Thank you so much, S.

Therapist 1: So it's hard to realize, but we've come to the end of our eight sessions. Today was a very beautiful session. It's hard to end things when they're so beautiful. Maybe better to end when you're happy?

S: Well, it's hard to end something that's been so helpful.

Therapist 1: Let me just say on my behalf, it's always this great privilege, as a physician, to become this intimate with people. It's not always . . . I guess . . . maybe it's something only doctors and cab drivers get that privilege to hear so much! . . . It's an honor and on some level this has felt like a sacred experience, because you've all shared so many meaningful experiences in here. You've shared sadness and hopes and dreams and for that I'm extremely grateful. I'm grateful to you for sharing with us and with each other. It's always sad for me to see these things end, but I'm sure we'll see each other again, even if it's just in the hallway.

Therapist 2: I just want to add to what Therapist 1 has just said. This has been . . . I have felt equally as honored to sit with you, and just as you've shared with us these really intimate experiences and stories of how cancer has impacted you . . . one of the things about these groups is that we mutually learn. You have all really impacted me by my sitting here. And I'm going to steal S's word about hero for a moment, if that's ok. Last week we were talking about courage, and both of you shared that both of you said you didn't feel courage. You know, I can't imagine how much courage it took to sit here and share what you said and for that you all are my heroes.

Therapist 1: We will not forget you.

L: Well you all created an environment that made it comfortable. So thank you.

Therapist 1: Thank you so much everyone.

APPENDIX 2

Transcripts of Two Full Courses of a Seven-Session Individual Meaning-Centered Psychotherapy Intervention with Two Exemplar Patients Conducted as Part of a Randomized Clinical Trial

NOTE TO READERS

The following transcripts were derived from audio recordings conducted of two entire seven-session individual meaning-centered psychotherapy (IMCP) interventions with two exemplar patents during a randomized controlled trial. Institutional review board permission was granted to publish these de-identified transcripts for educational and training purposes. The therapist conducting these interventions is Dr. William Breitbart (one of the authors of the IMCP chapter in this textbook that this appendix is intended to supplement; see Chapter 3). The patients are identified only as "Patient." Professions, places, and other potential identifiers were changed to help preserve patient anonymity. We have also kept the language intact, including erroneous use of language, in order to keep it genuine and authentic.

PATIENT 1 IMCP TRANSCRIPT

Session 1: Concepts and Sources of Meaning—Introductions and Meaning

Therapist: Okay, we're recording now. I hope you know that.

Patient: That's fine.

Therapist: Uh, let me start then. Welcome, I'm (name); I'm one of the psychiatrists here. You're participating in a research study.

Patient: uh-huh

Therapist: This research study compares two different kinds of counseling interventions for patients with cancer. You got randomized to the intervention that's called meaning-centered uh psychotherapy, meaning-centered intervention. And that's actually an intervention that we developed a few years ago, and we've been studying it in a in a couple different random controlled trials. We've done two of them already. One in group and one in individual format. And uh this is now a larger study of the individual format. So you're randomized to the counseling intervention that focuses on meaning. This is a handbook for you to use, to write down notes, to give you an idea of what's coming. To sort of re-read at your leisure, it's also basically a guide for you. Um, there are some practical issues. You have here some information, um on uh what to expect. We're going to have seven sessions

Patient: uh-huh

Therapist: of the intervention. And I'm going to go over the content of the seven sessions, what to expect. And just like today when you did an assessment you filled out those that battery of measures. We're going to ask you to do it one more time after the 4th session, and one more time after the last session. And then (name) or another member of the team will still be in contact with you so that a couple months later we can ask you to fill that out again. And this is a number to call, if you need to reach me, this is my information, my assistant's name is (name).

Patient: okay

Therapist: and this is uh sort of a schedule for you to hold on to if you need it, you may need it. I put down today, April the 12th as your first session at 8 o'clock. And we can plan out all the sessions or we can go week by week. We have a little leeway; we have to do 7 sessions within about 10–12 weeks. And maybe some time when you're traveling or can't make it or something comes up, or I often travel myself. And we could sort of re-visit the time as well. (Name) told me that mornings were best for you.

Patient: Mornings are best for me. Uh uh, the reason uh I came in today on a Tuesday is because I have treatment so it's just easier.

Therapist: We're going to be involved in doing this meaning-centered psychotherapy that, there's going to be 7 sessions, each uh, once every week, we'll skip a week or something, reschedule as things come up. Uh, and each session has a particular topic. The goal of the whole entire intervention is to introduce to you that the notion that meaning or being able to sustain meaning in your life despite having cancer, that that will help you maintain a sense of well-being, spiritual well-being, hope, good quality of life, it will buffer against things like depression and anxiety, and that's what our research shows, that if we can help patients sustain a sense of meaning when they're going through this cancer illness, that we can have these better outcomes in those areas. A sense of well-being, a sense of spiritual well-being, a sense of meaning, um, maintaining hope, um, better quality of life, actually a little bit less symptom distress, uh less anxiety and depression, so that's the goal. The way we try to do this in the intervention is to have a series of sessions like these that are divided into 2 parts. The first part is a little of an educational thing where we introduce you to an idea related to meaning.

Patient: Mm-hmm

Therapist: the second part of it involves an exercise, and experiential exercise where you write down a couple of answers to uh stimulus questions that are meant to have you think about the topic, the idea, and understand it in a in a better way, in a way that makes sense to you.

Patient: okay

Therapist: Cause a lot of these things are theoretical, and until you can describe them and you and I can talk about them as a real experience that you've had in your life, that helps you connect to what we're really talking about. And so the first session is an introduction, you and I getting to know each other a little bit.

Patient: uh-huh.

Therapist: me hearing a little bit about your cancer story, and me introducing the idea of meaning.

Patient: uh-huh.

Therapist: and um and actually a definition of meaning we try to figure out together, what does meaning mean. Uh, and then the rest of the sessions, the second session focuses of how cancer may have affected meaning in your life.

Patient: uh-huh.

Therapist: and the big bulk of the sessions, the heart of the sessions are really introducing you to the idea that there are some specific sources of meaning in life that are available to all of us. And when we go through difficult times, suffering experiences, we sometimes lose sight and get disconnected from these sources of meaning. So we want to remind you and reconnect you to these sources of meaning and for you to be able to use them as resources in your life and coping with cancer. And then finally at the end we want to sort of have a session where we recap everything and give you an opportunity to review what you've learned and think about what the next steps are. What lies beyond, you know, this intervention. Does that make sense?

Patient: yes

Therapist: Okay. Let's start out a little by getting to know each other. I told you my name, but again I'm Chief of the Psychiatry Service, I developed this a few years ago and again we've been studying it. A lot of this work, uh, on meaning, has come from; I adapted it from the work of a psychiatrist named Victor Frankl.

Patient: uh-huh.

Therapist: I don't know if you've ever heard of him or read his books. Um, so one of things that we're giving you as a gift . . .

Patient: Is it this book?

Therapist: Is this, *Man's Search for Meaning* the book that he wrote. As you go through this therapy, what you'll probably notice is there's a lot of what's in the therapy that's also in this book. But this book has two parts, the first part is an account of his survival in a concentration camp, and uh it's not meant to imply that having cancer is like being part of a concentration camp. . . .

Patient: Okay.

Therapist: but it's an inspirational thing for some people, but its offensive I think for some people to think this is like being in a concentration camp. We're not trying to send that message. But just the idea that uh any kind of limitation that's imposed either by a situation that Frankl went through, or limitations that are imposed by a cancer illness in terms of physical limitations or the limitations of what you had hoped to accomplish in your life or how long you thought you would live and things like that. Those limitations cause suffering. And if we're able to connect to sources of meaning, we can overcome that suffering, we can transcend it. We can take the suffering experience and find something about it that we can turn into uh a triumph. Take something that might be from the outside look like a tragedy and turn it into something that's really a triumph. So we're giving you this book for you to be able to look at it. One of the things I'll ask you at the end of today, is to when you get a chance you know look over any notes you've written for during this session, but also try to take a look at . . . read parts of the book, whatever parts you can get through, um you can start with the concentration camp part, most people do.

Patient: Mm-hmm.

Therapist: The second part of the book really talks about Frankl's ideas about the importance of meaning in human behavior. He basically says that a very basic motivating force of human behavior, human psychology, is the need to find meaning in life. Some people find meaning in their life through their religious life. Some people find it not through their religious life, but through the process of making meaning in their life. We're human beings, we're human creatures, so we by definition create, and we're here to create a life. We're born with a responsibility to create a life. When you think about the word responsibility you should also think about your ability to respond to being alive. It's a play on words.

Patient: Words, yeah

Therapist: But it's, how do I respond to being alive? And we usually respond by trying to create a life. And ideally we try to create a life of meaning and identity, and some kind of direction. We want to move. We kind of want to move, this way . . .

Patient: Forward

Therapist: Forward. We grow up, leave the house, have a career perhaps, get married, have children, we have an expectation of a life trajectory.

Patient: right

Therapist: And then there are things that are sort of are obstacles that get thrown in our way, which cause suffering. We're limited in that trajectory.

Patient: right

Therapist: um, so before I get more into the idea of meaning. Let me hear just a little bit, about your dealing with cancer, and what's been going on. I know you have breast cancer, but I don't know many details about it.

Patient: um, I was, um diagnosed with metastatic breast cancer in uh of December of 2008. And um, uh, I uh I was uh referred to Dr. (name) at Sloan by a friend I worked with at the college um (name) knew.

Therapist: what kind of work do you do?

Patient: oh, uh, what I used to do.

Therapist: yeah.

Patient: I'm an educational psychologist.

Therapist: uh-huh.

Patient: And um, so I was dean of freshman studies, programs at a local college.

Therapist: oh

Patient: And I was an adjunct at (name) University. Teaching in the graduate program in teacher Ed and Ed psych. So I had a very full life.

Therapist: I hear you

Patient: I was working 15–16 hours a day. Uh, I have two children. They're adults they're 32 and soon to be 27.

Therapist: are they married? Do they have kids?

Patient: One daughter is married, she has a little girl. The other daughter recently moved out with her boyfriend.

Therapist: Are you married?

Patient: I'm married.

Therapist: How long?

Patient: 35 years

Therapist: okay, do you think that'll work out?

Patient: yeah (laugh)

Therapist: okay.

Patient: I had this very full busy life, running programs, and teaching, and when I was diagnosed with metastatic breast cancer I immediately went to the computer to figure out what that was. Cause it didn't make sense to me that you could be diagnosed with stage IV breast cancer and not have gone through stages I, II, and III. It just didn't seem logical.

Therapist: so when you were diagnosed, uh, it went, you were diagnosed the cancer had already popped up in . . .

Patient: Oh, my lungs.
Therapist: lungs
Patient: My spine, and my brain.
Therapist: your brain as well?
Patient: and that
Therapist: and for an educational psychologist the brain is an important organ.
Patient: yes (laugh). And so um the brain was the one that kind of really threw me.
Therapist: That's the one that got you.
Patient: the rest of it, it's not like I didn't care, but I thought so I approached my illness as life changing. I uh, went to the president and told him I could no longer serve in the capacity that I used to serve. I did this before even treatment. I mean I just, I said I have to change. My life can't continue as it was, it just has to change. And where the focus was on my work, I changed the focus to my family. My daughter was getting married in May of that, May of 2008. I asked everyone at the college to pray for me that I would live long enough to see her married. And um, and I just I just stopped, I took a 4-month leave of absence b/c I felt that um, I didn't know what kind of strength I was going to have. And uh, I had my first stereotactic radiation procedure on (laugh) the anniversary of my father's death, January 18th, 2008.
Therapist: this was radiation specifically for the head?
Patient: right, I had . . .
Therapist: so isolated lesions.
Patient: two lesions uh
Therapist: was that really fatiguing, that treatment?
Patient: no, not at all. The video that they showed was frightening. Um I immediately wrote to the doctors and
Therapist: they should change the video
Patient: that they really needed not to show that video anymore (laugh). I'd be happy to talk to anyone who had to go through that procedure b/c the video was just horrifying.
Therapist: was it the mask?
Patient: Oh, well first of all the contraption that they put of this man's head. And it was not done at Sloan, it was done in Boston. So they don't even use the same apparatus.
Therapist: frightening.
Patient: better not to show it.
Therapist: you had an okay result from it?
Patient: I had an okay result from it. Um uh, my daughter married. Dr. (name), who is my physician, said to me, now that you've seen your daughter married are you going to ask me how long you have to live? And I said "no."
Therapist: no
Patient: my feeling was I wanted to be sure to be there for her wedding. And every day after is . . .
Therapist: and everything else is gravy.
Patient: is a gift. And that's the way I approach my life.
Therapist: gotcha
Patient: uh-huh.
Therapist: are you working now?
Patient: no, I am after 2008; I had 3 additional radiation procedures in um uh, . . .
Therapist: to the brain?
Patient: to the brain, and um uh November, I'm sorry in September, in December, and then again in um October. In October I decided it was time to retire for the college. Not retire, I mean I went on long-term disability. Um, uh, but I'm also on SS disability. So I and last February the uh the radiation oncologist said there were two new lesions and he wanted to do whole brain radiation, and I told him "absolutely not."
Therapist: gotcha. Are you on any medicines now?
Patient: I'm on um Tykerb and Xeloda.
Therapist: Xeloda
Patient: and Herceptin every three weeks, and . . .
Therapist: so you're on pretty active treatment still.
Patient: and Zymeta every 6 months.
Therapist: okay and how are you feeling?
Patient: overall, good. You know, I'm tired, when I'm tired I sleep. I don't walk as fast as I used to. Um, I uh, I would like to lose weight b/c I know that it's taxing on my body. And by the same token I feel that you know, um, I don't know. How much detriment can it do to me, really?
Therapist: right, let's go through this your workbook again.
Patient: okay
Therapist: so you can see this is an overview of the sessions.
Patient: Uh-huh
Therapist: and we're going to try to introduce you to the idea of meaning, as I mentioned to you a chunk of what this intervention, the inspiration really for the intervention was reading Frankl's book myself and learning about his ideas about the importance of meaning in human life. And he wasn't writing about cancer patients, he was writing about everyone. And I read that and said "You know there's

something here that can be helpful for cancer patients." And there are a couple things about Frankl's work that are important for you to know, and maybe you want to make a note of this as well. Maybe put it over here.

Patient: Okay.

Therapist: so the basic idea, the first one is that Frankl said that life has meaning, and that life has meaning from the first moment of life to the last moment of life. Uh, life never stops having a meaning.

Patient: I think this one (pen) is out too.

Therapist: that was doesn't work either?

Patient: nope

Therapist: Here's a pen that works. So, life never ceases to have meaning. If you ever feel that life has no meaning, its b/c you've become disconnected from it. It's like a set of keys that you've like misplaced and you can't find. Uh the keys haven't ceased to exist. They are just misplaced, where you can't find them, and so you have to search for them.

Patient: okay, that's a nice analogy.

Therapist: The second basic concept is that meaning is a basic motivating force for human behavior, that we as human beings have a need, a drive to find meaning in life as part of our nature. The third basic concept is that we have the freedom to find to make meaning out of our lives. We have the freedom, the free will, we have the freedom to find meaning in our existence; so no matter what the circumstances, situation we can find some meaning. We have the freedom to choose the attitude we take towards suffering, limitations, obstacle, and uncertainty. Now there are two kinds of suffering, right? Avoidable and unavoidable suffering. What kind of suffering is avoidable? If you have pain, there's no need to suffer with pain. You ah, you need to take pain medicines, or you need to do something about that. But some suffering is unavoidable. There are certain experiences in life, certain situations in life that are unavoidable like the fact that life is finite, and that we have limitations, and uh that there are obstacles that cause suffering in life. Even if suffering is unavoidable we can control how we respond to it, how we can choose how we think about it and the attitude we take towards it. The fourth basic concept is that Frankl felt that there were some specific sources of meaning in life, right? There are specific predictable sources of meaning in life, and uh they're listed in this table, right? I'll start here in the beginning. Most people derive meaning from life through dedicating themselves to something and dedicating their lives to someone, so usually through work or through love, right? Through work or through love. Um, and uh we'll talk a lot more about these sources of meaning throughout the entire 7 sessions. This is going to be the main focus for you to learn to be you know really facile with this notion of these sources of meaning. Uh, I'll always remind you during the course of our sessions, ah this is an experiential source of meaning. By experiential source of meaning, we're talking about deriving meaning from uh connecting to life and experiencing in life, with all of our senses and emotions. So, sight, hearing, touch, taste, love. So art, beauty, nature, food, and love, right? All sorts of love, family love, loving your children.

Patient: children

Therapist: and love of your fellow human beings. Uh love of your husband, romantic love, every other love. The second source of meaning is the creative sources of meaning. How we engage in life, and what we make out of our lives. And usually work is one of the main things that we make out of our lives, but there are others, besides work, there are still things we care about in the world, that we can engage in, right? A third source of meaning is the historical source of meaning. Now meaning exists in a historical context. Meaning in my life, meaning in your life has a particular flavor or character of nature because of the legacy we inherited from our family. You know, the values that we inherited, the experiences, our heritage.

Patient: uh ha

Therapist: and there's the legacy that we try to create by the life we live and the legacy we try to leave behind for our children, and their children. And finally when you confront suffering, right? You can always, you can derive meaning from suffering from the attitude that you take towards the suffering experience. And what allows you to overcome that, suffering experience, is to use these other resources to help you have it, to help you overcome and transcend these kind of suffering experiences. Uh but the important element of that also, no matter what you cannot control, you can always control how you think about what's going on and the attitude you take towards it. We call that the attitudinal source of meaning.

Those are the sources of meaning that Frankl talks about. So what I want you to do with the remaining time we have today is talk a little bit about this idea of meaning and what it really means (laugh). And do a little exercise to try to get that. Now, you can see here, you can come up with a couple definitions of meaning, that we use in our work, but before we go into that, do you have an idea of, do you have a definition of meaning that uh that you've kind of been using in your life that sort of strikes you or comes to you when you're thinking about this idea of meaning?

Patient: well, I think uh, meaning in life is uh, is a dynamic dimension of who we are.

Therapist: so it's related to identity.

Patient: it's related to identity, it's um uh it's ever changing.

Therapist: that's right,

Patient: um

Therapist: so from the beginning of life to the end of life, so when I'm a baby my life has meaning, and now as an adult, when I'm 90 years old my life will having meaning, but it changes overtime.

Patient: right, it's it's uh, and uh um, I think that as we go through different stages of our life, uh meaning takes on a different focus. So that um, at one point meaning for me meant being a successful professional, my family was always important, but um, but I don't think that I valued being with them as much as I value it now. Um, and so that's why I said it's dynamic, b/c you're always taking in and evaluating. . . .

Therapist: so if you would think about those sources of meaning we talked about, you might move from one source of meaning to another as being more important at one point in life than another. Right now the source of meaning through life and love of your family, that's more important than work.

Patient: right, um, but I also think there's this great meaning, I mean I think there are layers of meaning and I can't imagine that the meaning of my life would be as meaningful if I did not believe in God.

Therapist: so God is a source of meaning.

Patient: meaning for me. Yeah, you know faith.

Therapist: Faith. And when you think about meaning and God, do you see God as having created a particular meaning for you in your life that you need to try to find and obtain? Or do you believe that you have a big role in creating meaning in your life and that the relationship between what God might have in store for you and what you're creating, there needs to be some kind of relationship. Have you thought about it that much?

Patient: Well, I think of God as a benevolent father.

Therapist: Hmm.

Patient: in that uh um, he gives us the ability to become the people we are meant to be, um but I do believe in free will and I do believe in choice. I don't believe there's a divine plan. . . .

Therapist: right and that you just lay back.

Patient: . . . that I'm just kind of going through. You know, um . . .

Therapist: So you believe, you have free choice that you need to make meaning, you have a responsibility.

Patient: I have to make meaning, and that my decision to leave my active life at the college, and . . .

Therapist: and focus on

Patient: and focus on family and life now, and not worry. . . . I always, I was a planner. I planned 15–20 years out to my life figuring out where I wanted b/c I was goal-directed. Well, I'm still goal-directed, but not quite in that same venue. But you asked a question earlier about faith . . .

Therapist: Mm-hmm

Patient: and being challenged with cancer, and um, I would describe myself as a devout catholic, but one of the things that struck me was that um when I was first diagnosed and I asked people to pray for me. I had friends from uh, Jewish friends that said to me that they were praying for me, and I had Muslim friends saying that they were praying for me, and so its kind of interesting in that I um my concept of God has changed. You know my path to God is through Catholicism, but it just seems to be all roads lead to heaven, so that there are different roads that everyone takes. But the commonality is the prayer.

Therapist: right.

Patient: and the belief in God and whether we identify ourselves as Catholic, Muslim, or Jewish. That's to some extent I feel like it's a human identity. It's not really relationship with God.

Therapist: it's a connection between human beings?

Patient: Yeah, it just makes us who we are as unique people.

Therapist: Right, yes, and when I use the word transcendence? I'm often referring to the realization that we're connected.

Patient: right.

Therapist: to each other and to something greater than ourselves. Which is not necessarily God, but it can be God. But also it's all these other people in our lives and to a great deal all humans. Let me go over some of the definitions.

Patient: okay

Therapist: that we've been using, and I don't know you can give me a sense of which one makes a little more sense to you. Um, when we use the word meaning, we're talking about a sense that your life is meaningful, is full of meaning. As opposed to what does it mean to me to have cancer? It's not "What does that mean?" It's more like living a life that is meaningful, that's full of meaning.

Patient: right.

Therapist: and our goal in this therapy is to help sustain a sense that you're life is full of meaning. Okay?

Patient: okay

Therapist: So having a sense that one's life has meaning. This is the definition, one of the definition's we use, having a sense that one's life has meaning involves that conviction that you're fulfilling a unique role and purpose in a life uh.

Patient: That's a gift.

Therapist: that is a gift. Like that, what I told you before human creatures have a responsibility to create a life.

Patient: Mm-hmm

Therapist: create a life of meaning, and identity. That's very related. In creating this life, ideally you want to live that life uh you want to live that life by fulfilling your unique role that only you can fill in your life. You have to be the author of your life. Ideally. . . .

Patient: right

Therapist: it's not always possible in a very tight-knit Jewish or Italian family.

Patient: (laugh)

Therapist: and uh that this life is a gift that some people think about as a religious concept, but it's the idea that here you are, you've been given this gift of life, how do you respond to it? What is your responsibility?

Patient: Mm-hmm

Therapist: this life comes with a responsibility, right? To live to your full potential.

Patient: right

Therapist: uh, and if you're able to do that, you can achieve a sense of peace and contentment which is often experienced as meaning, my life is meaningful.

Patient: Mm-hm

Therapist: and a lot of people. Frankl would say the goal of life is not to be happy (laugh), but to feel that you are living a meaningful life . . .

Patient: Life

Therapist: . . . and have a sense of peace and contentment. When something good happens you're happy, when something sad happens you're sad. But the bedrock of your life is to feel that you're living a meaningful life.

Patient: mm-hmm

Therapist: and if you're able to do that you can even transcend or rise above your own individual concerns through connectedness, with other people. With things that are greater than yourself. It's this connectedness that allows us to transcend our own existence. So one definition is basically a thought or a belief that my life has meaning. Uh, and that's one definition we use. Another definition that's a little bit more of an emotional experiential definition is that meaningfulness or having a life full of meaning refers to moments that make life worth living. When you feel alive the most alive, and so it's the experiences that you might have when you felt most alive, those are the experiences that are innately the experiences where you feel dso fully human and alive and the universe comes together. You know? Uh, like a peak experience or a very powerful, meaningful experience in your life. Do you have any thoughts about these two definitions?

Patient: oh, I think I probably

Therapist: you like the combo of the two? You think the first one more?

Patient: this is more of my orientation, the one about thinking and a belief that our life has meaning.

Therapist: Us academics, we academics like this one more.

Patient: okay (laugh).

Therapist: So again as I mentioned to you, you know when we go through the sessions, the 7 sessions. A big chunk of it will be reviewing these sources of meaning, okay?

Patient: okay

Therapist: and how cancer has affected meaning, and then a kind of a wrap up. Now when we talk about historical sources of meaning, our legacy that we inherited, the legacy that we live, the legacy that we leave behind, one of the things I'm going to ask you to think about whether there's something you want to do in the form of writing something down or putting together a collection of photos or collecting recipes, something that you want to take from here in your mind or in your heart and make it concrete and real, externalize it as sort of we sometimes call it a legacy project.

Patient: legacy, right

Therapist: but, and some people actually do that, some people get really fancy, they make videos and things like that. Some people say at the end of my life that my life that I live, that my children see me live, that's my legacy, that's the legacy I'll leave behind, that's my legacy project, what I've done with my life. And that's perfectly okay too. So these are in the sources of meaning. So uh, one of the last things we'll do today

Patient: okay

Therapist: Is I'm going to ask you to write down a few thoughts and experiences of moments in life when you felt most alive, some of the most meaningful moments in your life. You can list one, two, three, you may have more, seems like you've led a very rich life. Write down a few experiences, moments when you felt your life was particularly meaningful, when you felt the most alive. Take a few moments to write that down and then we'll discuss that a little bit, and then we'll be able to wrap up.

Patient: Okay

Therapist: Okay? Take your time.

(*Long pause so patient can do assignment*)

Patient: okay

Therapist: okay? Why don't you share that with me?

Patient: okay, well the first is my daughter's wedding.

Therapist: ah ha

Patient: um, I couldn't believe how great I felt, how wonderful everyone looked, it was a perfect day, I mean it rained, but it seemed to stop raining when it needed to. And it was just a, everyone from the family was there. It was just um, it was a celebration of life.

Therapist: right.

Patient: so you know that really um

Therapist: and we find that milestones in life are often very meaningful moments.

Patient: Mm-hmm

Therapist: b/c they often represent um progress along this trajectory this life that you hoping to create and fulfilling your life to its full potential and I suppose for you being a mother and being a grandmother.

Patient: Mm-hmm

Therapist: is one of the things that you saw as fulfilling your full potential.

Patient: right, yeah, I mean it was you know um.

Therapist: so, that gives meaning to your life also. And in terms of sources of meaning right, it relates to, it relates to who you are, you're identity. I'm all these things, but I'm also a parent, a mother, and now a grandmother. Um, and it falls into these creative sources of meaning through uh, through experiencing the roles and the joys of life.

Patient: Uh-huh

Therapist: through the joys of love, and family. And is also related to this historical legacy, sources of meaning, right?

Patient: Mm-hmm

Therapist: uh, you know, it's a continuation of the chain of events and traditions uh that started long ago, and your grandparents and parents. Your parents were there for your wedding.

Patient: me

Therapist: and you're there now for your daughter's wedding. So there's a continuity, a legacy. And uh there's now the potential, I guess, does this daughter have a child?

Patient: Yes, she's the one who has the daughter.

Therapist: that's the next one probably

Patient: right, no actually that was the next one. Cause I was trying, I mean I was trying to put different aspects of my life

Therapist: sure, so you can see how a lot of these meaningful events uh, and moments of meaning uh, sometimes is one source of meaning and a lot of times is multiple sources of meaning that flow together to create a meaningful moment.

Patient: um, walking in the park with my friend (name). (Name) was my first instructor, he was my mentor, he sat on my dissertation committee, and for years every Tuesday and Thursday we would walk through Central Park, and just talk, and you know um, it's really the appreciation of the most simplest things in life. Walking through the park, seeing the seasons, and changes in the seasons, enjoying friendship and company.

Therapist: right, exactly. So again, this is also primarily experiential source of meaning. You're experiencing nature and the seasons. And your connection to this mentor. It's not always just through love, but here you have friendship, a different kind of love.

Patient: right

Therapist: and mentorship. In Jewish tradition you respect your teachers as much as you respect your parents.

Patient: Mm-hmm

Therapist: that's what you're taught?

Patient: right

Therapist: But here you are in nature, you're appreciating the beauty of life. Right?

Patient: and really for him, particularly with him, it's really kind of interesting in terms of how our relationship evolved.

Therapist: right b/c it's connected to work too.

Patient: oh yeah.

Therapist: right, and so its I guess a creative source of meaning. This relationship and this experience, really fostered your you're your growth and development through your mentorship and friendship in your work, I'm sure that it enhanced your . . .

Patient: oh yes, absolutely.

Therapist: it gave more meaning to your work too. Cause it's not unusual for us to not only get profound meaning from our work, but to also develop some important lifelong friendships, connections.

Patient: and the third thing that I wrote, um, was uh, a few years back we took a cruise to Europe.

Therapist: ah-ha.

Patient: and um, we went to France, and uh, ah Italy and uh Malta, and Tunisia, and uh, I called it the Roman Tour cause that's the way I felt. I was going to Carthage and I just felt like I was taking a historical tour. But, um, just knowing that a church that we saw was built in you know 900 AD.

Therapist: right

Patient: And LOOKING at what someone created and that you had the ability to see it. Who walked on these streets before us?

Therapist: right

Patient: and then when we went to the Sistine Chapel, I mean

Therapist: right

Patient: I remember just sitting and just looking and saying "I can't believe I'm here."

Therapist: right, so there was this element of a source of meaning through beauty. But this one strikes me more as legacy, right?

Patient: right

Therapist: the historical context of your life. People from here, this is my heritage and these are the people, some of the people came before me and created things. And this is, and its still here and they're remembered in some way. And I'm part of that whole continuity of not only Italian culture perhaps uh and civilization, but human civilization.

Patient: right

Therapist: and uh this is part of what I inherited and I am part of that whole continuity that will go on past me too. And somehow I will live on in what I create and what I leave, perhaps, not in this form of buildings

Patient: right

Therapist: but in the form of work and how I have impacted on people uh, you've probably had a lot of students . . .

Patient: oh, yeah, you know I didn't want to write

Therapist: and your family

Patient: my work, I worked with freshman.

Therapist: right

Patient: so I saw, and I ran the Honors program. So I saw them come in as I came in, develop as undergraduates, move on to graduate school, move on to profession. Yes, and I've always said to them, I used to say to them that we never truly appreciate our current relationships until we remember them fondly.

Therapist: right.

Patient: so yes, I got great joy out of my work with my students.

Therapist: one of the things you didn't put down, which uh some people put down are uh events that are perhaps, tragic in some way or sad, like the death of somebody or uh loss. And perhaps this will come up at some other point, but not only not only beautiful events, but that experiences that can lead to profound sense of meaning, but even difficult events can make one feel uh, a better appreciation for life and the meaning of life. But that might come up later.

Patient: okay.

Therapist: alright. Well, thank you for doing this.

Patient: thank you

Therapist: I'll just remind you for next week.

Patient: okay

Therapist: We're going to talk about how; we're going to focus on your identity.

Patient: Mm-hmm

Therapist: we're going to use identity as a surrogate for meaning, because you derive your identity from all those things that give your life a sense of meaning. We're going to talk a little bit about how cancer has affected meaning in your life. And we'll do 2 exercises, we'll talk about how you would've answering the question "Who am I?" before your cancer, and then we're going to talk about how you would answer that question now with cancer.

Patient: so do you want me to?

Therapist: you don't have to do anything. You can think about it.

Patient: think about it?
Therapist: I mean if you want to you could prepare and write down some answers in your homework page.
Patient: okay
Therapist: but your main homework for next week is to try to if you get a chance to start to read *Man's Search for Meaning*.
Patient: to read this?
Therapist: um, don't feel bad about homework. It's not like in school.
Patient: no, it's okay (laugh).
Therapist: (laugh) you know it's no pressure. If you don't read it, you can read it next week. But if this seems more interesting for you to try, great! But you'll find this very helpful over the course of the entire thing. If you get to read some of it, it reinforces some of the concepts we've discussed today . . .
Patient: are you going to be collecting these at the end.
Therapist: no
Patient: okay.
Therapist: these are for you to hold on to.
Patient: okay, great.
Therapist: and we'll see each other next week.
Patient: oh, not next week.
Therapist: oh right the 25th? Which is a Monday?
Patient: Monday
Therapist: here at 8. I hope to, I promise not to be too late.

Session 2: Cancer and Meaning—Identity Before and After Cancer Diagnosis

Therapist: Good morning.
Patient: Good morning.
Therapist: Alright, well, so I'm glad we had a chance to just go over the dates, and I'll double check on the May 2nd date.
Patient: okay.
Therapist: so this is Session 2. And I just wanted to check in with you about how things were going since the last time I saw you.
Patient: um, well I uh I've been reading his book uh.
Therapist: I meant more with your medical stuff.
Patient: oh (laugh).
Therapist: I know you're getting chemo next week, is it?
Patient: yeah, yeah, I'm doing well, you know, um tired, but um I really don't have any complaints.
Therapist: so things are going okay?
Patient: things are going fine.
Therapist: and you mentioned your husband.
Patient: yeah, my husband has a host of medical issues.
Therapist: I see.
Patient: um, from um, kidney stones to um.
Therapist: and he's the driver?
Patient: no, I'm the driver.
Therapist: you're the driver.
Patient: (laugh) Uh, so I have to be you know uh mindful of his appointments and
Therapist: so you have to juggle his appointments and your appointments?
Patient: yeah
Therapist: so you're both back-and-forth from the doctors.
Patient: right. In fact today I woke up, and the humidity was very bad today.
Therapist: yeah
Patient: so I actually woke him up and said you have to come with me to the city
Therapist: because?
Patient: because I would've taken the bus, but I didn't want to feel take the bus so I drove in and I said to him just find a place to sit, and . . .
Therapist: and what was your concern with the humidity?
Patient: I had a really bad headache. . . .
Therapist: you get headaches?
Patient: and then bus, it was just too much and I wanted to drive in, so today he's waiting for me, as opposed to me waiting for him (laugh).
Therapist: okay, so he's waiting for you downstairs?
Patient: yeah, but its fine.
Therapist: we'll finish up sometime today.
Patient: he knew you know.
Therapist: and where do you come in from?
Patient: we come in from Queens.
Therapist: and how long a ride in?
Patient: um, about 45 minutes.
Therapist: that's a long ride.
Patient: yeah
Therapist: So I interrupted you had some thoughts about . . .
Patient: oh yeah Frankl.
Therapist: Frankl yeah. And maybe you started to read the book.
Patient: yeah, I'm about a 3rd a way through, it's uh, and it's uh interesting b/c when um, when I was in school. You know when I was studying, and even when I was working, my focus was always to read things quickly so that you know I could understand it. And now that I have a lot of time, its more of a reflective reading, than it is you know. . . .
Therapist: I hear you.

Patient: So uh uh I'm fascinated by um his choice uh that you know uh to honor his mother and father he decided that he you know wouldn't take the opportunity to migrate to the US to safety, and um and um, and how he put family first. It was kind of an interesting and then the hardship of his life in the concentration, I can't even imagine.

Therapist: so you were struck by his choice?

Patient: I was struck by his choice, yeah.

Therapist: yeah

Patient: you know that um sometimes uh what seems to be an intellectually sound judgment is averted for other things, for family. So that was, that was very telling for me, cause when I was diagnosed with um stage IV, I had a very active professional life, and it was, family at that point was you know, uh kind of a demarcation of my life, I went to work and I said I can't do this anymore. I have to take care of my health. I have to put my family first. And so I guess I I identified with his choice, when given, and it certainly wasn't the same thing, when given that life changing event how you kind of re-evaluate, realign things. And there's a spirituality about him that I find uh kind of, I understand you know you know when he talked about his wife was probably dead and it was her 24th birthday and um, but that he felt that she was close to him you know, I understand that.

Therapist: mm-hmm, yeah, so you've only begun to read the book and you've been struck by a few things already.

Patient: Mm-hmm

Therapist: and um, this choice issue, uh you were struck by it, and you identify . . . can relate to it personally.

Patient: right

Therapist: and you can even relate it to part of what happened when you got your cancer diagnosis.

Patient: right

Therapist: everyone always talks about you mentioned a point, a life changing event some people refer to that as a crisis, right?

Patient: yeah

Therapist: and everyone always talks about how in Chinese, the Chinese symbol for crisis is danger and opportunity.

Patient: right.

Therapist: What people don't talk about it that the word crisis from the Latin refers to choice.

Patient: choice, right

Therapist: and so uh really uh, our life is full of choices, everything in life is a choice, we're constantly making choices, and that's actually the choices we make in our life is how we create our lives. Some choices are bigger than others.

Patient: right

Therapist: some are more major than others. So um the idea of family was very important to you and that's what you picked up in Frankl's choice.

Patient: yeah

Therapist: um, that he made a decision based on uh he had the opportunity to leave Austria, right?

Patient: right

Therapist: Vienna?

Patient: yeah

Therapist: but only on the condition that he would leave, he couldn't take his whole family. . . .

Patient: family, right

Therapist: he couldn't take his parents. And so he made the decision not to go uh b/c of that experience, he had finally the piece of

Patient: the rock

Therapist: you know part of the 10 commandments that turned out to be . . .

Patient: honor thy . . .

Therapist: the um

Patient: the third one

Therapist: the commandment to honor thy father

Patient: father

Therapist: and mother uh, which resonates with me a lot too b/c if you think about um the sources of meaning that we talked about very briefly last week, I don't know if you recall, we covered a couple things last week.

Patient: Mm-hmm

Therapist: it was a very, it was a lot to do in the first session right?

Patient: (laugh)

Therapist: but we talked about various sources of meaning too.

Patient: Mm-hmm

Therapist: and maybe we can review that again if you'd like, but one of the sources of meaning is um the historical context of meaning and the legacy that you inherit from your ancestors parents, grandparents, and the legacy that you create with your life and the one you leave behind uh so obviously connecting with uh, connecting with his parents, and that he didn't feel that he could be whole if he was not making that choice of leaving uh Austria without his parents, uh for him it wasn't a choice he could make and still be who he was.

Patient: right

Therapist: and still live a life reflecting what was important to him and what was meaningful to him right? So when you got diagnosed you were you were involved in a very active and fulfilling work life?

Patient: oh yeah.

Therapist: Which is another source of meaning. You know creative sources of meaning through dedicating yourself to work and things like, causes like that. Um, but then you, when you got your diagnosis of stage IV breast cancer right in the middle of I guess a busy and meaningful work life you stopped that was crisis point for you.

Patient: yeah, right

Therapist: and you made a decision, you made a choice, what was exactly the choice? You said it was something about your family.

Patient: oh, I um, well I was directing many programs, had a very long work schedule that really pulled me away from the family. And my feeling was that, I used to joke I used to joke at work a lot that on my death bed am I really going to think this was important? You know, you know, little daily crisis that come up the people attribute you know as being, this needs your immediate attention and so I would joke to everyone, well the five things I'm going to remember on my death bed is not going to be one of these so it can't be really that important in the focus of my life.

Therapist: So if I can can clarify what you're saying, you're saying that at work when you would run into problems the way you would try to deal with the I guess the stress of the, the difficulty of a problem is you say "Okay, when I'm at my death bed is this something that I'm going"

Patient: I'm gonna think about

Therapist: think about, so there's no need to get so worked up about it?

Patient: Right (laugh).

Therapist: Gotcha, I gotcha.

Patient: (laugh) so um, so when I was when I thought I was facing you know um, a kind of

Therapist: death?

Patient: an immediate death like . . .

Therapist: is that what you thought?

Patient: oh that's what I thought I mean that's what I cause . . .

Therapist: you heard the news and you thought I'm going to. . . .

Patient: Well I said that maybe I have six months, maybe I have a year, um you know maybe if I beat the odds I'll have three years. You know maybe if I really push it, I'll have 5. You know but I was thinking of my life span at most being 10 years. And even initially I didn't think that. So I, when I heard the diagnosis was um uh Christmas, Christmas Day.

Therapist: hmm

Patient: I was seeing doctor uh um (name) on the following day at Sloan, and so I thought to myself, everyone had gone to bed and it was very quiet. I thought to myself, well okay on my death bed (laugh) now that I'm really thinking about my deathbed "How important is my work?" I mean in my scheme of my life, you know, I've now given the college at that point some 30 years, so I think its time to close this chapter of my life. It was that, without having spoken to a doctor about treatment, I just face the diagnosis itself was enough, and so I uh, I called my boss and uh said to her um "You have to find me a replacement." I'm I'm not coming back to do what I used to do to run the programs. I'm not going to put up with the stress. I uh at that point I was 54, uh 53 actually and I said I can retire at 55, I have 2 years. I've gotta find something for me to do for the next 2 years, that does not require me to be there every day and does not require me to uh be stressed. I have to put my family first, and that's if I have 2 years. So it was uh, it was a definitive moment, and I didn't talk to anybody about this. I didn't talk to my husband about it. You know, alone, alone on Christmas Day and thinking ok what am I going to do with the rest of my life? Not knowing what that meant. And so the college was very supportive, and uh I uh I the next 2 years I basically did a lot of program evaluation, but I didn't have the daily contact with the students. Didn't have the responsibility of budgets, and you know uh. . . .

Therapist: Mm-hmm

Patient: So it was you know for me, it was um it was kind of you know a refocusing of my life. And my life became my family. Um, where . . .

Therapist: so it's interesting, part of what we're trying do in this treatment is uh teach you something about the importance of meaning in life and we're trying to teach you a way in which you can sustain and enhance a sense of meaning even in the face of cancer. And part of uh what we hope will be a resource for you in for you to identify and uh think about the various sources of meaning in life. And so you'll see the structure of the 7 sessions, the heart of it are exercises and discussions of the sources of meaning but even just in this discussion you're already talking about many of sources of meaning, and part of what my job is to um guide you through the 7 sessions but also to identify for you to highlight for you when you're talking about stuff that really relate to specific sources of meaning. So just in this discussion you've talked about almost every source of meaning so um we've talked a little about the importance of your work, on the creative source, and then we talked a little bit about your family, and your, we talked about legacy right? And how important um how that story about honor your father and mother you related to. Family is really love, right? And um what we call experiential sources of meaning. Um meaning you get from the people you love the most, and the closest to you. But um, you also describe something really important which is one of the most difficult sources of meaning to understand the source of meaning that comes from the attitude you take towards suffering, and um, simply put, suffering, is any experience you have in which you confront some type of limitation. Something that prevents you from moving forward in the trajectory of your life, that's a suffering experience, death is the ultimate limitation. And so there you were, a day before seeing Dr. (name), and you got this diagnosis and you thought to yourself, you were staring death in the face, you were aware of this ultimate limitation, and so what you did is you made a choice another way of choice is deciding on what attitude to take. So the attitude that you take towards suffering, the choice you make about how to handle a suffering experience is another source of meaning. And so you took a particular attitude and you yourself made a choice in the face of the ultimate limitation of death right?

Patient: right

Therapist: I'm going to change my priorities. I'm going to focus on what's really most meaningful to me, what I anticipate will be most meaningful to me, in the next phase of my life. For you it was to cut back on the work, your work involvement. You're still being involved I guess, right?

Patient: yeah

Therapist: But cutting back, and sort of paring it down to the essence of what it was in your work that maybe was enjoyable for you and focusing on your family. And you may or may not have gotten to the part of uh the book Frankl talks about where where the concentration camp is taken from them and they have no control over anything.

Patient: yeah

Therapist: and the only thing they have control over is their . . .

Patient: self

Therapist: is their mind and how they think, and the attitude that they take.

Patient: yeah

Therapist: uh and so you're story's beautiful uh cause it really exemplifies all of the sources of meaning and uh by the time you're finished with these 7 sessions of meaning-centered psychotherapy uh you're going to be able to say this is this source of meaning, and this is this source of meaning. And one of the things that I think it helpful about that is that you can always go to that well to remind yourself. Because part of what happens when you go through experiences of illness, of cancer illness, you suffer and you get perhaps a little demoralized, depressed at times. Uh you may, you may lose your way a little bit, have a sense of "Oh gosh, I don't have that will, that sense of meaning." And uh as we talked about last week, um one of the big core principles of the of the therapy and of the notion of the importance of meaning, is that meaning never ceases to exist, that meaning in your life never ceases to exist, nor the search for meaning in your life never stops. And um, you may feel like you don't have it, but it's not because it's not there, it's because it's been misplaced, when you become disconnected to it, from it. So um, knowing what the sources are helps you, kind of gives you a map of where to go. The other thing is that it's important to also note that you can also be flexible about where you, what well you go to to derive meaning. Sometimes it hard to get it from one source, you can move to another source, you know, you may be blocked in one way, then you can move to another way. Let's say for some reason, are you still working?

Patient: no

Therapist: no, so that's a good example that's a source of meaning that's not there for you right now. And so you know you can move to other sources of meaning that can fill you up, you know, love, family, experiential source of meaning. The way you think about things, the attitude you take, your legacy, historical context of meaning in your life. Those become more more uh important, when one source of meaning kind of gets blocked. Um if you think about last week, uh do you let's see do you this was last weeks?

Patient: This was last week's

Therapist: So last week we talked a little bit about the sources of meaning, so I was just talking a little bit about them, do those sound familiar to you?

Patient: oh yeah, you know I definitely um

Therapist: what did you think about the first session?

Patient: Well, um I you, when I did the exercise I put down all positive things. Since you know um

Therapist: Uh-huh

Patient: suffering also can be uh can provide you a source of meaning. And um . . .

Therapist: yeah

Patient: And um it's something I don't usually acknowledge.

Therapist: yes

Patient: I mean it's there, I know it's there. It's not something I readily think about.

Therapist: Mm-hmm

Patient: um in terms of um, providing the impetus change and most of the changes I've made in my life have came out of a suffering mode.

Therapist: that's very typical by the way. The things that give meaning to life, when we talk about them usually are very important events in people's lives. For instance, important transitions, some of them are very happy some of them are very tragic.

Patient: yeah so you know.

Therapist: so was there something negative you left out last time?

Patient: well um uh. There were, I'll tell you what the most recent was, that was. So um my husband was diagnosed with thyroid cancer, and he had thought that I was very brave when I was diagnosed. I don't know why people attribute bravery to cancer, it's just, maybe it's my life orientation, but I don't think there's anything brave about what I'm doing. I'm just living. I'm no more brave than anyone else, as far as I'm concerned.

Therapist: you don't believe that you have courage?

Patient: I don't believe that I have extraordinary courage. I think we all . . .

Therapist: okay

Patient: you know it's it's

Therapist: how about non-extraordinary courage?

Patient: Um, yeah I just think it's my life I'm propelled to go forward. So it's maybe it's my psychological orientation to life, but you know it's, you know . . .

Therapist: it's your attitude.

Patient: it's my attitude, right. So if the road is blocked one way, I'll just go another direction.

Therapist: there you go.

Patient: I'll get there somehow. Nonetheless, so when (husband's name) was diagnosed with thyroid cancer uh, I was completely devastated, um, never having been devas–, never having been, I don't think I was completely devastated quite the same way when I was diagnosed for myself. And so . . .

Therapist: So are you saying you were more devastated when you're husband . . .

Patient: with his . . .

Therapist: when he was diagnosed.

Patient: and so um, what I said to him was, it is easier to be the patient than to be the caregiver.

Therapist: interesting.

Patient: Because as the patient I was preparing myself for my own death. Not really thinking about anybody else. It was you know it was kind of me, myself and I going forward. But as the caregiver, thinking about losing him made me appreciate how he felt about me.

Therapist: How much he loved you.

Patient: and how much he loved me.

Therapist: how much he cared for you.

Patient: how much he cared for me.

Therapist: how important he was in your life.

Patient: how important he was to me.

Therapist: and how much you loved him.

Patient: and how much I loved him, right. And so um, that really you know. . . . I told him that. It wasn't anything that I kept. I said to him, I had a uh I had a new appreciation for the depth of his love for me. Um in the face that I might lose him. So it was kind of a . . .

Therapist: so the love that you and your husband shared was it was so much more, you appreciated it much more; you valued it so much more. It was so much more profound.

Patient: right.

Therapist: was it a little bit like when you love somebody, and something happens then that causes them to suffer. If you're a strong person even if you're not maybe. If you're a strong person like yourself uh, you want to take on the suffering for them because you know you can handle it. You know, spare them, let me take the burden. Is that how you felt?

Patient: yeah, well, um

Therapist: I got the cancer he doesn't need to get the cancer?

Patient: well, it was like we don't have to share everything (laugh) you know? I could've done this alone.

Therapist: right

Patient: but um, so that was one thing that really

Therapist: yeah

Patient: you know, struck me about last week, was that um. When I think about those things that propelled me to to make changes um for the most part it was, suffering or an event that I may not have had any control over, but that I made a change in who I was based on what was happened you know, something as simple as my cousin getting into a car accident. And losing who she was as a result of that car accident, so it made me think that you know, I can't control what the future is, but I can certainly impact on today. So it's more of an appreciation of the moment as opposed to the future. For someone who always planned everything, this was kind of a life changing event for me.

Therapist: it was, you know everyone always says live for the moment, uh it's sometimes hard, it sounds corny sometimes, and uh you never know what they actually mean, but it sounds like you . . .

Patient: oh yeah

Therapist: had a real, for the first time maybe

Patient: oh yeah.

Therapist: you had an understanding.

Patient: oh yeah, she's my age, she was 40 and very vibrant and going home and got into this horrific car accident that left her disabled and her life changed in a second. And so while it didn't happen to me . . .

Therapist: right

Patient: uh and so while it didn't happen to me, you know

Therapist: right

Patient: I was a witness to it. It made me think about you know um the clichés of ceasing the moment, really aren't clichés if you really understand what's behind . . .

Therapist: right. The other cliché which is also true is that we're all very connected in profound ways and you this affected you b/c you are connected to this person.

Patient: right, so those were the two things um that I think . . .

Therapist: So going forward, don't hesitate to bring up the negative stuff as well as the positive.

Patient: yeah

Therapist: that's always on everyone we're dual creatures you know.

Patient: Hmm mm

Therapist: there are always two things going on, there are always two things going on. We're never of one single mind.

Patient: um (laugh)

Therapist: there's always a duet with . . .

Patient: a duality

Therapist: A duality

Patient: and the other thing that struck me was this historical source.

Therapist: yes?

Patient: um b/c I've been preoccupied with tracing back my ancestries so that I can create a book for grand-daughter so that she knows from once she came.

Therapist: yeah

Patient: so it's been my new mission.

Therapist: you're new mission is to make sure you're grand . . ., do you have more than one?

Patient: one, one daughter . . .

Therapist: that your grand-daughter knows where she came from.

Patient: yeah, yeah

Therapist: So what was the book about?

Patient: Oh so, I've done some research on my uh on both my mother's and father's side. Ironically I reconnected with my my father's family after 30 years and know more about his side of the family than I ever knew. Had I not been concerned about you know acknowledging the past to give to my grand-daughter for the future, I probably would've never reconnected. I'm wondering what phase in my life I'm you know, I'm thinking about Erikson's phases of life.

Therapist: Mm-hmm

Patient: and I'm trying to figure out, I guess I am I really in; I'm solely in that 6th stage right now, you know?

Therapist: that's generativity.

Patient: right (laugh). You know, I'm just kind of

Therapist: that's a good place to be.

Patient: yeah, I guess it's a good place to be and that I'm very fortunate um again going back to um uh you know uh to family. I'm very fortunate to be in a place where I am.

Therapist: Mm-hmm

Patient: not to think that cancer was a blessing, cause I don't think of the cancer as a blessing, but it was just kind of the opportunity for me to go to this new phase, and I think that's why I kind of um enjoy Frankl's work because um . . .

Therapist: what did you think about the uh definition of meaning that we came up with, that we talked about last time? Did you have any thoughts about that? Or did any of it resonate with you? Or did you think you wanted to change it, you know? You want to modify it for yourself for us?

Patient: um, no, I think I'll need to think about it some more.

Therapist: okay.

Patient: um, I . . .

Therapist: well, we did talk a little bit about the sources of meaning right, we kind of reviewed that.

Patient: right.

Therapist: and uh I did touch a little bit upon one of the basic concepts of the sources of meaning, which was that, you know life life has meaning, never ceases to have meaning from the first moment to the last moment. If you feel you've lost meaning its not because its not there, it's sort of become disconnected from us. And uh and the other concept is that we have this drive, this basic drive to find meaning in our existence, right?

Patient: yeah, I um I think you know I kind of want . . .

Therapist: you've started making notes for the next one?

Patient: oh yeah yeah yeah

Therapist: okay, we'll do that in a sec.

Patient: I kind of. I would say the challenge I face now is that uh, I've kind of immersed myself in family. And my uh my difficulty is that I keep saying to myself, there's gotta be more to to what I'm doing, than what I'm presently doing. There's gotta be more to my life than what I'm presently doing.

Therapist: right now?

Patient: right now. So you know maybe it's kind of what you said before about you know when one source of of meaning . . .

Therapist: one source of meaning becomes kind of blocked

Patient: . . . gets, right. Then you kind of try to remember . . .

Therapist: all the others.

Patient: What else did I enjoy doing?

Therapist: yeah

Patient: uh so I I, I don't miss working but I I do miss the intellectual stimulation from working.

Therapist: Mm-hmm. I'm hoping that our meetings with be intellectually stimulating.

Patient: (laugh)

Therapist: so that it will feel like work. It'll be just like work.

Patient: well, there's gotta, what am I going do in the . . . maybe this is common for people who have cancer, but living for the moment is wonderful.

Therapist: Mm-hmm

Patient: but you also have to think about the future.

Therapist: that's right

Patient: (laugh). And so I, in some ways I have I still have this 10 year clock that I see in front of me.

Therapist: Mm-hmm

Patient: and I'm trying to I'm trying to bust the clock.

Therapist: sure, and you're also trying to live fully with whatever time you have left.

Patient: right, so that's what I'm hoping this will do.

Therapist: It involves a little bit of planning.

Patient: yeah, right

Therapist: Today's exercise focuses on how cancer has affected meaning in life. And this idea of meaning and um the definition of meaning that um we came up with, the two definitions, I think. Your manual is better than my manual.

Patient: this is having a sense of one's life has meaning, involves conviction.

Therapist: yes, right. So the first definition that we kind of proposed was that having a sense that your life has meaning involves um, involves believing that your living a life that in which you are fulfilling a unique role or purpose, right? A life that comes with responsibilities to reach your full potential, and through that trying to achieve a sense of peace or connectedness to um people or other things that are greater than yourself. And so one of the things that is related to meaning uh is this sense of identity. If you're trying to, if meaning is derived from living a life in which you fulfill your unique potential, a lot of what meaning is about is creating yourself. I might have said that your responsibility as a human creature is to create a life of meaning and identity. So your identity is very much connected to the things in your life that give you meaning. Uh, and so one of the reasons that we developed this intervention is because clinically we noticed that when people are develop cancer, and they go through some of the challenges of cancer illness and treatment, they kind of lose a sense of meaning and even lose a sense of their identity, the things that you know made them who they are. Um, people stop working you know, if I were to stop working I would have a big problem in terms of my identity.

Patient: (laugh)

Therapist: fortunately, there are other things in my life that contribute to my identity. So cancer has an impact on a person's sense of identity which is so much related to meaning. So today's session we're going to focus on in our experiential exercise as well on how cancer has really affected meaning in your life. And I think this is the exercise for today. Are these notes from this thing . . . ?

Patient: Mm-hmm

Therapist: oh, you made notes already!

Patient: (laugh)

Therapist: you're good.

Patient: (laugh)

Therapist: you're good. So they're really two parts to the exercise today. And I don't know if I made it clear last time, I might have told you . . . but the first one talks about um answers that you would've, ways you in which you would've answered the question "Who am I?" I guess before cancer. And then the second part of the exercise is how has cancer affected the answers to those questions, "Who am I?" So did you already do the exercise?

Patient: no

Therapist: do you want to take a few moments to kind of. . . . so I think the biggest problem when I've done these exercises, this exercise with groups of people is uh people start answering the first question already with the impact that cancer's had in their life. So often can't see the contrast, but uh if I'm trying not to do that as much, b/c I'm often not as clear.

Patient: um, uh.

Therapist: So if you want. . . .

Patient: when I, okay, um do you want me to write them down?

Therapist: whatever you want to do. You can take a few moments to write down a few notes that remind you of what you want to say.

Patient: so who who who am I prior to cancer?

Therapist: yeah, how would you have answered that question "Who am I?"

Patient: uh

Therapist: and we gave you some examples

Patient: right

Therapist: like um, I'm somebody who. . . . It can be roles that you've played. Or it could be qualities that you've had.

Patient: (laugh)

Therapist: I think most people reflect the roles that they've had. But uh.

Patient: well, why don't I tell you how how I would answer it? I mean I can write it down but um

Therapist: this is before the cancer?

Patient: before the cancer. Uh, uh I am a workaholic, uh, I am uh I am I'm enjoying . . .

Therapist: maybe you should write that down. Cause maybe you can reflect on it. So you're a workaholic?

Patient: I'm a workaholic.

Therapist: yeah

Patient: um uh, uh uh I have a full uh life in terms of my professional development. Um uh, and yet I am, and yet I was unsatisfied with what I was doing, for I did it so long I needed a change. Uh, I enjoyed teaching and yet have no time to teach because of my work. And so I had to give that up.

Therapist: is also part of your job.

Patient: it's right. So I I used to teach uh at Fordham, I loved it, but it was just, I couldn't I couldn't handle the demands of work in a changing psychological environment that wasn't to my taste.

Therapist: would you have said before cancer, that you were a teacher?

Patient: no. I never thought of myself as a teacher. I always thought of myself as a counselor.

Therapist: as a counselor?

Patient: right I'm a counselor.

Therapist: you are a counselor. Why don't you write that down?

Patient: okay. Um, and I and I

Therapist: but you would've loved to be a teacher?

Patient: I would've loved to be a teacher. Well, I taught but I wasn't a teacher.

Therapist: meaning what?

Patient: um, uh I um I taught graduate classes, uh graduate students, I taught graduate students how to be a teacher, yet I had never taught in a classroom. Uh, I taught it from an educational psychology perspective. And so I I taught them to think about teaching, but I never thought of myself as a teacher. I was kind of you know . . .

Therapist: so it's kind of a those who can do, and those who can't teach?

Patient: No no no

Therapist: and you were, you were a teacher who didn't teach, but taught people how to . . .

Patient: think

Therapist: how to think about teaching

Patient: teaching

Therapist: but there must have been a little bit of teaching going on there.

Patient: well, it was, but I didn't think of myself as a teacher.
Therapist: gotcha.
Patient: you know if you asked me who are you . . .
Therapist: exactly.
Patient: I may have said I teach at University
Therapist: but you're not a teacher
Patient: But I'm not you know.
Therapist: and what did "I'm a counselor" mean?
Patient: oh, I'm a counselor, um, uh, everything I did, every interaction um I had with program development, with advising students, I used to counsel students who were on academic probation. I never gave that up even when I did my little side job um in two years I never gave up helping students think about themselves, and see their potential. So I always, I was always um . . .
Therapist: So you were a meaning-centered counselor?
Patient: yes, I always wanted them to think about taking who they were, how they define themselves and think about um what they would like to do and how we could make that possible. And so every program I developed was about enhancing one's potential, so I would always think about myself as a counselor. And of course in terms of how I would define myself, I thought of myself as intelligent, sensitive um.
Therapist: so you're intelligent and sensitive?
Patient: intelligent and sensitive right?
Therapist: sensitive
Patient: Which of course kind of um goes with the roles that I played.
Therapist: but not particularly brave or courageous?
Patient: no, not particularly brave or courageous (laugh). No um, maybe overly optimistic
Therapist: can you put that down?
Patient: yeah, um, which I think works, b/c if you're not overly optimistic um they you sometimes you deny the potential of what might be.
Therapist: right, so if you want to get to here in life, you kind of have to shoot way up there.
Patient: right
Therapist: if you fail at least you end up where you want to be.
Patient: yeah, kind of it's like a default. Um, you know I I would um so that's how I . . . and of course I was a mother and a daughter, and a wife.
Therapist: you can write that down.
Patient: (laugh). I'm thinking of my husband saying "I always come last." (laugh)
Therapist: I was just about to ask you about the order.
Patient: yeah
Therapist: Is the order in order of; is this particular order meaningful in any way?
Patient: uh yeah. Uh I think that uh, my children have always have come first in everything. In every decision I've made.
Therapist: you only have one grand-daughter?
Patient: I have two daughters.
Therapist: and you have two daughters, thanks for reminding me.
Patient: and uh and so everything that I have, since they've been born everything I've done, I've put them first. Um, uh, who I am as a mother comes in large part in how I was as a daughter, how my mother taught me.
Therapist: so you're legacy
Patient: Right and how my grandmother, because my grandmother also raised me, you know their interaction with me fueled how I was as a mother.
Therapist: what did you get from your mother and your grandmother?
Patient: um, my mother . . . my mother strength of character
Therapist: strength of character
Patient: and conviction.
Therapist: conviction
Patient: yeah. Um
Therapist: these are characteristics
Patient: right
Therapist: as opposed to the values?
Patient: right
Therapist: maybe virtues, right?
Patient: virtues right.
Therapist: these are the virtues you aspire to.
Patient: Yeah, right.
Therapist: You inherited.
Patient: right, to thy own self be true, you know.
Therapist and *Patient*: To thy own self be true
Patient: right, um two things, to thy own self be true, and treat others as you would have them treat you.
Therapist: the golden rule.
Patient: two things that I really and still . . .
Therapist: write that down too, those are the values and virtues you got from them.
Patient: yeah
Therapist: Those are very important, and you are very beloved by your mother.
Patient: oh yeah, still am.
Therapist: you still are? They're alive?
Patient: my mom is alive; my grandmother died a few years back.

Therapist: but she still loves you.

Patient: oh yeah, my grandmother still loves me, and um from my grandmother um (said while writing: "to thy own self be true and um"). And from my mother, from my grandmother, I um I learned love.

Therapist: love?

Patient: love and compassion um

Therapist: she wasn't Italian was she?

Patient: she wasn't, yeah (laugh)

Therapist: (laugh)

Patient: you know everything my grandmother did was for family.

Therapist: so it was mother and then granddaughter? Oh, mother, daughter ...

Patient: and then wife

Therapist: and then wife, and then grandma?

Patient: oh, well, I

Therapist: did you include grandmother?

Patient: ah, I think. . . .

Therapist: it's a new role for you?

Patient: it's, well, that's after cancer, this is before cancer.

Therapist: I'm sorry, okay. Thank you for the technical correction.

Patient: right uh uh, and wife, it's in the 3rd position but it's not really last, it's really kind of.

Therapist: Mm-hmm

Patient: It's really like a circular role that I have.

Therapist: circular

Patient: I don't think of it as you know linear.

Therapist: linear.

Patient: uh

Therapist: I'd put that down too. It's circular.

Patient: right

Therapist: it's a whole.

Patient: it's a whole, right, because well it's actually in the 2nd position in terms of a linear life, cycle. Um, I did not have a strong male figure in my life.

Therapist: growing up?

Patient: growing up. My father died when I was 4. And so I have no recollection of my, no I have a recollection of my father

Therapist: you have a visual kind of

Patient: but I don't have ... a lot of it I think if kind of um a fantasy of life that I would have had with my father, I mean the two memories I have of my father are very limited. So I I never had a strong male presence in my life. And grandmother had remarried um, my my grandfather, not my mother's father, but he was an alcoholic and a gambler, and for a large part of my youth they were separated. Um, I remained in contact with him, but I understood the frailties of his character.

Therapist: so it's three Italian women?

Patient: Three Italian women, right. And I had a great grandmother, who was also ...

Therapist: wow

Patient: so I had real connections with generations. Um so when I talk about being a wife, um and they were all widows. They were all widows at a very ...

Therapist: young age.

Patient: ...young age. So I when my husband and I got married, I jokingly said to him. You know this is really unchartered water for me. . . .

Therapist: this is a dangerous move on your behalf.

Patient: (laugh). That's right

Therapist: on your part.

Patient: (laugh) that's right. Um, and you know I was very honest with him. You know about, you know kind of my. . . .

Therapist: about the, not the (last name) curse, what was your maiden name?

Patient: well, yeah I called it the (maiden last name) curse

Therapist: curse

Patient: b/c it was my great grandmother's maiden name was (last name), and her husband died when she was um 37 and my grandmother's first husband died when she was 33. And my mother's, my father died when my mother was 27. And I married at 22, so I said to (husband's name), now you're really looking at ...

Therapist: 25

Patient: 3–4 years, I said after that I think we're okay.

Therapist: it keeps getting shorter.

Patient: well, no now of course it's 35 years and counting. And so I told him he's out of the woods.

Therapist: so this is a major achievement in the legacy of your family.

Patient: oh yeah.

Therapist: you've had a husband who's lived.

Patient: I feel like I've broken the curse, whatever it was.

Therapist: you've broken the curse

Patient: you know um ...

Therapist: you've broken the curse.

Patient: I've broken the curse.

Therapist: maybe it was him.

Patient: maybe it was him. Uh, maybe he broke the curse.

Therapist: maybe.

Patient: well, actually he did break the curse, because he lived (laugh).

Therapist: there you go.

Patient: um

Therapist: so if we were to, so those are really wonderful answers, they relate to um work right, sources of meaning through your creativity, they relate to experiential sources of meaning through love, and family, and their historical sources of meaning with legacy and all the virtues and values that you've inherited. And uh and I think the story about your husband, then again that's another example of how uh through experience of suffering losing a father, grandfather, all that, not having something, not having a father figure in your life, that you probably whether you realized it or not picked a really great guy.

Patient: oh yeah

Therapist: who had a chance of living (laugh)

Patient: (laugh)

Therapist: and not leaving for any reason. You picked good stock.

Patient: yeah yeah, I did. He's a good husband, a good man.

Therapist: that's wonderful.

Patient: good father.

Therapist: so uh now with the cancer uh, how would some of those answers change . . . ?

Patient: change

Therapist: you think? Or would they be the same?

Patient: uh, um, oh no, they've changed.

Therapist: they've changed?

Patient: oh yeah, they've changed in that . . .

Therapist: the notes you made about how they've changed.

Patient: yeah, what I wrote was uh, I am a loving, thoughtful, intelligent woman who is a daughter, a wife, a mother, and a grandmother and a friend. Uh, I enjoy doing special projects for others as much as I enjoy their company in ordinary days. And so I'm looking at the differences in the in the dynamic and I think the change in the order really has to come with uh my acknowledgement of the fragility of life. Being a good daughter for my mother now who's become important to me b/c I kind of interesting I acknowledge that I am a good daughter, but I want her to know how important she is in my life, you know that she's not on the periphery of you know now what seems to be a very vibrant life you know very full.

Therapist: which is an impression she could have got when you were this career woman.

Patient: right

Therapist: so busy

Patient: right

Therapist: workaholic. When you're a workaholic you don't always have the time or the energy, focus of attention to let the people you love, like your mom know how much you love her

Patient: right

Therapist: and how much you value her.

Patient: yeah

Therapist: This is an example of how cancer has altered your priorities.

Patient: yeah

Therapist: and opened up an area of love, meaning through love and family. Made that even bigger and richer and more important, is that right?

Patient: yeah um that's what I wrote . . . cancer

Therapist: yeah?

Patient: Life changing event. Focus on family, not work. Um . . .

Therapist: you don't even need me, I mean you just . . . (laugh)

Patient: well, I do need you (laugh). But in order for, I guess for me in order for me to get the most out of our sessions.

Therapist: yeah?

Patient: I need to think about you know uh, and I didn't write this before this morning.

Therapist: Mm-hmm

Patient: I didn't give this

Therapist: okay

Patient: I mean I gave it thought, but I didn't, I didn't want to I didn't give it thought prior to today. Because I had to leave it up to today.

Therapist: that's okay because that's why we're here.

Patient: Yeah, I think that cancer really uh, in some ways it put the breaks on things for me.

Therapist: on?

Patient: put the breaks on what I once held as valuable and . . .

Therapist: realized was not that valuable.

Patient: well, yeah you know it was like okay. Um, I kind of think of work as as one would think of high school. Something I did, that's in the past um . . .

Therapist: you were the prom queen

Patient: yeah you know, I didn't believe in proms, but I mean I was kind of . . .

Therapist: you were the valedictorian

Patient: No I wasn't even that. I was just a . . .

Therapist: you were the editor of the schoolbook, the yearbook? No?

Patient: I was non-defined as a high school student.
Therapist: no, but I mean in terms of work?
Patient: oh, my work, my work, I was . . .
Therapist: if you were to compare work to high school
Patient: I was I was editor of the newspaper.
Therapist: editor of the newspaper
Patient: right. To be honest I was probably more a journalist who got hired as the editor, but I was you know . . . and now, and now I'm amazed at how fast life goes by and how you really need to make simple things meaningful.
Therapist: what sort of simple things?
Patient: um, gardening.
Therapist: so you're now a person who appreciates simple things like gardening.
Patient: gardening, going for a walk
Therapist: going for a walk
Patient: um I have this wonderful 18 month old baby who I would actually think of myself as um her teacher.
Therapist: now you're a . . .
Patient: now I'm a teacher
Therapist: and now you're a grandmother
Patient: and now I'm a grandmother
Therapist: and your role as a grandmother and your role as a teacher are linked you say?
Patient: oh yes, absolutely. I mean everything
Therapist: like the book you got her.
Patient: like the book I got her, like, just you know it's wonderful to be with an 18 month old baby who finds joy in looking at the lines in a parking lot and telling you that they're yellow, you know. and then you know looking at the sky and saying you know blue and just you know so you know or she sees a bird and she you know, she'll tell you know that the bird is flying and you can see kind of the joy this child gets out of everyday things, and to be able to witness that I mean. . . .
Therapist: So you were saying you see yourself as a teacher of this child.
Patient: oh yeah
Therapist: but in some ways this 18 month old granddaughter
Patient: oh is teaching me
Therapist: teaching you uh the joy of simple things that you would've maybe not noticed cause you were so busy getting to work and from work.
Patient: right
Therapist: uh, the yellow line in the parking lot, the bird, the way the light shines through the trees, the beauty of some flowers in the garden. Um there's so much beauty around us isn't there?
Patient: oh yeah. And she really you know . . .
Therapist: and she can see it because that's her world right?
Patient: right
Therapist: she's just discovering the world and through her senses that's what uh that why they call it an experiential source of meaning. The word sense in French "sense" means meaning and so we derive meaning through our sensations our sensory system, we see, and smell and feel, and touch, all the sensations of being alive and in the world, and you know just the smell of the baby and the skin, and holding your husband at night, being close in the warmth indoors, and or you know a really great shower or something like that.
Patient: right, really silly simple things.
Therapist: living, living is uh really living every, living for the moment, I would say living for every sensation, experience, is an incredible source of being alive, its those moments we feel alive and innately feel so meaningful.
Patient: yeah
Therapist: so this was a result of cancer, and a result of having a granddaughter
Patient: had I . . .
Therapist: with cancer. Now that you have cancer, having a granddaughter.
Patient: and really kind of thinking about that clock, that I I have to um let her know who I am.
Therapist: right, so the clock, time, you're as Heidegger would say "You're being (existing) in time and you're more aware of time now. And time brings a sense of urgency to living."
Patient: right
Therapist: and apart of what you want to do besides enjoying being alive and experiencing, feeling more fully alive every day is you want to convey some important lessons in life to your grandchildren.
Patient: mm hmm
Therapist: have you already done that with your children?
Patient: oh yeah
Therapist: they know who they are
Patient: they know who they are
Therapist: they know who they came from
Patient: they know who they came from. They know. They don't know they don't know as much as. . . .
Therapist: as you've recently discovered.

Patient: as I have recently discovered.

Therapist: so it's interesting, what do you make of this exercise here? Are there big differences, or do you think um, there are some differences, right? Some things are still the same about you.

Patient: oh yeah!

Therapist: absolutely, right

Patient: yeah

Therapist: but the big difference is that you've moved from this workaholic to a person who's for all these other areas of meaning opened up in very profound ways.

Patient: yeah and I, I think who I am today um, who I was in terms of being a workaholic, and organized, and multitasking and everything else, really gave me the ability make the transition to now.

Therapist: right, so we're almost done. But let me just, we've been talking a lot about this book that you gave your granddaughter and how important it is for you to teach your granddaughter where she came from, and how your kids know quite a bit, but they don't know the new stuff that's going on. The next session really is focusing, session three focuses on exactly this issue of your legacy . . .

Patient: okay

Therapist: and uh the legacy that you've been given from your great grandmother, your grandmother, your mother, and I guess you'll tell me about some of these things you've discovered about your family maybe next week. Your family story, your story, and the legacy that you want to leave behind. One of the things that I want you to think about over the course of the 7 sessions, and we might have a chance to for you to talk a little bit about it and if you've actually done anything about it we can discuss it in the 7th session. Is that um to create what we call a legacy project, there may be something that you would like to do, it could be concrete, or it doesn't have to be concrete uh, some people either write down stuff or create an album or uh make a tape or write a letter. Some people get really kooky, nuts, they put together a compilation of music, they make a video, whatever, it doesn't have to be fancy. But it sounds to me like you've already got the makings of something that you wanna create that can be lasting for your family. Something about who they are, and where they came from. Um some people who go through the treatment say I am my own living legacy, the way I've lived my life is my legacy project, I am my own legacy project. Your mother, grandmother, grandfather didn't create a legacy project, I don't think, unless they handed you some recipes or something like that.

Patient: not really.

Therapist: no, so the life they lived still lives on for you. So to get technical, to really get down to the essence, it doesn't have to be something you externalize and make into something that you can hold in your hands, but think about it, whether you want to do something like that . . . yeah just to think about that and we'll go over it in the next session.

Patient: oka

Session 3: Historical Sources of Meaning—Life as a Legacy That Has Been Given; Life as a Legacy That One Lives and Will Give

Therapist: So how are you doing?

Patient: good

Therapist: anything new happening?

Patient: no, not really. It's been a fairly quiet week. Not much has changed. Uh.

Therapist: you had chemo today?

Patient: yeah

Therapist: went okay?

Patient: yeah

Therapist: you don't get sick afterward?

Patient: no, well it's Herceptin, so . . .

Therapist: Herceptin

Patient: So I don't really have a reaction, other than being tired, but you know.

Therapist: makes you tired

Patient: yeah

Therapist: how long have you been on it now?

Patient: um, four and a half years, four and a half years

Therapist: wow

Patient: yeah

Therapist: so you tolerate it pretty well.

Patient: yeah, not the first treatment, but ever since (laugh).

Therapist: that's good. So do you buy Revlon products because. . . .

Patient: No (laugh), no, I buy Clinique.

Therapist: Clinique?

Patient: yeah

Therapist: Este Lauder?

Patient: Well, Este . . . I buy Clinique because of a skin reaction.

Therapist: wow

Patient: I have sensitive skin.

Therapist: I think Revlon money went to developing Herceptin.

Patient: Oh, did it really?

Therapist: yeah at UCLA. So what did you think about last week's session, or?

Patient: um, well I was uh, um . . .

Therapist: anything left over, something you thought about that you thought gee I wish I had mentioned that to Dr. (name)?

Patient: um, no. I mean, I think. I think I've given legacy a lot of thought.

Therapist: you've given this week's topic a lot of thought?

Patient: yeah, yeah

Therapist: Let me just give you my thoughts about last week

Patient: okay

Therapist: I thought it was very interesting, last week's session. And I thought it was very remarkable that you focused in on choice, from the section of Frankl's book that you had read. And how you related that to your own experience with cancer. That it was a time to make certain choices about how you were going to spend your time

Patient: Mm-hmm

Therapist: and how to devote your energies, and how to focus your attention and caring towards. And it was ah, and the cancer diagnosis was an impetus for you to rearrange your priorities a bit, or at least be more aware of your priorities. And rearrange how you spent your time.

Patient: Mm-hmm

Therapist: and so that was to me a very interesting part of last week. And it think that the other thing that was striking is that uh when you looked at when we looked at the things that give your life meaning, um gave your life meaning before the cancer, things that gave your life meaning after cancer. Who you were before, who you are now after the cancer. The essence of who you are has not been changed really.

Patient: No

Therapist: the essence of who you are is preserved. So you're somebody, just so you know (laugh), you're someone who's been able to integrate this cancer experience into a sense of who you are. And you haven't allowed it to define you. You know, you're still the same person, you have this in your life

Patient: Mm-hmm

Therapist: that you're trying to deal with the best that you can. But you've integrated it into your life. So you've been able to reform yourself. You had this event, with the cancer; it caused these shockwaves you know. The ground kind of like an earthquake, you know . . .

Patient: yeah

Therapist: yeah, earthquake. Ground opened up, something like that. But you managed to reform your life you know that you had beforehand and enhance it a bit, by going back to what basically gives your life meaning, which is your family, uh the things you care about, some aspects of your work.

Patient: Mm-hmm

Therapist: so this idea of integrating, being fully integrating, reforming, that's another way of saying you have manage to remain whole.

Patient: yeah, but you know, I, this is true, but

Therapist: but there's a but

Patient: But there's a but

Therapist: let's hear the but

Patient: and the but is, um, I've never really experienced some of the devastating effects, or impact cancer can have on one's life.

Therapist: you feel you did not experience

Patient: No, I mean, I did not have a mastectomy, I never, I mean I did have the stereotactic surgery on my brain. So I can't minimize that.

Therapist: A little minor, a minor procedure?

Patient: well, not a minor procedure, um

Therapist: hmm

Patient: My body, except for my brain, my body never really changed. You know so I didn't you know, I have a friend of mine, well she's not really my friend, but I know of her. She's had surgery upon surgery, just, who she was prior to cancer physically is not who she is now. And that you know I was thinking um actually I was thinking as I was sitting out there and I thought about this before. I don't know if I would be as whole

Therapist: Mm-hmm

Patient: if I had had experienced other things happening to me. That doesn't mean I lamented. I take who I am today with an air of caution.

Therapist: gotcha

Patient: you know that um

Therapist: b/c you anticipate that things could happen?

Patient: oh yeah, I mean I'm not uh. I feel like I'm in the honeymoon of my cancer experience, uh and like all honeymoons you enjoy them (laugh). And you enjoy being able. . . . I said to (name) it took me 40 minutes to walk from the Breast Center to here.

Therapist: hmm

Patient: She said you were taking your time, enjoying the scenery. And I said "No, that's about the pace of my walk now." I said, as I was walking, I was watching other women, much older than I, but walking with canes, and I thought to myself "Well it's taking you 40 minutes, but it's not like your walking, and you're not walking with the assistance of anything." And um you know that might be you some day, but it isn't you today, so just enjoy the walk and you know, I'm glad I had said to you that I could definitely get here by 10, because I'm a good judge of what I can physically do now. So yes, cancer has impacted the speed in which I do things.

Therapist: so I hear exactly what you're saying, you're saying that um, on some level you feel lucky that you haven't had all of the uh things that could possibly, the physically sequela of what could have possibly happened or happened with breast cancer. And so you feel perhaps your ability to remain whole hasn't been challenged as much as perhaps some other people have been challenged. But you kind of brushed aside the brain metatases and the stereotactic, so um, was that not a challenge at all, or?

Patient: oh the first one was a challenge. Um, you know, I was devastated.

Therapist: you were devastated?

Patient: yeah, you know that they were . . .

Therapist: because you use your brain a lot.

Patient: well, I used to (laugh). I used it a lot more than I am using it nowadays. But uh, well actually I can't say that. I'm probably actually using it more now, because I challenge myself to do things instead of responding to what other people want me to do. But um, uh yeah I was shocked and then um, when it came back because the doctor had said to me there was no evidence of disease from the neck down. Uh but that there was progression in the brain, I was you know kind of taken aback. But then ironically you know the 4th time when um the radiation oncologist had presented the fact that he was suggesting whole brain radiation, that's when I said to him, "Oh no, we're not going there." I I don't have any of the um physical debilitation that's described in the literature that would necessitate whole brain radiation and uh there are chemotherapies that can address the issue, and before we go the whole brain route, this is where I am. . . . Its funny the 4th time it was like okay so now you have to be more active in this than you've been in the past. In the past when they said to me you have to have stereotactic, I said okay you know, but now it was like I'm not going there.

Therapist: so you've had it a few times?

Patient: I've had it 4 times. Well, I've had it, yeah I've had it 4 times, and this would have been the 5th, and I said no.

Therapist: Mm-hmm

Patient: I'm not going to go whole brain. So um luckily, I've responded well to um the chemo and uh everything is stable which means basically there's no growth. And possibly there's some shrinkage, but they're not really sure. But its okay, it's you know . . .

Therapist: right. So one of the things that uh I'm hoping we can accomplish in the 7 sessions we have today is to give you a sort of awareness and a vocabulary around um issues sources of meaning uh sources of meaning that can be resources for you. That I've believe you've used already just as we've discussed in the first two sessions when I pointed out ah that's a creative source of meaning, that's an experiential source of meaning, that's an attitude that you've taken towards suffering, that's a source of meaning. Those are the things that have allowed you to maintain your sense of being whole . . .

Patient: right

Therapist: and who you are still. Uh and so this is a way of, it's like I guess swimming lessons you know, you're a natural swimmer I think, and without this therapy you've managed to stay . . .

Patient: Afloat

Therapist: Afloat. And we're going to make you into more aware of what it is that you've been doing that manage to keep you afloat and make you into an even better swimmer. So if you do encounter rough waters ahead you've got this knowledge and these skills that you're aware of. Uh, I know that I, when I go see patients in the hospital, I see them with fellows. The fellows see the patient and then I'll see the patient. And I'll go in and do an interview, which is very different from what they do. Uh and you know interesting things happen when I'm talking to patients in the hospital, and the fellows and then the fellows walk out and say "Wow that was so different than." And we try to analyze what I've done, because when I do it I don't think about it so much because I do it naturally. But in order to teach it the fellows need for me to explain what it is, first I did this, then I did this, then I did this. And the more that I'm aware of what I do, the easier it is for me to teach others how to do it, but the easier it is for me to remember uh to do it, I do it better next time because I know what I'm doing.

Patient: right

Therapist: So this is what this is all about. And today's session, um, today's session is about one of the other sources of meaning. We talked about the various sources of meaning, experiential sources of meaning, uh is how you experience the world through your sensations. I might have told you the French word for meaning is "sens."

Patient: right

Therapist: sensation, sensory system, so every, you know we're human beings and we have all these senses, right? Sight, smell, touch, whatever. And when we encounter the world using our senses we experience the world in a way that makes us feel so alive, the food we eat, the smell of the flowers, the touch of someone who loves you, touching you know stroking the hair of one you care about. Um, so uh love is a big source of experiential meaning, music, whatever, beauty, art. Things like that. Um, uh so then there are created sources of meaning. We have thing responsibility to create this life, a life of meaning, I life of identity, a life of direction, and so it's its in the way that we make a life, through the things we care about in the world, through work, thought things that, we're fully engaged in life.

Patient: Mm-hmm

Therapist: And so work is a big sense of meaning. You mentioned other things. You like to garden, right?

Patient: Yes

Therapist: right, so that making things grow, that's a created source of meaning. And a third source of meaning is the attitude you take towards suffering, and I might have mentioned to you anytime we encounter a limitation, something that constrains us we suffer. So how do we find a way to overcome these limitations? Is through the attitude we take towards the suffering and that attitude is informed by created sources of meaning and experiential sources of meaning. Those are resources, so the way we can transcend a limitation is by remembering and choosing to stay connected to things that give our lives meaning. Love and the things we care about, and the work in our lives.

Patient: Mm-hmm

Therapist: and the third source of meaning is this historical source of meaning. The notion that meaning exists in a historical context, it doesn't exist, you know, it doesn't exist in isolation.

Patient: right

Therapist: you're part of something greater than yourself. And there are moments when you realize that, and moments when you don't realize that. And actually when you realize that you are part of something greater than yourself, that's what I mean when I talk about transcending things too.

Patient: Mm-hmm

Therapist: it's like being connected to something greater. The way you overcome limitations is to understand that you are connected to something greater, um, when you were talking about walking here

Patient: Mm-hmm

Therapist: and seeing these other people you understood that these people, that you're connected to these other women, some of who are walking with canes and other, you are part of something greater. You understood that that could be me, right? And that wasn't just an idea like I could get worse or something like that, but it was also like I'm no different from that person, we're connected, we're related, and what could happen to them could happen to me. And so you felt this, you experienced this connectedness. And it's through being connected to, when you are a self transcended, in other words when your concerns are not merely for yourself but recognizing that you are part of something greater than yourself. That allows you to overcome obstacles, but also puts you in touch with the fact that not only are you connected to all human beings, all women on the upper east side of Manhattan, you are part of a whole line of human beings who came before you in your family, and that you are part of a continuum right?

Patient: yup

Therapist: you're part of a continuum. So today's, uh and that gives you special meaning to your life, what you do with your life. Uh so for instance, I'm the first, I'm the first child in my family ever to go to university. There other aspects of my family background that makes what I do so much more meaningful.

I don't want to spend the time talking about me. But you know there are things in my family history that make what I do so much more powerful or meaningful because of the people I came from.

Patient: right

Therapist: so today's session focuses on the legacy you inherited, the legacy that you live everyday and that you will leave behind for the next generation, for your kids, your grandkids, and things like that, how you will be remembered, etc. And you said before, just in the earlier part when we were talking about, you gave this session a lot of thought over the week.

Patient: mm hmm

Therapist: right? So let me have you, tell me what you were thinking.

Patient: um, on my mother's side of the family, um all the women married young, they were also widowed young, but they were also widowed young.

Therapist: I remember that, I remember that, you told me that last week right?

Patient: I had knew my great grandmother

Therapist: we were talking about how brave your husband was to marry you.

Patient: yeah right (laugh). So I knew my great grandmother and I knew my grandmother and of course I knew my mother. But even as a young child I would question each of them about their own childhood, b/c it was always important for me to know their story.

Therapist: right

Patient: because I, there was an awareness, really, and I can say this, even as a child there was an awareness, that um and probably because of death, but there was an awareness that this was a temporal state. That my ability to ask them questions was not something that I would always have at my disposal um . . .

Therapist: I see, so you were aware of death as a young person

Patient: oh yeah

Therapist: because of your father . . .

Patient: my father died when I was 4.

Therapist: 4 and your grandfather died young.

Patient: oh yeah

Therapist: so you had an understanding that life is finite.

Patient: oh yeah

Therapist: that you didn't have your mother, and grandmother, and great grandmother around, you weren't going to have them around

Patient: around always, right

Therapist: always to ask them questions about your life. I think the, I see that you made

Patient: yeah, I did my homework

Therapist: you did your homework, right. So um the exercise that I think

Patient: well the um the exercise is actually kind of a um. Today's exercise really . . .

Therapist: you did it as part of the homework.

Patient: I did it as part of the homework.

Therapist: okay, so uh maybe we can talk about it.

Patient: I can refine it, because . . .

Therapist: no problem.

Patient: this was

Therapist: these were your notes.

Patient: these were my memories

Therapist: right, so I think when you look back on your life and upbringing what were the most significant memories, relationships, etc, and so that's what you were starting to talk about right. So go ahead, I interrupted you.

Patient: It was really this kind of interrelationship that I had with them. In that it really wasn't about, I guess it's kind of a heightened awareness, but it really wasn't about who they were to me, I mean I knew who they were to me, but I wanted to know who they were. You know that was that was very important, and so um with my great grandmother uh, when I was little, my great grandmother was the one who was always cooking and in the kitchen. Um, she was always preparing, her way of, and she had a routine. So I think what I learned from her is that its okay to have a ritual to do things b/c there's comfort in that ritual.

Therapist: explain that a little more

Patient: when I would come home from school, from elementary school, from 1st, from kindergarten to 1st grade, 2nd grade, our ritual was she would make me a cup of soup. Now it didn't matter whether it was summer, winter, fall, every day I came home there would be a cup of soup, and I had to have the soup, and I must have complained, although I didn't remember complaining, I must have complained about having the soup as I started to get older, so she would invite my friends that lived on the block to also come in to have a cup of soup. And then after the soup it was time for them to leave and I had to take a nap. And it didn't matter that I wasn't tired but I had to take a nap, I had to rest, and cause she would say to me that "When you rest, you think better" (laugh). Kind of an interesting way of thinking about incubation, and how you know if you get away from something for a while then you'll, but so she taught me that as a child. And then uh it was only a half hour nap, and she would tell me "You can get up at 4." And then I would do my homework, and then um we would have dinner, and we always sat as a family for dinner. So there was a, there was a, there was comfort in that ritual.

Therapist: there was a ritual

Patient: but it was a ritual, I mean we . . .

Therapist: there were family rituals and traditions.

Patient: right

Therapist: really around caring for the young in the family.

Patient: right, yeah, and so that's what she imparted, I mean

Therapist: loving and caring.

Patient: right the loving and the caring.

Therapist: what was the important part for you? Was it the ritual? Or the caring, the loving that came through? Or maybe the way it was combined?

Patient: I think the way it was combined. You know, we, she uh she showed me by doing.

Therapist: she showed you how much she cared for you and loved you and valued you by what she was doing.

Patient: right so it was always.

Therapist: and she was ahead of her time. She understood that if you after school when you learned all the stuff you took a nap you could in your sleep in your nap sort of integrate some of the stuff. So she was a neuroscientist ahead of her time.

Patient: yeah (laugh), you know I'm sure she must have done that with her own children.

Therapist: ah ha

Patient: or maybe this is what she did as a child

Therapist: do you think that is what her mother did with her?

Patient: well, I don't know, cause I I didn't really question my great grandmother that much. It was my grandmother that I really learned to ask about more.

Therapist: Mm-hmm

Patient: My great grandmother would encourage me when she was baking to come and knead the bread. And so at Easter I was making an Easter bread and as I was kneading it, just the action of doing it, I thought of my great grandmother.

Therapist: Mm-hmm

Patient: you know in the way that she would knead the bread and she showed me how to do it. Um.

Therapist: right

Patient: so it was never um, she respected the fact that I was a child and that I needed rest, but she didn't think there were things that she did that children shouldn't do. So she engaged me in the doing of life.

Therapist: she brought you into the family of women in your family.

Patient: right, that this is what we do.

Therapist: yeah, that this is what the women in the family?

Patient: the (maiden name) family

Therapist: the (maiden name), you are a (maiden name) woman.

Patient: yes, this is what we do.

Therapist: and this is what we all do.

Patient: yes, this is what we do.

Therapist: you're part of the club.

Patient: yeah I'm part of the club.

Therapist: you're part of the family.

Patient: and you know

Therapist: La Familia

Patient: and I did that with my girls.

Therapist: you did that with your girls

Patient: Um when they were, when they were 3 we had a ritual of having a baking party at Christmas time and all there friends would come, first it started out small of course, but at 3 it was time for them to learn you know measuring and . . .

Therapist: 3?

Patient: 3

Therapist: like you

Patient: yeah, so it was you know I encouraged them, and I'm sure they will encourage their children.

Therapist: so this is being passed down

Patient: right

Therapist: and after you're gone when your kids are baking Christmas stuff they'll remember you.

Patient: Right and the baking party when you talked about things that you do. All there friends still talk about their fond memories of the baking parties.

Therapist: Mm-hmm

Patient: And as each of them has started to develop their families, they too want to start the baking parties. So it's . . .

Therapist: so you've not only have influenced your own family, you've taught others the importance of family . . .

Patient: and sharing

Therapist: rituals, family sharing and sharing.

Patient: yeah

Therapist: that's another value

Patient: oh yeah. I mean . . .

Therapist: you're talking about values in your system. In your family.
Patient: yeah
Therapist: there's the value of a of tradition, there's a value of . . .
Patient: can I write this down?
Therapist: sure
Patient: may I? Thank you.
Therapist: there's a value of tradition, there's a value of um bringing the children into the process of what of what we women in this family do in concrete ways to nurture our children and to show them we love them. It's one thing to say you love somebody; it's another thing to show someone how much you love them in concrete ways. Here's your soup sweetheart. . . .
Patient: yeah
Therapist: come lie down take a nap. Um
Patient: yeah I mean there's . . .
Therapist: Let's bake this bread together.
Patient: There's always a gentleness about it.
Therapist: there's a gentleness.
Patient: you know, um you know not overbearing. Uh
Therapist: you know some people might say you know this is women's work; it's not like what you ended up doing in your career at John Jay and all that. But uh and some people put values on it, but clearly this had enormous, this was very treasured, very valued by you.
Patient: yeah
Therapist: Is that true?
Patient: oh yeah, absolutely, and I did bring it to my work.
Therapist: oh, you brought it to work too?
Patient: Oh, Absolutely, you know when we would have meetings um I would always bring refreshments. Um, I ran the deans' list, which of course was you know a very large party. Uh um, and a friend of mine would joke with me, cause I felt that each person that was on the deans' list should be honored for being on the deans' list, and I represented that honor of being you know, yes you were all on the deans' list, but each of you have an individual accomplishment. I used to um get a single yellow rose with baby's breath and my friend would laugh at me because he said to me "You know, florists can bring the roses and put them in the vase, you don't have to do that." I said "I know, but I feel like I'm acknowledging them by doing that." I don't have to tell them, but you know, um when someone is being recognized among the mass sometimes they lose their own sense of individual accomplishment. And I wanted them to feel that sense of accomplishment. So they would joke at me, you know that I was the mother of the freshman, you know that I took time for each individual student.
Therapist: so you were.
Patient: but I wasn't being, um it was it was how I was raised.
Therapist: exactly, so were you raised with that recognition?
Patient: everything was celebrated.
Therapist: but individually you?
Patient: yes.
Therapist: uh
Patient: yeah, at Christmas time . . .
Therapist: were there other kids?
Patient: no, but at Christmas time, each of us had our moment to open gifts.
Therapist: Mm-hmm
Patient: we weren't all . . .
Therapist: you didn't do them all together?
Patient: no, we you know so if it took us half an hour to open gifts doing it that way. It was giving, I know it was a silly, I mean I'm thinking as I'm saying, I'm thinking well I really haven't given this a lot of thought. But it was really you know, even when my girls were little each one had there, you know we would take turns.
Therapist: their moment
Patient: But each would have their moment. You know, and it was important, it's still important to me.
Therapist: right, cause each life is unique
Patient: Right
Therapist: your life is unique, the life you create for yourself and for your family. It's . . .
Patient: It's special
Therapist: uniquely yours. It's special, yeah.
Patient: yeah
Therapist: and um, what you, it was important for you to prepare the flower for each one of the young people on the deans' list, because that was your way of showing your love for them, or your . . .
Patient: my love, my acknowledgment . . .
Therapist: your acknowledgement.
Patient: of what they accomplished.
Therapist: right, yeah um
Patient: cause I think sometimes, sometimes particularly in the administration you get tainted by the sameness of the academic year.
Therapist: right
Patient: but for the person that's experiencing it that may be the first time that they've

ever been acknowledged for something that they've done.

Therapist: and you learned the value of that from your family.

Patient: oh, absolutely.

Therapist: this is part of the legacy that you inherited.

Patient: yeah

Therapist: so um things become more meaningful when they move from being an idea and a concept to being concrete, right?

Patient: Mm-hmm

Therapist: Like I may have the idea that I love you,

Patient: right

Therapist: but unless I make it real, it almost, when you make it real it takes a life of its own. It's a, when I give you that card or a flower, or that soup, or a diamond ring whatever. It becomes much more real, and concrete. And it becomes a symbol right? A symbol of what's of what the feeling of love.

Patient: right

Therapist: and the profound meaningfulness of what you're engaged in. It probably gave more meaning to um what you did with your girls. It gave more meaning to being a mother. What you did with the deans' list kids, gave more meaning to your role of the dean of students right?

Patient: well, I was the dean of the freshmen.

Therapist: dean of freshmen.

Patient: right I mean it, um, yeah I lived what I, I lived my role.

Therapist: You lived you role, there you go, that's what you should write down.

Patient: I lived my role, yeah, um yeah.

Therapist: that's the true essence of being

Patient: right

Therapist: to live your role.

Patient: you know, I uh, it wasn't a part that I played.

Therapist: Right, and that's a value you learned at a, that's something you learned from your family. To live. When your great grandmother made that soup, she was living her role.

Patient: right, you're not passive about it.

Therapist: Right, she lived her role. That's so interesting.

Patient: yeah, so I you know when I was doing this exercise, um, you know I thought about my relationships, although, I put my, I put my, what I said was what I learned from my mother was I was the most important person in her life.

Therapist: mm

Patient: uh, I think, I think, part of that may have been a little too much you know. So I learned to respect distance, you know that you can love someone but you should not be overbearing with that love.

Therapist: you want to allow them the room to become . . .

Patient: who they want.

Therapist: who they want to be.

Patient: yeah, that you know.

Therapist: were you given that freedom?

Patient: no (laugh).

Therapist: okay, but you took it?

Patient: But I understood it.

Therapist: did you eventually take it?

Patient: did I eventually take it?

Therapist: I understand it was a struggle.

Patient: oh

Therapist: because there was so much love.

Patient: yes, but I did I um

Therapist: did you eventually make your own in your life?

Patient: I demarked my limitations.

Therapist: you did?

Patient: yeah, uh and then and then I think in the last couple of years um, I understood that I was not I was not my mother's child. In terms of, her will was not my will.

Therapist: exactly

Patient: that we had two separate identities. But in order for me to do that I had to pull away from her.

Therapist: yes, we all have to do that

Patient: and now, and now, I've you know I've always accepted who she was. It's funny because we're talking about mothers, and I'm thinking about Mother's Day, and I was looking at Mother's Day cards.

Therapist: Mother's Day is coming up.

Patient: yeah, and the Mother's Day cards are kind of interesting because they said "You're easy to love." Well, they really should say something more like um "I love you for who you are" as opposed to "You're easy to," cause I don't know too many mothers that are easy to love. I mean because I think part of what we do it try to you know separate and individuate and to become who we are, as opposed to not an image of who they are.

Therapist: exactly.

Patient: but what I learned from my mother was that um I learned who I was to her.

Therapist: hmm

Patient: as I said before she's a very strong person with strong convictions.

Therapist: so I would say you've learned a couple things from her, right. You learned how much, you learned from your mother how much you were loved right?
Patient: right
Therapist: and you learned who you were to her. The importance of your importance to her, I guess and to her identity she was a mother . . .
Patient: right
Therapist: and you helped her fulfill her identity. But you also learned the importance of how to become a mother who can convey love and nurturance to a child, but you also learned the importance of giving your children the space to become who they were. And is that what you did with your kids?
Patient: yeah
Therapist: so you did that slightly differently.
Patient: oh yeah
Therapist: because you learned that from her.
Patient: I mean I learned that from her, being on the other end.
Therapist: on the receiving end (laugh)
Patient: (laugh) and there were three other people that were important in shaping me. Um uh, my friend (name) who was like a sister to me. We were very close. And she had a horrific accident when she was 40 years old. And uh and in that event, I mean we had always been close, I realized how fragile life is. That we can't take things for granted.
Therapist: right
Patient: you know, I mean even though there was an awareness that you know you have to make the most of a relationship, um I think that's what I learned from her.
Therapist: yeah well, I think you learned that you learned that lesson repeatedly in your life from what I'm hearing. You learned that as a 3 year old when your dad died. You came from a legacy of a family where death of a you know a father, husband, grandfather, this occurred often. So that taught you that death is real, life is fragile, your best friend (name)?
Patient: (best friend's name)
Therapist: experience again, life as human beings is frail, fragile. But did you also learn from (best friend) that while, and from your par—, mother, grandmother, great grandmother did you also learn that even though life is fragile that terrible things can happen, did you also learn about courage and resilience?
Patient: oh yeah absolutely, um I would say resilience.
Therapist: resilience.
Patient: I would say resilience, and um
Therapist: and I would say that your great grandmother for instance, part of what helped her be resilient was her relationship with you. That she could cook you soup every day, and she put you to bed, that gave her meaning and purpose in life. You know she couldn't do that for her husband.
Patient: right
Therapist: you know. What was your great grandfather's name?
Patient: oh eh (name)
Therapist: (name)
Patient: (name)
Therapist: (name) come have some soup.
Patient: right
Therapist: go take a nap you worked hard.
Patient: right
Therapist: she did that with you
Patient: right, yeah, and she was a character
Therapist: are you, is your name, are you named after anyone?
Patient: No, I'm named after my father.
Therapist: you are named after your father.
Patient: his name was (name) so.
Therapist: (name). And does that mean anything to you to be named after him?
Patient: Its funny you would say that, because that's how I took this exercise. Um, I actually went back, well, I actually knew what (my name) means, it means "noble."
Therapist: Noble
Patient: and so
Therapist: so you actually, when you did the exercise, you said okay (name), what does that mean? "Noble."
Patient: yeah, like
Therapist: like from the Latin.
Patient: (name)
Therapist: (name)
Patient: right and I knew that, I mean I've known that for a very long time. Um, and so for me it meant that I had to live up to that name you know that I had to be noble in what I did as opposed to . . .
Therapist: (name) means noble?
Patient: right
Therapist: mm hmm
Patient: but it terms of being . . .
Therapist: then what's Patria?
Patient: Patria, I don't know.
Therapist: it means father doesn't it?
Patient: right, Patriarch.
Therapist: Patriarch

Patient: um, but in terms of being named after my father, um I always perceived that as my mother's way of holding onto my father knowing that he was sick. That um I was carrying his legacy.
Therapist: I see. So she named you that before he died right b/c you were 3 years old.
Patient: oh yeah
Therapist: so you think she named you that in anticipation because he was frail and ill?
Patient: well, that's what I always thought, you know.
Therapist: and you carry his . . .
Patient: I carry his name.
Therapist: and you said his legacy
Patient: and his legacy yeah
Therapist: and what is his legacy?
Patient: my father, um my father was a carpenter, uh very good with his hands.
Therapist: so in your family people do things with their hands
Patient: yeah
Therapist: to show love
Patient: yeah to create
Therapist: to keep people alive, to create.
Patient: right
Therapist: and for their work.
Patient: and I think I have my father's temperament. I know that I don't have my mother's temperament, so I definitely must have my father's.
Therapist: which is what?
Patient: mild.
Therapist: mild, mild mannered
Patient: mild mannered, um, you know my mother would say that if my father was in a room and someone was hiding in a closet, they could count the number of words that my father would say in the room. And then my Aunt corrected her one day and said "It's because you don't stop talking." (laugh)
Therapist: (laugh). So he was a man of few words.
Patient: right, yeah
Therapist: but we don't know if it's a function of the fact that the women in the room . . .
Patient: no, I think he was a basically you know quiet, but um, but when you said the origin of your name, yes she named me after him.
Therapist: when you took it to be noble or patriarch how did you, what did you make of that?
Patient: um that you would have to uh be honorable, I mean I don't, I knew what noble meant, but not as noble as someone in an aristocratic role.
Therapist: of course, honorable.
Patient: that everything you did had to have honor to it.
Therapist: and what do you mean by that?
Patient: um, uh for me it would be um treating others as you would have them treat you.
Therapist: recognition that we're all connected.
Patient: yeah
Therapist: so the golden rule.
Patient: the golden rule
Therapist: treat others as you would have them treat you, or don't treat others as you would not want yourself treated.
Patient: yeah you know, above reproach, that what you do . . .
Therapist: being honest
Patient: being honest, yeah
Therapist: being mild mannered
Patient: well being mild mannered.
Therapist: humble. Sounds like your father was a humble man.
Patient: yeah I would say so, um you know . . .
Therapist: humility
Patient: I didn't really know the man. Um.
Therapist: didn't know him?
Patient: I have an image of him, but I don't know if it's accurate.
Therapist: what's your image?
Patient: um, just someone who was very kind hearted, you know and helpful, not overbearing. Um
Therapist: he would've put those little flowers in vases himself.
Patient: yeah he would've made the vase (laugh)
Therapist: what would he have done?
Patient: he would've made the vase
Therapist: he would've made the vase
Patient: you know, um, uh when they didn't have much money when they first married he made the bedroom furniture because that's what he could do. You know . . .
Therapist: Special
Patient: so it was special right, so it terms of . . .
Therapist: that's probably where you were conceived.
Patient: well, probably, I don't imagine I would . . .
Therapist: I doubt they were at the Waldorf Astoria
Patient: yes, I don't think they went traveling anywhere. But I mean there was something um and I guess he too put himself into what he did too. I come from a family of people who go the extra effort you know.
Therapist: do you think you slept in a crib or a?
Patient: he made my crib
Therapist: that he made?

Patient: yes, he made my crib.
Therapist: mm hmm
Patient: he made my crib, and my children used that crib
Therapist: used that crib.
Patient: and unfortunately um the crib was destroyed in a house fire.
Therapist: but it was used for another generation
Patient: it was used for another generation yeah. And that, it bothers my older daughter more than the younger one, but um that for me is important you know, things that people used before.
Therapist: absolutely.
Patient: so when I was born my great grandmother made my christening gown and I used it for both girls.
Therapist: wow
Patient: But my daughter decided she didn't really care for the gown she wanted to buy a new one. And I said that's fine you know. And she said to me "Are you upset?" I said no you have a right to make a choice; I'm not upset you know.
Therapist: so you wore the christening gown?
Patient: well, I wore the christening gown, yeah.
Therapist: no I'm saying she got a new one for her little girl, so you wore it.
Patient: no I didn't wear it.
Therapist: you didn't fit into it?
Patient: no, I didn't fit into it, no. And then um you said important events right? Well, it's really um, I would say probably besides the things that are the most obvious, my wedding and my children's' birth, graduating with my PhD, that was, you know that I did for myself.
Therapist: so when you talk about your mother and you
Patient: that was me
Therapist: that was your accomplishment.
Patient: right that was on me, you know
Therapist: and are you also like me, someone who's the first person in their family to get a PhD?
Patient: oh yeah
Therapist: So you're a symbol of an evolution of a family of an immigrant family, where people came from the old country and had . . .
Patient: hairdressers
Therapist: huh?
Patient: they were hairdressers.
Therapist: hairdressers, people who worked with their hands
Patient: hands, right
Therapist: and you were this new generation who was going to work their mind.
Patient: so that I
Therapist: I guess on some levels that was perceived as progress, I don't know (laugh)
Patient: well, yeah I mean they were all . . .
Therapist: what do you think? progress?
Patient: um, yeah I think so.
Therapist: Mm-hmm
Patient: I think so. I think for me it was symbol that you could become who you were meant to be . . .
Therapist: yeah
Patient: but not necessarily at the expense of who you were you know.
Therapist: exactly. You can become who you're meant to be but you will never cease being someone who carries the legacy of your origins
Patient: right
Therapist: yeah
Patient: and I would, as much as I think I've accomplished I look back to my great grandmother who came here from Italy, and the bravery that she showed in making that trans-Atlantic trip, I mean you know I'm not so sure I could go . . .
Therapist: yeah, you're not sure you could take that same risk
Patient: no
Therapist: did you do any of the exercises that look back on things that you're most proud of? I guess that PhD is something you're proud of.
Patient: well the PhD is what I'm most proud of, you know, and my work at John Jay. Um, it still continues the programs that I developed. I'm having dinner this week with two of my students who have gone on in their professional lives, um, but still want to remain in contact with me. And each of them is doing some aspect of mentoring and for me that meant a lot.
Therapist: Mm-hmm
Patient: I'm actually in contact with a lot of my students. You know, so I've lived a good life.
Therapist: Yes and actually being a teacher you by definition you're passing along lessons to the next generations. Are there other things, are there things that you've learned, we've already kind of touched on a lot of them. Some of these values that you've learned and traditions that you've passed on to your kids as well. Um, the crib, your crib, the baking at Christmas, the christening gown, things like that. Are there other lessons, values and lessons that you, that you want to pass down to others? Or that you have already?
Patient: um.
Therapist: I think you've already talked a lot about that already.

Patient: yeah, I can't think of anything else.
Therapist: besides the one's we've talked about?
Patient: yeah, I mean I think I've really um . . .
Therapist: yeah, you've talk about. Um, how do you want to be remembered, you think? You've said you've lived a good life.
Patient: I've lived a good life, yeah
Therapist: yeah
Patient: um, how do I want to be remembered? Um, I don't know I guess as someone who was uh thoughtful, um and patient, um not too opinionated, uh you know someone who loved them. I want them to think of me in loving terms.
Therapist: yeah, some combination actually of your great grandmother, and grandmother, and your mother and your father.
Patient: yeah, when I think of them . . .
Therapist: and the lessons that you've learned from them, the good ones. . . .
Patient: and the not so good ones you know um, you know I jokingly would tell my girls, um when they wanted to discuss something, that they're something as a mother, I run a benevolent dictatorship, and I wanted them to understand that, that they're some things that we are not going to discuss, or you know so that. I guess I guess what I'd what them to know is that I had a strong sense of myself, and that I was true to who I, you know how I interacted with them was really who I was.
Therapist: yeah you mentioned that you lived a life that was true to yourself.
Patient: right, yeah, you know that the essence of who I am . . .
Therapist: and that's what you want for them too
Patient: that's what I want for them too. I want them to be themselves.
Therapist: yeah so you want them to remember you as someone who lived the life that they wanted to live for themselves.
Patient: right
Therapist: created a life of meaning.
Patient: I did what I wanted to do.
Therapist: Right and you did it fully?
Patient: um,
Therapist: as fully as you can?
Patient: I think so.
Therapist: yeah?
Patient: yeah
Therapist: okay, are there other things you wrote down that we didn't discuss
Patient: no, I think that was about it.
Therapist: okay, so there's some homework.
Patient: for 3?
Therapist: (laugh) this is an interesting exercise I think, do you find it interesting?
Patient: yeah
Therapist: so you've told me all these things about your family. Do other people know it? Like your girls? Your kids?
Patient: um, yeah I think that they know some of it. I'm not sure if they know all of it.
Therapist: so the homework is to really think about really whether you would like to share the stories that you told me. I think the story that you were conceived in the bed that your father built is that would embarrass them wouldn't it?
Patient: that probably would embarrass them, um
Therapist: I have a story, my grandfather on my mother's side died, about a year or 8 months later we had an unveiling of the headstone, and um my parents are survivors of the holocaust from Eastern Europe, and they were in a displaced person's camp after the war. And my father lived in the men's barracks, my mother lived in the women's barracks, and there was a man there whose name was Mr. (name) and he was butcher. And he had several digits on his hands missing because of the butchering.
Patient: butchering right
Therapist: and he was chatting with me, he was telling me all his ailments, because at the time I was a physician already. And he said to me, I said "These are very interesting stories, Mr. (name). He said "I have a story that I don't think you know." I said "What's that?" He said on the night that your parents were married in the displaced person's camp, your father lived in the men's barracks, your mother lived in the women's barracks and they didn't have a place to sleep on their wedding night, so my wife and I gave them our bed, so you owe me more than you realize.
Patient: (laugh) very interesting
Therapist: (laugh) so
Patient: yeah I actually had never thought about the fact that I was conceived on the bed that my father made.
Therapist: see it takes me (laugh)
Patient: really (laugh)
Therapist: it takes the warped brain of Dr. (name) to come up with that.
Patient: (laugh) um
Therapist: so think about whom would you share the story with you think? You have some grandkids too right?
Patient: I have one, she's young
Therapist: how old, 3?

Patient: she's, no, she's 18 months.
Therapist: ah you have to be 3 in your family.
Patient: In my family you have to be 3. Uh, but I do have a book for her.
Therapist: ah.
Patient: that I'm preparing.
Therapist: a book about your family?
Patient: yeah. It's a . . .
Therapist: is that going to be your legacy project?
Patient: yeah I think so.
Therapist: good
Patient: uh. I mean I've worked on it, but I haven't really been diligent about it, but um . . .
Therapist: and it might be really nice to do it simply, to make it less burdensome for you. To do in simply, almost like a children's book.
Patient: well it's a book, it's actually a . . .
Therapist: it's a children's book?
Patient: it's a children's book. It was ______ my AARP.
Therapist: ahh, so it's something . . .
Patient: it's about who I am
Therapist: ah ha. And can you put in there stuff about your great grandmother, grandmother?
Patient: yeah
Therapist: I love it
Patient: yeah
Therapist: okay, any last thoughts about today's session cause we're kind of coming to an end . . .
Patient: no, um
Therapist: was this interesting for you?
Patient: yeah
Therapist: you learned something?
Patient: well, yeah, I learned a lot actually. And I think there are things that you think about but until you actually say them they don't become concrete.
Therapist: that's what I was talking about.
Patient: right, and so it's ah
Therapist: until you say them or put them in some kind of form, you know concrete form . . .
Patient: to share
Therapist: mm hmm, share, right, that way you share.
Patient: right
Therapist: they live beyond you, just like the beauty of the furniture your father built, that crib especially.
Patient: oh, I was heartbroken when it was destroyed in the fire.
Therapist: but hey you remember it.
Patient: but yeah. It was . . .
Therapist: the fragility of life, everything is finite
Patient: yeah, everything has a time. So . . .
Therapist: but as long as you remember it and your kids remember it, it exists. So next week I think we're meeting at 9 I guess.
Patient: 9 right
Therapist: and the session is on encountering life's limitations. This one, this is about the fragility of life and the finiteness of life.
Patient: mm hmm
Therapist: we've been talking about that this week, and this is just a continuation of that.
Patient: (laugh) I'm looking at what you consider to be a good death. Closing your eyes and going to sleep (laugh).
Therapist: okay so we'll talk about that next week.
Patient: right
Therapist: Show up next week, don't let the topic scare you.
Patient: no no no. Thank you
Therapist: We'll see you next week
Patient: at 9 right.

Session 4: Attitudinal Sources of Meaning—Encountering Life's Limitations

Therapist: Okay, good morning
Patient: good morning
Therapist: so let me see, we've done 3 sessions, this is the 4th session. I guess this is mid-way, right?
Patient: right
Therapist: this is the middle session. And I just wanted to check-in to see how things have been going in general, with your health?
Patient: oh, um, its okay, this week was a little rough for me. But uh its I you know this was Mother's Day this week. So uh, one of the things that I do on Mother's Day is I go to the cemetary, and I visit all the graves, and there are many graves, and uh I clean the graves, and you know I prepare them. As I was sitting at the last grave, I did 7 that day, I was in the cemetary for about 4 hours, as I was cleaning the last grave I thought about Victor Frankl and how difficult it must have been for him to not have the peace to go to the cemetary to visit the graves of his mother and father and wife. And I just, you know, I just it struck me you know how important that is to me, me personally you know to connect with a, to have real meaning to connect with someone that you loved. And my husband and I often talk about it, that we think we're the last generation to go to cemetary cause I don't really see my daughters as embracing this you know uh. But the whole sentiment of honor thy father and mother really transcends life.
Therapist: hmm, interesting. So you're thinking that this tradition of going to the cemetary and

visiting the graves of some of your relatives—some of the people that we talked about last week right?

Patient: right

Therapist: your mother, your grandmother, your great grandmother, are they all buried in that cemetary?

Patient: well, my mother's alive.

Therapist: I'm sorry (laugh)

Patient: that's alright (laugh), but my you know my grandmother, my great grandmother, my father.

Therapist: Right and we were talking last week, the last session was about legacy right?

Patient: right, yeah

Therapist: so you're thinking a couple of things. One is you know Victor Frankl didn't have that

Patient: right, he . . .

Therapist: he didn't have that ability to do this in a physical, virtual way.

Patient: virtual way, right

Therapist: he didn't have a grave site to go visit.

Patient: yeah.

Therapist: um, you know my parents are also Holocaust survivors and one of the things that comforted my mother when my father died or when her parents died was at least her parents had a proper grave site and a headstone, so many people didn't right?

Patient: right

Therapist: but then you also mentioned you think you're the last generation maybe that would engage in ritual of actually going to the cemetary. And you think that, that saddens you or that?

Patient: yeah it saddens me, I a well . . .

Therapist: what does it mean to you that your kids may not do this?

Patient: I don't think they um, I think that they will find comfort in remembering me without having to go to the cemetary, which may be the way to really go. But it's still a tradition that I find great comfort in.

Therapist: so it may be that they may remember people in the same way that Frankl remembered them. In terms of memory and uh

Patient: yeah, not to have to physically go somewhere.

Therapist: not to have the physical representation.

Patient: I think it's more of a matter of not so much remembering the person that passed, but really the comfort the person finds by going to the cemetary.

Therapist: so you find some comfort?

Patient: oh yeah

Therapist: well, it's interesting the last session we had was about legacy, and legacy you inherited and the legacy you leave behind, things like that.

Patient: yeah

Therapist: uh and one of the things in the homework last week possibly was to share some stories. So did you go alone to the cemetary, or did you go with?

Patient: no I went alone

Therapist: you went alone

Patient: yeah. I um, I visit many graves, and my husband does not, well he wants me to hurry, you know

Therapist: so he waits in the car?

Patient: no he comes out, but you know its "Oh you've cleaned enough." I mean I really I have a trough, I have a rake, I really make it nice and presentable. And I take my time. You know, I don't rush. And I guess it's because I've always gone to the cemetary, I mean from when I was a child, I used to go. So this to me is you know, I don't know, I call, I saw I'm going to visit my relatives, because I actually have more relatives buried in the cemetary than alive in terms of aunts and uncles. For me it's a source of comfort.

Therapist: so when you're there you clean up those grave sites.

Patient: graves, right.

Therapist: do you say anything?

Patient: oh yeah you know kind of catch up.

Therapist: you tell them stories

Patient: I tell them stories, you know.

Therapist: of your life.

Patient: well you know what's happening. I say a prayer. I find that, I think they've prayed for me, so I thank them.

Therapist: you thank them for praying for you about, what your health?

Patient: yeah, yeah, um

Therapist: you tell them about your health.

Patient: oh I think they know. I think they were with me for the surgeries. Um, you know, so I remember them that way. You know, not that I want to join them (laugh); I'm okay where I am.

Therapist: I hear you

Patient: but I you know, I don't know is it mystical? I have a friend of mine who says to me that he wishes he has faith, because he just feels afterlife, that's it.

Therapist: and you have a different belief.

Patient: I have a different belief.

Therapist: yeah, your belief is what?

Patient: my belief is that you join your family. You know, that there is an afterlife.

Therapist: so there's a way to transcend death.

Patient: right

Therapist: and what helps you is what you believe

Patient: oh yeah. That my life isn't going to be, my physical life is going to be over, but my spiritual life will continue.

Therapist: you know one of the things that my mother did, mother and father did, which caused a little bit of conflict in my own family and marriage. Uh is my parents went ahead and bought cemetary plots for me and my wife and for my brother and his wife without consulting anyone. And of course my wife's parents had bought the cemetary plots for her, and so we could be buried in two different places.

Patient: places (laugh)

Therapist: we can be alternated, but has anything like that _____ with you. Is there a spot there for you?

Patient: oh yeah my grandmother one Christmas, she must have been I don't know 94; she died when she was 96. And one Christmas day at dinner she said to me "Listen" she said "I just want you to know that when I die I'm going to go in the (name) grave and there are 3 spots left, one is for (cousin name) which is a cousin, and the other two are for you and (husband's name). She said "Um, I want (husband's name) to be buried on top of grand-dad" which is my grandfather, and she said . . .

Therapist: is that how they do it in your family. Kind of stack them up?

Patient: yeah, stack, I guess its 9 graves, and um . . .

Therapist: several levels

Patient: several levels.

Therapist: like an apartment building.

Patient: like an apartment building. She said "I want you on top of me and I want (husband's name) on top of granddad."

Therapist: this is all underground?

Patient: this is all underground, yeah. So I said to (husband's name) "Wow," I said "Now that's a Christmas gift I never thought I'd get." (Laugh).

Therapist: it keeps on giving.

Patient: yeah (laugh)

Therapist: did you visit that site?

Patient: oh yeah

Therapist: did you look at that and go "hmm."

Patient: well, he said to me, but not last time cause he didn't come with me. But he has said to me "So where exactly am I going be?" And I said . . .

Therapist: this is (husband's name)?

Patient: my husband yeah, and I said "You're going to be on the left, and I'm in the middle." And he said "Good, because that means I'm not near your cousin (name)." Cause she'll be on the other side (laugh). I said "Yeah."

Therapist: but you had no preference of being on top

Patient: well, there were only . . .

Therapist: only one space

Patient: there's only one space. He doesn't have much of a choice, but uh

Therapist: well, it's really interesting this story and you probably know from the homework and from what we've discussed that this next session focuses on what are called attitudinal sources of meaning.

Patient: Mm-hmm

Therapist: and what's that all about really is that in life uh we suffer, we suffer. And there is some suffering that's clearly unavoidable

Patient: Mm-hmm

Therapist: and there's some suffering that's avoidable, right? And uh so if you've got pain or other physical symptoms, those are not, that's suffering that you don't need to endure, that can be avoidable, the pain medicines and things like that.

Patient: right

Therapist: there's suffering in which there are solutions. So there's no inherent value in the suffering necessarily, but in life we also encounter suffering that's unavailable. And they're a lot of different ways to understand what suffering means to people. I'd be curious what you what you think suffering is, how you define it? Or how you think of it. Frankl thought of it and a lot of other people who worked in the same sort of area of existential psychiatry, philosophy, really saw, really felt that suffering occurs anytime that you encounter any sort of limitation, you have this trajectory in your life, you're creating a life, that's one of your big responsibilities, our responsibilities to create a life of meaning, and identity, and direction, and for most of our lives that direction is forward and upwards. But when we encounter some kind of limitation in that trajectory, we suffer, its encountering a limitation, and the ultimate limitation is death. And so the ultimate suffering is anytime we think about the finiteness of our lives, the reality of the finiteness of our lives. There's really one certainty in life, and that's we live and then we die. What's uncertain is how long we live and what we do with our life, and the goal really is to live as fully as possible for as long as we have. To try to live that life with meaning and purpose and identity and love, and uh joy and those kinds of things, and heartbreak. And this idea from suffering, we derive meaning from not just from good things that happen but also bad things that happen. And in the I think the 2nd session where we talked about how cancer affected meaning in your life, uh or even in the first session when we talked about sources, you know of meaning in your life, meaningful moments in your life, some of them related to experiences that were quite tragic. The early death of your father, right?

Patient: Mm-hmm

Therapist: that resulted in a, in a in an adjustment in your family, an opportunity to be raised by some incredible women who taught you great life lessons of courage.

Patient: Mm-hmm

Therapist: um and so the challenge often is how do you overcome suffering how do you transcend suffering. If you can't transcend suffering, that can bring an added dimension of meaning in your life. Um, and you can really, one of the ways to do that is through the attitude that you take towards the suffering, and you actually highlighted an attitude another word for attitude is choice, what you choose to believe. For instance you know, so you were saying you know a friend who's not particularly religious and this and that, but you have faith, I don't know if you chose to have it, but that's the attitude that you have.

Patient: right

Therapist: and that helps you transcend the limitations of death, the attitude that you have. How would you describe suffering would you see it in similar terms, or is there more to it for you?

Patient: um, well, I think they are different degrees of suffering.

Therapist: different degrees

Patient: yeah, well I think there's physical pain

Therapist: Mm-hmm

Patient: um and as you said you know there's medication that can be treated, but I think there's also I think what medication really does it may lessen the experience of the pain, but anyone who really has a debilitating disease, you know may not feel the pain, but they're still suffering knowing that . . .

Therapist: cause they know what the pain means

Patient: means right

Therapist: the pain means something bad about their disease

Patient: yeah the physical being, so I think there's certainly um a physical element to suffering.

Therapist: and an emotional element of suffering from physical pain.

Patient: emotional . . . pain right. And I think that people who suffer alone uh who have no one to share what they're feeling

Therapist: yes

Patient: suffer even greater

Therapist: yeah

Patient: I think that when you have the ability to say to someone that you love or who you're close with, "I really don't feel well" or "I'm scared" that ability to share I think helps you deal with the suffering differently, you know . . .

Therapist: that's an excellent point. And if we go back to the various sources of meaning, uh the experiential sources of meaning through love, through the created sources of meaning, through the work that you do and who you care about, what you care about in the world. The historical sources of meaning, the legacy that you, the courage and perhaps the lessons, and the realization that the connection you have with generations pasts and generations in the future all three of those sources of meaning, what you're saying, is that all three of those sources of meaning can help you um when you're encountering the suffering of life's limitations, when you suffer because you're facing death. And those sources of meaning help you transcend uh the limitation of death and help you develop an attitude that uh comforts you and allows you to transcend death. So all those sources of meaning help you with this attitudinal source of meaning. Having the having the helpful attitude, being able to choose a way of viewing death that would be different if you really didn't have much in the way of those other sources of meaning.

Patient: right

Therapist: and so lots of times what happens is when you're ill and you get debilitated and you lose site of you become disconnected from these other sources of meaning, its helpful to reconnect with them, rediscover them, these other sources of meaning, so that you can utilize them in helping you transcend the ultimate limitation.

Patient: yeah I think it's really important that when you don't feel well that you share not feeling well as opposed to trying um to hide it or trying to spare the people that ... you know, I think you know, if you're having a bad day it's okay to say why you're having a bad day. So that when, so that when you have another bad day, you can say to yourself "Well it really isn't as bad as that other time" or "You know, this is a little worse." Or you know um, uh ...

Therapist: yeah

Patient: and I think it also helps the people that know you um I mean an example is yesterday I had terrible pains in my stomach, diarrhea just awful, I was at my daughter's house and she said to me "You're not feeling well?" and I said "No", and she said "It wasn't the food was it?" And I said "It was the medication." So she said uh ...

Therapist: did she make Mother's Day lunch ...

Patient: yeah, she made a Mother's Day dinner ...

Therapist: she was worried she might've poisoned you?

Patient: yeah (laugh). And so I said "No no no," and she said "Well, I have Imodium AD, do you want to take it?" And I said "Yeah, if you have it." So she, I didn't say anything, but we had spoken about how sometimes the medication backs up and sometimes I react to it, and she was sensitive to know what I needed. So that's why I said that I think it's important, um, maybe I share too much, I don't know.

Therapist: no, it's really interesting. So um one of the things that I wanted to ask you today is whether you shared your whole life story, the whole family story, uh with other people, and you can tell me whether you did or didn't.

Patient: Mm-hmm

Therapist: either with the living or the dead. I don't know ... (laugh)

Patient: (laugh)

Therapist: at the cemetary. But it certainly sounds like you share other, other stories; you share how you feel with a lot of other people.

Patient: yeah

Therapist: so you don't isolate yourself.

Patient: no

Therapist: you find it important to keep connected and relating to people you love. So you're focusing on experiential sources of meaning, but you're also, what's the word, you're also relying on the support of other people.

Patient: yeah I actually this it's a protecting myself from being isolated.

Therapist: yes, you're protecting ... that's what I really wanted to say, you're trying to protect yourself from being isolated.

Patient: right

Therapist: and uh to be part of, what you understand that you're connected in powerful ways to lots of people, especially you're immediate family.

Patient: yup

Therapist: and uh its, that's really what transcendence means. Transcendence doesn't necessarily mean going up and over, it's realizing that you're connected to lots of other people and something greater than yourself, and you rise above your own personal concerns and your connect with others. And it's almost like going around it or enveloping the thing that you fear.

Patient: yeah

Therapist: going lots of different directions. Did you actually share what we talked about last week with anybody about the family? Stories and the little of rituals of your family or especially around food, and soup was it? A lot of soup?

Patient: well they know the soup story, but I did talk to my husband about last week, and um uh and I said to him you know when you asked me about the origins of the my name?

Therapist: yeah

Patient: I said, sometimes I feel like I miss the most obvious things, you now um and of course I knew that I was named after my father, but I was really looking at the meaning of my name you know and how I always felt that it was so important as opposed to be named after my father and my grandmother.

Therapist: remind me of the meaning of your name.

Patient: noble

Therapist: noble

Patient: noble.

Therapist: I think they're both very important actually

Patient: So you know, um, and in terms of you know ...

Therapist: that's the impression I get from our sessions, you are quite a noble person.

Patient: Thank you. I'm glad I'm living up to my name.

Therapist: and how do you understand being noble?

Patient: um, forthright uh if I had to put it in a word I would say forthright.

Therapist: and what do you mean by forthright?

Patient: honest
Therapist: honest
Patient: yeah, honest, honest to yourself, honest with others. . . .
Therapist: authentic
Patient: authentic, right
Therapist: courageous?
Patient: yeah you keep saying courageous, I don't, no its not . . .
Therapist: do I keep saying that?
Patient: you do say, you've asked me if I'd define myself as being courageous, and um its not a . . .
Therapist: you relate more to humility?
Patient: well . . . I think honest, I mean . . .
Therapist: a realist
Patient: a realist, yeah, I'm definitely a realist.
Therapist: definitely a realist.
Patient: I don't sugarcoat, but I always look for the sweetness in something so, there's a . . .
Therapist: you don't sugarcoat, but you look for the sweetness . . .
Patient: in life right.
Therapist: cause there's usually something sweet.
Patient: there usually is something sweet, yeah
Therapist: there's a passage in the Frankl book where eh they're in the concentration camp and you know things are just so terrible, but uh in the evenings when the sun sets uh Frankl describes how even in the camp when they are able to enjoy the beauty of the sunset.
Patient: right
Therapist: even in that horror they are able to experience something sweet.
Patient: yeah, so that's what I would say, I don't sugarcoat but I . . .
Therapist: and that's an attitude
Patient: oh yeah
Therapist: that's an attitudinal source of meaning. The idea that you can choose to see things as being more complex and to see the possibility of something sweet or beautiful even in a difficult situation.
Patient: yeah I would say in terms of sharing . . .
Therapist: so you told your husband the story about that you had missed that about your father. And so what else did you say to him about it?
Patient: No, that I seemed to have done that a lot in my life where um the simplest explanation is usually the best, but I usually go for something beyond that. And sometimes I miss the simple explanation.
Therapist: and the simple explanation here being named after your father, what did that mean to you when you realized it?
Patient: oh well for my mother, I thought it was really you know to honor my father to name me after my father, and it turned out I did it with my second daughter, I named her (name) after her father. In fact he was convinced it was going to be a boy, she was going to be a boy, he wanted to name him (name) after my father not given the Italian name, but um we never discussed a girl's name, because for me there was no doubt that she would be named after her father. So I guess I was honoring the tradition in Italian families, you name the first child after the husband's father, so (name) . . .
Therapist: whether they're alive or not.
Patient: whether they're alive or not, right, and so (name) my first daughter was named after . . .
Therapist: (name)
Patient: well, no his name was (name), but we had an (name) and (husband's name) didn't want an Alexandra or an Alexis so we named her (name), and her name means "little faithful one." And (name) actually means "freedom." The derivative is really freedom from Francis. So um, I didn't think of it as I was actually following the tradition of naming children . . .
Therapist: yeah this honor thy father and mother is something that resonates in you very powerfully
Patient: yeah
Therapist: you've brought it up a few times. And I think, why do you think it's so powerful for you?
Patient: um, well, you know I never thought of things in terms of legacy, but I think part of it really is . . .
Therapist: it's help . . .
Patient: it's the acknowledgment of someone else's life.
Therapist: it's the acknowledgment of the continuum of your existence.
Patient: yeah, right
Therapist: the legacy you've inherited, it's it gives profound meaning of your life. That you are someone who has come from this family. And you've done with your life what you hoped that you could do with this life for a variety of reasons, but also to create um a legacy for the future for your child and perhaps your work.
Patient: and it terms of, other things have happened this past week that goes back to other sessions. And I actually met with two of my students that graduated almost 10 years ago from college, and they were thanking me for being so supportive to them. And uh I said to them "Do you realize" I said um "My work

with you and what you've done in terms of what you're doing with your own life is part of my legacy." I mean that's . . . I didn't tell them in great detail, but I said to them you know "We don't really realize how we impact other people's lives, but we do."

Therapist: we do

Patient: um and um

Therapist: that's part of your legacy too.

Patient: and they said to me "Well, thank you for choosing us." And I said "No, I didn't choose you, you actually chose to come into the program" I said "I sent letters. You took the initiative of responding to the letter. Had you not taken the initiative, none of the other things would've happened." And both girls are having difficult parts in their life for different reasons. And one of them was saying she thought she failed, she was in law school and she didn't finish and she flunked out of law school. And I said to her "(name) you really need to look at what really happened with law school. You went across the country" she went to California because she was getting the tuition. I said "You realized when you were first there, because you said it to me, that um you couldn't you were so lonely." I said "One of things you should consider is that law school failed you. In that it wasn't the place for you to be in California. You're a very bright, smart, intelligent woman; you told me the work wasn't hard." Um, and I said to her something that you know Frankl said directly or indirectly that "You have to find enjoyment in your life." I said "So forget about you know failing and that defined who you are now, and think about what you enjoy doing. And use that experience to build bridges to what you want to do. You know you're 31, you're not 90. And even at 90 you can do new things."

Therapist: transforming. Transformation is building bridges.

Patient: right, so uh yeah and then, so I have his book really, as I told you I take a lot of time reading the book, but its something I'm really enjoying.

Therapist: good. Did you take a peak at what we were going to do this week?

Patient: Yes, I did it. I did my homework.

Therapist: okay

Patient: so telling the story of my life, uh, um . . .

Therapist: we had talked a little bit about whether you shared that with anybody.

Patient: Yes, I did

Therapist: you did?

Patient: Yes, I did. I shared it with my husband.

Therapist: mm hmm

Patient: and I've shared, I really have shared this most of this with everyone that I know. You know, maybe I didn't think of it as, but I took great pride in what I did, in everything that I did. If I didn't it wouldn't have made sense to have done it.

Therapist: mm hmm

Patient: But what I wished to have accomplished, that was interesting.

Therapist: let's see here . . .

Patient: You know being a mother um uh I had two miscarriages before I had my daughters. So being a mother for me was really a gift of life, and how you shake that gift . . .

Therapist: so for instance, in the exercise last time it was, the legacy you inherited, and the legacy you live and the legacy you leave behind, and one of the questions was "What was one of the things you're most proud of?" and "What are one of things that you wished you might have done?" "How you would like to be remembered?"

Patient: Right and um certainly pursuing the PhD was important.

Therapist: so you were starting to talk about the miscarriages . . .

Patient: oh yeah when I had the two miscarriages back to back the fragility of life you know um was certainly um uh certainly heightened by awareness of how things can go wrong in a pregnancy.

Therapist: sure

Patient: and that not until you're actually holding that baby is you know do you have the baby actually.

Therapist: right

Patient: um, and so being a mother to me was always a very important role, and being a grandmother is different, but also important, because again its mentoring a child um . . .

Therapist: and it's a good example of how you're identity is so connected to what gives your life meaning.

Patient: yeah, and then of course pursuing the PhD. Um when I was a child, I struggled with reading. And for me I never really thought of myself as a good student. I always worked hard, but you know I always thought I could've worked harder. And to get the PhD was really a validation that the struggle I had with reading probably wasn't academic, it was probably emotional. Not addressed until after I was an adult. But it certainly gave me a compassion when I worked with students that had failed in college that you know the failure doesn't define who you are, its just what happened to you. And who you are is still something that you can create for yourself.

Therapist: that's correct

Patient: So for me the PhD was you know beyond a professional accomplishment.

Therapist: it was something you're very proud of.

Patient: yes, it was a personal accomplishment.

Therapist: and the thing that you're most proud of about it is you were able to accomplish it even though it was quite difficult.

Patient: No, what I'm most proud of is uh, I pursued it even though I was labeled as a child that had difficulty with reading and comprehension, so you know I kind of . . .

Therapist: you transcended the limitations

Patient: yeah (laugh), I immersed myself in the library.

Therapist: so there a lot of limitations you know we're talking about death as the ultimate limitation, but we're born into this world we have a certain genetic structure, and we have a certain body, and the brain, our IQ may be this or that, or we may have problems with dyslexia or this or that, or eye color may be brown instead of green or blue, or we're born into a specific family, in a specific town or city in a specific economic situation, and so those are the facts of our lives that we're born into, but as a human being we can create a life that isn't defined by those . . .

Patient: limitations, well, I don't know if it's defined as limitations. . . .

Therapist: those limitations that you . . . yeah

Patient: but um . . .

Therapist: you can transcend those limitations

Patient: and then of course the last thing I'm most proud of is my work at the college, you know the programs that I created that are still you know

Therapist: yeah

Patient: and how the kids that came into those programs how their lives, you know they've gone into social work, they've pursued PhDs, and these are inner-city kids who really thought they were coming to the college to be cops.

Therapist: right

Patient: you know, and I had them look at what did that mean for them, you know, so um . . .

Therapist: you helped them aspire to something perhaps more greater than they thought they could accomplish, and more true to what they wanted to accomplish.

Patient: right, so that for me, and then I looked at what I wished to accomplish

Therapist: Mm-hmm

Patient: um, and then uh, I took the uh NY state licensing exam for Psychology twice and I failed it, uh and uh, I wished I had taken it again to pass it, not so much that I wanted to practice, but I wanted . . .

Therapist: this is the clinical licensing exam for Psychologists?

Patient: Psychologist, right.

Therapist: was your PhD in clinical psychology?

Patient: No, it was, it's really in educational psychology

Therapist: and do they a specific exam for that?

Patient: well, it's the general . . .

Therapist: it's the same exam for clinical psychologists

Patient: right

Therapist: and what's involved? A lot of studying?

Patient: a lot of studying. I did it at a time when I was working and you know I really didn't . . .

Therapist: how close did you get?

Patient: oh, about 5 points.

Therapist: 5 points, not much.

Patient: no it wasn't much. But when I failed the second time, I said you know what I don't really want to practice, it was more why am I putting myself through this?

Therapist: why did you?

Patient: because I thought that when I retired it would be, I wanted to go into family practice. That's what I thought. And I particularly wanted to work with children who had difficulty in school.

Therapist: and that license would help.

Patient: and that license would help

Therapist: it would permit it.

Patient: yeah

Therapist: can you do it without the license?

Patient: probably

Therapist: You can? And is that something you would still like to do?

Patient: well, because I get disability I can't work

Therapist: ah

Patient: but I could volunteer

Therapist: that's not exactly true, because you're on disability you can't earn above a certain amount of money. You can earn a certain amount of money, but not above.

Patient: oh, I didn't know that.

Therapist: I think so

Patient: I thought we couldn't work, but anyway

Therapist: but you could volunteer
Patient: but I could volunteer, that has, but I'm really busy right now with (granddaughter's name), so uh, I can't, but it's something I could do in the future.
Therapist: so that's something you still have in your mind, that's something you could still do and still become.
Patient: oh yeah
Therapist: there's still time to become.
Patient: yeah, I don't, um, my uh my clock isn't that important to me anymore.
Therapist: your clock isn't that important to you anymore, explain that
Patient: my time left on earth.
Therapist: Mm-hmm
Patient: you know the ten years that I was told that I was going to have. You know, do I know that it's going to be 10 years? No, I jokingly said when I was first was diagnosed in trying to comfort people who were really upset that I had stage IV cancer. I said to them you know, "I know, I don't know anymore, I don't have any more information about the hour of my death now than I did before I was diagnosed."
Therapist: A lot of people think they do.
Patient: yeah well
Therapist: but you saw that as being still quite uncertain.
Patient: right, and it is
Therapist: and it is
Patient: you know, so I don't worry about uh . . . cause even filling out the questionnaire, there are some questions about . . .
Therapist: sure
Patient: are you concerned about your death?
Therapist: right
Patient: and the answer is no, I mean maybe if I was on my deathbed I'd be concerned about my death, but I'm not concerned right now you know. Um, I always wanted to learn French. When I was in high school my mother made me take Spanish because she thought it would be useful.
Therapist: and you know Spanish?
Patient: (laugh) I could tell you to open the window (laugh)
Therapist: right
Patient: that's about it.
Therapist: but you wanted to learn French, why? You wanted to travel in France?
Patient: I wanted to travel in France.
Therapist: and you wanted to have liked a French boyfriend?
Patient: no
Therapist: ah, no (laugh)
Patient: No, but I always wanted to learn French
Therapist: travel
Patient: yeah, I always wanted to learn French really
Therapist: to do what? You love, love . . .
Patient: I just thought the language was beautiful.
Therapist: because the language was beautiful
Patient: um, and I want to travel to Sicily.
Therapist: Sicily
Patient: uh, I want to see the town where my family came from . . .
Therapist: yeah
Patient: Pesaro. And I want to earn a degree in American History, I've always fascinated with that. So it was interesting cause when I did it I thought well, I'm not going to take the licensing exam cause it's really not that important. I mean I wish, take the licensing exam.
Therapist: right mm-hmm
Patient: But I actually can still learn French.
Therapist: Yes, you can.
Patient: and uh, I can take classes in American History.
Therapist: Yes
Patient: And I plan I plan
Therapist: you can go to Sicily.
Patient: I plan to go to Sicily for our 40th anniversary. Which is . . .
Therapist: Is it coming up soon?
Patient: No, 5 years from now
Therapist: but you have your 35th anniversary
Patient: Yeah
Therapist: did it just pass?
Patient: No, it's October.
Therapist: October, hey that sounds like a good trip
Patient: (laugh)
Therapist: what's so magical about the 40th?
Patient: um, nothing, it just gives me 5 years to plan on, to hold onto something that.
Therapist: Oh, I see, so it gives you something to hold onto.
Patient: Right, you know and if I say if I do it on my 40th anniversary then I'm not saying I'll be dead in 5 years.
Therapist: true, but then of course you could do that and then you could . . .
Patient: do something else
Therapist: yeah, the next time.
Patient: yeah, uh so that's what you know
Therapist: That was that was; you did a lot of thinking about the last the last session. So uh

today, we have about 15 minutes or so left, maybe a little more.

Patient: okay

Therapist: maybe we can do the exercise that focuses on limitations. And uh, having visited the cemetary and seeing your gravesite and all that, probably this is good timing to do this particular exercise. Uh, I think there are three questions huh?

Patient: right

Therapist: so the first question is what are some of life limitations and losses and obstacles you've faced in the past, and how you've managed to deal with them?

Patient: Well, you know um

Therapist: I guess these two are similar, right?

Patient: Right

Therapist: Are you still able to find despite ... okay this is the second question.

Patient: right

Therapist: Are you still able to find meaning in your life despite the awareness of the limitations and finiteness of life? And then, I think this is the most probably difficult one, What would you consider a good meaningful death? And how would you imagine being remembered by your loved ones? Want to take a few minutes to think about those? And you can spend more time on one than the other.

Patient: um, well, I think life's limitations, loses and obstacles ...

Therapist: you actually talked a little bit about that

Patient: I talked a lot about that

Therapist: yeah

Patient: um there's always another road.

Therapist: right, so you've encountered lots of limitations and obstacles in your life, from your father dying young to all sorts of other issues. What are some of the other big ones?

Patient: Um, well, certainly the diagnosis was an obstacle. Losses, my grandmother.

Therapist: yeah

Patient: great loss. At work, um, uh at work I should have left the college um I should've left the college after I completed my degree and gone somewhere else.

Therapist: To a different school?

Patient: To a different school. Uh, I really should've gone into, um I really should've pursued you know my field, which is educational psychology. Teaching it as opposed to teaching it part-time. And the obstacle I faced there was that um the administration really wasn't concerned with students and I knew it, but I stayed anyway. And then the administration changed and then it just went from bad to worse. I left; I left at a good point in my life, because I wasn't finding it fulfilling anymore, that particular place. But I've coped with everything just in terms of um looking at it as you know a new path for me to follow.

Therapist: so you took a particular attitude.

Patient: right

Therapist: you saw it as an opportunity not just an obstacle or a crisis.

Patient: right

Therapist: uh, crisis's are crossroads, a moment for uh a moment to make a choice.

Patient: choice yeah

Therapist: and so when you're stuck, when you're stuck you have to make a choice.

Patient: yes, and I've always relied on myself. I think one of the questions is "Are you in control of yourself?"

Therapist: right

Patient: the answer is "Yes." I make the decision, um, um, and ...

Therapist: And would you say that the like that you were talking about before you utilize some your support system

Patient: absolutely

Therapist: to make these decisions too, or no?

Patient: No

Therapist: No

Patient: No, I use them to maybe talk about why I've made a particular decision.

Therapist: you make a decision then you try to get a little bit of support for what you want to do.

Patient: right (laugh)

Therapist: that's good.

Patient: um, uh, and in terms of you know, well we've talked about the diagnosis. It's you know it is what it is; I have faith in the doctors and the treatment. And as I said to you before, because I've responded well, it's probably easier for me to have this view of cancer and the impact ...

Therapist: the attitude.

Patient: yeah. Uh you know I haven't gone through many of the debilitating issues revolving around cancer, uh ...

Therapist: I was thinking about you and what you've gone through with the cancer, and correct me if I'm getting this wrong but you've had this stereotactic brain radiation, not once, not twice ...

Patient: four times

Therapist: not three times, but four times, and you still view yourself as not having had any debilitating?

Patient: No, no I mean it was a procedure, they did it, I've responded to it.
Therapist: you weren't that ill during the thing?
Patient: No
Therapist: so it was almost like an abstract idea
Patient: yeah
Therapist: oh I have this, and they're just going to take care of it.
Patient: yeah. It's um, when I'm in that machine
Therapist: yeah?
Patient: I think of it really as their treating the body, but they're not treating the mind, and no um, I have the ability to um think about other things
Therapist: right
Patient: . . .while I'm in the machine, so its, in some ways it's not me, its or . . .
Therapist: right, I understand. You think about the situation you're in, uh, you control how you, you choose that way you want to think about what's going on in that machine. The treatment is affecting my brain, but not my mind.
Patient: Right
Therapist: Is that what you're trying to say?
Patient: yeah, yeah
Therapist: And what's central to this whole uh source of meaning the attitude you take towards a suffering experience, is the knowledge that no matter what's going on, that limits you or that you cannot control, not matter what the situation is. You always have that last vestige of control. In terms of how you think about what you're going through. You choose your attitude.
Patient: that's my . . .
Therapist: and that's what you did.
Patient: right, so when you asked me . . .
Therapist: in that stereotactic machine.
Patient: yeah, right, so when you asked me if I think of myself of courageous? I think of myself as I'm going through life. Are we, do we think of that as having great courage? I guess so, you know.
Therapist: ah, you're breaking down.
Patient: well . . .
Therapist: how is it courage in any way shape or form?
Patient: well, cause you're choosing to live as opposed to choosing to vegetate.
Therapist: Right, you know there's this poem that my mother loved by Rudyard Kipling called "If."
Patient: "If" yeah
Therapist: "If" you know that one. And you know, I don't know if that ran through your mind when you were getting that stereotactic brain radiation four times, but the first time is "If you can keep your head about your while all others around you are losing yours" you know that's what you try to do, you try to keep your head about you even though they were radiating you.
Patient: right you know so um so yeah, that's how I feel, and it terms of . . .
Therapist: so courage is the attitude
Patient: courage is the attitude yeah I guess courage is the attitude. That's good, courage is the attitude. Right it's not the act, it's the attitude.
Therapist: right
Patient: and in terms of a good and meaningful death, uh . . .
Therapist: what do you think about death? What are you feelings about it?
Patient: um
Therapist: how do you understand it?
Patient: well, I think of death as you know there a term about a "peaceful death" that you find.
Therapist: yes
Patient: There's no, it's not traumatic in terms of going from a physical to a spiritual life, I mean that's the way I interpret it, and so I have I have always told everyone how I've felt about them. So I don't feel that I need to say goodbye in a in a, well I don't say that now cause I may say that when I'm on my deathbed. I don't feel the compelling need to right all the wrongs.
Therapist: right
Patient: I've lived a good and honest life.
Therapist: right
Patient: If I'm angry with somebody I tell them I'm angry and I tell them why I'm angry, and then we talk about it and then we move on and that's it.
Therapist: forgive them
Patient: And that's it, right. Well, for the most part. Uh, ah, so when I think about you know a good or meaningful death I think of it more in terms of as a peaceful death, knowing that I've done everything that I could do. Now that doesn't mean I'm not uh I'm not dreading it to some extent.
Therapist: Mm-hmm
Patient: because I don't want to leave the people that I love.
Therapist: there's a sadness
Patient: but there's a sadness to it. And it terms of how people would remember me . . .
Therapist: so when you think about it, go to meaningful death, does it the main characteristic is that it would be peaceful.

Patient: right, yeah
Therapist: without a struggle.
Patient: without a, yeah I don't think I'll struggle. You know when its time I'll go. Um, I don't believe in extraordinary measures to keep oneself alive, and I've said that to them.
Therapist: Do you have some notion, idea of um where you want to die, under what circumstances; you want to die in your own bed, with family around you?
Patient: no
Therapist: you haven't thought that through that far?
Patient: I don't need to.
Therapist: so it would be okay to die in the hospital
Patient: yeah, you know maybe when it's more imminent I'll give it more thought.
Therapist: Uh-huh
Patient: but you know it's not something I think about nor dwell on
Therapist: right
Patient: and I would imagine that people will remember me for who I was you know, uh
Therapist: forthright?
Patient: Well, I hope they think of me as being fun, and you know, fun
Therapist: fun
Patient: and enjoyable.
Therapist: joyous.
Patient: yeah, and uh, you know um and I think they will, I mean I you know, um there's a saying you live each day as if it's your last.
Therapist: Mm-hmm
Patient: it's basically, when I go to bed at night I say my prayers and I thank god for giving me another day. And um, you know, and I think what this uh what this therapy has done is it's given me a consolidation of my ideas, they were very loose ah, I hadn't given it a lot of thought.
Therapist: it helped you consolidate, some of the lot of things you had been thinking about.
Patient: in a meaningful way. That you know um maybe I should work on a legacy project as opposed to.
Therapist: That's the thing to consider about the legacy project. I think that's your homework.
Patient: right, oh, is that my homework?
Therapist: yeah (laugh).
Patient: (laugh)
Therapist: so you're thinking maybe you should?
Patient: yeah you know that uh
Therapist: there's a line in that same poem "Let me dream, but let my dreams not be my only master pieces."
Patient: right
Therapist: in other words there's something very important about taking a thought and putting it into . . .
Patient: something concrete
Therapist: concrete, yeah
Patient: yeah, so, I think that's what . . . you know, so that's my homework.
Therapist: that's your homework. Let me see if we covered everything. Yes, okay, I think we covered everything.
Patient: great (laugh)
Therapist: so
Patient: well, this is good cause I'll have an extra week then
Therapist: you'll have an extra week, yes.
Patient: So
Therapist: do you have a sense of what that legacy project's going to be about?
Patient: um
Therapist: I know you don't have to have it all worked out
Patient: well I have an um, I thought I was going to do it for Mother's Day, but I didn't.
Therapist: Uh-huh
Patient: I was going to write letters.
Therapist: letters
Patient: to different people
Therapist: okay
Patient: about how I felt about them, and how I felt about them in relationship to me.
Therapist: and you might suggest to them, please visit me at the . . .
Patient: (laugh)
Therapist: don't be the last generation
Patient: it's funny because at one of the graves, my cousin on Saturday asked me, they looked at the headstone, and they looked at some numbers and they said to me, do you know what that means? There were two letters it was EE5762. And (name) said to me "Do you know what that means? Is that significant?" And I said "That's the plot number." And so I can put down "visit me" with the plot number (laugh). "See you soon."
Therapist: there you go. And just the last piece of business is that um you can take a peak maybe over the week to look at Session 5, which is creative sources of meaning.
Patient: okay
Therapist: you know, uh love is very important in all of this work.
Patient: Mm-hmm
Therapist: I find it interesting that the word "live" is basically um very similar to the word "love" but there's an "I" in it.

Patient: right

Therapist: so living is basically how "I" love, is how I spend my life loving. And, but creative sources of meaning is more a source, is related to that but its how, it's the life you've created for yourself and how that's given you meaning. And of course your relationships are part of that; it's a little bit more the experiential sources of meaning. You know ...

Patient: okay

Therapist: love is like, who do you love? And what do you love in the world? And the creative sources of meaning is what do you love in the world?

Patient: what do you love in the world?

Therapist: what's given you love from your engaging in life?

Patient: okay great

Therapist: Okay, so double check on the next time. So we're still going to meet next week?

Patient: Next week is, no we're not going to meet next week. Next week, today's the 9th right?

Therapist: oh, today's the 9th, we're not going to meet next week, we're going to meet on the 23rd.

Patient: The 23rd right

Therapist: okay very good

Patient: great, thanks

Therapist: thanks

Session 5: Creative Sources of Meaning—Engaging in Life: Creativity, Courage, and Responsibility

Therapist: So, how have you been?

Patient: good

Therapist: how have things been since last time?

Patient: good, I've been this legacy project a lot of thought, and ...

Therapist: have you thought of a legacy project?

Patient: well, um kind of, I have two things that I am working on. One is this book for my granddaughter.

Therapist: for my grandchild, a grandmother's gift of memory.

Patient: right, it's a, they're prompts in terms of one's life. Um, this by the way is my great grandmother she was the one who traveled from Italy to the US with her brother. So I'm putting together a book for my granddaughter so that she will have it.

Therapist: so this is a book, so she will know who her family was

Patient: yes, who her family was, and who her grandmother is um.

Therapist: this is an interesting one.

Patient: oh, that's our wedding picture

Therapist: this is you?

Patient: this is me, and my husband, his parents, and my grandmother, my mother and grandfather.

Therapist: wow, handsome people

Patient: yeah, so uh, I'm putting together you know different things that she would be able to know who I am. I started it with the thought that I might die before she really knew me. Because I had the privilege of knowing my grandmother and my great grandmother, and I have vivid memories, but not knowing whether or not she would actually remember me, I thought that would be a good way of of her knowing who I was. And then I stopped for a while, because I decided that maybe if I finish this little legacy project my work would be done and that would be it. So um, I stopped, I mean it was kind of interesting, but I'm continuing. And then the other thing that I got was uh this is a book again with prompts, and this is okay, but I think really my project is going to be more about, I'll use some of the prompts because they're good, but it's not ordered in the way that I would want to order it.

Therapist: Mm-hmm

Patient: you know, I thought about ordering it in decades

Therapist: and this is for your kids?

Patient: um this is for my kids, uh, I jokingly told a friend of mine about the project, and I said what I really want to do it to write everybody a letter, and so at my funeral there will be an envelope with their name on it and there'll be a letter from me to them telling them why they were so important to me, and uh and she said to me "Suppose somebody comes and there's not a letter for them, how are they going to feel?" I said so then I'll have a general letter about my life you know, what was important to me. I said but there some people that have touched me, and I felt that was important. I she said "Well, I don't know if you should do that." And then she told me a story. Her father was a seaman, and um he died in a boating accident off of Cape Cod, but his letter to his wife came two days after he died and she said it was a difficult thing for the family. So I'm still working on this, its coming together I think, but it's ...

Therapist: yeah, the good thing about a funeral is if you didn't do something right (laugh)

Patient: they couldn't complain.

Therapist: who are they going to complain to? You know so you might as well do it your way.

Patient: (laugh) yeah I'll see.

Therapist: and let the chips fall where they may.

Patient: you know, um

Therapist: what are they going to do to you?

Patient: well, nothing, I mean they could, I probably um . . .

Therapist: your intentions aren't to hurt anybody, your intentions is to thank people, or to say something meaningful to important people.

Patient: yeah, and so

Therapist: if somebody wasn't important enough to get a letter from you it wasn't your fault it was their fault.

Patient: (laugh) she said to me well what are you going to do if they die you know pre-decease. I said "Well, then I'll tear up their letter." You know.

Therapist: give it to their kids or something.

Patient: um, but I think that well I think one of the things we talked about last week is you know a good death. And um, I'd rather not think about it. I'll face it when I have to, but you know, you know a good death to be would be going to sleep and not waking up in the morning.

Therapist: that's a good death

Patient: that would be a good death. Um . . .

Therapist: painless

Patient: painless, right. But um, I don't think that's a reality so um.

Therapist: you don't think you'll be that lucky?

Patient: no. (laugh)

Therapist: you think you'll be more aware of it in a way.

Patient: yeah, yeah, I think it's harder to be aware and say goodbye, than to not to be aware you know.

Therapist: But even thinking about what you were planning to do at your funeral, thinking about your funeral, implies a level of awareness and a level of courage to prepare for that and face that and respond to it in a creative way.

Patient: right, you know I've already said to my family . . .

Therapist: By telling people how much you care for them

Patient: I don't want them to wake me, I don't want a wake. I just want to go to mass, and from the mass go to a burial. And my sister-in-law said to me "That's not fair to your family, the wake is really for them to be comforted." And I said "Well, they can decide not to abide by my wishes and not have a wake, but if you're asking me what I would prefer, this is what I would prefer." If they choose not to do that, and do something because it's more difficult for them to let me go that way. That's okay, but the truth of the matter is I'm gone at that point, so you know."

Therapist: it's interesting. So was your sister-in-law also the one who told you not to do the letters?

Patient: No no no, that was a friend.

Therapist: So you're friend and your sister-in-law are highlighting your responsibilities to other people.

Patient: right

Therapist: as opposed to your responsibility to live your life and have your life end the way that you want it.

Patient: right

Therapist: it's a dichotomy between caring for yourself and caring for others. And that's kind of interesting cause that's part of the focus of this particular session, the 5th session, where we talk about the created sources of meaning, we're going to talk about things like courage and caring and the life that you've created for yourself.

Patient: I like the idea of the letters, cause for me its personal it addresses not so much what I've accomplished, I think that's done in other things, but more about why they were so important to me.

Therapist: right, its consistent with what we've been talking about, these are people whose love and caring and who's relationship with you has been a tremendous source of meaning in your life. And you're trying to express gratitude I guess and highlight the importance, the meaningfulness of that relationship in your life.

Patient: yeah I think so.

Therapist: well, it sounds like you're making great progress

Patient: progress?

Therapist: in the legacy project. So just as a reminder, this is the 5th session we have gone through 4 sessions already right?

Patient: Mm-hmm

Therapist: If we were to go I think in the, where is it, in the front, oh yeah here we go. So if we go through the sessions, you know, we've done the first 4 sessions. Introducing the concepts of meaning, and sources of meaning and how cancer has affected meaning. And we talked a little bit about your legacy, the historical context of meaning, and meaning through encountering life's limitations, the ultimate being dying and death. And we have uh we actually have a few more sessions left. We have three more sessions left. Today's which focuses on creative sources of meaning, the next one, the 6th, which focuses on the experiential sources of meaning, and the last one where we kind of review everything. And if you remember the sources of meaning are you know the experiential, creative, uh historical, and attitudinal.

Patient: Mm-hmm

Therapist: we've kind of hit the historical and attitudinal sources of meaning, and we're going to focus the last couple of sessions on two really very primary uh sources of meaning, meaning through creativity, through your work, through the things you dedicate your life to, dedicating your life to someone something, you know basically care, caring, who you care for, what you care for. So there are kind of two aspects of these creative sources of meaning. One is we talked in the beginning, I think the very first session, as a human being you have a responsibility to create a life of meaning, and identity, and direction, self-transcendence, understanding, which you need to give to other, you achieve the most in you life by giving and caring for others. Self-actualization that you become who you are by the act of giving to others. So uh this exercise focuses on that whole basic statement, so for most people creative sources of meaning really relate to their work. You know work is the primary way they think about creative sources of meaning. But creative sources of meaning also come not only from the work that you do to make a living, but what you do in your life in terms of how you engage in the world. You know who you care about and what you care in the world, the courage it takes to create a life despite the vulnerabilities, the risks, the obstacles, the tornadoes that can happen in life.

Patient: yeah

Therapist: you know it takes some courage to get out there every day and try to live a life in the world.

Patient: Mm-hmm

Therapist: and also this notion of responsibility. What do you mean that I have a responsibility to live a life? And responsibility, whenever I get a chance I try to play word games that really reveal the true meaning of words. Responsibility's not just you know I have a responsibility to do this, I have a responsibility to do that, but it's really more my ability I respond to being alive, how do I respond to being alive? By creating a life, a life of meaning, a life of caring.

Patient: Mm-hmm

Therapist: right, and so we talked about identity, we talked about sources of meaning. This is going to be uh more of what is my responsibility, how do I respond to being alive by creating a life of caring, a life that involves courage and commitment to something. My life's work or things I care about in the world. So one of the subtitles for the session, I think is "connecting with the world?" "Connecting with life." So creative source of meaning is actively, I'm sorry "engaging in life."

Patient: Oh, actively engaging in life.

Therapist: Not connecting, but engaging in life. Through getting in there, engaging, encountering life, and trying to create a life. And I think there are two exercises that we have for today. Actually there are three. How many do you have in there?

Patient: This one? There are 4.

Therapist: you have four, okay.

Patient: right

Therapist: We might cut it down, we'll see.

Patient: okay

Therapist: so the first one involves courage and commitment to live a life

Patient: Mm-hmm

Therapist: so the first exercise, do you have the same one?

Patient: right

Therapist: living life and being creative requires courage and commitment. Can you think of times in your life when you've been courageous, taken ownership of your life, made a meaningful commitment to something of value to you?

Patient: oh well

Therapist: you already wrote it down.

Patient: yeah, I do my homework

Therapist: you do your homework.

Patient: (laugh) my life's work at the college was really my commitment to helping students develop their own potential in every aspects of their lives. All the programs I developed, I mean that sounds very altruistic. But there's a feeling that I've always had, that I was taking care of me by taking care of them. So I knew, when I went to John Jay I came from a private boarding school, an all girl's boarding school, and I went into this large public college, which wasn't large, but I thought it was large. And I realized how lonely it was, and I'm outgoing, so I can go into a room with strangers and kind of introduce myself, but it takes a lot of effort to do that, and it dawned on me maybe because I was in a small Catholic girls' boarding school, but it dawned on me very early on that people walk into a room and they don't introduce themselves to each other. And so you can sit 15 weeks, 4 years in a classroom with other people and never know who they are. Everything I did at the college I did from my own experience of being a student. I knew what it was like to be lonely. I understood how difficult it was to connect to professors. So I developed a mentoring relationship program. Honestly, it was very satisfying. I look back and say I did a good job. So I, and the other things that I wrote, beyond the program development, I took ownership of my life when I was 34 when I decided to pursue a PhD, I had been at the college for 17 years and I went into a friends' office and I said to him "Do you know I'm 34 and I've spent half of my life here. There's gotta be more to live than this. There's just gotta be something else for me to be doing." And so I took the work I was doing at the college and decided uh, I had finished the master's degree at CUNY, and decided that I needed to do something else. So I went home, and I don't know if it's a product of being an only child, but my major life decisions aren't something I've discussed with anybody in terms of this is what I'm planning on doing. Its more of this is what I've decided to do and I just want to let you know that this is where I'm going. So uh, I guess it's being self-assured. But eh, and I went home and said to my husband, I'm going to go on for a PhD.

Therapist: You were creating your own life, your unique life; you were going your own path.

Patient: my own path. Um, so I would say . . .

Therapist: and it took some courage to do that?

Patient: Oh, yeah, it took a lot of courage to do that.

Therapist: because what were the obstacles.

Patient: well, I had two young children at home, we had just bought a house in the country, a country home, money was tight, and it was you know I've given a lot of thought to buying the house, and buying cars, and I've done that, and here I want to do something for myself, and I'm going to do it.

Therapist: you wanted to invest in yourself.

Patient: right, and so that took a lot of courage. Um, but I also had a lot of support in that decision. It wasn't like I was doing it in isolation. And then . . .

Therapist: and it took a lot of commitment to get this PhD.

Patient: oh yeah, I mean I was sleeping; I was sleeping four hours a night. I was going to bed at 11 o'clock at night and getting up at 2 in the morning, working from 2 to 6 on school work, going to work working full-time, because my rule was that when I came home from class, I couldn't do anything until the children were asleep. And I couldn't give up Saturdays for them, and Sundays we used to have a study hall day and we would all sit around the table and we'd be preparing for the next work. So I engaged them in the process of you know, we're going to be doing this together, but we're actually going to be doing our own work.

Therapist: Just you and the kids?

Patient: Yes, me and the kids. So it was it was vigorous.

Therapist: that's an incredible example of courage and commitment.

Patient: yeah um, and . . .

Therapist: something that was valuable to you.

Patient: yeah, and it was . . .

Therapist: Did it turn out to be valuable?

Patient: oh yeah, mm-hmm, yeah

Therapist: what did it allow you to do?

Patient: oh, I I, I really wrote a lot of grants.

Therapist: So you entered the grant writing

Patient: I entered the grant writing. I became a middle states evaluator. I taught my daughter, who entered into teaching, I taught her at Fordham, I was her first professor in graduate school. And I had a lot of; I had a lot of . . .

Therapist: A lot of stories she'll have for her kids

Patient: I was anxious about doing it, cause I didn't know whether it was ethical. And uh, I went to the . . .

Therapist: Well of course the grade you gave her had to be . . .

Patient: Oh, I did blind review and I had somebody else um . . .

Therapist: grade her?

Patient: No, I had somebody else enter the information so I really didn't know whose number was who. And I had somebody else read them with me so that . . .

Therapist: what grade did she get?

Patient: She got an A

Therapist: (laugh)

Patient: (laugh). Um, but then most of them, they did a lot of work. And you know grading I think for me is more are they able to demonstrate that they learned something and it was meaningful and did they complete it in a professional way. So really I was probably an easy grader, but you know, it wasn't about, there was a standard that they had to meet and if they met the standard I didn't care how many "A"s I gave. Because each A is individual to that individual, it's not a collective group. So that for me was meaningful. And uh, in the second one, do I feel that I've expressed the most meaningful . . . yeah, I think that . . .

Therapist: what was it?

Patient: do you feel you've expressed what is most meaningful to you through your life's work and creative activities?

Therapist: so that's the one I don't have, but go ahead, that's okay.

Patient: oh, my job, yes you know certainly. I crochet, and so um I think that it's important to give someone that you love something that you've made, and I've done that to all of my friends who have played an important role in my life.

Therapist: it's like that letter

Patient: like the letter, right

Therapist: so you crocheted things and give them to people who you care about.

Patient: right

Therapist: who you have important relationships with you or have done something. What do you crochet?

Patient: blankets, scarves

Therapist: blanket, scarves

Patient: Yeah in fact the one that came to mind, the woman that I met at John Jay who knew Dr., well actually she didn't know him, she knew, she worked at Sloan for many years and she made the contact for me to get into Sloan. And she was leaving the college and I crocheted her a scarf of with uh beig and rose and I said to her the significance of the beig was there was a purity of who she was, she was very nostalgic, she shared a lot of her history with me, and though we didn't share nationality, you know we didn't share nationality or religion, there was a bond that I felt, kind of a maternal bond, and that was what the white signified to me was that kind of maternal bond that we had. And the rose we that um she was always hopeful, you know she always told me you know just go through it you will be fine. And she shared with me her cancer journey. And when it turned out that she was leaving, and I didn't realize that she was leaving I had made the scarf for her. But I sent it to her, and um there was a section where it was purely beig and then there was a section where it was purely rose, and then there was the blending of the two colors. And I said to her the blending of the two colors was significant for me cause it meant the blending of our lives.

Therapist: that's beautiful

Patient: (laugh) so actually you know what this has done for me this whole session, is it's there's a thread I see in my life that I knew was there but I was never really aware of it in terms of sharing what I've done with others and sharing the meaning, the significance that it has for me has made this be a very interesting endeavor.

Therapist: yeah, and by sharing a little bit more what do you mean by that?

Patient: um, I don't think that we do things haphazardly, there's meaning behind what we do, but it's not significant unless we share why we've done it.

Therapist: Mm-hmm

Patient: so for example, my daughter and son-in-law just celebrated their 4th anniversary, and I wanted to give them something from the baby to celebrate their 4th anniversary, and so I gave them geraniums.

Therapist: geraniums

Patient: geraniums, and I explained in the card that the geranium is the flower for the 4th anniversary, and the significance of the geranium is that it gives comfort, it gives one comfort, and there's a there's a, well its comfort and patience.

Therapist: patience

Patient: and I said and both of those things we need in a marriage.

Therapist: right

Patient: So I've always tried to not only give a gift, but there has to be a reason behind why I'm giving you that gift. Otherwise . . .

Therapist: even the scarf, the colors you chose, the geranium, all that there's meaning behind the gift . . .

Patient: yes, there's a significance for me

Therapist: Yeah, there's a message in it.

Patient: right

Therapist: there's a message of love and caring and wisdom.
Patient: yeah, I guess so.
Therapist: There's a thread of wisdom of things that you've learned of value, and one of the things I think you've learned of value is sharing and caring and the realization that you're so connected to not just your family, but a lot of people.
Patient: a lot of people
Therapist: most people
Patient: a lot of people, yeah
Therapist: yeah
Patient: Um, and my responsibilities
Therapist: yeah who are you responsible to, and for and whatever.
Patient: and for. Certainly I'm responsible um; I'll do responsible for first cause I think that's . . .
Therapist: okay
Patient: I'm responsible for myself
Therapist: yeah, you got it!
Patient: that's who I'm responsible for.
Therapist: you got it, you got the insight.
Patient: (laugh) and who I'm responsible to is you know to my mother, to my daughters, to my granddaughter, to my family, to my friends, to society you know um . . .
Therapist: so that's really interesting, you've delineated responsibility for and to and for is yourself
Patient: right
Therapist: and it's only if you take responsibility for yourself that you can then . . .
Patient: be responsible to others.
Therapist: be responsible to others.
Patient: right yeah, and its something I haven't given a lot of thought to but . . .
Therapist: when you thought about the comments you got about the cards, or the comments that you got about something else . . .
Patient: oh my funeral.
Therapist: the sister-in-law said something
Patient: right
Therapist: what did your sister-in-law say?
Patient: oh, she said that I couldn't it would be selfish of me to not have wake.
Therapist: wake
Patient: right
Therapist: so you didn't particular feel responsible for making them happy about it.
Patient: right you know, and it was really, so I'm responsible for myself for my actions for what I think.
Therapist: and for creating your own life.
Patient: and for creating my own life.
Therapist: and the responsibility to, tell me the distinction there
Patient: Um, I'm responsible uh to others to be honest and truthful to be and I distinguish between honest and truthful in that the honesty is really more about my response to them how I feel about them, so I have to be genuine about you know if I'm happy or I'm unhappy, if I approve or disapprove. I'm responsible to tell them how I feel about something that they've presented or their doing. It's my responsibility to them, whether they like it or not that's for them to decide, but I I need to tell them how I feel about something and truthful uh uh I'm trying to think of an example where honesty and truthfulness may not always be similar, um . . .
Therapist: you're talking about honesty in the way you respond to them.
Patient: right
Therapist: in an authentic way. Truthful often has to do with the actually words you use . . .
Patient: I chose, right
Therapist: You chose to express yourself.
Patient: right, so I yeah . . .
Therapist: and some truths are very harsh, is that what you're trying to say?
Patient: You have to temper things sometimes.
Therapist: Mm-hmm
Patient: you know and um, and I think that's my, um I think that's what I was thinking of. I feel responsible to love them if I you know, and to do the things that I think express that love. Um, ah I had a friend of mine, well actually it was my mother's friend who was dying of cancer and my mother just couldn't bring herself to see him, and one day she said to me "He died." And I said "Well, ma, he told you 18 months ago he was dying, when did you think you were going to see him?" And she said "Well, I just didn't think he would go so fast." And I said okay well "I understand that it was hard for you to go see him, but if you really wanted to go to see him, you would've." So um, I tried to say it in a way that I wasn't going to make her feel bad, but I mean you can't postpone something cause you're not able to do it, sometimes you just have to suck it up and do it.
Therapist: yeah. It was hard for your mother and she didn't realize it perhaps how hard it was.
Patient: Yeah well, my mother doesn't take anybody's death well, she's always surprised.
Therapist: she's had a lot of losses
Patient: she's had a lot of loss, right. And to my husband, who's been just a terrific life partner

its my responsibility to him is not to allow his physical difficulties to um to invade the possibilities of what he can do, and so I have to try to keep him back up. That I feel really responsible for, I can't allow him to just wallow in kind of self-pity you know.

Therapist: That might be one of those cases where you've made a lifetime commitment of a life with someone and the idea of being responsible for yourself kind of extends to him too cause you're partners, in some couples you know you don't know when one ends and then other begins.

Patient: right

Therapist: that's sometimes how I feel about my son, I don't know where I stop and he starts.

Patient: he begins, yeah (laugh)

Therapist: Is it a little bit of that?

Patient: yeah yeah, um, and uh I think that's really my responsibilities.

Therapist: that was incredible, that was great.

Patient: and uh unfinished business, tasks I want to do, undertake, um, well I've always wanted to learn French, basically because I wasn't allowed to take French in high school, I had to take Spanish.

Therapist: they forced you?

Patient: No, my mother told me that I needed Spanish in the world.

Therapist: She was a utilitarian person in the world, she was practical, she looked at the demographics in New York, and said Spanish/French I think Spanish will be more useful.

Patient: right (laugh)

Therapist: but French was more appealing to you in some other way, and what way was that?

Patient: yes, uh, I well, I've always been a student of history

Therapist: student of history

Patient: and so French just their sense of independence, their social commitment to each other, I don't know there's a saint Our Lady of Lourdes is in . . .

Therapist: oh, let me see, there's a saint?

Patient: There's a saint, Saint Bernadette.

Therapist: Saint Bernadette, and there's a place called Lourdes . . .

Patient: Lourdes, in France

Therapist: in France

Patient: and so as a child I was always very devoted to Our Lady of Lourdes and Saint Bernadette, in fact my confirmation name is Bernadette and so I always felt . . .

Therapist: I see, and is that how you got so committed to that cause of your confirmation name or you chose that name?

Patient: I chose that name, um . . .

Therapist: something about that attracted you?

Patient: something about her, she was a peasant girl, just an ordinary child, and she lived an extraordinary life.

Therapist: what did she do with her life, I don't know the story?

Patient: well, she became a sister in a French order, and she did a lot of good works. And uh she devoted her life to God. And I thought that to learn her language would be to honor her.

Therapist: I see

Patient: It's something I . . .

Therapist: Have you ever visited Lourdes?

Patient: No, it's something else I want to do.

Therapist: Is that something you want to do?

Patient: Yeah

Therapist: now my understanding of . . . is you wrote that down?

Patient: I wrote that down

Therapist: what did you write?

Patient: I wrote down to learn French and visit Lourdes.

Therapist: Okay, my understanding of Lourdes is a place where people go for contemplation, and prayer and . . .

Patient: and miracles

Therapist: miracles.

Patient: right

Therapist: really related to I guess also some things about health especially.

Patient: health right

Therapist: Is it exclusively for health?

Patient: Well, it's for mental conditions, it's for . . .

Therapist: love?

Patient: it's for love, yeah.

Therapist: Please bring back this love . . .

Patient: yeah

Therapist: It's for health, so you want to go to Lourdes?

Patient: But I don't want to go to Lourdes for health.

Therapist: why do you want to go?

Patient: I just want to go because um I'd like to go to the place where she was.

Therapist: it's more a devotion to her.

Patient: It's more of a devotion, well to the blessed mother. Right, so that's why faith for me is very important.

Therapist: Faith

Patient: and in terms of miracles I feel that I am a miracle, I'm here.

Therapist: it's already happened

Patient: It's already happened.

Therapist: Your miracle has already happened. In that you're here . . .
Patient: I'm here, I have good quality of life, I've lived to see my granddaughter born and I don't worry about dying.
Therapist: You don't fear death?
Patient: No, I don't think, it's nothing to fear, it's a natural progression.
Therapist: Do you feel you have unfinished business?
Patient: Unfinished business, I'm sure there's unfinished business
Therapist: there always is.
Patient: I just don't you know, is there something um is there is a burning desire for me to do something? The answer would be just to be with my granddaughter and see my children. Enjoy what my grandmother enjoyed in terms of a long life.
Therapist: Your grandmother enjoyed a long life?
Patient: She was 96 when she died.
Therapist: 96, that's a long life.
Patient: that's a long life.
Therapist: And did she have all the miracles and blessings you have?
Patient: yes
Therapist: She had a loving family
Patient: She had a loving family, she had good health, she was strong . . .
Therapist: She overcame a lot of obstacles and had courage and commitment like you?
Patient: yeah she was a widow at a very young age
Therapist: Is her confirmation name Saint Ber . . .
Patient: No, her name was (grandmother's name).
Therapist: (grandmother's name)
Patient: (grandmother's name), that's my middle name.
Therapist: that's the Virgin Mary.
Patient: That's the Virgin Mary right
Therapist: that's what you meant by the Holy Mother.
Patient: So yeah, I um, and the other things that I, and so time is the obstacle for me, but that isn't really an obstacle cause you can do things you know you can make time, it's just a matter of just doing it.
Therapist: Do you think you'll get to Lourdes?
Patient: Yes
Therapist: do you have the ticket already?
Patient: No, I want to learn French first
Therapist: really?
Patient: I want to be able . . .
Therapist: Don't you think you'll be able to learn French a lot quicker in France on the trip?
Patient: Probably, but you know I was in Greece for 3 weeks and I never learned . . .
Therapist: You didn't learn Greek?
Patient: No, so I think . . .
Therapist: You probably learned how to order food in Greek
Patient: No, I had a friend who was Greek, she ordered for me. But uh, I just . . .
Therapist: Does anyone want to go with you; do you want anyone to go with you to Lourdes?
Patient: My husband
Therapist: Mm-hmm. Does he speak French?
Patient: No
Therapist: Spanish?
Patient: No
Therapist: Italian
Patient: A little, not much
Therapist: Do you speak Italian?
Patient: No, I took it in college, but I'm not really fluent. I understand it more than I can speak it.
Therapist: So really it is a big precondition that you learn French before you do this?
Patient: No, it's just something I'd like to do.
Therapist: It's just a . . .?
Patient: Something I'd like to do.
Therapist: Sounds like a plan
Patient: And I don't have . . .
Therapist: Please don't go to Lourdes before we finish our sessions.
Patient: No (laugh), no, I won't be going for a while. And uh that's, does it sound strange that I don't have any unfinished business?
Therapist: No, it's not strange at all. It sounds like you've been doing what you want to be doing and you've pursued things you've wanted to do.
Patient: yeah
Therapist: and you gave all the people that deserved crocheted things crocheted things.
Patient: yeah
Therapist: and it sounds like you tell people who you love that you love them all the time.
Patient: yeah I do.
Therapist: and you're right, nothing's ever completely finished in our life.
Patient: No, you know, um, it was funny cause when I left the college I threw out all my, I didn't throw out all, I threw out a lot of my professional books and publications and I got a letter from middle states and they asked me to serve on a committee in September. And this is the first time I'm doing something of my training in 3 years.

Therapist: Well, it's been a great session. I want to give you a sense of what's coming up.

Patient: okay

Therapist: the next week, we're focusing on experiential sources of meaning. Uh, meaning through connecting with life, and basically through experiencing life, and we experience the world and life through all of our senses. You know, through our eyesight, our smell, touch, taste, hearing, uh you name it. And for most people the most important source of love, experiential source of meaning is love, people we love, but there are other experienced in life that are profoundly meaningful and joyous, music, humor, beauty, food, gardening, whatever it is.

Patient: right

Therapist: Uh and so next session we'll focus on experiential sources of meaning. And I think there's a little exercise that you can.

Patient: This one?

Therapist: Yeah the homework, and you can look at that again like you do, you're good with the homework. And I think our next meeting is something like . . .

Patient: I think its Monday. Oh no, it's not, its June 6th.

Therapist: So we'll see each other next week at . . .

Patient: 8?

Therapist: at 8, I'll make sure to set the alarm.

Patient: okay (laugh)

Therapist: Thank you

Patient: Thank you

Therapist: I'll see you then.

Session 6: Experiential Sources of Meaning—Connecting with Life Through Love, Beauty, and Humor

Therapist: So this is session 6, good morning.

Patient: Good morning.

Therapist: So we had a little break, we had Memorial Day weekend or something. Did you do something, did you go away?

Patient: oh yeah, we have a house in Newburgh. And uh uh my sister-in-law and brother-in-law and one of my daughters came up. So we spent a nice weekend together, you know it was lovely, we sat around, and talked.

Therapist: and how long were you up there?

Patient: About 4 days.

Therapist: and how are things medically?

Patient: um, fine, I uh, I'll go to the doctor next Tuesday. And uh I assume then I will start the next round of CTs and PET scans, and whatever else comes about. So it's like a holding pattern until you go through it and find out that you're okay and then you move on.

Therapist: yeah

Patient: But I don't have any physical difficulties.

Therapist: symptoms, okay, so do you remember session five? And I see that you did your homework for this session.

Patient: I did do my homework. Do I remember session five?

Therapist: Do you remember session five when we were talking about creative sources of meaning, through the life that you created, and the job?

Patient: Well, it actually. I started to work on the legacy; I really have been working on the legacy project

Therapist: you have been?

Patient: Yes, for the last week and a half. And uh really full steam. I spend almost every day doing something on it. What's interesting is I was kind of stuck on the first decade of my life.

Therapist: remind me of what your legacy project was going to be.

Patient: Oh, it's a well it's really a three part project I think.

Therapist: it's a how many part?

Patient: 3 parts

Therapist: 3 parter.

Patient: basically because it seemed to me to be overwhelming just to do one.

Therapist: exactly

Patient: And so the first part was to look at my family history, and to write about the family history. Stories that were told me about how my family migrated from Italy to the US, and then the life they created once they were here. So I have been taking out old photos so that I could include in the legacy of the family. And not to isolate my husband from this project, I've taken on the legacy of his family.

Therapist: You've included both families.

Patient: So that my children have the sense of who the family, what the family did when they came here. And the life that they created, and how subsequent generations have built in that life you know. And yet the values, I mean its interesting the values, there's a thread of values that you can see throughout the whole I guess last 120 years that I've known about. So it's kind of an interesting endeavor.

Therapist: Yeah, in terms of sources of meaning, when you talk about creative sources of meaning, the session from last time, sort of the life that you create part of the life that you create involves, not only do you have the historical facts of where you came from, your legacy and what you leave behind, but uh when you create a life you create not only an identity, but you also create a set of values.

Patient: right

Therapist: and you also, these values are important because they're sort of the markers, standards by which you evaluate your life and how much you have been able to live up to those values. So it results in a sense of self esteem

Patient: yeah

Therapist: which uh which uh is an important source of meaning having some self esteem. And uh, does that make sense in terms of what you were thinking too?

Patient: well, it's a very reflective process

Therapist: yes

Patient: you know, particularly when you look at the life span of the pictures you know.

Therapist: right

Patient: so it's a and I was talking to my daughter about it yesterday at lunch. I was looking at pictures of my great grandmother and I thought all that she did when she was 20 you know, she migrated to the US, she got married, she had her first child when she was 21, the second one at 23, the third one at 26, and then by 36 she was a widow.

Therapist: hmm

Patient: and it was beginning of the depression. Well, no actually it was the market crash, she had 3 children, and she had a house and a business. And she had the secure the safety of her children and herself, and my daughter said to me, she said, there was no social um network, no social programs that would have supported her and so . . .

Therapist: safety net, no social safety net.

Patient: So she had to do that, and I said well I guess, and she said well if that happened now she would've gone on welfare. And I guess there's something to be said to that, but I'm really focusing on how strong she was in character to you know like muster up whatever she needed to do.

Therapist: well, certainly there were people in that time that . . .

Patient: family.

Therapist: who failed, and people who couldn't succeed, and couldn't endure the situation and lost their businesses, and you know lived on the street, lived in Central Park, or . . .

Patient: So there's a pride that is associated with that. You know

Therapist: Absolutely.

Patient: and I was saying to my daughter (name) there's a sense of history that we have to impart, you know, I have to impart to you and you have to your daughter and to future generations, so that the uniqueness of their lives isn't lost.

Therapist: right, so there's a value that you were trying to convey in what your grandmother did when as a 36 year old widow with three kids and a business on a verge of a depression. She had to find a way to survive, there was some sort of value you were trying to convey it was a matter of pride and courage and perseverance, and taking care of your family.

Patient: yeah you take care of your family you know and you do what you need to do, and you don't focus on difficulties that you encounter you know you.

Therapist: giving up is not a choice.

Patient: so that's the first part of the legacy project. The second part is really about my life, and so um, uh not to get bored and not to get stuck I um focus on different things, different days, and I I didn't really think much about my first decade of life, I mean I didn't give it a lot of thought . . .

Therapist: right

Patient: until I started to write about it. And then it's taken me a long time. I'm not really quite, I'm at the end of 63, but it's not really to a place where I can say I can move onto the next decade.

Therapist: How do you mean, you feel like you're pretty young still?

Patient: No no no, in thinking about what my childhood was like, and all the meaningful things.

Therapist: Oh, I see, you're still writing about that decade

Patient: yeah

Therapist: and you haven't quite finished with the . . .

Patient: cause I didn't realize how important it was.

Therapist: That's interesting, and what made it so important do you think?

Patient: Well, kind of um, why did it make it so important?

Therapist: It was a time in which you were so closely linked to the past generation wasn't it?

Patient: yeah, um, I think it was the value, I mean I really didn't . . .

Therapist: it's where you learned all your values.

Patient: It's where I really learned all my values, you know that I can look back now and say I guess this is true for many people that lived during the 50s and 60s, there was kind of an innocence during that time where I didn't need any gadgets, it was about social interaction, it was about the joys of playing, and you know simple little things that we would do as kids, you know go to mass on Sunday morning. I had a block, and on the block there were about 30 kids and we were like a family on that block. Um, and so we I learned at that point not only to, I learned independence, I was allowed to be independent even as a child in terms of going out in the morning, and who's house I was going to go visit and what we were going to do for the day. Yeah I checked in, but I always felt safe, I think that was the other thing, I always felt safe, and when you feel safe I think that builds your self-assuredness.

Therapist: yeah

Patient: So it was um, you know . . .

Therapist: We all need a safe place, and often it's back in a place when we were younger.

Patient: Yeah, and the other thing that happened, is my niece, this was part of my conversation with my daughter yesterday, um my niece is gay and her significant other has had a very hard life, she's young, but has had 4 children. She has been on public assistance, they had a house fire, she's in a shelter, um, she was relocated from NY to Philadelphia so now she's away from her family. And I was talking to my daughter about the impact that you know the difference between my life, and her life and my granddaughter's life, and the lives of these children, who . . .

Therapist: these kids.

Patient: and I don't think they ever feel safe. You know and so um it's an acknowledgement of the richness that I've had and that I've enjoyed. And now she's facing cancer so you know there's . . .

Therapist: this woman?

Patient: yeah, it's just you know. Cause my daughter is a little harsh about this girl and the choices she's made in her life, and I said "You know you're coming from a place of privilege you know where everything for you is a norm in terms of safety." You know.

Therapist: yeah, and you know one of the sessions one of the sources of meaning is the attitude you take towards suffering or limitations in life and how you overcome challenges. And this situation with your niece's partner lot of challenges to overcome. And the story you told about your grandmother?

Patient: great grandmother, yeah great grandmother.

Therapist: Yeah, uh with the depression?

Patient: right

Therapist: yeah, that was also overcoming an obstacle, or limitation. And the courage that's involved and the attitude that's necessary, you know "I'm going to make this, I cannot fail, I choose to overcome this." Take this tragic situation, make something . . .

Patient: and I spoke to the girl on Saturday, and um I asked her how she was doing and she said to me "I find Philadelphia to be very hard because I'm alone," but she said "For my children it's been a much better place for them."

Therapist: there you go

Patient: and I said well . . .

Therapist: is she there with your niece?

Patient: no, my niece is . . .

Therapist: they're separated?

Patient: yeah, they're separated. But she comes, there's a van that takes them up to New York, whenever she wants to come to New York. So they see each other once a week on the weekend for about five hours, so it's a strain in their relationship and she was telling me "You know we're fighting all the time." And I said "Well, it's a hurdle, I mean the distance," but I said "You have the phone," and uh . . .

Therapist: ways to overcome it.

Patient: "You talk about it," you know, and I said "You talk about the cancer too." I said "Don't sit in your room and think about the impact this is going to have on everybody. Share it, share it with your children when you feel comfortable, share it with (niece's name), share it with your family." I said "You're not burdening them, but you have to talk about it."

Therapist: Stay connected to everyone.

Patient: You have to stay connected, and I said "And the pull that you're feeling is that you're not sharing because you want to protect them, but they want to help you so you're pushing them away, but its not a time to push." I said actually "It's a time to embrace."

Therapist: and I think the session today on, well the session yeah today is on experiential sense.

Patient: connecting.

Therapist: yeah connecting, love and connectedness, so . . . and then there was a third part to your legacy project . . .

Patient: the third part is my is my letters to the people who were most important, who are most important in my life. And so I've decided to write it in the present tense.

Therapist: that's where you are.

Patient: That's where I am right. And um, you know so it's been ah I don't know what aspect of it you would like me to have completed?

Therapist: well, whatever you know

Patient: But when it is complete, I will give it to you.

Therapist: yeah the idea is to suggest it to you and you've obviously have taken it up. We have I think one more session after this. We've shared a lot about the legacy project already, if there's anything that you've got, share next time, great.

Patient: okay

Therapist: but even just talking about like this, what more you have planned, or whatever that's fine. It would be my privilege to see it someday. Let's go on to this session. I think it looks like you did the homework from last time.

Patient: mm hmm

Therapist: On this session, this session like a lot of the sessions after the first introductory sessions each one focuses on a different source of meaning, so the historical sources of meaning through legacy you inherit, legacy you live, legacy you leave, and this is the legacy project you're talking about. And then a source of meaning through encountering and overcoming limitations, and the big one being death obviously. Uh, and then the one last week we talked about creative sources of meaning, was it called engaging in life, the last one? Where you . . .

Patient: Yes, engaging in life. Actively engaging in life.

Therapist: Exactly. So it's basically your work and the life that you created. Not just the work you do, but also the life you create, the values in your life that you create, etc. The courage to overcome obstacles, the a your responsibilities in life, we talked a little bit about that right?

Patient: mm hmm

Therapist: this one's a little bit more fun, I think, its experiential sources of meaning. We we derive meaning through experiencing life right?

Patient: mm hmm

Therapist: and uh the French word for meaning is "sense" "sense" like sensation and lots of times you know we might say "I need to make sense of this." Which means I need to figure out what this means.

Patient: right

Therapist: So sense and meaning are often used interchangeably. And uh when we talk about experiential sources of meaning it's through the experience of life through all our senses, through touch, through smell, through taste. And so when you engage in life right? You're using all your senses

Patient: mm hmm

Therapist: and you're experiencing life with your senses. And the most common source of meaning, experiential meaning, is through love, through all sorts of love, love you have for your children, love you have for your husband, love you have for your parents, all sorts of love. I throw lust in there sometimes too.

Patient: (laugh)

Therapist: love of nature, love of food, love of beauty, love of humor, love of reading, love of art, all sorts of things that really get your juices going. It's feeling alive. It's the and there's almost nothing that makes you feel more alive than loving and being loved. You know. And uh, and it's sometimes people think what's the meaning of life, what's the secret of the meaning of life. And it comes down to something very simple, I think its all about love and living life fully, sometimes really rather simply. You know your parents, your grandparents, your great grandparents didn't have cable TV or the Internet, and this and that, but there were some simple joys and things that just gave their lives meaning. They weren't fancy people, accomplished people, but their lives were meaningful because they had some basic things that they could appreciate.

Patient: mm hmm

Therapist: And uh so that's what experiential sources of meaning are. So when you go back to Victor Frankl and his that book *Man's Search for Meaning*. What could never be taken away from him was the attitude that you know he took towards whatever situation he was in, how he thought about it and also how he felt about it. And one of the things that sustained him was his love for his wife.

Patient: right

Therapist: Um, of course you know love, and that's why when you lose someone you love that so hard. Or when you stop loving somebody that's hard, when somebody stops loving you that's hard, and you still love them. And sometimes you wonder what does it all mean, what does life mean? You can see what a life blood for meaning love is, is when you lose it or it's in danger.

Patient: oh yeah

Therapist: yeah. When you say "oh yeah" is that because of a reason?

Patient: um, well yeah, when my grandmother died, I was uh I took her death um you know

Therapist: her death was particularly hard

Patient: very hard, yeah

Therapist: because of love?

Patient: yeah, but um but its part of life

Therapist: sure

Patient: but you know it's, it was significant, it is significant.

Therapist: did the love for you grandmother ever cease?

Patient: No

Therapist: And do you feel like you've lost her love?

Patient: no

Therapist: Not really

Patient: it's just changed.

Therapist: it's changed

Patient: it's just different

Therapist: it's different. So in the immediate the loss feels so permanent and all that

Patient: right

Therapist: but in the process of grief you understand it's never really lost, it's just changed.

Patient: yeah

Therapist: so you did a little bit of the, what did you think about the homework and the exercise I guess? This is the exercise we're going to do today. List three ways in which you connect with life.

Patient: It's funny because I did the exercise and then I actually read the 6th session

Therapist: mm hmm

Patient: And um you know it says I guess it says quote in terms of uh being transfixed, and you know and I guess the truth that you see in someone's songs, you know a philosophers quote, and I guess what I wrote in terms of love. It's very simple, "Everyday with my husband." Um, you know uh is is uh wonderful.

Therapist: so a way in which you connect with life and feel most alive through love is everyday with your husband.

Patient: and then when I read this, I thought of course I like a lot of songs, so um what song would remind me of that, so I came up with "How Sweet It Is" by James Taylor.

Therapist: ah ha

Patient: I said I think those lyrics are lyrics that I would think about in terms of you know one's love you know um. And then uh . . .

Therapist: it's a love song.

Patient: It is a love song . . . "How sweet it is to be loved by you."

Therapist: "how sweet it is to be loved by you." And so when you think about you and your husband . . .

Patient: right

Therapist: a big part of how that love makes you feel connected is how much he loves

Patient: yeah

Therapist: and how beautiful it is, and sweet it is, and safe it is

Patient: its just you know

Therapist: to be loved by you

Patient: by you

Therapist: and he's loved you for a long time

Patient: yeah, 3—, well, I guess 37 years.

Therapist: and you've been married?

Patient: We'll be married 35.

Therapist: And it was love at first sight?

Patient: No, not at all.

Therapist: Not at all?

Patient: Not at all.

Therapist: What was?

Patient: Uh we were in college I was a freshman in college. And uh, I mean its funny, so I went to a public college. I graduated high school early. I had gone to boarding school. And it my . . .

Therapist: An all girls' boarding school

Patient: Yeah, an all girls boarding school. And in my sophomore year a friend of mine wrote a note to her friend and her mother found it and in the note she mentioned that she was getting high. And she brought it to the principal and my name was mentioned somewhere in the context of the note but it had nothing to do with them getting high. And my mother, who was a policewoman, decided that . . .

Therapist: Your mother was a policewoman?

Patient: yeah, yeah. That she was going to take me . . .

Therapist: I did not know that. You neglected to mention that . . .

Patient: Yes, my mother was a policewoman.

Therapist: with a gun?

Patient: with a gun. Uh, my mother was a policewoman with a gun. And decided that I had to, I could no longer stay at boarding school, that for the rest of my sophomore year, despite me telling her I had nothing to do with, I don't even know what this is about. So, um on the way home, on her birthday March 3, 1970, on the way home I told her "I would never forgive you for this." Um, which of course is not true, but it did take about 35 years for me to forgive her for this. But anyway . . .

Therapist: Really? It took you 35 years for you to forgive your mother for . . .

Patient: for taking me out of boarding school and not believing me that I had nothing to do with it . . .

Therapist: for not believing you.

Patient: um

Therapist: and you not forgiving her, how did it affect your relationship?

Patient: oh, I severed it. I severed it psychologically.

Therapist: there's a disconnection.

Patient: oh yeah, for a long time there was a disconnection.

Therapist: on my

Patient: so of course I was in the motherhouse of the sisters of St. Joseph for about 8 years of my life, and now I was, so the home that I knew I was taken away from and brought back home. And anyway I went to a public high school . . .

Therapist: the punishment was taking you out of that school.

Patient: Right. Um, I um, I went to a public high school where I was like I did not belong to this environment at all. It was 1970 everybody was wearing jeans and ty-dyed shirts

Therapist: ty-dyed shirts

Patient: and I came from a Catholic boarding school where I wore a uniform every day, I had never worn pants, so it was like completely foreign. So anyway I decided to graduate high school early because I couldn't take being in a public high school any longer, and I went to John Jay and in my freshman year I took religion and I lost my religion notebook. And (husband's name) worked security, so I went to find out, cause in my mind if you lose a notebook somebody would return it and bring it to "lost and found." Kind of naïve but nevertheless. So I went to security to get my religion notebook and he was the security guard and he said to me "Nobody had returned the notebook." And I said to him "Well, you didn't even look. Go to lost and found and open it up and see if they returned it." So he opened it up and uh, he said "No, there's no religion notebook here." So I said "Well, I'll come back next week."

Therapist: So right away you know he's a guy who takes orders.

Patient: well, no, he's a guy who dismisses anybody that makes a silly request (laugh).

Therapist: okay

Patient: So I went back and he opened it up and he said "No, there's still not a notebook here." And the third week I went back cause it was the end of the semester and I was fretting about my notebook and what I was going to do. Um, and uh and this time I brought my mother. And he said to me "So now you bring reinforcements?"

Therapist: with a gun?

Patient: (laugh) and then we really didn't, I mean I knew about him, in fact somebody suggested I date him, and I thought "No no, I don't want to have anything to do with him." And then I worked in security, I used to serve subpoenas for a law firm and one day they sent me up to Lennox Avenue and I walked out of the subway station and I saw all the broken glass and I went back to the attorney and said "You would not send your daughter to where you sent me for the subpoena. I'm done." And he said to me "Well, I can't pay you for today." And I said "Not only do you not have to pay me for today, you don't have to pay me for last week. This is it." And I walked out. I went to John Jay's personnel office and asked if they had anything on campus and they said I could work as a secretary for security, and I said to them "Oh, I don't think so." And he said "No no, go in and . . ." To make a long story short what happened was we were both working for security, I was a secretary he was a supervisor and a friend of ours was having an engagement party and (husband's name) asked me to go to the engagement party and I said yes. And despite the fact that I thought he was a jerk, I gave him a second chance. And uh you know 37 years later we're . . .

Therapist: so what's so sweet about how he loves you?

Patient: um, he just loves everything about me

Therapist: he adores you

Patient: when I'm silly, when I ask him something for the 4th time that day, uh you know uh, he said he likes the way I, he just said this to me recently, he said to me "I like the way you make our bed every morning with the comforter as if we were going to have company even though its just you and I."

Therapist: mm-hmm
Patient: you know um, so it's every day.
Therapist: it's emotional for you?
Patient: yes, yeah it is.
Therapist: did you think you were going to find this kind of love in your life?
Patient: yeah (laugh)
Therapist: you did.
Patient: yeah, cause although my mother and grandmother were both widowed, my great grandmother, were both widowed very early in their lives they loved their husbands you know completely. So yeah I guess for me this was this is how it works.
Therapist: gotcha, so you had confidence were going to have . . .
Patient: a good marriage, yeah
Therapist: you love him a lot, or did I take number 3?
Patient: I'm sorry?
Therapist: did I did I take you number 3 when I asked you, how sweet it is to love him?
Patient: No, I saw that all as number 1, I see it as a mutual a mutual.
Therapist: so that's what you mean by everyday with him?
Patient: everyday yeah
Therapist: the love you have for each other
Patient: yeah, um and number 2 um is kind of connected, it's spending time with my family both my uh uh both my immediate family as well as my extended family. And I thought about what what would in art would I think about in terms of an expression of that.
Therapist: mm-hmm
Patient: And the first thing that came to my mind was Norman Rockwell's uh Thanksgiving.
Therapist: mm-hmm
Patient: you know I said that would express just . . .
Therapist: so everyone together, one place, enjoying a meal together
Patient: sharing our lives
Therapist: sharing your lives
Patient: happy stories
Therapist: political arguments
Patient: political arguments, yes we have a divided house
Therapist: you do?
Patient: yes in terms of democrats and republicans
Therapist: democrats and republicans
Patient: yes, I
Therapist: like our government
Patient: I think I'm basically in the minority right now, but that's . . .
Therapist: really?
Patient: yes, I live in a republican household.
Therapist: I see
Patient: yeah, my family is democrats, but I've married into the republicans
Therapist: I see. Have they turned tea party yet?
Patient: My one sister-in-law has, yes
Therapist: oh boy (laugh)
Patient: um, and I mean there's just humor, you have to kind of laugh.
Therapist: you have to laugh
Patient: And so my number 3 was uh talking to my friends, I have wonderful friend, and uh, and the song that came to mind was "Up on the Roof" by Carole King. Uh you know that when life gets you overwhelming sometime you have to go up and share it with somebody.
Therapist: so you have really close friends who you can share all of your all of your life with, the good and the bad and the ugly.
Patient: yeah
Therapist: it's critically important to have at least one person that knows everything . . .
Patient: yeah I do have
Therapist: all the secrets
Patient: I do have one . . .
Therapist: even the ones that your husband doesn't know
Patient: doesn't know. Yes, um, yeah I do have one friend, I have actually . . .
Therapist: a couple
Patient: I have a couple, but I think (friend's name) probably knows the most about my inner thoughts. And then with beauty, I had gardening as my first.
Therapist: gardening
Patient: yeah, uh I just love to be in the garden uh, planting walking through a garden um . . .
Therapist: what's beautiful about the garden?
Patient: the vibrancy well I guess there are a few things, but the vibrant colors, um
Therapist: so the product of what grows is really beautiful
Patient: grows, yeah, um, the . . .
Therapist: flowers mainly?
Patient: flowers um flowers and springtime trees that flower. Even the garden in winter is pretty, there's serenity about life.
Therapist: Is it a lot of work to garden? To bend down a lot?
Patient: oh yeah, there's a lot of work. I like to plan and weed.
Therapist: That part's nice too?
Patient: I like the weeding cause it's like you know you're uh
Therapist: You're very close to the earth right?

Patient: and there's just something about you have a plot of dirt that's full of weeds and uh you have to decide, I mean some weeds are actually pretty so you leave cause there, I said to (husband's name) "Well these are either weeds or wildflowers, which one would you like me to think of them as?" (laugh), uh cause he'll say to me "You didn't get everything," "Well, those are my wildflowers, those aren't really my weeds." But there's just a sense of you go in and then you have to um clean it up to make it look the way you want it to. So it's kind of like your life, you present it with this and you decide what you want to keep and what you want to nurture. So gardening for me is is um a thing of beauty. Um, and then I wrote taking pictures of places um that I've visited um and um and taking pictures isn't really an adequate way of thinking about it but its not only places that I've visited, but places where I'd like to visit. So seeing in photographs things that you know . . .

Therapist: So like the world is a beautiful place

Patient: oh yeah

Therapist: and uh you so for you I guess the idea of seeing the world maybe traveling or at least remembering places you've visited or imagining or looking at places you'd like to visit. The world seems there's a lot of beauty . . .

Patient: it's majestic

Therapist: It's majestic, and so some of the pictures involve places like where?

Patient: Oh the Grand Canyon

Therapist: So places of natural beauty

Patient: Natural beauty yeah, well, the Grand Canyon

Therapist: And cities too

Patient: yeah um Paris is beautiful, I mean it's just

Therapist: and is that a place that you have pictures of visiting?

Patient: I didn't care for London

Therapist: gotcha, Paris is prettier

Patient: right, Paris is prettier

Therapist: so some of the pictures you have of Paris are of what?

Patient: well the Seine.

Therapist: the Seine

Patient: I have pictures of Notre Dame, the Eiffel Tower, and we went, we were on a cruise, we went to Provence, I can't remember the town's name. And it was very old and very quant and we were walking on this cobblestone street and there was a marketplace and I have such a pretty picture of this marketplace you know with the umbrella's it was lovely, very quant. And we've been to Malta, Malta was beautiful.

Therapist: Malta was beautiful

Patient: yeah, Malta was beautiful, we also went to Tunisia. We went to Tunis, and uh we were standing, our guide said to us this was Carthage, and he showed us the ruins, and I said "Oh my god" the history of you know. And then we went to Italy, and Rome was magnificent.

Therapist: so the world's a beautiful place to travel.

Patient: yeah, for me I had to pinch myself that I was actually here.

Therapist: that gives you sense of how connected you are to people around the world too.

Patient: Yeah it's lovely. And my third thing, I know it sounds silly, I really enjoy the sunset, no matter where I am.

Therapist: it's not sunset I mean it's not silly.

Patient: its just you know, I like the way the sky looks at different points of the year. And you know it's something I take note of. I actually thought to myself as I wrote it, I say "Well why don't you ever take note of the sunrise?" And it was "Why is it the sunset rather?" And I thought "I don't think the sky is as vibrant."

Therapist: huh?

Patient: the sky is not as vibrant at sunrise as it is . . .

Therapist: it's really interesting, some people are sunrise people

Patient: are they?

Therapist: you know they get up real early

Patient: I am, I do I get up all the time

Therapist: you're an early riser?

Patient: Yeah

Therapist: and they, some people who get up really early and they . . .

Patient: they watch the sunrise?

Therapist: yeah their ritual is to watch the sunrise, and then they are like busy at work when the sunsets, something like that. A lot of people are more sunset watches. But the association that I have is do you have any other thoughts about why sunset rather than sunrise?

Patient: well, I think it's a sense of completion.

Therapist: Mm-hmm

Patient: and uh and well for me it's a sometimes in the sky you can tell how the day is going to be the following day.

Therapist: I see

Patient: Particularly in the summer time if its orange you can tell its going to be hot the next day. So I just think it's, I would say you're satisfied with what you've done for the day and you're looking forward to tomorrow, but you take time to appreciate today.

Therapist: yeah, so you put it in terms of very similar to my association which was that you know in terms of life the cycle of our lives, we're born, we have a life and then we pass away we die, and we talk about sunrise may be the birth, sunset the last years of our lives, the sunset of our lives.

Patient: yeah the sunset of our . . .

Therapist: And uh and sometimes it's hard to think of it as a beautiful experience, but if you think of it in terms that you just described of being able to look back at a life that you've accomplished something, that you're pleased at how you've used your life then it can represent something beautiful.

Patient: and humor, my daughter (daughter's name) has a wonderful sense of humor

Therapist: what was that?

Patient: my daughter (daughter's name) has a wonderful sense of humor

Therapist: not you?

Patient: oh I do too, but she, I enjoy her humor

Therapist: is (daughter's name) the one who keeps asking who said to you if you're great grandmother hadn't the social . . .

Patient: no that was my daughter (other daughter's name), the older one

Therapist: Okay, so (daughter's name) has a great sense of humor

Patient: great sense of humor, she uh, I just like, I like being with her, she finds everyday things to be funny. So and then . . .

Therapist: so she's not like a joke funny person?

Patient: no, she comments on . . .

Therapist: she's an observer . . .

Patient: she's an observer, she makes interesting comments. You know I told her, well I've done this all my life, when things aren't easy for me to take I try to find something to make them to make whatever I'm going through to be more palatable for me.

Therapist: yes

Patient: and so I see my sense of humor in her. So I guess that's why I you know. When I was in the college I would have a line of people who would come in and you know they would give me sad stories, and there was this one woman in particular, she was always crying and she was always coming in, and I looked at her one day and I thought she reminds me of someone I wonder who she reminds me, it sounds terrible. But in the movie *Batman* I thought she could be the Penguin's wife.

Therapist: I see, I don't think Penguin had a wife in the movie, but if he did . . .

Patient: yes, but if he had a wife she could be the wife.

Therapist: gotcha

Patient: and I looked at her and I smiled, and she smiled back and I broke whatever ranting she was going through for that minute and I thought okay "This actually works me for me."

Therapist: there's actually a human being in there

Patient: So (daughter's name) has my sense of humor in that way

Therapist: and humor is a very powerful way in which we all connect, there's nothing like that scene around the scene that you were talking about that Rockwell scene, the people sitting around, there's nothing like everyone laughing at something.

Patient: And then whenever I, well whenever I was going through anything difficult with the cancer the one movie I always put on was *Birdcage*.

Therapist: Birdcage

Patient: loved the movie

Therapist: the one with Robin Williams and Nathan Lane?

Patient: Robin Williams, right yeah. And then I wrote "life's events with family or friends" I mean I just . . .

Therapist: there funny things that happened

Patient: just funny things that happened, just silly things. We were driving to the baseball hall-of-fame and there was a cow, the cows had passed the road and the road was just littered with manure, and I didn't know, so I was driving and I thought well I'll go through it fast and of course the entire car reeked of manure . . .

Therapist: and it splattered?

Patient: oh it was awful and we were driving and we of course had a long way to go, and when we parked the car in the parking lot, people were looking around it was just hysterical. My brother-in-law said to me "I can't get back in that car." So we went to have the car washed, and it didn't help.

Therapist: it didn't help?

Patient: No, oh it was about a month before you could get the entire smell out. But it was just funny (husband's name) said to me he was about to tell me "Go through it very slowly" but he said "You gunned the car and went right through it." (laugh)

Therapist: So we've stooped this low, to manure jokes, manure stories (laugh).

Patient: (laugh) well, that's

Therapist: but that was funny
Patient: that was my humor
Therapist: so so can you relate to how these experiential sources of meaning, these love, beauty and humor, how they relate to meaning in your life?
Patient: well, I think there's a common thread. Being connected to family.
Therapist: yeah
Patient: what I said about gardening, those are individual pleasures, but the other pleasures sharing it with other people.
Therapist: Mm-hmm
Patient: and humor you know, I don't know, I think its all interwoven
Therapist: yeah
Patient: it's a . . .
Therapist: living life using all your senses
Patient: right, yeah
Therapist: not cut off from anything, you're just living fully
Patient: yeah
Therapist: it's like driving through the manure, full speed, that's why you did it because you're that kind of person.
Patient: Well . . . had he said to me drive through it, he saw it as well as I did . . .
Therapist: no, but you're an existentialist heart you know that you . . .
Patient: I embraced it.
Therapist: I embraced it; I'm going to plow right through it, high speed
Patient: high speed
Therapist: I'm going to have the full experience of driving through manure (laugh)
Patient: I'm going to gun it (laugh)
Therapist: so the next session is our last session
Patient: okay
Therapist: there's always a little bit of sadness about the last session cause you know we get to know each other a little bit and hear a lot about your life, but like everything you know um some things do some to an end. Part of next session is final reflections on what you learned in the 6 sessions about the sources of meaning and how they can be resources for you, and living your life fully despite your cancer. We talked already about how you've started your legacy project and how you've outlined it and I'll love to hear a little bit more next time. And then I think what we'll, the homework, is there a homework?
Patient: Mm-hmm
Therapist: yeah, uh so the homework, what's it's been like . . .
Patient: reflection
Therapist: yeah, the homework involves what it's been like for you to go through all this right? It would be nice if they gave you that . . .
Patient: here
Therapist: thank you. What's it like for you to go through this. Yeah, and I think the most important thing is, well these are important, but I want to talk a little bit as we end about your hopes for the future. List as many as you can.
Patient: thank you
Therapist: and I think we had a date for that?
Patient: yes, it's next Tuesday at 8.

Session 7: Transitions- Reflections and Hopes for the Future

Therapist: Here we go. Good morning.
Patient: good morning
Therapist: so, we've come to our last session. It's hard to believe huh?
Patient: yeah
Therapist: I haven't seen you in a week or two, how are things going in general?
Patient: Good, good, health is good.
Therapist: Medically things are okay?
Patient: I went to the doctor last week and she asked me if I was anxious about going through the next round of testing. And I told her "no" and she said if I wasn't anxious they would do it at the end of the summer probably because all the blood work seems to be normal, and uh I'm responding well to the medication.
Therapist: I see
Patient: And she said if anything call her, but if not everything seems to be fine
Therapist: they want to give you another month off?
Patient: uh about two months off, so . . .
Therapist: two months off
Patient: yeah, so you know its funny cause when she asked me she said "Are you anxious about not having the testing down?" I said "No, but now I'm anxious that you asked me." (laugh) But I was okay, you know.
Therapist: Yeah. Did you go away?
Patient: Yeah, we have a country house, so we have family that comes up, and it's was nice.
Therapist: Where is your country house?
Patient: Newburgh, Orange County.
Therapist: oh, it's towards the Catskills, or in the Catskills?
Patient: yeah, it's actually right before the Catskills.

Therapist: Yeah, I think when I was a kid we used to go up to that part of . . .
Patient: Monticello
Therapist: Monticello, Bloomingburg
Patient: Bloomingburg
Therapist: Past and then I think when I was a kid in our bungalow colony we had a baseball/softball team and I think we used to play some of the bungalow colonies in Newburgh. And I used to go up somewhere to get my haircut, Falls burgh, or South Falls burgh?
Patient: okay, yeah
Therapist: is that close by?
Patient: Its maybe about half hour, 40 minutes away.
Therapist: So . . .
Patient: north
Therapist: its north of you
Patient: North of me.
Therapist: Oh okay, so you're closer to actually Bloomingburg.
Patient: we're about an hour and 40 minutes from the city.
Therapist: and it's a house and a community?
Patient: No, it's actually . . .
Therapist: just on its own?
Patient: It's on its own, but it's on a main thorofair. We have a half acre of land.
Therapist: that's nice
Patient: and for me that's enough. You know its enough of the country, but not too much.
Therapist: I hear you, its not . . .
Patient: I don't have an estate.
Therapist: It's not a log cabin in the woods.
Patient: No no no, fully air-conditioned, you know.
Therapist: But it's a getaway for you.
Patient: oh yeah absolutely.
Therapist: Well you know we've spent six sessions over 8 or 9 weeks . . .
Patient: Mm-hmm
Therapist: So um, and uh before I turned on the tape you said "This has been an interesting . . ."
Patient: experience
Therapist: project, or experience.
Patient: yeah
Therapist: what we've been trying do is something we call meaning-centered psychotherapy and the focus of it has been to introduce you or make you if you've been aware make you a bit more aware of the importance of meaning in life.
Patient: Mm-hmm
Therapist: and introduce you to some of the sources of meaning. You know the whole concept of uh of our responsibilities as human beings is to live a life of meaning and identity, and direction and connection and transcendence and overcoming limitation. And in living this life trying to develop a sense of self-esteem and value, and the idea that we want to be, we want to live lives in which we are valuable, significant people, a valuable person in a life of meaning, a meaningful life, a life that has meaning.
Patient: right
Therapist: in a world of meaning, as opposed to a completely meaningless world. Maybe we create the meaning in the world ourselves or some people who are religious, say God might create that meaning.
Patient: Mm-hmm
Therapist: The idea of being a person of value in a world that has meaning. So in the process of trying to do that is trying to make you reconnect with that importance of meaning by reintroducing you to the sources of meaning through uh uh experiential sources of meaning, the way we're connected to the world using our senses and experiencing world, experiencing the joys of the world and sometimes even the tragedies of the world that make us feel alive. Through love, through art, beauty, food, through travel, all the things that make us feel alive and that we're living life, they invoked emotions in us right?
Patient: Mm-hmm
Therapist: And then experiential sources of meaning through the way that we make a life in the world, and feel connected to the world, engaged in the world through our work, through the things we care about, the people we care about. Through historical sources of meaning, through the legacy that we've inherited from our families and from others forever, the legacy of the life that we live and what we leave behind. And attitudinal sources, the idea that life is finite and we are constantly encountering limitations in life that cause us to suffer and death is just sort of the ultimate limitation. And that we have our ability to choose our attitude towards those limitations whether uh we allow ourselves to feel hopeless and helpless and have episodes of loss of meaning or whether we choose to overcome or we choose to take an attitude to the suffering that helps us connect to all the meaningful things in our lives that are represented by those sources of meaning. So all those other sources of meaning that sometimes help us transcend limitations is the loving connection of who we are in

the world, our legacy we leave behind. Those things help us transcend limitations, even limitations like that. So that's what this has been about. And we've talked a little bit about a legacy project and I have a feeling, I saw you scribbling there, I think you did something.

Patient: I did

Therapist: You did, so we'll talk about that in a minute.

Patient: okay

Therapist: But I'd be curious, I'd be interested in your reflections on what we've done over the six sessions.

Patient: I would say that coming into this I had a pretty good understanding . . .

Therapist: yes, I think so

Patient: of my life. And you know I took pride in what I had accomplished and had ownership of my decisions, but I think what this did for me is it helped me re-focus on not just, cause my inclination is to only look for positive things, so it helped me really re-focus on how are those stressful, difficult moments, how in fact did they shape my life.

Therapist: yeah, people don't usually see those moments as having value at all.

Patient: Right you know you try to think oh that was a terrible time.

Therapist: That was terrible

Patient: they actually were the impetus for me to move

Therapist: Yes

Patient: not being content with where I was so that I re-directed my attention. I mean I knew about it, I was aware of it, but I never really owed it as the strength that it had in re-shaping me.

Therapist: So the terrible moments . . .

Patient: yeah

Therapist: were powerfully important in your life because they really woke you to what was missing in your life and what you needed in your life, and they also helped you re-direct you towards very important things and accomplishing certain things . . .

Patient: like step up to the plate

Therapist: step up to the plate. You gave me I think during the therapy the weeks of therapy some examples of that related to your education I think, right.

Patient: right

Therapist: can you remind me of that one, if another comes to mind?

Patient: The one I actually wrote extensively about was actually something that happened to me when I was in 4th grade in the first year of my boarding school experience. You'll read about it . . .

Therapist: yeah

Patient: But basically what happened, I was accused of lying to a Nun and I hadn't in fact lied to her, and then she turned around and she slapped me. And I was never abused as a child, there was never violence in my house, and here I was 9 years old, actually 8, 8 or 9, and I was in boarding school and this authority figure challenged me and I slapped her right back. And I said to her "My mother doesn't slap me, you certainly are not going to slap me, nobody slaps me." And she ordered to my room and I didn't get to see my mother that day and another sister came over and gave me ice and we became friends. But that was really, I think about moment and I was um true to my own convictions you know, that in the face of you know what seemed to be this an authority that I should not be challenged, that I respected, when it became obvious to me that you know she was out of line, I went into action. And I can look at that and I can see other points in my life where when I was in college I was working for this department and the director of the department had heard that the kids had gone to a party and that they spoke pot and then he very uniformly fired everybody. And I wasn't involved in the party, I never attended the party, I wasn't even involved in the incident, but I was privy to what was going on, and I handed in my resignation and I wrote this scathing letter at 17 telling this man he was completely out of line. The incident didn't happen in school, it was here-say and that these students should have not been fired. And then of course I quite work and I went back to work when I was ready, but I stood for my principles.

Therapist: yeah

Patient: you know it was, and I hadn't thought about that in years since I started doing this. And I don't I don't think I really um thought of those, well they were pivotal moments in my life, but I didn't realize the impact that they had in kind of re-affirming in yourself who you are. You certainly can listen to whatever those people have to say, but you don't necessarily have to march to their tune.

Therapist: Right, it's a little bit more that you were defining yourself as opposed to being defined by others.

Patient: by them right

Therapist: And it seemed to indicate that you, well there were several elements in there, it was courageous right?

Patient: Yeah (laugh)

Therapist: (laugh) And you need courage to define yourself as opposed to letting other people define you. You need to have will. You're a pretty willful person, right? And you were not conforming to other people's ideas of what you should do, and so you were also very much being living your own authentic life. You were trying real hard, and when the rubber hit the road you were trying real hard to go in your direction, not somebody else's direction. You were trying to and I think succeeding in being the author in your own life.

Patient: Yeah and I you know, I . . .

Therapist: and it involves some self-esteem too.

Patient: Oh yeah, I would say I was also self-assured, but in a quiet way.

Therapist: there you go

Patient: you know um . . .

Therapist: So it wasn't really an immature, self-assuredness, you know naïve . . .

Patient: right. No, but it was, and then I think of even when I went for the PhD I had spent half of my life at the college, I was 34 and I thought "There's gotta be more to my life than this."

Therapist: Right

Patient: because I had reading difficultly when I was in elementary school, I never thought of myself as a good student, I thought of myself as a hard working student, but I never thought of myself as a good student, and I just thought a PhD you just had to be brilliant. And I had all these reasons not to go on and then and yet I said "Try it, give yourself a challenge, see if you can do it, if you can fine, if you can't do something else." So there was never a sense of defeat.

Therapist: you had ambition

Patient: yeah I guess I had ambition.

Therapist: And ambition is just a way of saying you have a will and a desire, which is good stuff to have in life.

Patient: Yeah

Therapist: That helps you create a life. It's the power, it's the fuel.

Patient: Yeah, and one of the reason I decided to do this was that I was feeling that I had lived, and I said it in the past tense, I had lived a meaningful life I wasn't sure I was still meaningful life. Well, I didn't feel as engaged as I was before and then I realized um I was busy before, but I'm actually more engaged in my life now.

Therapist: That's so interesting, now that you've been ill.

Patient: yeah

Therapist: You have been less busy with work.

Patient: right

Therapist: Yeah, they say sometimes they call it "business" "busyness" and when you're busy sometimes you're busy in a way that distracts you from . . .

Patient: living right

Therapist: what's really meaningful, or important

Patient: what's important, right.

Therapist: So you think that a little bit of what you have been going through in terms this therapy is helped you connect you with that realization.

Patient: yeah

Therapist: you were kind of doing it on your own without this therapy?

Patient: Um, well, no

Therapist: No?

Patient: No no, I was going through a process of lamenting the life I had and what happened was right before I got the call for this I got a letter from Middle States asking me to be an evaluator again, and I thought "I can't do that, um, I haven't been working in almost a year, I'm not really connected to that part of my life." And then kind of that little girl in me came out and said "Well, why don't you just do it. Why don't you call them and tell them you haven't been working and you are ill, and you'd like to make the commitment but there are so many unknowns and see what they have to say," and I did. I spoke to the woman who had written to me and she said that, she said to me she said "Do you have any loss of cognitive function?" and I said "No." She said "You know what you know; your illness hasn't taken that way from you. As long as you feel confident that you would be able to make the trip, why don't you do it?" And I thought "okay" I said "That's fine." So I signed up for it and I'm going down to Puerto Rico in September. And this opportunity came along and I said "You know I think I need to this kind of get me to the next step," because I was still I was still making excuses why I couldn't do it. "Well I don't really speak Spanish, so if they are talking to me and they want to express what they are saying I may not be able to understand them, or I might not get what they are actually trying to say to me." So then I called the woman who is actually doing the evaluation team, and she said to me that they are bilingual and if I really felt that there was something that I just was not able to ask or have them respond to they will find an evaluator. So I said to myself "Just got down, really it's enough, you know you've ruminated about this enough, just go and do it." So I feel like with the combination of the two I'm reclaiming my meaningful, that's its not that I've lived a meaningful life, it's that I'm still living a meaningful life. That life isn't over.

Therapist: that's right, life isn't over.

Patient: Right, you know.

Therapist: Life isn't over and there's plenty, and you can still live a meaningful life. I was struck by you referred to that "little girl."

Patient: Mm-hmm

Therapist: Uh that little girl represents the part of you right, that that is fully alive right?

Patient: yeah

Therapist: That has ambition and takes risks and goes for it. Is that right?

Patient: yeah, and . . .

Therapist: It's kind of interesting, that it's that little girl.

Patient: It's that little girl . . .

Therapist: Who is that little girl?

Patient: That little girl . . .

Therapist: It's you I guess

Patient: Well, it's me, but it was, well I was going to say 4 year old, but it was really older than that, it's this little girl who had death all around her and sadness.

Therapist: You had death all around you and sadness.

Patient: Yeah my father died, my great grandmother died, my mother was in mourning, they wore black all the time, and uh I ironically always wanted to wear white and yellow. You know I kind of rejected all the dark colors and . . .

Therapist: you were the life force in that . . .

Patient: yeah I was a life force. Yeah . . .

Therapist: you had death all around you and you were the life

Patient: yeah

Therapist: it was almost like your job to be alive for your mom.

Patient: yeah it was my job to keep her connected to life.

Therapist: you were that flame in the family.

Patient: yeah, it sounds ridiculous to say that but yeah I was.

Therapist: Mm-hmm, and for yourself.

Patient: and for myself that when things got you know difficult it was you know it was okay.

Therapist: and its something about being young where you're so vital, you know your optimistic, you haven't been knocked down, you haven't been told too many times that you can't do that, you haven't had a lot of failures you know you haven't had the world beat you down. Although you did have these terrible tragedies around you these deaths, and these losses.

Patient: yes, but I had them around me.

Therapist: but they didn't . . .

Patient: but they weren't me

Therapist: they weren't me, you were very much aware

Patient: right

Therapist: It wasn't you. You were still alive.

Patient: I was still alive

Therapist: And you weren't ready to pack it in.

Patient: No, I wasn't ready to pack it in.

Therapist: You were just starting.

Patient: Yeah, you know and so um when uh my mother wasn't athletically inclined at all and so whenever I asked her to do something she put me into competition which was kind of ridiculous, but um so when I asked her to ride a bike, I joined the Long Island Woman's Association, and rode an English Racer I mean that was my first bike. So it was like, it's kind of like the story when I told you about going through the cow manure.

Therapist: Right you could go slow or you could go fast

Patient: Yeah I just go fast. I, whatever it is I immerse myself in it and do what I can.

Therapist: What do you think it is that gives you that life's force, that will, what fuels that? We were talking a little bit about you know starting as a kid you were this sort of counterweight through all that loss and death you were this life-force in the family.

Patient: I think really . . .

Therapist: Probably to cheer people up a little bit.

Patient: But there was a lot of strength in my family

Therapist: A lot of strength

Patient: yeah, I mean I looked at these women and you know I was aware that there was a lot of hardship, but they endured, they survived. So it was . . .

Therapist: Did you have a lot of hopes and desires, things that you wanted in life, hopes, wishes, dreams?

Patient: I guess so. I've always been cautiously optimistic. I never thought that I'd win a million dollars, but I thought I might be able to earn a million dollars.

Therapist: There's a difference.
Patient: There's a big difference.
Therapist: and the difference is you earn it . . .
Patient: well you pursue it
Therapist: You pursue it, as opposed to having it come to you accidently.
Patient: come to you, right right. So yeah I think that in terms of hopes and desires I thought everything was possible
Therapist: You thought everything was possible
Patient: if you worked at it.
Therapist: and you got that from you. . . .
Patient: I'd say I got that from my mother.
Therapist: your mother felt that way? That was a value . . .
Patient: That was a value that she . . . yeah
Therapist: So you did do some kind of legacy project huh?
Patient: I did
Therapist: This is it
Patient: This is it
Therapist: Beautiful job, graphically. I just describe it, it says, the title of it is "A Meaningful Life" I guess by or about (patient name).
Patient: Right
Therapist: and it's a tree, a beautiful tree and it looks like it has four yellow fruits
Patient: Mm-hmm
Therapist: lemons I guess. I'm not sure if they are lemons . . .
Patient: (laugh) Well, I'm not sure . . .
Therapist: they could be yellow apples
Patient: they might be yellow apples.
Therapist: is that was that accidental the four, you think?
Patient: No, actually that was the graphic design. I could assign meaning to the four, but you know . . .
Therapist: You could, what would it be?
Patient: well the first would be my mother and father, and uh their things that they gave me that I inherited and provided before me. The second would be um my education and uh and the wealth that I've experienced as both a student and a . . .
Therapist: teacher
Patient: teacher. The third would be my husband and our marriage.
Therapist: your marriage, which you value so much.
Patient: which I value. And the fourth are my children and grandchild.
Therapist: there you go.
Patient: The design was by itself, but the tree was significant because as you'll read um my father planted crabapple tree. I was really looking for a crabapple tree.
Therapist: So this is like a crabapple tree
Patient: So for me it was more of a crabapple tree, and he planted the tree when he found out that my mother was pregnant.
Therapist: hmm
Patient: so the tree has always been a symbol of life.
Therapist: Pregnant with . . .?
Patient: with me
Therapist: with you, specifically you. So we have an introduction, so this legacy document is a story?
Patient: a story
Therapist: and it's the story of your life.
Patient: the story of my life
Therapist: your family's life perhaps, or my life?
Patient: And my family . . . both
Therapist: So it's the story of my life and it starts with early memories of your father and you great grandmother. Little pictures, beautiful pictures. Is that your great grandmother?
Patient: that's my great grandmother.
Therapist: And memories of your childhood.
Patient: that's my mother and I.
Therapist: that's your mother and you. And that academy . . .
Patient: Yes, the academy of St. Joseph.
Therapist: With the nun
Patient: with the nuns, yes
Therapist: with the infamous nun, Sister . . .?
Patient: Well, Sister (name) was the nun who . . .
Therapist: slapped you
Patient: slapped me yea
Therapist: oh and then your John Jay college years. And you, look this is you
Patient: that's me
Therapist: who's that?
Patient: That's (friend's name) he was my first instructor, and my mentor and uh he sat on my dissertation committee, my best friend.
Therapist: and this is you in your dissertation robes?
Patient: well, yeah, well those are the dissertation robes. That was actually the John Jay graduation.
Therapist: Graduation, so you wear specific robes because of your ranks
Patient: and my degree
Therapist: and your degree. Kind of beautiful with crimson and black and the shield, and you have a hat with a tassel, a gold tassel.
Patient: And that's (husband's name) and I when we first

Therapist: this is you and (husband's name) in the beginning.
Patient: in the beginning.
Therapist: Look how beautiful you are
Patient: yeah
Therapist: (patient's name) you were hot.
Patient: well, I don't know about that, we were happy
Therapist: you're beautiful
Patient: still are happy
Therapist: This guy's a lucky guy this (husband's name).
Patient: and that's, that's my girls
Therapist: these are your girls when they were . . .
Patient: when they were small, with my mother and grandmother and grandfather who were instrumental in raising them and helping me to accomplish everything that I wanted to.
Therapist: and interspersed here is your family life, and your education and teaching and stuff like that. (daughter's name)
Patient: she was named after
Therapist: (husband's name) right
Patient: and my grandmother
Therapist: and you're paternal grandmother (name). Her name means "freedom"? (daughter's middle name)?
Patient: No (daughter's first name) (laugh)
Therapist: and this is a new focus, and the new focus is the beginning of the cancer
Patient: cancer right
Therapist: breast cancer and your breast cancer experience. And your focus now is on your family. And your daughter getting married. (Daughter's name) is getting married, this is a beautiful picture of (daughter's name) getting married with a very tall husband.
Patient: Yes (laugh)
Therapist: where are you?
Patient: I'm over here, that's my mom
Therapist: you are here, your mom.
Patient: (daughter's name),
Therapist: that's (daughter's name)
Patient: (husband's name)
Therapist: (husband's name) ah-ha. That looks like a beautiful wedding.
Patient: yeah, it was
Therapist: where was the wedding?
Patient: It was on Long Island, it's called . . .
Therapist: villa villa
Patient: No, actually it was French
Therapist: it's French? The Versailles?
Patient: No (laugh) I don't remember. But it was in, it was on Long Island, it was very nice.
Therapist: it was nice
Patient: and that's us.
Therapist: this is . . . and your daughter
Patient: and my granddaughter
Therapist: was expecting in March, and you, this was during your illness right?
Patient: right
Therapist: And it was around the same that you needed to have a 4th stereotactic procedure on your brain.
Patient: that's when I decided it was enough
Therapist: it was enough
Patient: it was enough work, it was like you know
Therapist: and your granddaughter was born (grand daughter's name) October 7, 20XX. Since leaving John Jay you've lived a very full and productive life, family life, you engaged in helping your daughter raise your granddaughter on Tuesdays, Wednesdays, and Fridays. You go with her to the library, to explore the world.
Patient: Mm-hmm
Therapist: God has been very good to me and I treasure every moment that I spend with my husband, and family. This picture was taken a year ago on Father's Day
Patient: right
Therapist: a year ago from yesterday.
Patient: yup
Therapist: and you have (daughter's names), (son-in-law's name), (husband's name), Me, and your mom. It's important to treasure the past, enjoy the present and look forward to the future even in the face of stage IV cancer. I think you picked up a few things . . .
Patient: I think so too
Therapist: This is your family history
Patient: right
Therapist: starting with the background of your mother's family from Cesaro, Sicily, your great grandmother traveled to the states in 1906 to marry her husband, it was an arranged marriage, and then your grandmother, and then your grandfather, your mother. My mother's the strongest person I know; she became a NYC police officer in 1963. And she helped you with your children . . .
Patient: children, right
Therapist: Just like you're doing with your daughter
Patient: right
Therapist: and this is your father (father's name). This is a beautiful history, and then at the end you've got a family tree.
Patient: Mm-hmm

Therapist: And this is a very impressive family tree because you have pictures of a lot of people
Patient: yeah (laugh)
Therapist: which not everybody has. You've got a few more pictures on your mom's side than on your dad's side. She kept better records?
Patient: Well you know they . . .
Therapist: Oh, it keeps going
Patient: That's us now
Therapist: That's you now. And this is the future.
Patient: right
Therapist: What's coming down the pike. (daughter's name) is beautiful, (other daughter's name), two girls.
Patient: two girls
Therapist: (daughter's name) is the first
Patient: Mm-hmm
Therapist: she's the one with the child
Patient: right
Therapist: This is beautiful.
Patient: thank you
Therapist: this is a document of your family history, your history and your family history. What are you going to do with it you think?
Patient: Oh well, I'm actually going to work on it; I actually brought this for you.
Therapist: Thank you, I'll keep it.
Patient: I'm going to continue to work on it. In fact, I was focused on getting every detail and as a result it was taking me a tremendous amount of time to really get through this.
Therapist: Uh-huh
Patient: and then last night I said to myself "You don't need to get all the details for this" just this is a working document.
Therapist: yes
Patient: so make this your blueprint and
Therapist: Yeah, you have time.
Patient: you can add in things as you feel you need to.
Therapist: that's right, there might me more to come.
Patient: So that's what I did, I was up this morning and I finished it. I'm not sure if it's completely grammatically correct, in fact I found one error as I was going through it sitting outside. So I will send you if you'd like an addendum.
Therapist: No, actually I love things, between you and me; I love things that have slight imperfections in them
Patient: oh, okay
Therapist: cause I believe that's how life is, it's not perfect
Patient: okay
Therapist: I do a lot of writing and over the years, I've published, I've written papers obviously and published newsletters, and I things like that and I now edit a journal. And I learned this lesson when I was publishing this newsletter. This newsletter would come out every four months and inevitably someone would say to me "(name) did you realize there was a typo on this page" and I would be crushed and so what I decided to do was you know I need to embrace the imperfection of everything and I started to put typos in intentionally.
Patient: Oh really?
Therapist: at least one typo in intentionally, so the document went out with a typo that I knew about. And then inevitability people would say "Hey (name) did you notice there was a typo here?" And usually it wasn't the typo I put in.
Patient: (laugh)
Therapist: and I said "No biggie, I always put a typo in." So it's like that when you have a brand new car, the first scratch hurts
Patient: then afterwards . . .
Therapist: But I you already have another scratch, the other one doesn't hurt.
Patient: right
Therapist: So I encourage you, well, it's up to you; it's your legacy project
Patient: No, it's fine
Therapist: Then of course Mark Twain, who's a pretty good writer
Patient: Mm-hmm
Therapist: he would submit his manuscripts to the editor and he would get all kinds of complaints about his grammar and his punctuation, particularly his punctuation. And at some point he would submit his manuscripts and he would put every punctuation mark in English grammar at the bottom of the page, and said to the editor "use at your discretion." (laugh)
Patient: (laugh)
Therapist: He wasn't interested in the punctuation he was interested in what was there in the content. Now if you've got a typo that changes the meaning. . . .
Patient: Well, no, I don't think . . .
Therapist: if you have "I hated my mother" instead of "I loved my mother"
Patient: Yeah (laugh)
Therapist: there are two possibilities
Patient: right
Therapist: one is you actually have mixed feelings about your mother and the other is that it's a typo

Patient: right. And then the other thing I did was the feedback um

Therapist: oh, this is feedback

Patient: yeah

Therapist: So I'm going to read it, if that's okay. Okay, what's it been like to go through this learning experience. . . . Do you want me to read it, or would you like to read it?

Patient: Oh, it doesn't matter

Therapist: why don't you read it?

Patient: Okay, um, okay what has it been like for you to go through this learning experience over the last 7 sessions have there been any changes in the way you view your life and cancer experience having been through this process? And my response is. While I have thought many times about writing about the history of my family and my life the impetus for actually starting this legacy journal is a Memorial Sloan–Kettering Cancer Center Counseling Program I enrolled in 2011. I was introduced to the work of Victor Frankl, I found his book *Man's Search for Meaning* to be thought provoking. I have lived a good life and am blessed with a loving and supportive family, I have wonderful friends, and I have a very rewarding and personally fulfilling professional career. There have been times since my diagnosis and I've wondered how I could have lived such a productive life before cancer and what is the meaning of my life now. The reflections each week has made me realize how fortunate I am to continue a family tradition of nurturing the next generation by taking caring of my granddaughter (name) three days a week, to spend every day with my husband enjoying ordinary pleasures. And to enjoy the company of my immediate and extended family and to do the things that are important to me. To quote Carole King "I am more cognizant that these are the good old days, and try to live my life so that each day matters." Sorry . . .

Therapist: it's okay

Patient: everyday that I am alive is a gift of God, I do not take this gift for granted, particularly since my diagnosis of stage IV breast cancer in December 12, 2006, for me the diagnosis was a wakeup call to acknowledge that it was time for me to move away from my professional life and focus on my family. I have never appreciated how brave that decision was (patient crying). See I'm good, just as long as I don't talk about it.

Therapist: it's good that you talk about

Patient: until I participated in . . .

Therapist: just for the record I'm giving (patient) tissues because I'm a sensitive doctor

Patient: I never realized how brave that decision was until I participated in these sessions. Okay the next is not as emotional.

Therapist: this was the emotional part, that everyday you're alive is a gift from God? Or the courage?

Patient: I think everything

Therapist: everything is emotional.

Patient: everything, yeah if I think about it I get emotional. If I keep it on the back burner and just plow ahead, I'm okay. I guess that's where the strength comes in. Uh, do you feel like you have a better understanding of the sources of meaning in your life, and are you able to use them in your daily life, if so how? For me the historical sources of meaning is every present, I am fortunate to have known my maternal great grandmother, grandmother and paternal grandparents. I have reconnected to my cousin on my father's side to learn more about my grandparents and to share stories about growing up on the farm. Additionally, I have spoken to my mother at great length about her memories so that I could record them for my children and grandchild. I have encouraged my husband and his sisters to do the same for their family. With respect to attitudinal meaning, the acknowledgement of the significant roles of personal tragedies in my life, death of my father, grandparents, friends, illness and disappointment has had in motivating me to make choices is profound. In the past, I thought of meaningful moments as happy, joyous events and did not appreciate the . . . sorry (crying) . . . significant role suffering has played in motivating me to make choices, cause that wasn't completely over. Courage and attitude is important to remember and is something I've taken for granted and minimized. Of course I have no insight into how long I will live and how long I will enjoy a good quality of life. I am cautiously optimistic that with continued good response to treatment my life's work on earth will continue for some time. I acknowledge the reality that stage IV cancer is a serious medical condition and the life expectancy is usually 10 years from diagnosis. It is an interesting balancing act. Again the sessions have helped me to provide a way to appreciating the creative sources of meaning in my life. My work at the college was an extension of my personal life, I enjoyed working with the students, I enjoyed working at the college and creating new programs and engaging in a meaningful profession of student development. Because it was so personally fulfilling I look back on these achievements with fond memories and no regret for moving on to the next chapter of my life. I acknowledge that I am responsible for myself, but am responsible to my husband and family, is essential in maintaining a balance in family dynamics. I am learning to appreciate how important this is when interacting with my adult children. I think the focus on experiential sources of meaning is the essence of life, the ability to appreciate a sunset, or a magnificent, I spelled that wrong, view, provides a framework for understanding how beautiful life is, okay it should say, well it's a typo, in ordinary days.

Therapist: exactly

Patient: For me it is essential that I tell my family how much I love them and to demonstrate that love by doing everyday things like making dinner or laughing about the day's events. Okay, what are you hopes for the future? My hope is to continue to appreciate life fully and to recognize the people in my life that are important to me. I expect I will continue to work on my legacy project to work to create a journal of my life that included my family and my husband's family history. I am working to embrace a healthy lifestyle of eating; again it is important to remember that everything we do involves making a choice. A choice that God will guide me along a path that my faith will help me through any difficulties that I may face in the future (crying).

Therapist: take your time (patient's name)

Patient: The last sentence really resonates

Therapist: that last, this thing you're about to say is what you're preparing yourself for.

Patient: This is easier to type

Therapist: yes

Patient: I know that death is the natural end to life; I hope I have the strength to face it bravely.

Therapist: yeah, I think that if that little girl is beside you at that point, she'll give you some strength

Patient: I think so too

Therapist: it's that little girl

Patient: oh me!

Therapist: that little girl lies there in that bed with you

Patient: yeah I hope so

Therapist: she's in there you just have to call on her. That was emotional for you.

Patient: Very

Therapist: thank you for being brave and sharing that to read it. I guess I could've read it, but there was something that made say "Why don't you read it" I don't know what it was, maybe my instincts.

Patient: Well, I probably wouldn't have been as emotional if you have read it. I think I would've been okay

Therapist: The emotion, the emotion related to what? There are obviously certain parts that are emotional. The last sentence. Is the last sentence a culmination of what you learned here?

Patient: Uh

Therapist: or they've been so many lessons.

Patient: I think they've been so many lessons. I think I have a tendency of not thinking about this a lot

Therapist: about death

Patient: Death yeah. Um, it doesn't make sense to focus on something you have no control over . . .

Therapist: Mm-hmm

Patient: Unless of course you take your own life. Uh, so um and I think it's an absolute waste of time to focus on something may happen tomorrow, today, ten years from now, 20 years from now. That you miss so much of living by focusing on death.

Therapist: right

Patient: so rather than focusing on somebody else's, on my death, um, I I mean I have thousands of pictures of my family. I look at the pictures of my family, particularly in 1941 my mother must have been about 10 years old, she must have just got a camera and that summer she took hundreds of pictures of her family. And it was just before her grandfather died and her father died. And I look at those happy faces in those pictures and that's what you want to remember and what you want to be remembered for, the joy in your life. Now I say this all this acknowledging the fact that I have responded well to treatment, I don't know what the future will hold, I don't know if I will continue to respond to treatment. I can hope that when I don't respond as well to treatment and look back at these projects that I'm doing, and remember and draw strength from how I handled things before. When I was younger my mother would wake me up, it sounds torturous but it was funny at the time, she would take a little water and she would sprinkle it on my face to wake me up in the morning. So I think sometimes these projects this project in fact will be like sprinkling water to wake me up, this is something for you to remember, you know it's a new day.

Therapist: yeah um you make the point that you don't think it's a good thing to focus on dying all the time.

Patient: no

Therapist: but do you think there is something to be gained by examining for a moment and then learning something from it, like the other tragedies in your life, they were calls for action.

Patient: right

Therapist: and to have the courage to examine it briefly and say "What kind of lessons can I learn from this?" what does this teach me, it teaching me how important it is to live life every day, that's what that does. So you don't have to think about it constantly, but you have to be able to look at it and say what can I . . .

Patient: what can I learn from this

Therapist: learn from it, and I think that's what you did.

Patient: yeah, that's what I did. And again, it's much easier for me to think about it, and to write about, and to talk about it.

Therapist: okay whatever works.

Patient: I can be a, I'm emotional when I talk about it.

Therapist: Mm-hmm

Patient: because the fear of what lies ahead is profound

Therapist: Mm-hmm

Patient: um, but if I write about it, I can . . .

Therapist: you're a little bit removed.

Patient: its its

Therapist: well, you have some faith in God, looks like

Patient: yeah

Therapist: I don't recall if we talked about if you have a definitive idea of what happens after death, do you?

Patient: well, um, I'd like to think

Therapist: mm-hmm

Patient: we are rejoined with our loved ones

Therapist: but you're not thousand percent positive

Patient: well, no

Therapist: so there's a bit of unknown.

Patient: right

Therapist: and there's a bit of a mystery in a sense of its difficult to know for certain, what's ahead right, after death. So um, I kind of like the word mystery, because with mystery comes infinite possibilities.

Patient: rather than uncertainty

Therapist: Yes and so there are infinite possibilities including a lot of really pleasant ones and good . . .

Patient: yeah I'd like to think that I'll see my father again

Therapist: right

Patient: kind of catch up

Therapist: right

Patient: but I don't know

Therapist: right, it's mysterious

Patient: it's mysterious

Therapist: so there are infinite possibilities, and you have a choice as you said

Patient: right

Therapist: everything we do involves making a choice

Patient: everything we do involves making a choice

Therapist: including how we die

Patient: right

Therapist: and how we think about dying

Patient: right

Therapist: This magnificent . . . this is just a magnificent legacy document and. Thank you for writing down the feedback, reflections and feedback, your hopes for the future. And I think what's dramatic and noteworthy the hopes for your future really are to live your life fully, whatever life you have left you want to live that fully and meaningful.

Patient: yeah when I first read the 3rd question, I was thinking of it more as a to-do list, you know like what do you want to do, and I said well, that's not the question. The question is what are you hopes, not one of the things you want to accomplish.

Therapist: Right, yeah well, some people write different things. People say "I hope to be surrounded by my family, and not suffer" and things like that. But you focus on living.

Patient: yeah

Therapist: which is good

Patient: yeah

Therapist: well let me just say (patient's name) the kind of work we did together the kind of work I do in general as a psychiatrist at Sloan–Kettering bring me in a position of sharing very intimate things with people, people share with me their fears and the stories of their lives, and you know not the kinds of things you share with everybody. So I feel very privileged to be able to share that with people and I feel very privileged to have had this time with you to get to know you a little bit better, and to hear this incredible life story of yours which you have put down on paper. And I'm just so impressed with just you as a person.

Patient: thank you

Therapist: even before the cancer, but now that, in terms of what I have learned about you, and what I feel and see and interact everyday when we have our sessions.

Patient: mm-hmm

Therapist: but also just so impressed with how you've been able to take what we've been trying to do in the sessions and really used them to formulate, you've really reflected on the therapy in a way that has perhaps has helped you sort of reinforce and clarify for yourself what went on in therapy, but it helps me also in terms of the next patient. You know it focuses it, so this is going to be enormously helpful for me. And uh I feel sad that this is our last session, I'm going to miss you.

Patient: Thank you, I'll miss you too.

Therapist: But uh, you'll hear from us in about 2 months.

Patient: okay

Therapist: and I think what you need to hear from me is that while I, I meet a lot of people of course in my work, I don't believe I'll ever forget you.

Patient: Oh, thank you, thank you

Therapist: I don't believe I'll ever forget you, I think I'll always remember you.

Patient: Thank you, It's been um, it's been a, it's been very meaningful to me.

Therapist: That's the word, thanks (patient's name), thanks. We'll turn this off.

Patient: okay

PATIENT 2 IMCP TRANSCRIPT

Session 1: Concepts and Sources of Meaning—Introductions and Meaning

Therapist: Okay, we're recording. So thank you for doing this.

Patient: Mm-hmm

Therapist: I really appreciate it. I'm Dr. (name), like I said you can call me (name). Um, you're participating in a research study,

Patient: Yes

Therapist: so I appreciate that very very much.

Patient: Mm-hmm

Therapist: what we're doing is we're comparing a few different types of counseling for people who have cancer.

Patient: yes

Therapist: And actually you were randomized, you ended up getting, the therapy called meaning-centered psychotherapy. And actually this is a psychotherapy that I developed, so you're getting it . . .

Patient: Okay, I am lucky (laugh)

Therapist: So you're getting it from the guy who developed it, okay?

Patient: right

Therapist: And we've been studying it for a while, we've been working on it for 8 years or more. And we developed it and studied it in a group format, and we've studied it in an individual format.

Patient: right

Therapist: and we're now finished up doing a large trial of the group, and this year is the first year of the 5 year study of the 1-1.

Patient: 1-1

Therapist: So it's a research study, we're going to be recording these sessions.

Patient: Mm-hmm

Therapist: The main reason for the sessions to be recorded is I have people listening to make sure that I do the therapy exactly the way it's written in the manual.

Patient: right

Therapist: Now I have a manual and you have one too.

Patient: okay

Therapist: This is something that you get to take home and keep. And you can write in it, okay?

Patient: okay

Therapist: You can take notes in it and things like that. Uh, you can take notes and there might be a couple things you want to take notes about. For instance, this this is something for you to have

Patient: Mm-hmm

Therapist: It tells you a little bit about the therapy, where you have to come, you know and this is how to reach me. That's (name), my assistant, and my phone number. Um, and an email, although, I'll give you my card as well later so you can have that . . .

Patient: okay

Therapist: . . . and we're going to try to fit in 7 sessions.

Patient: Yes

Therapist: and as you just saw, we're trying to measure how well this kind of intervention helps with things like anxiety, depression, hope, things like that. As you might gather from the title, the name of the therapy, we're focusing on meaning . . .

Patient: right

Therapist: . . . and trying to help people sustain or even enhance a sense of meaning even in the face of a difficult time with the cancer.

Patient: Mm-hmm

Therapist: So there will be 7 sessions, after our 4th session, (name of RSA) will probably try to meet with you before or after the session and repeat the assessment.

Patient: okay

Therapist: and then after the 7th session, and then we'll catch up with you about 2 months after that . . .

Patient: okay

Therapist: . . . to do that again. So this is just information for you to have.

Patient: right

Therapist: this is a little calendar to help remind you and me of when the sessions are. So we're just having our first session on the 9th . . .

Patient: today's the 9th?

Therapist: I'm sorry, 10th. I'm bad with dates, you?

Patient: Mm-hmm

Therapist: So um and then perhaps what we can do to figure out when the next one is. Is this a good time for you?

Patient: This is a good time for you. I'm usually up and going at this time.

Therapist: So should we basically plan to meet again next week at this time?

Patient: Sometimes I may have to coordinate according to my schedule

Therapist: Absolutely

Patient: you know to make things easier.

Therapist: Absolutely

Patient: So I'll call, and when I know my schedule and then we'll go from there.

Therapist: But do you know if next Tuesday is okay? Or you don't know yet?

Patient: I have to discuss with the doctor.

Therapist: Absolutely, sure.

Patient: I need to recover from this chemo, before I take another dose.

Therapist: Sure

Patient: Cause it drains the daylights out of me.

Therapist: I hear you. So what I'll do is I'll ask (RSA name) to discuss with you when the next . . .

Patient: Mm-hmm

Therapist: So you can have this so that you can you can know for yourself when the things are.

Patient: of course, yes

Therapist: and I'll just put it back in for you.

Patient: right

Therapist: Now when you look through this what you'll see is there are a lot of quotes in here, but you don't have to read all the quotes. But there are going to 7 sessions and each session we're going to focus on a particular topic

Patient: right

Therapist: and each session has a section right. We're going to focus on . . .

Patient: Session 1, right

Therapist: We're going to focus on today. I'm basically going to be interested in telling you . . .

Patient: Context of sources of meaning.

Therapist: First things first I wanted to tell you about the therapy and what to expect over the next bunch of weeks. And then I want to hear a little bit about your story, and then we can talk a little bit about some of the concepts of meaning. Now each of the sessions involves a little bit of discussion, sort of meet, try to give you a little information about some concept related to meaning.

Patient: right

Therapist: And then there's a sort of exercise in which you answer a couple of questions to think about how better to understand that particular concept. So it's a way of learning.

Patient: Right

Therapist: And you can see there are 7 sessions, they all focus on meaning. How cancer has affected your meaning is the second session. And then in a moment I'll tell you a little bit about some of the basics of the idea of meaning and where it comes from. And then the rest of the sessions focus on the sources of meaning, what are the common sources of meaning in our lives. And then the last session is sort of a review.

Patient: Mm-hmm

Therapist: Okay, and then again each one of these tabs focuses on a session. This is the one we're focusing on today, but we'll get into that in a little bit. So (patient name) before we start getting into the idea of meaning and the various concepts of meaning, tell me a little bit about your story, you started to tell me a little bit about being tired and chemotherapy and things like that.

Patient: I found out, 2 years ago

Therapist: three years ago?

Patient: two years ago

Therapist: 2

Patient: I had this pain only when I'm on the train.

Therapist: Only when you're on the train.

Patient: Train, I couldn't sit still

Therapist: you mean on the subway?

Patient: In the subway

Therapist: and why are you on the subway a lot?

Patient: heading to and from work, I'm a registered nurse.

Therapist: You're a nurse, and where were you headed to work?

Patient: To Mount Sinai

Therapist: You work at Mount Sinai, mm-hmm.

Patient: and I told my son, I cannot sit still on the train because I have this pain in my back. He said "Mommy, you should see the doctor." I told him this in February, and in April I told him "You know what? This pain is bothering me." He said "Well you won't listen, Mommy go to the doctor today." So the doctor was down the street from me, and I told him, and I go to the doctor often. I told him "You know I have this pain only when I'm on the pain and I can't sit still." He said "Okay, let me examine you, maybe you should have a CT scan. You go tomorrow?" "Yes." And I had a scan the following morning, they saw a mass, and they sent him the report, they sent me to someone else, MRI, well it was cancer, and I came back to the doctors whom I work with and I told them what was going on. They did the biopsy, it was cancer, and like two months later I had surgery.

Therapist: At Sinai?

Patient: Mm-hmm and they referred me here to Dr. (name) chemo.

Therapist: So you have pancreatic cancer?

Patient: Yes

Therapist: and when they first diagnosed it, it was possible to do surgery.

Patient: Yes

Therapist: It was probably a good thing right?

Patient: Yeah, it was a good thing.

Therapist: That's what they said.

Patient: Mm-hmm

Therapist: And you had mentioned this to the doctor that you worked with. What kind of doctor do you work with at Sinai?

Patient: Sometimes I work with oncologists, hematologists, and this was a hematologist team that I felt comfortable with, they're so good to me

Therapist: I see

Patient: and he took over

Therapist: So you work in hematology/oncology, and how long have you been doing that?

Patient: 20 years

Therapist: 20 years, okay. So you had your surgery at Mount Sinai and you were referred to Dr. (name).

Patient: And with the past scans, he's said the cancer is back, so I'm back on. I had chemo and now I'm back on chemo again, but this chemo is not like the first one. The first one was a breeze, this one isn't.

Therapist: I hear you. So I think you were referred to Dr. (name) after the surgery.

Patient: After the surgery

Therapist: to get what's called adjuvant chemotherapy.

Patient: yes

Therapist: To try to make sure that you were disease free, and you had that for a period of time and then the scans had shown that it had come back. And where did it come back?

Patient: Right in my pancreas again

Therapist: Right in the pancreas again. And did it spread anywhere else?

Patient: It did spread, but I didn't go into details with him.

Therapist: you don't want to know about it?

Patient: I don't want to know

Therapist: Yes, I understand

Patient: I'm just hoping to do my therapy and get some respite; I don't have as much pain. I'm happy.

Therapist: You were having quite a bit of pain I guess before the surgery.

Patient: After the surgery, no more pain.

Therapist: Okay, and then it came back?

Patient: and then I had little pains.

Therapist: that's when they found out that you had some growths?

Patient: and um, sometimes I have the pain, sometimes I don't have it. It's not unbearable pain that I can't manage.

Therapist: are you on pain medicines?

Patient: I take pain medications, but I don't even need them

Therapist: Don't need them all the time?

Patient: I don't think I need them.

Therapist: every once in a while?

Patient: if I take a Tylenol, I could do two days without the pain medication, even though I don't take the Tylenol, but um, I know I have the pain medication in case I need them.

Therapist: Gotcha. Do you have any medical problems besides in addition to the?

Patient: High cholesterol, high blood pressure . . .

Therapist: the usual. Now, I detect a slight accent.

Patient: I'm from Belize, I'm from Central America.

Therapist: From Belize, now Belize sounds like a beautiful place.

Patient: I wish I was there this morning.

Therapist: Uh-ha

Patient: I told them, I wish I could sneak away for like a 1 week. We own a home in Belize.

Therapist: you have a home
Patient: I go home and I feel so good.
Therapist: everybody needs a place like that
Patient: I get into my hammock, no one knows that I'm home, and I am so on top of the world.
Therapist: So you have a place in Belize and there's a hammock in the backyard, the front yard, where?
Patient: On the porch
Therapist: On the porch and that's your favorite place.
Patient: That's my favorite place
Therapist: Is there a particular time of day that you love to be on the hammock?
Patient: Like 11 am in the morning
Therapist: 11 am in the morning.
Patient: I get into my hammock
Therapist: and what is it about the hammock, the porch and Belize?
Patient: It's quiet
Therapist: its quiet, the temperature is . . .
Patient: The sky is blue, clear
Therapist: clear
Patient: You can smell the salt in the air
Therapist: What do you smell in the air?
Patient: the salt
Therapist: the swaz?
Patient: the salt, the salt
Therapist: The salt
Patient: because we're in front of the sea. My house is far away from the sea, but you can smell the salt in the air
Therapist: because there's a little bit of a breeze
Patient: There's a breeze all the time, and there is a river, that when I'm standing on the porch I could just look at. And its just peace and solitude.
Therapist: a little bit later we're going to do an exercise, to help you try to understand what we mean by the word "meaning." And one of the definitions of meaning are moments when you feel most alive and you feel most connected to something greater than yourself. And it sounds like those are moments like that right?
Patient: Yes, there are birds. When we had the house built, like 14 years ago, it was like a conservation area.
Therapist: I see
Patient: And there were all sorts of bird, toucans, parrots, beautiful birds, and I would just sit there and enjoy every moment of it. But they've cleared it
Therapist: They've cleared it? They've built more houses?
Patient: To build more houses. But still the birds come.
Therapist: It's still beautiful
Patient: It's still beautiful.
Therapist: No you mentioned a son, and you said "We have a home." So who's in your family?
Patient: My mother
Therapist: your mother
Patient: she's not really my mother, she's my aunt, but she raised me since my mother died. In fact my mother would be 86 years old today.
Therapist: Today?
Patient: Today's her birthday. She died at 26 years old giving birth to my brother, who died on that same day.
Therapist: Oh my
Patient: They both died on that same day, and that was my birthday.
Therapist: So that day was your birthday
Patient: My birthday
Therapist: your brother's birthday
Patient: My brother's birthday and she died on that day.
Therapist: what day was that?
Patient: September 12th
Therapist: It's like everybody remembers September 11th, but you remember September 12th, don't you? How old were you when your mother died?
Patient: I was 2
Therapist: 2 years old, and your grandmother raised you
Patient: My Aunt
Therapist: I'm sorry, you're Aunt
Patient: My grandmother, well my mom had two sisters and a brother and her mother, and they've done the best they can. I don't think I could've been any better without these people.
Therapist: So this house in Belize, you're grandmother and aunt?
Patient: It's my house
Therapist: your house, she lives there?
Patient: with my husband. My aunt, my mom is here with me
Therapist: She lives here with you. And you're married?
Patient: I'm married
Therapist: How long? How long?
Patient: 39 years
Therapist: 39 years
Patient: this September
Therapist: This September, September the 12th?
Patient: September 23rd
Therapist: Okay and you have a son?
Patient: I have a son

Therapist: How old is he?

Patient: 31 years old

Therapist: Any other children

Patient: I had a 3-, he would've been 36 last March, he died at 21 years old in a motor vehicle accident, a hit-and-run.

Therapist: I'm sorry to hear that. So you've had some beautiful things happen in your life, and some tragic.

Patient: But you know all in all I sometimes evaluate my life; I've had a good life. These knocks that have happened in my life, I see them bring me meaning.

Therapist: these events

Patient: these events

Therapist: bring meaning in your life

Patient: meaning to my life. My son that died, (name), was my first child.

Therapist: your first child

Patient: And sometimes I say he was the best thing that ever happened to me.

Therapist: Of course, why do you say that?

Patient: because I had (name of son) and (name of son) was born with osteogenesis imperfecta. And I told myself that (name of son) had osteogenesis imperfecta, but that it would not consume his life. He was so smart, everyone loved him, he was wheelchair bound, fearless, when he was like 3 or 4 people would say "Oh why don't you just stack up those papers so he can reach up to the table and eat." I said "Why not, he will sit in the chair and he will eat. As long as he can reach his food, he can eat okay." And he said to me "Mommy, why do you raise me like this?" He was my first child, and by the time he was like a year and a half he was talking. I would talk to him all the time.

Therapist: special

Patient: He was very verbal, very. I said "You know (son's name) you have to do things for yourself, no one is going to do it for you. You have to say please, you have to say thank you. You'll be in and out of the hospital. These people are there doing things for you. But they don't have to do it for you; you have to do things for yourself too." He was just a good kid. He did everything for himself. He went to college, he drove a car, he cooks. He would climb up on my counter, and make a meal. He will leave something unusual on the floor "Mommy, your lunch is in the refrigerator." He will pack something at the door, it doesn't belong there, and I know that I should see what it is "Mommy, I left this for you in the fridge or on the table for lunch."

Therapist: So it sounds . . .

Patient: I was so so proud of him

Therapist: You should be proud of him. And in fact, this story you're telling me about (son's name) fits very much with what I'm about to try to introduce you to. This therapy focuses on meaning, meaning-centered therapy is based a bit on the work of a psychiatrist named Victor Frankl and he a lot about and wrote a lot about meaning. And there are very basic concepts about meaning. First of all, each of us has a responsibility; we have a responsibility to create a life of meaning, identity and direction. And so we create this life and it has a sort of trajectory, but all of us have to create this life within the context of the facts of our physical and environmental limitations. We're all born with certain, I'm born with a certain kind of intelligence, with a certain color eyes, I'm born to be just this tall whatever, (son's name) was born with osteogenesis imperfecta, and so its our responsibility to create a life of meaning, identity, and direction and self-transcendence, giving to others, and self-actualization, becoming who only we uniquely were meant to be. And we need to surpass, reach beyond our limitations. And your story of (son's name) is exactly that story of a person, a young man, I'm assuming that a lot of this was his own drive and will, but you nurtured that, you also had that same expectation.

Patient: I enabled him

Therapist: you enabled him, to become more than what he, what others might have said "This is your limit; you can't do more than that." And you also in your life in facing cancer overcome the limitations of what people say.

Patient: Mm-hmm

Therapist: Perhaps that's why you didn't want to know exactly where everything was because you didn't want it to interfere with your desire to overcome and transcend whatever limitations.

Patient: Yes

Therapist: So meaning turns out to be a very important part of what we need to create in our lives and Frankl basically said that one of the basic human motivating forces, that one of the most basic motivating forces of human behavior, human psychology is to find meaning in our lives, to search for meaning and to find meaning in our lives. Other big thinkers like Freud thought well we're all driven by our biological need to procreate to have children, libido, other people thought to get power. Frankl felt we're driven by the need to find meaning and create meaning in our lives. Frankl said there were several basic things about meaning. One is that our lives have meaning from the moment we're born until the moment we die. Our lives never cease to have meaning, they never stop having meaning, meaning in our lives may change but they never stop having meaning.

Patient: meaning

Therapist: We may feel that our lives have lost meaning, but it's not because meaning has ceased to exist

Patient: right

Therapist: it's because we have become disconnected from it. We've lost sight of it. It's like you've lost the keys to your house, you've misplaced them someplace. It's not like the keys don't exist anymore, you just . . .

Patient: can't find them

Therapist: lost them, you have to find them again you have to rediscover them again, you have to uncover them. The second basic thing is that we have this need to make meaning or find meaning in our lives, and the third basic concept is that we have the freedom to find meaning in our existence wherever we can from good things and from things that are at first glance seem tragic.

Patient: right

Therapist: and the fourth basic concept is that even when we suffer, even when something tragic happens, we have the freedom to find meaning even though suffering through the attitude that we take.

Patient: Right, right

Therapist: the way we think about the events or circumstances, so we have the freedom to find meaning even in suffering through the attitude we take towards suffering. So we can take a tragedy and turn it into a triumph.

Patient: Sure, I believe in that.

Therapist: Something like what (son's name) did, right. Frankl also said that there were some very specific sources of meaning in our lives.

Patient: Mm-hmm

Therapist: and part of what we're going to do over the next 7 weeks is we're going to go over and over and over again through variety of exercises these various sources of meaning in life, because these sources of meaning become resources of meaning. We can go to them like a well. Cause sometimes what happens is one particular source of meaning becomes blocked because of fatigue, from the chemotherapy. You'd love to go to Belize but you're in the middle of this chemotherapy, you can't make it, so some other, you know. . . . So there are multiple sources of meaning that we can go to as resources, and we can move from one source of meaning to another when we're blocked.

Patient: Mm-hmm

Therapist: so a simple way to think about these sources of meaning is the following. We get meaning, we derive meaning through our lives through dedicating ourselves to someone or something so when we dedicate ourselves to someone, we serve someone, we love someone that is a source of meaning. He called it an experiential source of meaning. That we derive meaning in our lives through love, through love and connected with people, with nature, with the ocean, the breeze from the ocean, the birds, the smell of salt, nature, other things that we can appreciate in the world you know the touch, of when maybe (son's name) would maybe kiss you or touch, his voice. . . .

Patient: Oh yeah, which he did every day.

Therapist: . . . right, his voice whatever. All of our senses or experiences source of meaning through love basically, through love, and though dedicating ourselves to something, that's usually our work. You get meaning from our work, our life's work, now our life's work is sometimes is mainly the work we do for a living.

Patient: Living

Therapist: like a nurse, I would say that's a kind of career that's more than just a 9 to 5 job. You're expressing a caring, you care about people, you care about the world and you express that through your work. And there may be other kinds of work you do in the world things that you, causes that you care about like charity, generosity, truth, justice, caring, compassion.

Patient: Mm-hmm

Therapist: Our lives exist in a historical context, you told me the story about your mother and your older brother and how you were raised. So meaning exists in a historical context, the meaning in your life is unique and special because of where you came from and who you came from.

Patient: From

Therapist: your history, your legacy, the legacy you inherited, and you also derive meaning in your life through the legacy that you live and the legacy you leave behind.

Patient: Mm-hmm

Therapist: what's your other son's name?

Patient: (son's name)

Therapist: (son's name)?

Patient: (son's name) (and then spells it out).

Therapist: (son's name)

Patient: I speak another language and (son's name) means my son.

Therapist: My son, what language is that?

Patient: that's Garufina

Therapist: Garufina

Patient: Uh-ha

Therapist: Is that . . .

Patient: When the Africans were brought to the Caribbean these people did not want to be taken as slaves from St. Vincent's so they drove them out and they ended up on the coast of Honduras on the coast of Central America, so we still maintained our language and culture.

Therapist: And you are from those people

Patient: Yes

Therapist: So that is a big source of your legacy and your identity, and we derive a great deal of meaning from our identity.

Patient: yes

Therapist: and that's related to basically who we love and what we do and where we came from, that's our identity. That's why I said when you create a life; you create a life you need to create of a life of meaning and identity.

Patient: yes

Therapist: And direction.

Patient: yes

Therapist: the direction has to do with when you're young; you're growing up and all that, you're moving forward. But when you're encountering an illness like yours, the trajectory kind of stops and people think okay there's no direction at all, I'm stopped, but that in fact what happens is you're moving now in lots of directions, you're still looking forward, you look maybe to beyond, what lies beyond. You also, you told me you lived a good life. You also look back and you're looking around you at the people who you're connected to. So you're moving in lots of directions.

Patient: I move in lots of directions (name) and when I inventory what I'm going through I tell myself I happen to have this diagnosis yes, the only thing that gets me down is the fatigue and the side effects of the chemo, otherwise I go about my business. And I think it's because of the way I've lived my life, I'm not a negative person, I try not to harbor that in my life, I do not look back, I move forward, in whatever, in wherever it may end. I look forward

Therapist: Right

Patient: And if there happens to be negativity around me, I'll be the first one to say you know what I'm not harboring that around me, I do not need it, keep it out.

Therapist: I was really talking about looking backward as a very natural and necessary part of trying to be able to continue to look forward and to live full everyday in some sense of peace, that I've lived a good full life, I've lived a meaningful life hopefully, and so I can keep moving forward with some sense of peace. I think we need that naturally without even knowing about it, maybe you did it purposefully, that is what I sensed when you told me "You know I've lived a good life." You took a look and you said "Yeah, it's not too bad."

Patient: It's not too bad.

Therapist: even though there were some tragic things in it.

Patient: there were some tragic things, and you know well I didn't have control over my mother and it hurt when my son died and to this day the police officers that were there came and they said "When we met your son we were shocked that he would drive, but we saw how he was dressed, we saw your other son and they spoke so well." And I said "You know, God is good." It was, whoever hit his car left, it would've killed me if they found him, because I would spend every penny I had to get him a death sentence or something. I tell myself . . .

Therapist: It would've consumed you.

Patient: It would've consumed me.

Therapist: And if it consumes you then you give up your life.

Patient: I give up my life to that

Therapist: to that, not to something better

Patient: Not to something better and I still have another son. And my other son was in the car with him, because my co-workers would bring me from work at nighttime, but he said "No mommy, you're not coming with your co-worker, I'm coming to get you." And I said "No I'm coming with my co-worker." And he called like 10 o'clock in the night "Mommy, I'm coming." I said "Be careful." At 10:30 and I'm downstairs at Mount Sinai and he's not there, I knew something has gone wrong, I just had that feeling.

Therapist: So it happened here in NY.

Patient: Mm-hmm. I knew something had gone terribly wrong, but I said you know God is good that they didn't find, he left because I didn't want to be consumed by that, as much as I would want justice for him. But he's at peace

Therapist: Yes

Patient: You know because I had another child to look to, he had a fractured pelvis, he had a fractured spine

Therapist: wow

Patient: thank god, he's up and about.

Therapist: (son's name)

Patient: (son's name).

Therapist: So those are the sources of meaning, and you're going to have this book so you can re-read this.

Patient: I will read it; I put my little notes in there

Therapist: You put your notes

Patient: I put my little notes in there

Therapist: So the exercise for today and its almost unnecessary because we've actually talked quite a bit about it. Let me see how much time we have, good a little bit of time. So people often find it difficult to understand what we mean by meaning, but I think you understand it intuitively. But we have two different definitions, the second definition is the one we've been talking about was that meaning refers to moments when that make life worth living, when you feel needed or alive, things from the past the way you look back on them you still find to be very important, in other words meaning in moments where you feel most alive. The other definition that we try to work with is having a sense that you're life has meaning involves a belief that you're fulfilling a unique role and purpose in life, some people think of this life as a gift, and this life comes with a responsibility like I said to live this life to your full potential. And if you're able to do that you can achieve a sense of peace, contentment, even transcendence through connectedness with something greater than yourself. Would you improve on the definition? Would you have your own definition? Or do you think any of these definitions make more sense?

Patient: I don't know if I could improve on the definition.

Therapist: Or modify it a little bit?

Patient: Personally I feel that my life has had a meaning, purpose, and sometimes I tell my aunt and my uncle, you know you guys did me well, but you made me too responsible. As I was their first child in the family, and I had everything it didn't only fall on my aunt that eventually took responsibility for me. My uncle, if I'm sick he would say "What's wrong with you?" If he has to take me to the doctor and my mom is there, he's going to pick me up and take me to the doctor.

Therapist: so you were surrounded by people who took responsibility very seriously, and you saw that that was something you needed to do.

Patient: and to this day, they're hovering around me.

Therapist: They are?

Patient: They are, my mom the one who raised me she's 88, she was the oldest and she is what's making me ache.

Therapist: she's what?

Patient: She's making me ache, my heart ache, she makes me hurt, because she looks at me and she's not saying anything. She's not saying much, at 88 years, she's very verbal and my mom is all fearless as I am. And I come downstairs at nighttime she says "Are you okay?"

Therapist: So you're heart aches b/c you see she's worried about you?

Patient: She's worried about me. "Are you okay?" she said "What's wrong?" "Ma, I'm just coming downstairs for something to eat." And I see her just sitting there sometimes just praying and talking to herself, and that makes me hurt.

Therapist: So you don't mind these definitions?

Patient: No, and that is one of the reasons I agreed to do this.

Therapist: to do this

Patient: personally for myself, I'm okay. I've known that at some time that I have to go. We all have to die.

Therapist: Is that true?

Patient: We all have to.

Therapist: I think so, I think you're right.

Patient: We all have to. Some people are afraid. When my patient, I would never let my patient die alone.

Therapist: You stay there with them

Patient: I would stay there; I would always stay there with my patient. I think I owed it to the human being.

Therapist: You are someone who feels so connected to other human beings. This is what we mean by transcendence.

Patient: Right

Therapist: To not be so concerned with just yourself, but understand that you're connected to people.

Patient: Yes, this is a whole, we need each other.

Therapist: Yes

Patient: and in whatever way, I have never let a patient die alone, him or herself, don't care what religion it is, I would stay there and say a prayer, because this is the end for all of us you know. And I know I have to go at some time, on my own terms.

Therapist: what does that mean?

Patient: um, I'm not in pain, but I'm not going to have pain.

Therapist: Okay, we're going to have a session later on where we talk about the limitations of life and the ultimate limitation of death, we'll have plenty of time to talk about what you mean by that, death.

Patient: Okay

Therapist: Let's finish today by doing this exercise, and like I say it's almost unnecessary, because we've already started to talk a lot about it I think. But if you could just take a moment and write maybe if you want to make a few notes for yourself, or you may already you don't have to write it out fully. Just one or two moments when life felt particular meaningful to you, something that helped you through a difficult day, or a time when you felt most alive. And it could as you say, it could be something very beautiful or it could be something really tragic and you've already talked about a lot of things both beautiful and tragic that you thought gave your life meaning. You actually talked about almost all of the sources of meaning today, you talked about love, you talked about your work, you talked about the attitude you took towards tragic events that gave your life meaning. And you talked about your legacy . . .

Patient: Because (name)

Therapist: and the Gari—

Patient: Garifuna.

Therapist: Garifuna

Patient: Garifuna

Therapist: ah, Garifuna. And the name of the people?

Patient: That's the name

Therapist: that's the name

Patient: The Garifuna

Therapist: that's the name, the Garifuna

Patient: and that's the language

Therapist: And they came from what part of Africa?

Patient: Oh God, I can't tell you now, but it's the Youroba, Y-O-U-R-O-B-A, Youroba people from Africa.

Therapist: I see, they are different from the Garifuna people or the same?

Patient: The same

Therapist: That's the people, gotcha.

Patient: The thing is (name) I'm into my family, and that makes me the happiest. I don't party, I don't drink I go to work, oh but we'll party at home. Everything's an event, you know if it's someone's birthday we'll make a cake, the kids come, my uncles' children, and I enjoy that just being there with the children. And I knock on wood every day, I'm the oldest and they all congregate at my house. And I say "We have good children, and for that I'm happy."

Therapist: right

Patient: I'm sick; they all know I'm sick. They come when I'm at the hospital, oh God, the nurses will say "Where are your children?" Because the whole troop comes and even neighborhood children, I keep them at my house, cause when I moved to the neighborhood 31 years ago it was all children, young children the same age as mine, and I didn't want mine on the streets so I would tell them you know what . . .

Therapist: come to my house

Patient: come to my house. They'll be fixing the irons, fixing the bicycles, out of the streets, but stay here get out of trouble. And it's been good. If they meet me on the street "Oh Ms. (name) you used to bring us to the porch." And they are all grown men now. If I'm out there at nighttime "Come one we'll take you home."

Therapist: So caring for all children gives your life a sense of meaning too.

Patient: Mm-hmm

Therapist: The idea of children is very valuable you view the, that's the next generation.

Patient: I had one yesterday that had a baby, she's in Belize, I had her there with me, her mother had a hard time. She said "I wish I could go to school or something." I said "You will go to school; I'll send you to school." And she's gone to school and she ended up having a baby. I said "There's nothing wrong with having the baby." So yesterday she had her baby girl and she called yesterday she had a C-section first thing in the morning. And I said to her, she said "I had a baby girl this morning." I said "Thank god just take care of yourself and her."

Therapist: Yeah, let me just got back to this exercise.

Patient: Mm-hmm

Therapist: I know you jotted down a couple of notes, but some of the things that you told me that fitted to this exercise are, lying in the hammock, 11 o'clock in the morning in Belize with the salt air, being connected to, speaking Garifuna, and being connected to these very proud people, and your family. Out of the tragedy of your mother's death and your brother's death you were raised by such loving aunts and uncles whatever, and the strength of your family, the strength of the legacy that you've inherited of your people, your family and the people that gave you incredible meaning to your life. It formed you to be a person who cares, who's responsible, who cares for others, so your love and caring extends not just to your family, your own children, but to children everywhere. And its through your work too, I'm sure that you feel that life is very meaningful when you're working and you're sitting like you do, sitting at the bedside of a patient who is dying and accompanying them as far as you can and maybe saying a prayer for them. So those are some of the experiences that you have told me already. Did you write anything else down?

Patient: No, feeling most alive with my family sitting, talking and caring

Therapist: and caring, or sharing?

Patient: caring yeah and sharing

Therapist: Yeah, and I think that hammock is important, everyone needs a place where they feel at home, safe, peaceful

Patient: peaceful

Therapist: yeah, to be able to just be.

Patient: Just be with myself

Therapist: With yourself, just be, alive. It's almost like time stops still, stands still. A lot of people talk about meaningful moments as moments that were so profound they felt so alive and they felt like they lost track of time. Time went slower or stiller or they lost track of it completely. I can imagine that happened in that hammock. We have to stop sweetheart because I promised you we would stop on time. One last time, there's a little bit of homework, but it's not terrible

Patient: Okay

Therapist: And I don't even think that they have it in your book here, maybe you can write it down, but I'm going to give you a book.

Patient: okay

Therapist: this is a good by that fellow, Victor Frankl.

Patient: mm-hmm

Therapist: there are two part to the book. The first part of the book describes his experience in concentration camp during the Holocaust; the second part of the book describes his ideas about meaning. You can read the whole book, or you can read just the part about meaning, or you can, however you'd like.

Patient: Okay

Therapist: by giving you this book we are not trying to compare having cancer to being in a concentration camp, but it's his story and the experience that brought him awareness to the importance of meaning.

Patient: meaning

Therapist: It's an easy book to read you may be fatigued and tired and may not be able to get yourself to read.

Patient: I can read a page

Therapist: yeah, but whatever you can do. It's okay to skip around if you want.

Patient: Mm-hmm

Therapist: But it's yours to have. There's a lot in here that helps reinforce what we, more explanations of what we're going to do the whole 7 weeks. But it's yours to keep and to read

Patient: Thanks

Therapist: and maybe next time when I see if you've read any part of it we can discuss it if there's anything you've read in there that you thought gee that was interesting or I didn't like that. Usually people say that "I've read something in there that was very interesting" you know. So that's for you.

Patient: Cause we had a dear friend from the concentration camp

Therapist: Uh-huh

Patient: and I never forget him. He told me he and his brothers and his mom. He saw his brother going into the chamber.

Therapist: right

Patient: He said "(name) I never forget the look." And sometimes when my mom is having a quiet moment, and I guess thinking about it he can just see that look on her face. But he was ever so good to me (name).

Therapist: Yes, now you know there's a lot in the literature about the Jewish Holocaust, but you told me the story of the Youroba and the Garifuna people, so there are so many cultures that have so many stories of Diaspora and slavery and all that.

Patient: Yes Yes

Therapist: So I don't mean to give you this as the only example of this

Patient: but you know this is a story also that is so dear to my heart. I never forgot him. When I came to the states he would say to me "This is just how people are so good, and that's why I have to keep sharing this."

Therapist: yeah, you have to tell your story

Patient: When I came to the states, I worked for this guy and he would say to me "Okay, I don't have enough work, I'm putting you on unemployment, collect your check, and Saturday and Sunday you work for me, and I'll pay you." And at the same token he was like "What did you do with the money? What did you do with the money?" "I'm taking it to the bank to save it." And he did.

Therapist: Let me just finish one more thing. Next week, next time we meet, I'm going to ask (RSA's name) to help figure out, we're going to have a continuation of the discussion of meaning and we're going to talk a little bit about what gave your life meaning. We're actually going to talk about identity.

Patient: okay

Therapist: And we're going to talk about your identity before cancer, and how cancer may have impacted on your identity and your sense of meaning. And that's going to be the next session.

Patient: okay (name)

Therapist: okay?

Patient: okay

Therapist: This is for you. Do you want our pen too?

Patient: No, thank you.

Therapist: alright, let's go.

Session 2: Cancer and Meaning—Identity Before and After Cancer Diagnosis

Therapist: Okay, so this is Session 2

Patient: two, right

Therapist: we won't mention what time it is on the tape, or people will think we're nuts.

Patient: (laugh) okay

Therapist: yeah, in terms of the schedule, I think I left my schedule with (RSA's name).

Patient: (RSA's name)

Therapist: Are we going to be able to do next week? The same?

Patient: I don't know about next week because I have to get a new schedule today, and I have to have chemo today.

Therapist: uh-huh

Patient: Next week is, next week. . . .

Therapist: We'll see. So what I'll do is have (RSA's name) call you

Patient: yes

Therapist: and we'll see when the next meeting makes sense for you

Patient: Usually I'm sick the week after

Therapist: Usually after chemo you're sick the week after.

Patient: I am so sick; I can't even get out of bed

Therapist: Mm-hmm

Patient: That is one of my problems

Therapist: of course

Patient: with the first chemo I did very well, but with this chemo I'm sick.

Therapist: the made a switch in the chemotherapy

Patient: Yes, but this is not . . .

Therapist: You're not tolerating this well?

Patient: tolerating

Therapist: the main negative effect is being very tired?

Patient: I'm tired, I'm weak, I can't do as much

Therapist: Right

Patient: which is not me

Therapist: right

Patient: I hurt, and I hate that the most I generally don't feel good

Therapist: you don't feel well

Patient: I do not feel well. This has made me sick

Therapist: and that's how you have been feeling this past week?

Patient: yeah

Therapist: You're getting chemotherapy today this will be which number?

Patient: the third one today

Therapist: the third one

Patient: last week I told them there was this fuzziness in my mouth, my mouth had been burning, okay I keep checking my mouth, I keep rinsing with the salt, so I know you know its not fungus its not anything, but my mouth had been burning, and I looked its like red inside of my lips. It's clearing now; it's not as bad as last week. The fluids help me, and I keep flushing it at home. But and I say I'm taking this chemo today, what will happen again? I can't seem to recuperate from the chemo.

Therapist: well, usually before you get chemo they check your counts right? And that's what they'll do today?

Patient: That's what they'll do today

Therapist: You're suffering from fatigue related to the chemotherapy.

Patient: I'm suffering from fatigue

Therapist: At least that, maybe making you sick in other ways . . .

Patient: I generally don't feel well, I do not feel well

Therapist: so they are going to have to check to make sure they are not making you more anemic or something like that.

Patient: You know, my counts are lower, but I just do not feel well

Therapist: yeah, do you get to see the oncologist today?

Patient: I get to see him today, and I'll tell him how I feel.

Therapist: Yes, yes, they're usually some things that can be done

Patient: I'll tell him how I feel

Therapist: I'll write down the name of a medicine that might help your fatigue.

Patient: I am . . . and I generally don't feel well in my stomach, but prior to this chemo I felt well.

Therapist: what was it like to get up so early to get here today to get here?

Patient: I'm an early riser

Therapist: You're an early riser.

Patient: I'm up at 4 am everyday because that was the time I used to get up to go to work.

Therapist: to work, I see (laugh)

Patient: So I get up, whether I'm here or in Belize I wake up at the same time. If I read or sometimes I go outside and wait for the sunrise, and then I go back in my bed and go to sleep

Therapist: when you're in Belize you do that?

Patient: Mm-hmm. I get up to watch the sunrise at least stay quiet, cause everyone complains I get up so early and make a ruckus. I have the lights on or I go into the kitchen and I wake the whole house, household. And then I say "Okay, let me just go and watch the sunrise and then get back into my bed."

Therapist: yeah, last session, they're several things that I remember about the session that were really noteworthy to me, they were memorable to me. One was how Belize and how everything about Belize, especially the feelings that you have, your hammock I remember, the wind, the breeze, your home there, everything about that makes you feel happy and alive. You smile broadly when you talk about that.

Patient: (name) when I'm in Belize I feel so well. Other times that I have gotten off of chemo I have spent in Belize. I come in three days prior to my appointments. In fact my son will say "Mommy, you seem to do so well in Belize."

Therapist: Yeah

Patient: "I bought your ticket, go to Belize tomorrow." I'm not complaining, my suitcase is packed, I'm gone.

Therapist: so do you think you'll go back for a little bit?

Patient: the first chance I get, I'm leaving.

Therapist: Yeah, the other things I remember about the first session we had together is, there were several things related to Belize, was the language that you speak, Garifuna

Patient: Garifuna

Therapist: Garifuna and the legacy and the pride of your ancestors. And then your Grandmother and your Aunt and all the women who raised you after your mother died. And then the tragedy of losing your son, and how you cope with that.

Patient: Part of me died

Therapist: Part of you died

Patient: Yeah

Therapist: yeah

Patient: but you know I say, I always say "God is so good." He moved me, and I think that everything was predestined. My two sons were in the car, the other one cracked his spine, broke his hip, but he shared with me. He's almighty; he could've taken the two.

Therapist: Right, and of course we talked about how all those things give meaning to your life. And uh we reviewed Frankl's ideas about the sources of meaning.

Patient: mm-hmm. I'm okay; I have some in my pocket

Therapist: you have some tissues? Okay. We reviewed the sources of meaning through experiential sources of meaning, through love, and all those feelings connected to your beautiful Belize and the breezes and the feelings you have. And the food, right? Through creative sources of meaning, through all that you do in your life, through your work and other things that you care for others and hopefully care for yourself a little bit.

Patient: I do

Therapist: yeah, and through meaning that you through meaning that comes from the attitude you take towards suffering experiences like losing your son. And what lessons you learned from that.

Patient: Yes

Therapist: and then of course the historical sources of meaning, legacy that you've inherited from your immediate family, all the great women in your family and your ancestors and the legacy that you live and leave behind. Those are the big sources of meaning. Is there anything that you that stuck you about the first session? That was important for you?

Patient: (name) discussing the first session reinforced that I have always searched for meaning in my life, and just discussing with you reinforced that I was doing what I was supposed to be doing in my life.

Therapist: Ah-ha. Can you give me a . . .

Patient: You know I have always had a positive attitude, even when it looks negative, I tell myself "There has to be something in it to turn it around."

Therapist: Mm-hmm

Patient: I am no nonsense I don't play any games with my life, or with anyone's life. I do not play games period, it's either a yes or a no, and when I say no I mean no. And I see that in my sunlight everyday and I'm, but I've always always tried to reach out to anyone who has touched my life in a positive way. Looking back that I'm ill, so many so many people have called my house "How are you doing, what can I do?" I have a co-worker, she called, I think if anything happens if I refuse to go to the ER she will come and drag me to the ER. We've worked together for like 15 years and one day she said to me "You know (name) I'm having such a time with my husband" she was a young woman, and she has just bought a home. She had worked on this unit like 15 years prior to my coming there, and I met her and her mother, and they were such good people. She met this guy, she got married, she said "You know what am I going to do?" I would tell her when I started working there I met this lady on the elevator and I said "good morning" and it was first thing in the morning. She was grinning from ear to ear, an older woman she said "Did you know I used to work here. And I've just retired." Just the two of us on the elevator, she said "You work here?" I said "Yeah, I just started working here." She said "Don't forget, they have a tax shelter here, you just started working here, get into it."

Therapist: Get into it she gave you some financial advice.

Patient: She said "I am so happy" and she was just bouncing in the elevator "I'm so happy." I said "Why?" She said "You know, I get three checks at the end of the month." I said "You do?" And she was just so jovial. So I got up onto the unit and I told my co-worker "Girl, I met this old lady on the elevator and she was just so jovial, and she told me she's getting three checks." And we were just laughing at the attitude of this older woman. And I said to her, my co-worker, "You've worked here for so many years, are you in this tax shelter business?" She said "No, what is that?"

Therapist: huh?

Patient: I said "You don't know?" She said "No." I said "We'll investigate we'll investigate" so I said to her "We'll find out what it is." So we call and we find out and she said to me "Okay (name) I'm getting into this." And I said "Okay, I'm getting into this too" and so we did. And she married this guy and he hoodwinked her. . . .

Therapist: Hoodwinked her

Patient: he waited until she was so established and knew her mother gave her money to help with the down payment for her wedding gift her mother gave her some expensive Italian furniture, she got her the china and like two years later he was so violent and mean to the girl, and she didn't say anything until one day I guess she couldn't take it anymore, she said "(name) I'm going through this with my husband." And I was just so angry, "What are you doing to do" she said "I don't know" I said "You don't need to take this. You do not need to take this. And you've told me, it's not my business, but you've told me b/c you trust me." I said "You know what, leave, your mom is there, you have your mom and you have your brothers."

Therapist: So at work you took care not just of patients, but of your co-workers.

Patient: we took care of each other.

Therapist: you took care of each other, and she also told her how she should take care of herself the way you would take care yourself. You heard about this tax shelter, you're going to do it you told her. Were you able to take a peak at that book?

Patient: Oh yes

Therapist: You looked at the book?

Patient: Mm-hmm

Therapist: so you did

Patient: yeah, I'm reading the book

Therapist: Anything about it that struck you?

Patient: it's interesting

Therapist: Mm-hmm

Patient: How he overcome all those things he went through

Therapist: yeah, which is something you know about, something you know a lot about.

Patient: yeah, and I say that comes from my parents, the women that raised me.

Therapist: uh-huh

Patient: the women that raised me. And I think it's funny earlier on in my life we had sons, I had sons and my siblings. My uncle has 10 children and we had always stayed together and they had sons also so everyone would come to my house and I said to my mom, you know we have to be careful of how we raise these boys because they may hate women, because we're strong women

Therapist: I see

Patient: we are strong women and we have to be careful, because I was always afraid, I didn't want to be too harsh on them because I know the women in my family.

Therapist: You wouldn't want your boys to hate women.

Patient: huh?

Therapist: You didn't want them to get the wrong idea about women

Patient: That women are hard

Therapist: I'm sure they love women

Patient: And now my son says sometimes you know "Mommy, I look at myself and I think about you, you're stubborn." And he won't give and neither will I, and then I look at myself, I said "Oh my God, he reminds me so much of myself."

Therapist: there you go

Patient: cause we're always clashing.

Therapist: that's right

Patient: because he won't give and neither will I

Therapist: well you know if life, we spoke about in the first session that our responsibility is to create a life of, to create of lives, and to create a life of meaning, what's also really important int here are values, right?

Patient: Yes

Therapist: Our life has to; we try to create a life that has meaning based on values

Patient: values

Therapist: and you're not just trying to live your values in your own life, but you're trying to teach your values to your children; that's part of the legacy that you leave too. So that's very important to you to leave a legacy. The other part of what's important in creating a life is creating a life of identity. Who am I, right? And the second session focuses on identity, and how it relates to meaning. Usually the things in life that give us meaning, the people, the roles etc., you can just skip to session two here. The things in life that give meaning are usually the things that contribute to our identity. So today's session focuses on identity, and just before we go into the session today you know when you in the beginning of Frankl's book when he talks about the experience that they he had in the concentration camp and he talks about how in the camps they took everything away from him and they controlled everything that he did. The one thing that they were not able to take control of was the way he thought about things and his attitude. And he describes a scene where even in the camp he and some of the camp inmates were still able to appreciate the beauty of the sunset. I was thinking about that when you told me about what you do in Belize at 4 o'clock in the morning, you get up and then you watch the sunrise, and then you might go back to sleep. Even if you're feeling as bad as how you have been feeling this past week on the new chemotherapy, you're still able to appreciate the sunrise, the beauty of the sunrise you're still able to connect to that source of meaning, that beauty, and nature, the universe. And I know you're a religious woman, the creator of the universe.

Patient: Mm-hmm

Therapist: So um, so this exercise, this session focuses on two exercises really to answer the question who am I. These are the sources of meaning that I just went over with you again.

Patient: Mm-hmm

Therapist: this book is for you to have if you want to skim through it.

Patient: Mm-hmm, I skimmed through it.

Therapist: Good, you know even before or after we do a session. There are two parts to this exercise.

Patient: Mm-hmm

Therapist: One is answering the question who I am before you had cancer, and the second part of the exercise is to answer the question "Who am I" after this cancer experience. So why don't you take a little bit of time and write down a few answers to the question "Who I am" before this cancer experience started you know, and then we'll discuss that, and then we'll do the "Who am I" after.

Patient: Mm-hmm

(Pause for patient to do assignment)

Patient: okay

Therapist: okay, do you want to start? Actually let me take this, I'm going to ask you later if you can, but go ahead

Patient: Pre-cancer, I love life.

Therapist: so you're somebody who loved life

Patient: I love life

Therapist: who loves life.

Patient: I don't love life partying and what have you, that's not me, but I just love my little life and taking care of me, I work every day, I take care of my family. My husband, my mother, my son, sons, when it was two, my extended family, I just love them, my friends.

Therapist: So if you were to put that into a role, your identity of who you are, you're somebody who's a care . . . who takes care, caregiver?

Patient: Not as a caretaker, I just love these people
Therapist: ah-ha, you're a lover
Patient: these are my family
Therapist: you're a person who loves her life and her family. Not as a caretaker
Patient: not as a caretaker
Therapist: is there a way you love them besides caring?
Patient: you know I care for them
Therapist: yes
Patient: I have many friends that I've met here in the United States since I came here. Very good friends, my patients, when they leave the hospital I would give them my phone number, "You call" they would call and check.
Therapist: so what you're saying here is you're somebody who loves your life, and who loves your family, and its just a way of being you don't have to do anything, any specific action to retain this part of your identity, you don't have to be super energetic you can be super fatigued and still love.
Patient: I wake up in the morning and I feel good. I have no complaints, I go about what I have to do, likewise when I don't feel like it, then I don't feel like it, I'm not doing it.
Therapist: right
Patient: you know, but for no other reason than I'm giving myself a break, and I'm good at it, I indulge myself, and I live like that every day. If I encounter someone in the morning, I don't know what their reason is, but I don't know what their reason is but don't give it me, cause that's not what I'm about this morning period.
Therapist: So is that part of you a person who gives themselves a break, that falls into what loving yourself, I'm somebody who loves life, loves my family, loves yourself. So part of loving yourself is giving yourself a break?
Patient: Oh yes
Therapist: and
Patient: and that's how I live my life everyday
Therapist: And forgiving yourself, for being human, and not just a robot.
Patient: Right
Therapist: Okay, did you write down a few other things?
Patient: I believe, I always think positively
Therapist: Mm-hmm
Patient: Let's come to an agreement and try to solve whatever the problem is, you know there should be no negatively, and sometimes its hard cause things happen sometimes you can't see your way out of it, but something good will come out of it, if you make it that way.
Therapist: So you're someone who is positive, optimistic, but you're someone who's willing to work hard to make the positive or optimistic outcome come through.
Patient: And I do this because I say you know there is a supreme being, who is not only for me, but for you also, and he is just good. People are just good.
Therapist: So God is not just your own personal God, he's God for everybody.
Patient: Everyone
Therapist: And so that makes everyone very similar to you in the sense, well you're connected to everyone. So you're someone who understands that you're connected to . . .
Patient: Yes, we're all connected
Therapist: To everyone and everything that God created
Patient: (name) I would get on the train with my son; he was b/c of the brittle bones he couldn't move around much. And when he was smaller we would travel from Queens all the way to 81st street to come to the museums. I would get on the train or the bus, we're coming, nothing keeps us or nothing stops us.
Therapist: Mm-hmm
Patient: and New York City children, they're rambunctious they're rude, they curse, but they are also good. Who would be the first one to say to me "M 'am do you need help?" It is these children, it is these children. So I say you know "People are good, they are innately good, it's just that some fall behind."
Therapist: Mm-hmm
Patient: not all of us are the same either for whatever reason, but people are just good in New York City. They are just good. You don't try to find the bad in them.
Therapist: So you're someone who tries to find the good in others.
Patient: And maybe because, and sometimes I tell myself it's because of my experiences, I was blessed with this child. Prior to me having this child, I had a good life with my parents and I lived in a small world because my father was here, my mother died, but my father didn't remember that I was alive, that he left me behind. And I always said that throughout my life, my aunts, neither my uncle as I was growing up had said or have I even heard saying "Where was her father? He wasn't there, he wasn't missed." They just took over, and my grandmother's cousin had died she left 4 children and my grandmother as poor as she was raised these children and as I grew up they

were there. They weren't my mother's siblings, but they grew up together, they're just about, so my father, I didn't miss anything. I did not miss anything growing up.

Therapist: right

Patient: and I found out I grew up. When I had this child, prior to that I would go about my business without saying hello, I would say "Good morning" I was raised but I didn't care, but he made me see life differently.

Therapist: so you're a mother, you're a mother

Patient: He made me see life differently. As I go about to the doctors, oh my god, he would be sick, he would be okay, he would fall in the house, he would just stretch in the bed, and then he would break himself.

Therapist: You started to say something about when you're mother died you father kind of forgot about you. Did he disappear?

Patient: He was here.

Therapist: he was there?

Patient: He was here in America.

Therapist: In America, so you didn't have him in Belize with you. So some people might have felt, some children might have felt like I lost my mother and my father, and um, my mother recently died, my father died about 8 years ago, and one of my friends said to me "Oh (name) I'm so sorry now you're an orphan."

Patient: Mm-hmm

Therapist: an orphan

Patient: Mm-hmm

Therapist: I said "Excuse me," he said "You're an orphan, I'm so sorry, you're an orphan," I said "I don't feel like an orphan, an orphan is someone who is deprived of love and caring of a mother and father. I had that for so many years."

Patient: So many years, right

Therapist: I'm not an orphan, but did you feel like an orphan?

Patient: No

Therapist: You didn't because you had this love.

Patient: and I knew that my father was somewhere, because occasionally I guess whenever he remembered, he would send, but I guess my parents welcomed when he sent, and they would say you know "Your father sent this." They never spoke of him, but I didn't miss him.

Therapist: So you did not feel like an orphan?

Patient: No

Therapist: Mm-hmm

Patient: No

Therapist: So that is not your identity, I am not an orphan? You're thinking about it.

Patient: I didn't feel like an orphan. Recently, like 3 years ago one of my nieces was in trouble and got in the foster care system and I took her.

Therapist: Uh-ha

Patient: and they said "You know you did such a good job with her, we want you to foster." And there was this other child, her father died and her mother died, and I said "I will take her," and they said "Why do you take her?" I said "She has no one." And my husband was home when she came, where was I? Somewhere, I think I was at work. And from the first time I saw her, I loved her. And till this day I love her. And she's a good kid, and I would sit and talk to her, and I had to send her back.

Therapist: She was difficult?

Patient: She would go to school, she would come home in time, she's a good kid, but I said to myself, her mother was sick for years as she was discussing with me, and she was used to fending for herself.

Therapist: I see, very independent.

Patient: very independent, but she would fight

Therapist: very oppositional

Patient: Very oppositional, and I said to her "You know what, you and I will get along but I can't put up with that behavior. Because you will go to school and they'll call me and I'm at work and I can't come to get you. And it's not right for you to allow people to possibly injure you or mane you, or something you know. I do not like that behavior."

Therapist: Was that difficult for you?

Patient: Very difficult.

Therapist: yeah

Patient: and I told her "As much as I want you to stay with me and I love you, I do not like this behavior."

Therapist: Do you feel like you were trying to take care of your own family and yourself, protecting them and protecting you a little bit? And maybe also doing what was right for her? Or was it a choice, did you have to make a choice between?

Patient: Its not that she had to make a choice

Therapist: you I mean

Patient: Me? No. But it was just, even to the house, she would come and fight. I said to her "This does not happen here, and I will not allow you to do it. Even with my neighbors, I've lived here for so many years."

Therapist: Do you regret the decision you made?

Patient: Yes

Therapist: You regret that decision?

Patient: Oh yes, everyday.

Therapist: that you sent her back you mean?
Patient: That I sent her back
Therapist: wow, what do you feel in retrospect that you should've done?
Patient: She should've stayed; she should've stayed with me
Therapist: should've
Patient: But, now that I'm sick, I wouldn't want her to go through this again.
Therapist: So this was recently? The last few years?
Patient: Uh, it will be three years.
Therapist: 3 years
Patient: She still comes
Therapist: she still comes, so you have a relationship.
Patient: She still comes, and I know she's hurt
Therapist: how old is she now?
Patient: 17
Therapist: Mm
Patient: and I know she's hurt that I had to send her back, and it hurts me also
Therapist: Yes, I can imagine
Patient: Because it's not like me to give up.
Therapist: It's not like you
Patient: It's not like me, but it was just her behavior
Therapist: Mm-hmm, do you think it was giving up? Or were you trying to make the best decision that you in a difficult circumstance?
Patient: (name), I was trying to make the best decision, but it hurt.
Therapist: Yes, it hurt.
Patient: It hurt
Therapist: But it sounds like, you made a decision, it hurt, but you're trying to stay in touch and still communicate that you love her.
Patient: I told her
Therapist: At a little bit of a distance
Patient: "If you ever need, come here."
Therapist: yeah
Patient: That's all I can offer you.
Therapist: and it makes it harder because of your experience when you lost your parents and people, but you were a different child, than this here.
Patient: It was
Therapist: yeah, did you write down anything else?
Patient: I believe that there is a good and just God. Cancer has not affected my life, mostly.
Therapist: So are you moving into the second part?
Patient: Uh-ha, to the second part
Therapist: So the question is, how has cancer affected the way you would say "Who I am?" and how?
Patient: It has not affected who I am.
Therapist: Mm-hmm
Patient: I live the same way
Therapist: Mm-hmm
Patient: I deal with this cancer on a daily basis
Therapist: yeah, so you you're still somebody even with the cancer, you're still somebody who loves their life, who loves her family.
Patient: I can't eat as much
Therapist: huh?
Patient: I can't eat as much, but I eat what I want.
Therapist: So you're somebody who loves to eat
Patient: and I love to eat good.
Therapist: So let me ask you, just as a way of trying to, one of the things that we want to do in this treatment, this counseling therapy is to teach you the sources of meaning so that you can go to them as resources, so loving your life, your family, eating all these kinds of things, which one of the sources of meaning, those are examples of experiential sources of meaning right. Through love, through relationships, through all your senses, use of all of your senses, food, things like that. The second part that you wrote, what was the second?
Patient: Cancer has not affected . . .
Therapist: No no, I mean the second thing you wrote after you love your life, someone who loves life?
Patient: I believe there is a good and just God.
Therapist: Oh, you said you had a positive attitude that was the second thing . . .
Patient: I always think positively
Therapist: You always think positively, right, that's an attudinal source of meaning right.
Patient: Mm-hmm
Therapist: You choose the attitude you take towards life, towards suffering, towards anything adverse.
Patient: Mm-hmm
Therapist: and the other part has to do with God? You believe that . . .
Patient: First of all in my life there is always God. Like I said he is not only for me, he is for us, he's good. He's good; he's just, um . . .
Therapist: Is God a source of meaning for your life?
Patient: He is, I had a disabled child, and God was there for me every step of the way. Like I said, having (son's name) I would look at him and I would say "You know what? This is not going to keep me back." And despite the hardship I went through, I went to school; I took care of him to the best of my ability. And he said to me "Mommy you take such good care of me." When I found out I was pregnant I went to nursing school, and I told my brother "I'm not going to nursing school, I'm just going to have my baby." And it so happened that he has

these brittle bones, and this is the same child that would say to me "Mommy, you take such good care of me"; he was like 11, "Why don't you go to nursing school?"

Therapist: "Why don't you go to nursing school?" he gave you the idea

Patient: Because every time he goes into the hospital, I would go, I move, I was pregnant and I was literally at the hospital. He would have a bed, I would have a bed, he would get a tray, we would be in a private room. He didn't want the nurses taking care of him, so he said "You have to come take care of me." The only time I didn't have to do much when he's in the, when he had surgery, nurses would give him the medications, and I learned everything that they did there. He said "You should go to nursing school" "Who's going to take care of you?" "I will."

Therapist: So you've also been talking today in this exercise, you've been talking about creative sources of meaning through your work in nursing through caring; when you talk about God as being a source of meaning, that's very much related also to the attitudinal sources of meaning.

Patient: Yes

Therapist: the attitude you take towards suffering is very much for you a function of your belief in God and what you see is God's plan for you?

Patient: His plan for me

Therapist: Yes, and then I think you also talked a lot about losing your mother, your father being in the states, trying to bring this niece of yours into foster care. And this is your historical sources of meaning as well you know you legacy and how it influences what you do in your life and the things that you want and the values that you inculcate in your children, your son, and the attitudes that you inculcate in your sons. And the legacy that you want to leave behind. And I think what's most striking about this exercise, is that for you there was, we didn't have to go through a lot, it was clear to you right away that cancer really didn't effect who you are as a, didn't change who you are as a person. And that's the main, that's one of the main points of this exercise, to try to show people that you know cancer can sometimes make you feel like oh I'm too weak, I can't be a nurse, I can't do this, I can't do that, but see you derive your identity and a lot of sources of meaning not so much through things that you do physically its through your attitudes, and through your feelings, and through your . . .

Patient: spirit

Therapist: spirit. And so that's unaffected by anything physical that can happen when you have cancer. So the main essence of who you are as a person, the main sources of meaning in your life are really unchanged with cancer, they're still available to you to give your life meaning.

Patient: Mm-hmm

Therapist: Next week we're going to talk a little bit more about legacy and the historical context of meaning. And we've done quite a bit of that over over I think this is this is what we're going to work on next week. And what I'm going to ask you to do, and we've already done so much of this, but it will be a little bit more specifically we'll focus on this. It's your legacy, you've already told me about all the women in your life who helped raise you, I want to hear more about your ancestors that came to Belize and all that, and the kind of things that you hope to are your legacy, um, the kind of legacy that you would live and give and leave behind. So if you get a chance you can think about these a little bit, you don't have to write down the answers . . .

Patient: Okay

Therapist: but, cause we can always do that here. But we'll, think about those answers.

Patient: Okay

Therapist: and then, I think (RSA name) will contact you later, probably today's going to be a busy day for you with chemo. Are you usually there most of the day?

Patient: I'll be there most of the day

Therapist: Most of the day, so probably (RSA name) will give you a call tomorrow.

Patient: cause I have to see the doctor, then wait for my chemo.

Therapist: wait for your tests, blood test results and things like that. So um, (RSA name) will contact you and we'll set up the next appointment

Patient: alright

Therapist: and I'll be there, thanks (name)

Patient: okay (name)

Therapist: thanks

Session 3: Historical Sources of Meaning—Life as a Legacy That Has Been Given; Life as a Legacy One Lives and Gives

Patient: This is the Session 3 homework, I couldn't find it. Session 3.

Therapist: yeah, that's the one

Patient: When you look back on your life and upbringing, what are the most significant memories, relationships and traditions?

Therapist: So this session, Session 3

Patient: Session 3

Therapist: is about legacy. It's about the historical context of meaning in your life, in our lives, and if you remember if you look at the sessions, we've done the first session which was an introduction to sources of meaning and how cancer has affected meaning. So the next three sessions, are really going to, next one, two, three, four sessions, are going to focus on the various sources of meaning. We derive meaning through creativity through our work, through what we care about, through the life we create, through experiential sources of meaning, through the way we interact with the world, through the way we experience the world. And then through the historical sources of meaning, through the legacy we inherit from our families and the legacy we leave for our children and everyone else. And the meaning we derive from the attitude that we take towards suffering, being able to transcend suffering. So before, so we've done the first two now this one we're talking a little bit about historical sources of meaning, the legacy that you've inherited. We've talked a little bit about this in each session actually, but today we'll focus more on that. Before we jump in, I'm sorry you weren't feeling well last session, how are you doing today, you went to urgent care, right?

Patient: Yes, no I didn't go to urgent care. Since I was here already, I told my niece just take me to

Therapist: The clinic

Patient: that we should just go upstairs so they can check my vitals.

Therapist: oh, okay

Patient: And I thought I felt well, I told her lets go on the train and as soon as we got up here I was feeling lightheaded again.

Therapist: and so when you got to the clinic there . . .

Patient: They did my vitals, it was okay

Therapist: Did you need some fluids?

Patient: But they said that, I needed some fluids, and after I got the fluids I went home. My husband said "You know, I came home, I stayed here with you and you were out." When I woke up I felt somewhat better. I just don't have any energy, I want to do something, but I just don't have any energy.

Therapist: So did you, were you scheduled for chemo last time?

Patient: no

Therapist: No, just a check-up?

Patient: Mm-hmm

Therapist: And when is your next chemo? Today?

Patient: Supposedly today, but I told him, I had a scan on Friday, I told him I'm going to read my scan today, and I'll decide whether I'll have any chemo. (Name) prior to this chemo, this one, I felt perfectly well. I had some pains I understand I would have some pains. But I felt perfectly well, but this chemo it does not make me feel good

Therapist: right

Patient: and I don't feel good about it, and I can't figure out what it is.

Therapist: Well, you've been feeling very ill on the chemo.

Patient: I have been sick with this chemo, I can't do a thing, I can't do anything, I don't have any energy.

Therapist: so your quality of life has not been good on this chemo.

Patient: No no no no no, I'm not trying to be difficult

Therapist: It's just very hard for you to tolerate this chemo

Patient: I'm not tolerating this chemo, I can't do a thing for myself they have to do my laundry.

Therapist: right, so you want to have a discussion with the doctors about whether . . .

Patient: I have told him already

Therapist: about whether you want to continue chemo or maybe change it to something else that maybe is not so difficult.

Patient: We discussed this the last time, I'm telling myself if I change this and take the oral meds, then what?

Therapist: Mm-hmm

Patient: But this has been a bitch, I cannot do, this is not me. It's like everyone says "What is going on, this is not like you." I try, try, I can't I told them last week take me out to the mall, I sat there at the mall, I didn't know what the devil I did, I know I made a phone call. By the time I got home I didn't know where my telephone was or what I did. I don't know. I don't know. But I attribute this to just not feeling well, and I was just trying, I just wanted to leave my house just to be out there for a little bit. And I sat on the bench, I made one phone call, I don't know if I didn't put it back into my bag, I thought I put it into my pocket, I must have put it in my pocket,

I thought I dropped it in the car, but its not in the car, unless I dropped it somewhere and I don't know.

Therapist: hmm

Patient: Or maybe I got up and left my phone where I was sitting.

Therapist: Or your phone, right. So you'll have a discussion today.

Patient: I'm going to discuss it with him today.

Therapist: Good

Patient: (name)

Therapist: I know from experience very often very often they will have to change the chemotherapy because someone is just not tolerating it well.

Patient: I am just not . . .

Therapist: If it's working very well, they'll want to try to convince you.

Patient: That's why I said, I'm going to see, I'm going to read my scan from March, I'm going to read my scan on Friday and then I will decide.

Therapist: You want all the information

Patient: Because prior to this I didn't want to know. I didn't want to.

Therapist: Mm-hmm

Patient: The other one I felt well, I didn't read my scans. That's not like me; I just didn't want to be bothered with it, cause I have all the records of my scans and what have you. But this one . . .

Therapist: You want the information because you want to make a decision about the chemotherapy.

Patient: I want to make a decision, you know.

Therapist: I understand

Patient: This is how I run my life . . .

Therapist: You've only really wanted the information that was necessary to make a decision.

Patient: Yes

Therapist: Before you probably didn't want to know whatever, because you knew you needed to take the chemotherapy.

Patient: I knew I needed to take it.

Therapist: You knew, so you had enough information.

Patient: I had enough; I knew I needed to do the chemo

Therapist: right

Patient: I told him you know, um from the first chemo most likely you won't need radiation, because that was what I was most fearful about the radiation and um for the first month I didn't ask for any of the scan cause I knew I needed to do um do it, and I felt well, there were those days that I didn't feel well and maybe within 2 days to 3 days I'd be up and about.

Therapist: right, so today will be an important discussion

Patient: Today, today, today

Therapist: So let's focus on this for a minute, do you, I know you were feeling ill last week and all that, but the first two sessions do you have any when you look back on those two sessions, anything that struck you about the first two sessions, or something that you thought maybe was important that you learned, or something you thought that gosh I should've mentioned this or that?

Patient: Not really, not really. I headed on to Session 3.

Therapist: we're on Session 3

Patient: And um, I always reflected on my grandmother, my grandmother was an only child.

Therapist: An only child

Patient: Only child, her parents' only child. And um, she was not much into traditions, but she was into her family, I guess earlier on she always had her cousins, I guess back in those days she used to say, when her dad, her dad was from Honduras. That's Spanish Honduras, and when in the war they came, and like families came, so they were able to get land and they all lived close by as neighbors, and when her cousin died she took her child and she raised them. So basically everyone in the neighborhood where my grandmother's house was a family, and there were older as I was growing up and in those days my grandmother was the farmer. And every time someone would have a baby my grandmother would come and do the traditional things with the baby.

Therapist: what's that?

Patient: The umbilical cord, she would bring the embers of the fire and with a rag and warm it up and put it on the baby's umbilical cord until it falls off.

Therapist: ah

Patient: And she would also bring food. And for every baby that's born there, my grandmother would do that. And she would take me on.

Therapist: Mm-hmm, so there were two big things that were done every time a baby was born. She would make this preparation that dealt with the umbilical cord it was a special procedure to make the umbilical cord fall off from them . . .

Patient: Heal and fall off . . .

Therapist: heal and fall off. And how long after the baby was born would this kind of thing be done?

Patient: this would be done like um within the first week.

Therapist: within the first week

Patient: and then my grandma would do this for like 2 weeks.

Therapist: she would come back every day.

Patient: she would come back every evening.

Therapist: evening and do this

Patient: Mm-hmm

Therapist: So it's a way of caring for the umbilical . . . and what would be done with the umbilical cord?

Patient: I don't know you know . . .

Therapist: I think we have my son's someplace

Patient: I didn't hear this from her, some people would keep it. I kept my children's until they were old enough and then they threw it away. Sometimes they would, that umbilical cord would fall off and there was a process they would do and they feed it to the child.

Therapist: Oh, is that part of the cooking she did?

Patient: Is that part of the?

Therapist: You said she cooked.

Patient: No, my grandmother wouldn't do that. But I think the parents, the parents would do that. I heard that some people, they'd go through a process and they'd do it, they'd feed it to the child or the parents would just keep it. At our house, it's not fed to the child, it's kept.

Therapist: right, so this session is about is about legacy. What do you understand by the term legacy?

Patient: passed on from one to the next

Therapist: what sort of things passed on?

Patient: Well, traditions

Therapist: traditions

Patient: family history

Therapist: family history

Patient: stories that have been in our family.

Therapist: what type of stories?

Patient: as a young child, for example this tornado that's happened in . . .

Therapist: Joplin, Missouri

Patient: Yes, I was telling my husband at home sometimes they would see the funnel and the older men would go despite the storm and the rain to the beach. But all those older men in our neighborhood would go but I never knew what they do, I was a child. And from our doorway, I could see straight to the sea. And I would see these people, they would call each other and they would say that there's a funnel starting, but I never knew what they do. So as I was talking to my husband this week, the past couple of weeks, I said to him you know what these men used to go to the beach, but I didn't know what they did. He said "They're chopping" they would go with axes, and I don't know what they did.

Therapist: they would go with axes and they would chop

Patient: Yeah, I didn't know what they did

Therapist: They tried to chop the funnel?

Patient: Yes, but I don't know. And then we wouldn't have the storm anymore.

Therapist: interesting, magic

Patient: and I, we were talking about this with my husband, and I said I need to ask my uncle what they do, what was done.

Therapist: yeah, what are you imagining?

Patient: (name) I could remember far back to when I was 3 years old, I remember, I remember because I would be there with my parents. I would be there in the thick of things with them. I remember my aunts working in the valley and my uncle did not want me to go apparently and I remember my uncle coming to get me to bring me back home. And one of my aunts had to come to take care of me. He said "I don't want her here" and they came to take care of me at home.

Therapist: so for you legacy means the things you inherited from your family, the histories, the stories, maybe the values

Patient: the values yes

Therapist: the attitudes towards life

Patient: yes

Therapist: wisdom

Patient: Most of all that attitude . . .

Therapist: life lessons

Patient: you know my life's lessons, because my parents kept me um, I wasn't parented by one person until I must have been 6, then my aunt and her husband really took me with them, but prior to that I was parented by everyone at the house. And it's been good things. I had an uncle, I had some much hair and prior to going to school sometimes I didn't like my hair like this, I didn't like the way my grandmother did my hair, I would tell him "You know, do my hair." And to this day, he's still alive he'll say "Oh, I had to do your hair and I had to tie the back of your dress." "Yes, I remember those things."

Therapist: So you remember the caring and the love.

Patient: I remember that. And my grandma would always take me with her to all these traditional things. She would not partake, but she would just be sitting there. They had drums, it was Garifuna drums, oh and then they'd beckon to you. And I just liked to sit there and listen to that, and that's one of the reasons why I always want to go home. I had a friend who was a teacher and he had discussed the curriculum of his school with me, and he said you know, this was like 20 years ago, "I want to institute those drums" and I said you know "You should."

Therapist: something about the drums

Patient: Mm-hmm because um the children then the tradition, some of the tradition won't die, because the children learn to sing the songs and they'll learn to beat those drums. So he said: "You know when you're here some morning come by and before classes start at 8 o'clock in the morning they would have a drumming session." And I see a difference in the kids, they were just so calming.

Therapist: So legacy isn't just what you inherit from your grandparents and ancestors is what you leave for the future generations.

Patient: yes

Therapist: and the drums beckon you home

Patient: It beckons me home and I'm so happy when I hear those drums.

Therapist: and you want those kids to have that feeling too to know where their home is.

Patient: Yes, and now . . .

Therapist: and home is the same place for all of you.

Patient: Yes, and little children now in the neighborhood where my house is, and those little children would come from school and they're singing and they beat those drums, or if they pick up a container they'd be sitting there singing and beating those drums.

Therapist: and I bet you that if you're beating the drums and your singing those songs you're home even when you're not in Belize. Is that right?

Patient: Yes

Therapist: your home is being connected to . . .

Patient: all these things

Therapist: all these things

Patient: because as a child

Therapist: and that gives your life meaning

Patient: Yes, my uncle, there was a, my uncle is so traditional, at home we spoke Garifuna language, my uncle didn't want us, because there's a broken English spoken in Belize, and my uncle didn't want us speaking that broken English even though we knew how to speak it. And he wanted us to be able to speak our language fluently.

Therapist: Garifuna

Patient: Garifuna, and the older men at times he would invite all the older men to come to the house, and they would be chanting and singing. I was never, till this day I can't sing in Garifuna

Therapist: You cannot?

Patient: No, but I love it, my sister does, and I would say "Sing for me" they would say "Oh, you can't learn it?"

Therapist: So there are some special songs that are in Garifuna that are very meaningful?

Patient: Mm-hmm

Therapist: Do your, does your son know it?

Patient: Some, my oldest son spoke Garifuna fluently. He went to NYU and he said "Mommy, the teacher was discussing Belize, Central America, and I told him I was Garifuna." And he said and the teacher was amazed and spoke to him in Garifuna. And he said you know I was able to discuss our culture with the whole class. And he was so happy, so happy. But the younger one, he likes the music, he plays the music. He understands Garifuna and, but he doesn't speak as much of the language. But if I say something to him, when I'm talking to him in Garifuna he understands very well. And so my nieces, they know how to speak it, even this one here.

Therapist: she's very sweet. She came to tell me you were sick. So let's actually do the exercises, it looks like you actually tried to do some of them . . .

Patient: and I did this, last week

Therapist: oh okay, because you were in preparation of coming.

Patient: Yes, uh-ha

Therapist: So I think the first part of the exercise today was to sort of think about, talk about, when you look back on your life, upbringing, what are the most significant events, memories, relationships, traditions, you actually have been talking about that, that had the greatest impact on who you are today. Specific memories, I guess you have been talking a lot about these memories and relationships and traditions, how they have had an impact on you today. Are there things that you wrote down that you didn't mention?

Patient: Uh-ha, going out with my grandmother in the evening.
Therapist: Uh-ha
Patient: visiting the sick, doing tradition things like the music, so sometimes going out to gatherings where older men would tell stories and sing traditional songs.
Therapist: Yes
Patient: and drums. Today I got home often to listen to the songs and the drums.
Therapist: So what impact does these memories and traditions, what have they had on you?
Patient: Um, that tradition is so important and we cannot lose and we need to carry it on through our children, through the family members. And even here, I am as the oldest in the family, and there is 12 of us, I make sure that we all gather with the children, to keep up this tradition. And my nieces and nephews are in and out of my house, luckily my husband likes these things also and he supports me you know. We've kept in alive.
Therapist: You've kept it alive.
Patient: And we would make the food, sometimes they wouldn't like it but some of them they like, and the songs and the dancing so even when my son's friends come they like the music also.
Therapist: Do you have recordings of it?
Patient: huh?
Therapist: Do you have recordings of it? Tapes?
Patient: At home, Mm-hmm.
Therapist: You play that
Patient: And its calming (name). It calms me.
Therapist: So its not, its not, I know there is a lot of CariTherapistean music . . .
Patient: It's not like reggae and . . .
Therapist: you know a lot of dancing. This is different, how would you say, more spiritual?
Patient: To me
Therapist: yeah
Patient: you would have to hear it to figure out if you liked it or what you'd like from it. But it's basically drums and different rhythms.
Therapist: Drums and different rhythms, not too many words?
Patient: And then sometimes it's just the drums or and then they're singing the songs.
Therapist: More chanting.
Patient: Mm-hmm
Therapist: More African roots
Patient: African roots right
Therapist: So did this play a big role in making you who you are as a person? All of these memories and traditions?
Patient: it does yeah, but I would say for those people, some people don't like it, and then I wasn't raised like that. My grandmother didn't even know how to dance, neither does my parents, but the children liked this, and then we would bring it home. We would bring these drummers to our house, and my parents know how to sings the songs especially my aunt and my uncle, because they weren't raised like that either, because my grandmother was very reserved.
Therapist: so you taught them something, you taught them something about their own traditions.
Patient: Mm-hmm. And as I would tell my uncle "You guys weren't raised like this." Neither was your grandmother, she didn't expose you to this, but they know the songs, the love the music. When they're here with us, they would dance with us despite me telling them "Oh, you can't dance." And um neither does my aunt, my mom don't know how to do this. And then we bring the drummers home, even here, I don't have those drums here and I keep saying I will buy my own drums. So um . . .
Therapist: Is it possible to buy these drums?
Patient: Uh-ha, and bring them here. I have a grandnephew, I told my niece you know you have to take him to these places where they can practice practice these drums. And she does and he loves it. And my niece is a foster mother to some Spanish children. So she took them also, so they know how to sings the songs and how to beat the drums. And I said "Do they understand what they are singing?" But the children love it.
Therapist: One of the things that that we'd like you to do or think about, its not an absolute requirement, we don't want it to be a burden, but one of the things we'd like you to think about doing, by the end of the 7 sessions you know to maybe have thought about or even created some kind of project, a legacy project, something concrete you know, that represents your legacy and something that you'd want to pass on to your the next generation. It strikes me that, and some people put together an album of photographs, some people put together recipes, some people get very fancy and they make a video or audio and they tell their children what they want them to grow up to be. And some people make a collection of their favorite music. One person, one patient actually planned his funeral and said this is the music I want played at the funeral kind

of thing, it was an interesting thing. But um, sounds to me like these drums and the music is an interesting part of your legacy.

Patient: I have told my sisters, when I die, all I want is, I told them you know when I die just bury me, no fuss, but I want this music.

Therapist: You want this music.

Patient: I want this music.

Therapist: do you know what songs?

Patient: I have told them which songs, I have told my sister which songs, and I want those drums.

Therapist: Physically?

Patient: Physically

Therapist: So you want to get those drums?

Patient: They have those drums; my sister knows how to access those drums

Therapist: Interesting

Patient: I did that for my son because my son loved those drums. So after his passing I had them bring the drums to the house.

Therapist: You want them to bring the drums to the house.

Patient: and I want them to bring the drums to the church, because that is . . .

Therapist: Do you listen to it now?

Patient: huh?

Therapist: Do you listen to it now.

Patient: Mm-hmm and I listen to it every day.

Therapist: You listen to it every day?

Patient: Yeah, we play it at our house

Therapist: I would love to hear it by the way, anytime

Patient: Next time I come I will bring I'll bring some of that music, so you do hear it

Therapist: I would love to hear it. Let's do the second part of the exercise. When you reflect on who you are today, and your different roles you know what you've done with your life, being a nurse, a parent a daughter, all that, and your accomplishments. What are the things that you're most proud of in terms of all those things?

Patient: (Name)

Therapist: and what are some of the lessons that you've learned from life that you want to pass on to your kids?

Patient: Most of all . . .

Therapist: what are you most proud of?

Patient: I'm most proud of mothering.

Therapist: Mothering

Patient: I'm most proud of mothering

Therapist: You did a magnificent job, especially with your disabled child.

Patient: He, most of all, sometimes the doctors would call my house "Why is he like this." Because generally I would tell him you know "No one owes you anything out there. You have rights, but everyone has rights, um, most of all I want you to be pleasant." Even though he'd raise hell, he doesn't want this and then the nutritionist would do whatever she can. "You guys don't cook like my mother" they would call and say "Bring his food." But he would say please, he would say thank you. And I'd tell him, "Whatever you don't want anyone to do to you, you tell them, I don't like it you don't do it to me. But there's a way of saying things." And I was so proud of what he became, he had an accident first, and I said to him you know what "You put that vehicle away because you're going to do." He said "Well, that's not how you brought me up; you brought me up to be confident."

Therapist: courageous

Patient: "You never said that I can't do anything. How dare you tell me that you're not getting my vehicle repaired?" He said "You don't have to get it repaired, I'll repair it myself." That's why (name) it hurt me, part me died when he died, but I have no guilt, and at times we would discuss he says you know he would discuss dying, that I'm dying.

Therapist: with him

Patient: with him

Therapist: because of his condition

Patient: Mm-hmm. Cause I would be telling him "You're in this vehicle you have to be careful getting in and out of this vehicle." He would just be going down the street senselessly, and everyone in my neighborhood knew him. And um, we would talk about death and dying and he would say "The day that I can't do anything for myself, mommy, just let me go. Do not ever put me on a ventilator just let me go, mommy," because he was so independent.

Therapist: hmm, and you were proud of him when he, when you said to him you know "Put that car away, you're going to end up in an accident." He said "That's not how you brought me up" and even though he died in an accident you felt like you had raised him to be independent, and he was independent, he really learned that lesson and if he hadn't learned that lesson he wouldn't have lived his life with the joy he lived it. Is that right?

Patient: you know he would not have lived it. He was a presidential student, he went to Washington, he went to meet the president, he went to meet the governor. That was the way he was brought up, and in his wheelchair, in his wheelchair. He, I think he stayed at the Hilton, he said to me "Well, I want to live someplace nice in Washington." I said "Okay, make your reservations, go ahead," and um he met, god what is her name, one of those senators from our neighborhood, he met her there . . .

Therapist: Hilary Clinton?

Patient: and she gave him a scholarship of about $2500 or something. He said "Mommy I was on the elevator and I met Quincy Jones." (Son's name) was just someone who you met him and he made an impact. "I met (celebrity name), mommy, and he invited me to come to his party," and he loved food. I said to him "Did you go to the party?" he said "Yes, I did." He said "Mommy there was so much food, I ate; he said there was so much food mommy and all those drugs they had there, I went home you know I went to my hotel." I said "How can you go and infringed on these people?" He said "Well he invited me." But that was on impressionable he was.

Therapist: So these values, he was proud, confident, he had courage, he was independent, he was unafraid, he stood up for himself.

Patient: oh yes

Therapist: even though he couldn't stand very well

Patient: I would normally would say to him, you don't stand but your mouth does. Because I would go to work, he could eat off of my floor, he would tell the brother "Mommy and daddy are at work, so we'll take care of everything here." And it's not just (son's name) that so I'm proud of, I'm proud of all my children.

Therapist: yeah

Patient: We had all these boys; we had 8 of them in the beginning. And they would be, and mostly because of (son's name), he'd want them over like every weekend. And as they became big boys we had king size quilts, cause we didn't have enough beds and they would all be on the floor, they would cook in the night, but the kitchen would be clean.

Therapist: so some of these lessons came from you.

Patient: Oh yes

Therapist: yeah, so the so it was not just be independent, courageous, stand up for yourself, it was also sharing,

Patient: Sharing

Therapist: and loving

Patient: loving

Therapist: and caring. Like you got from your . . .

Patient: my parents

Therapist: and grandparents

Patient: and today all these children, they're such good children. They are you know, in today's world and for black youths, I am so proud of them. I am so so proud of them. Like I tell them "Listen if I get sick, you guys make sure that I get cleaned up, wash me up, don't be afraid of me, just before anyone comes here you make sure I'm taken care of."

Therapist: pride, pride and dignity.

Patient: and my mother, when these children come, they take my mother to the bath. My mom was sick one day and it was just my youngest son there, he got her undressed, he washed her, he took her to the doctor. And my doctor says you know "I'm so proud of him, he took care of his grandmother, changed her to put her into the scanner and he got her dressed again before he took her home. (Name) how many of these children these days would do this." I said "That's how they were brought up." I am so proud of them.

Therapist: and being proud is important to you.

Patient: oh yes

Therapist: Being able to stand up and being proud of yourself.

Patient: and I am so proud of them. (Name) they are in and out of my house, aunt (her name) you need anything, are you okay. My husband tells them sometimes "Oh guy you should just knock before you come upstairs." I said "Just leave them alone, if I'm here naked they can see me, I don't care. They have seen me since they were babies." But they don't stop, they come. And like I was telling my mom, one of these children, that I would go to with my grandmother to do her umbilical cord like three weeks ago, she's a matron in the hospital at home, she has been calling and calling and calling, and she said "I'm coming to NY to see what's going on with you." And she came, and I said "You know can you imagine, I went with my grandmother to for her to do her umbilical cord and she's a grown woman now." And she came to see how I was going. And I'm so proud (name), I am so proud.

Therapist: you know what's interesting is one of the first things you told me when you were talking about your past legacy, what you inherited from your family, the traditions and the tradition you told me about, at least the one that strikes me, the drums, the singing the language this is all very beautiful, but the tradition you told me about that I think is most striking to me is the tradition of your grandmother taking care of, in an almost holy way the umbilical cord, and if you really, you don't have to think about it too much because its pretty clear, the umbilical cord is what connects one generation to the next, mother to the child.

Patient: child

Therapist: So what the tradition is about a connection, treating it as holy and treating it with respect and a lot of attention. And its interesting, its two parts, one part is making sure that its almost preserved in some way, but also the other part is it comes the process of the umbilical cord becoming unattached from the baby is done with incredible care and love, recognizing I think the fact that when you're a mother and you launch the next generation your children to be independent and to live on their own. That has to be a nurturing process a one that allows them to be disconnected from the umbilical cord with a lot of love that they take with them. And maybe the most important thing in your life, you talk about being a mother as your biggest accomplishment and the lessons you want them to learn with dignity, independence, etc. Sounds to me like the greatest legacy you inherited and the greatest legacy you give, you give is love.

Patient: that's right

Therapist: Enormous love. And home, home is the place of where love and who you are, where you came from, your identity, the people you're connected to that's where home is. Home is the source of love.

Patient: Yes, yes. Yesterday, we had a friend, when I moved to my house, 31 years ago, I met her and I said to her "What's wrong with this child?" She said "You know, I had him at a babysitter, I don't' know." I said to her "You don't know what happened to this child?" his face was black and blue. I said to her "I'm not working, you don't take him over there anymore, tomorrow you bring him to my house. I'm going to watch him."

Therapist: Ah, she should've taken him to daycare or something

Patient: Yes, well, she didn't afford the daycare. I said to her "I'm going to watch him; you don't take him there anymore." He was just a year and a half. She said "Will you watch him?" I said "Yeah I will, bring him to my house, bring his clothes" and she brought him to me. Um, I kept him and through the years, he has been in and out of my house. So yesterday she called to say "(name) is in Boston." I said "I know." She said to me "I don't know how much to thank you," she said "I'm so worried about him." I said "No, he's out of a job now, but he'll get a job in a short time." And she said "(name) I am so worried about him because he's in Boston." I said "Don't be fearful because he's with his brother." She said "I don't know how to thank you; (name) has turned out to be so good. And he's had a child now, that he is so careful with and want to have this child in his life." I said "Well, maybe b/c he didn't have a father." I said "Well," I said to her "He couldn't be anything else, he could not be anything else."

Therapist: Another child you loved.

Patient: Yes

Therapist: So we're going to have to stop soon.

Patient: Mm-hmm

Therapist: I want to talk a little bit about the next session, Session 4. Meaning through the attitude we take towards suffering, the limitations in life. And actually part of what we talked about, one of the biggest limitation in life is death. We already talked a little bit about the music that you wanted at your funeral. So this is I guess the homework, just to think about, no this is the homework from Session 3, let's see Session 4, this is the exercise we're going to do for Session 4.

Patient: okay

Therapist: You can think about a little bit for next week.

Patient: excuse me

Therapist: and then we'll do that next week. I don't know if you set a time, do you want (RSA's name) to call you? Or should we try next Tuesday?

Patient: She'll have to call me because I don't have a schedule.

Therapist: okay, so I'll ask (RSA's name) to call you.

Patient: Today is the last day of my schedule so far, maybe they'll give me a new schedule today.

Therapist: okay, we did everything

Patient: okay

Therapist: oh, one of the things, the homework for today, besides looking at that, is you probably do this all the time but to discuss to share some of this legacy to discuss it with some people in your family.

Patient: they know how I feel

Therapist: I know they know how you feel, you share it every day

Patient: every day

Therapist: yeah, okay
Patient: cause when the time comes for me, the only that I am really concerned about is my mother
Therapist: yeah
Patient: and now she knows that I don't feel well.
Therapist: I see, so she's a big concern of yours. So we'll talk about that next week cause it fits in with next week's session.
Patient: alright
Therapist: okay.

Session 4: Attitudinal Sources of Meaning—Encountering Life's Limitations

Therapist: Good morning (name)
Patient: Good morning
Therapist: So this is Session 4, and uh, I just wanted to say hi
Patient: Hello
Therapist: thanks for filling out those forms.
Patient: Mm-hmm
Therapist: how have things been going since the last time I saw you
Patient: Well, things have been on an even keel, but last Friday I have had tremendous pain, that I have had to take the pain medication.
Therapist: I see. You have been trying to hold off on taking the pain medication?
Patient: I had been holding off and the pain would go away.
Therapist: Uh-ha
Patient: But it's totally out of control
Therapist: Does the pain medicine help?
Patient: it does
Therapist: okay, where have you been having the pain?
Patient: in the back
Therapist: in your back
Patient: On my . . .
Therapist: abdomen?
Patient: right upper quadrant
Therapist: right upper quadrant, mm-hmm
Patient: but the pain medication has helped, I took it last night and I haven't had the pain
Therapist: good, what pain medication are you taking?
Patient: Oxycodone
Therapist: Okay and how are things going with the chemotherapy?
Patient: Not good, they have had to stop the chemo because it's not working and the mass has grown.
Therapist: hmm
Patient: So they offered me phase one chemo. I have to wait for two weeks, but I do not feel good about that chemo.
Therapist: You've been thinking about whether you want to do that
Patient: I don't think I'm going to do it. I'm not going to do it, I'm pretty sure.
Therapist: yeah, what are you thoughts about it?
Patient: I'm beginning, other than the pain, I feel well.
Therapist: yes
Patient: I do not want to go back into that again
Therapist: Into the whole process of chemo, and feeling so tired and sick?
Patient: The first chemo I did well, I couldn't complain. But that Folfiri and Folfox I couldn't tolerate it, I felt terrible, that is the worst I have ever felt in my life.
Therapist: So your quality of life was not that great while you were on that. You're feeling better now, except for the pain.
Patient: I'm feeling better now, except for the pain.
Therapist: and the pain can be controlled
Patient: and the pain can be controlled.
Therapist: Absolutely
Patient: I don't ever want to feel like that again, because of the fear of the unknown
Therapist: Yes, m 'am
Patient: I am not taking the chemo, and put myself into that, I'm not.
Therapist: the fear of the unknown is the fear of what that chemo would do?
Patient: It'll do, but me into not feeling well. Oh goodness (name) I did not feel well and I told the doctor "I do not feel good about this chemo, neither do I feel well from it," and I told him all the time. I'm not trying to be difficult, I'll try it for myself, okay it didn't work.
Therapist: yeah
Patient: I don't think I'm going to do it.
Therapist: so today's session focuses on encountering life's limitations and the attitude that you take towards suffering or these limitations and the ultimate limitation is death right? That's the ultimate limitation. Um, so finding a source of meaning through the attitude that you take towards limitation like death even, that's the big topic of today and a lot of exercises for today. So when you think about not taking chemotherapy, you must have thought about what the consequences would be right in terms of whether the . . .
Patient: (name) throughout my life I know that I'm here for one purpose, to go through this life and die, and I will die my way

Therapist: There you go.
Patient: on my own terms. I don't want to suffer with pain, and when that time comes I know what's available to me in the medical field.
Therapist: Yeah
Patient: You know, start my drip and let me go. I have lived my life. Some die younger, some die of an old age. I'm 61, I have more to live for, I have a lot to offer, but this may be the time for me to go, I am accepting of that.
Therapist: I see, so you're attitude is one of acceptance.
Patient: I accept it
Therapist: and your attitude your whole life has been to have one purpose in life which is to live your life as fully and as meaningfully as possible for as long as it lasts. And you also saw death as a part of life.
Patient: It is a part of my life
Therapist: As your attitude
Patient: I have been very careful, meticulous with my life, I'm not going to endanger myself for no reason whatsoever. But I'm going to enjoy every moment of my life.
Therapist: You're going to what dear?
Patient: Going to enjoy every moment of my life
Therapist: You're going to enjoy while you're alive
Patient: Oh yes
Therapist: Yes, that's another attitude that you're going to enjoy everything while you're still alive.
Patient: and I intend to
Therapist: And that helps you feel alive when you're alive.
Patient: that helps me feel alive
Therapist: there you go. So that's a big part of the discussion today. But I see that you brought in some pictures, cause last session we were talking about your legacy and the legacy you inherited, the legacy you live and the legacy you will leave behind. And I think we even talked a little bit about a legacy project.
Patient: Mm-hmm
Therapist: And of course this is the 4th session, we're going to have 7 sessions so, we're about half way through, half way through, and so you've already begun a little bit to think about and maybe do some things about your legacy project you say right?
Patient: um (name) I said my legacy for, I live my legacy everyday.
Therapist: Yes, absolutely, what do you mean by that?
Patient: for example yesterday, my aunts, my mother's sister that raised me didn't have any children and her other sister had one they brought us up together and they would not see and the Diaspora that I come from taking care of children. So my aunts would, children would always be at my house, my uncle has 10 children, so we were raised together, but if there were children that needed a pencil that needed breakfast, my aunts were there. And we had raised these children since she was 7 months old, and she heard that I was sick and she came, she's been coming. and yesterday I guess she wanted to vent she said "Aunt (name), I'm 36 years old now, I don't know my mother's likes, I don't know her dislikes, she's told me about a meal she made last week and serve it to her husband. And he said "this is good, where did you learn to make it?" and she said "oh, my aunt would always make that." She said to me "You have paid my tuition, you have sent me to college, my mom has never offered." And now the mother's going blind, and she said to me "She's called me and I've helped her, but I just can't get it together with her." I said, she said "You have never brought us up like that, you have been firm, you have taught us that we have to be independent, to take care of ourselves" and she said "I'm not working, but I know how to spend my money and I have a little that I can offer someone, but I have to also take care of myself. you had taught me that, and I have to be first," and I said to myself yesterday, because it hadn't been long since I did this, and I said to myself . . .
Therapist: yeah, it hadn't been long since you did the exercise.
Patient: yes, this I don't have to write my legacy on paper
Therapist: exactly
Patient: this is it
Therapist: You live it everyday
Patient: and I sat there and I listened to her, and my son came in from work and they were just talking because my son that died had broken his jaw, and for that Thanksgiving he said "Mommy, I want my Thanksgiving meal." I said "How are we going to do that?" He said "Just put everything into the blender, including the collared greens." And we were just talking about that yesterday and oh my goodness it was hilarious. And she said "Auntie when I come from work he would just be standing here at the door waiting for me to see what I brought from work." Cause she said "Do you know sometimes he would call me with a

whole list of things" because she used to manager Burger King. And she said to him "I don't own Burger King I just manage it." She said "Those are days I think of and laugh." And I said "Those were some days when you guys were growing up here, it was crazy, but it was just fun with these children." I said "This is my legacy, when this child can just come."

Therapist: Yeah, it's very interesting, so when you talk about legacy, you live your legacy every day. You're the link between the legacy you inherited from your grandparents, grandmothers, great grandmothers . . .

Patient: Aunts

Therapist: . . . and aunts. You're taken you've incorporated their values, the values of dedicating yourself to the people you love, and taking care of others and serving others. You're taken these values, and live them every day in your life and you teach them to the next generation, so you're the link between past generations and future generations. And you live those values every day, the values of living life meaningfully through dedicating yourself to someone, through love, through experiential sources of meaning, love, through dedication to others and through keeping the memories alive of people who have passed. You know people are often confused cause we say the legacy you inherit, the legacy you live and the legacy you leave behind. They don't know "What do you mean the legacy I live?" And you've got a very nice example, of the legacy that you live. The legacy that you live is playing the role of being the link between generations.

Patient: I have my nieces every weekend including the 18 month old, so my sister's grandson came, and they all had um, my husband bought potato chips and what have you from the store, he came. So I just saw them sharing everything and the grandson came, and he says "No" he reached out to the other one's hands and said to her "I don't want what I got, this is what I want." Reaching out to pull it out of her hands, I said to him "No, that's what she got and she didn't complain, you ask her whether she wants it or not." I said "Well, if you don't' want what you got you either exchange it or don't eat it." So I was telling them about this incident yesterday, my son and my niece, and they said "Oh, he doesn't know you, he wasn't brought up here. He's not here as often as we are in this house. And know that if you're here, he's not going to pull that off." I said "Yes, he doesn't know."

Therapist: Yeah, its also the sense I get from everything you've said from the first day we've met is that you are very much aware, you're very much aware of being part of a continuum of your family. You're part of something much greater than yourself, you're part of a whole line of people, your family, your ancestors, your children, the children of your relatives, you see this as starting way before you and continuing way after you.

Patient: It started before me; my grandmother raised her cousin's children after she died. And they were very good I couldn't ask for uncles or aunts, and I came here (name), I came into this country illegally, and my father was here and my father didn't know and my brothers didn't know and my father was furious when he found out. And I said "I don't care, you don't know me. I have been raised by my aunts and uncles." He's been here all my life, I didn't know him until I was 13, I didn't know him, he didn't know me.

Therapist: Right, so we're going to talk a lot about attitudes overcoming obstacles and limitations. And you learned, you learned a lot about overcoming obstacles. And your attitude has always been "You don't know who I am, I come from a long line of people who don't give up, and we do what we need to do to get, we do what we need to do to get the things that are important."

Patient: To do what has to be, to do what has to be done.

Therapist: To do what has to be done and to become who we have to become. Just like your son, with the osteo imperfecta.

Patient: Despite his disability

Therapist: Despite his limitations, that's the best example that you've talked about, well one of the striking examples of overcoming limitations.

Patient: I used to tell him, you know "You are, in the English language you're disabled, but you're most certainly are not unable."

Therapist: You're disabled but not unable. In Garifuna they don't have a word for disabled?

Patient: Yeah, in Garifuna there is. Danimat.

Therapist: Danima?

Patient: Danimat

Therapist: Danimat

Patient: ah-ha, for disabled

Therapist: There is a word

Patient: There is a word

Therapist: and what does it mean? Does it mean unable?

Patient: Ah-ha, mm-hmm
Therapist: So you even had to change that
Patient: Mm-hmm
Therapist: You had to even change that
Patient: Mm-hmm
Therapist: so that the correct attitude was implied or imparted
Patient: Mm-hmm
Therapist: So you brought in some pictures was that part of something that related to?
Patient: This is our house in Belize
Therapist: Oh, this is the house in Belize. It's pretty.
Patient: This is our house in Belize. It is pretty.
Therapist: Where is the hammock that you talk about?
Patient: I always have a hammock.
Therapist: there it is
Patient: This is on the porch
Therapist: On the porch, is the porch on the top?
Patient: The porch is ah-ha, here
Therapist: up there on the top floor
Patient: There are two sides, this is the front, this is the side where the porch is.
Therapist: So there are almost two kinds of porches right?
Patient: Mm-hmm
Therapist: and a nice kitchen, nice rooms, you get a little bit of flavor of what's going on outside. It's beautiful. Does anyone stay there during the time when you're not there?
Patient: we have someone that stays there . . .
Therapist: who kind of keeps the place up?
Patient: keeps the place up
Therapist: Did you share some of this with anybody? I know you were talking about this young girl who came and you shared your recipes.
Patient: They know, they know of this
Therapist: everybody knows?
Patient: They go home and . . .
Therapist: you were talking about after doing this homework a lot of this was on your mind, and you were communicating this to this. . . .
Patient: I didn't share the homework with her, but I was amazing that she pointed out sharing "Auntie this is how you brought us up."
Therapist: She shared it with you.
Patient: And I said to myself, "Why would she talk about this." You know cause this has been on my mind recently about this legacy you know, and I said to her you know "Just keep it, always with you. Remember, I did the best I can, to enable you guys, and you have to pass it on to somebody, to your children you know always have somebody in your life. Just give a helping hand, that's all you have to do, and pass it on."
Therapist: So let's move into today's session, you already the exercise yes. This is Session 4, so you know when we started we were talking about the sources of meaning, and uh this is the next one coming later. We've gone through, we've talked a little bit about what does meaning mean, and how cancer has affected your identity and meaning in life. The interesting thing was that there was more that was the same than changed really.
Patient: Mm-hmm
Therapist: but um, trying to find . . . there we go, so there are 4 sources of meaning, we talked about the historical source of meaning, legacy, today we're going to talk about attitudinal sources of meaning, the next two sessions are going to focus on creative and experiential sources of meaning. Creative sources of meaning are meaning you get from the work that you do, and your dedication to things you care about, people maybe you care about in the world. And experiential sources are of meaning are sources of meaning that come from being connected to life versus from love, dedicating yourself to people that you love, and experiencing life through beauty and food, the breezing on your hammock in Belize, and all those things. And attitudinal sources really focus a lot on the self-esteem that you get from being able to overcome obstacles in life, limitations. And a lot of that comes from the fact that no matter what you cannot control in life you always have the ability to control the attitude that you take towards the situation. And um you have choice no matter what attitude to take, and you had a choice about whether you were going to come here legally or illegally, you had a choice of raising your son as a disabled person or as a person who is able. And so any, and here you are, you're encountering the limitations that chemotherapy has placed on your life, and you're making choices about how you want to handle that. The attitude you take towards whether you are going to take chemotherapy or more, what's more important to you quality of life versus the length of life etc. So um, what a lot of people find is in order to overcome or transcend some of these limitations in life, the attitude that you take is supportive by your ability to find meaning from other places in your life so you can have the strength to make the proper choice, to make the choice that's right for you, to take the

attitude that's right for you. And that comes from all those other sources of meaning, from all the love in your life, from the values you inherited through your family, from your desire to live, you told me "I want to feel alive when I'm alive." To still experience life

Patient: Life

Therapist: yeah and what's more important is living life meaningfully, not living life . . .

Patient: just laying down and sleeping, that's not me

Therapist: In terms of time . . . yeah. So today's exercises focus on these issues of limitations. So there are three exercises and I think you already started in your homework to look at them. The first one, I guess there are three and maybe we can go in order, the first one was "Since your diagnosis are you been able to find meaning in your life, despite the fact of your awareness of the finiteness of life?" I think you have that.

Patient: Which one is this? "Since you're diagnosis what are the specific limitations or losses you have faced."

Therapist: Okay, actually this one is different, so use this one.

Patient: The first one is "What are some of life's limitations or losses or obstacles

Therapist: that you've faced

Patient: that you faced in the past and how you cope?" And I wrote about one. Some life limitation is my life was coming to America and going to my father without papers. I had to do medial jobs and was always afraid even when taking my son to the doctor's. Coping I worked along with my husband, and always we always had money to do what was necessary for us.

Therapist: Okay, so this is what are some of life's limitations, loss, or obstacles you faced in the past and how did you cope with them at the time? So this one was mainly about your son?

Patient: this one was the most significant to me.

Therapist: And the obstacles with your son were what?

Patient: We didn't have papers here and it so happened that he was disabled.

Therapist: right

Patient: and I didn't want to tell anyone that I was in this country illegally by then my father filed the papers, but it was quite different the way it was done then than now, because I would have, maybe after three months now I would have had working papers, so I wouldn't be fearful, but those days no it was a longer process. So we had to work, my husband and I, and we would save our money and pay for all the care we got.

Therapist: hmm

Patient: We never had Medicaid.

Therapist: So your husband was your main source of help here?

Patient: Mm-hmm, when I couldn't work my husband did. He has always worked, always.

Therapist: Did you reach out beyond your own nuclear family for help too?

Patient: No, my brothers were there to help; my brothers would always say "Do you need help?" I said "No" because my husband provided.

Therapist: so really it was an awful lot of dedication and hard work, and focus on your son and his needs and doing whatever was necessary like you said before the attitude was "We are going to overcome this. I am going to do; my husband and I are going to do whatever we need to do in order to give our son a chance at a productive life." And you dedicated yourself this way, all this hard work, to raise the funds to get him care because your attitude was care was going to do what for him it was going to?

Patient: well, he had brittle bones . . .

Therapist: yeah

Patient: . . . and sometimes he would break out of nothing, just stretching in the bed. And my husband had a job that had insurance, okay, and he would be in the hospital. Within this time, he had been in the hospital and they said it was child abuse, because they hadn't done any testing. So I took him to a bone specialist in Queens and he did a bone biopsy and that's when the diagnosis of osteogenesis imperfecta was confirmed. And we remained that doctor (name) until he died. And that doctor was like a parent to me, he said "From now on, if he gets sick you call me." Sometimes he would come to the house if I tell him you know he's in so much pain, I don't want to lift him up, or if I would take him the office for X-rays and if he needed to be in the hospital he and I would literally be admitted to the hospital. Cause he's in so much pain, he doesn't want anyone touching him, the doctor said "Let his mother come in here and take care of him."

Therapist: Did it take a little bit of courage to do what you did with your son?

Patient: I don't think it took courage.

Therapist: and commitment

Patient: (name) I loved him dearly.

Therapist: So it was love, it was love that motivated you.

Patient: Yes, because some people suggested "Oh give him up, put him in a home." I would not do that that was out of the question. He could sit, he was still able to move around, and talk, oh my goodness.

Therapist: So you're attitude was that "you could do it, and you could do it better than anyone else."

Patient: I think I did it better than anyone else. Cause the doctors would be calling my house "Mrs. (name), what did you do to him, how did you bring him up like this?" I think it was something that every parent would do to for their children or to their children. I just raised him how I raised the other one, and they are as different as night and day. Because (son's name) would come up to my room every night, he sleeps late, he would do his homework, I don't have to say to him "Do your homework." And he would clean the house he would say "I don't want my grandmother cleaning." Of course he would cook, climb on top of the counter to cut what he has to cut up, climb from the wheelchair to the counter do what he has to do, climb come back down to the wheelchair to the stove and cook his food. Leave my food there for my lunch, clean the kitchen, clean the floor, you could eat off of my floor. And then he'll come up and he would shower, and he'll come into my bed, "(son's name) I have to go to work tomorrow, stop picking at me." But that was just the way I lived with him. He said "Mommy, I love you." And he said that to me every day, every day.

Therapist: So this was the biggest obstacle that you ever had to overcome.

Patient: Mm-hmm

Therapist: You mentioned there are losses too, and obstacles. I guess obstacles would be coming here illegally.

Patient: which was a breeze

Therapist: was it a big obstacle?

Patient: After I got here then the obstacles started.

Therapist: Oh really, what happened? You couldn't do this? You couldn't do that?

Patient: You couldn't you know jobs.

Therapist: A driver's license?

Patient: You couldn't get a drivers license. And then I had this child then he was disabled and then I had to take him to the doctors.

Therapist: You didn't have insurance?

Patient: well, my husband worked then and we had insurance

Therapist: Your husband was not here illegally?

Patient: He was also

Therapist: Also illegally

Patient: But those days they didn't ask any questions if you had a job and you had insurance, it's not like now.

Therapist: So he managed to get a job with insurance

Patient: Mm-hmm

Therapist: What did he do?

Patient: He was a parking attendant at a garage on 47th and Madison.

Therapist: Interesting. Let's do the second exercise. I'll read it out loud. Since your diagnosis what are the specific limitations, losses you have faced and how are you coping or dealing with them now? Are you still able to find meaning in your life despite your awareness of the limitations and finiteness of life? That was a little bit more like the one I had.

Patient: Since my diagnosis having to stop working, and feeling sick after chemo, worrying about my scans, uh what is this I wrote down, dealing with it has been praying, believing that God will always be with me, talking to my friend have been how I cope.

Therapist: With the limitations? Having cancer and chemotherapy.

Patient: Because I have plenty of friends, and they call they call they call they come.

Therapist: So part of overcoming limitations is again, and the attitude you take towards being able to overcome these limitations is fed is the source of it, the strength of being able to do that comes from these other sources of meaning. Through your connectedness with others with your friends, through the love of your friends, but then you also mentioned God. Tell me a little bit about that. Is it a matter of God's love? God gives you strength? You feel very connected to God.

Patient: (name) however, whatever religion calls it, I believe that there is a God. That is my belief, and I believe that God has been good to me throughout my life. There has to be someone that's directing all of this and however we call it, we call it God, I believe he's there. And I believe that he's always with me.

Therapist: How do you how do you express your belief in God, or how do you practice your belief in God in your life. Are you somebody who belongs to a church, or anything like that, or you pray or something like that?

Patient: I belong to a church. If someone invites me to a church or I go to some services, I enjoy it. Okay, but every day in my life I have been good to everyone I've met, if you're nasty I'm going to be nasty and tell you exactly where to get off, but it's not in my nature.

Therapist: So it's not a Christian thing then. It's not like Christ is very important in your life, because Christ would say "If somebody's nasty to you, you love them back."

Patient: Mm-huh

Therapist: It's not like that?

Patient: Mm-mm, I'll tell you where to get off, but I will be good to you.

Therapist: You're going to be?

Patient: Good to you

Therapist: Okay, so when you look of God, is Christ involved in this?

Patient: Well, if it's Christ, if he's God . . .

Therapist: Not really. It's less specific for you.

Patient: It's less specific for me, but I also think, I also feel that because I've had a good life

Therapist: Yes

Patient: it's not even in my nature to be just nasty to people, just be good, just be civil, just be human.

Therapist: So you believe in a God that's sort of a creator, and a designer of life, that God has a destiny . . .

Patient: For every one of us

Therapist: . . . in store for every one of us. So things are already . . .

Patient: Predestined

Therapist: predestined or . . .

Patient: And I believe, we're supposed to enjoy this life, we don't know when it will end, not to do anything to harm this life or this time we have. Just live it.

Therapist: You believe in some sort of afterlife?

Patient: I don't think so

Therapist: not really

Patient: I think you have one chance here on the face of this earth and that's it.

Therapist: And that's it

Patient: And that's why it's so important to enjoy every moment.

Therapist: right, enjoy every moment. So this relationship that you have with God and it sounds like if I were to give you a choice of whether you're religious or spiritual or you know an athesiast, agnostic whatever. You would probably use the word spiritual maybe.

Patient: Spiritual yeah

Therapist: yeah, so this relationship the presence of your understanding, your sense of God how does that give you strength? Or does it?

Patient: Because if I'm down, for example when my son died, I thought I was going to die, I thought I was going to lose my mind. But I would sit and talk to God to take this pain to take this feeling away from me.

Therapist: So you talk to God, a little different than prayer or no?

Patient: Sometimes I would pray.

Therapist: you would pray too

Patient: Sometimes I would be sitting on the train or on the bus.

Therapist: And ask for your pain to be relieved, the grief

Patient: the grief. Because sometimes I wouldn't think about him, and the next moment it would come to my mind and it wasn't a good feeling. And it took a long time; it took a long time . . .

Therapist: For the pain to get lighter

Patient: for the pain to get lighter, because discussing it sometimes I think that his death hurt me as much then as it do now.

Therapist: when you talk about it

Patient: It's easier.

Therapist: you'll never forget him, you'll always remember him

Patient: never, and now that I'm sick my son and I were talking on Saturday he said "Mommy, what are you going to do? Maybe you should try the treatment." I said to him "Be aware that I am okay with my diagnosis, I'm not afraid. I have someone to go to."

Therapist: I was just going to ask you, whether you felt that you might see your son again after you die.

Patient: I hope I do

Therapist: You hope you do. You used the word to your son "I have some" when you were talking to your son you said you were unafraid, you said "Remember I have someone to go to." You meant your son who had died, so the idea that you will be reconnected in some way, maybe not to see him, but reconnected.

Patient: reconnected, mm-hmm

Therapist: And that makes you less afraid.

Patient: It does make me less afraid. ON the other hand, I didn't want him to feel that I didn't want to take the treatment because I want to go to this one and leave him.

Therapist: right right right, of course. Yeah, you didn't want to be in a position of saying "I prefer to be with your brother."

Patient: But I've told him from the gut my diagnosis "Listen, this is not an easy cancer to deal with, I want you to be fully aware. This is not an easy diagnosis to deal with; we don't know which way it will go." But I have told him listen I have seen so many people die that I'm not fearful.

Therapist: when you say you have seen some many people die you mean in your work? In your family?

Patient: In my work, in my family.

Therapist: In your work as a nurse.

Patient: and in my family too, in my family. I was with my brother at night and in the morning at 5 am my niece called me, "Auntie you should come, my dad is sick." And he must have been dead already cause they woke up, his wife got ready to go to work, and when she turned around he was lying down in the same position, so she looked at him, he was dead, he had a heart attack in his sleep. She couldn't take it; she says "Auntie, my dad has died." And I thought that, I don't know I went crazy, I don't even know how I felt. And my brother's house was around the corner from mine, and when I got there he was just lying there. And my brother was so full of life like myself, we liked the same things, at least mostly the same things, and it happened to the other one. My older brother had had lymphoma, and one weekend he was sick I say "You know you have to go to the hospital. Go and I'll meet you there." He said "No, don't come." And I told him you know "Call our cousin have him take you to the hospital." And Monday morning I went there and he said "No don't stay here go to work." And I went to work, but I couldn't take it and I went to the hospital, he says "You know what I going to let them start my drip and I want you to go home." And by the time I got home, the hospital called. So it could not be a bad thing.

Therapist: No, so let's go to this last one because that talks a little bit more about I think it's the same in mine as yours. What would you consider a good and meaningful death?

Patient: Meaningful death

Therapist: Yes. How can you imagine being remembered by your loved one?

Patient: a good meaningful death is not dying alone, and I know I'm not going to die alone. I know for sure that my loved ones will remember the times we had. Enjoy it as a family, a community, that as the oldest sibling in one's family, I have been a sister always guiding, loving, providing, assisting, and that's what I have been.

Therapist: And that's what you want to pass on this sort of.

Patient: And that's what I want to pass on. That's my legacy.

Therapist: That's your legacy. Repeat that last part, that you were what? Your legacy is what? That you were always a?

Patient: I have been a sister

Therapist: sister

Patient: always guiding

Therapist: guiding

Patient: loving

Therapist: loving

Patient: Providing

Therapist: providing. So a meaningful death is to not die alone in other words the focus really is on connectedness, love, experiential source of meaning, so even in death to be connected.

Patient: to be connected

Therapist: and in death being connected not only to people surrounding you, but the values that you've lived in your life . . .

Patient: my legacy

Therapist: to be a legacy your legacy is what's important. That's gives your death meaning too.

Patient: meaning too

Therapist: your life and your death

Patient: Mm-hmm. My brother was at home with one of my uncles and I called him, he was at home this Sunday. I said to him "When are you going home?" He said "I'm going home next month." And he's been the one bringing me here. He said "And I'm going home in 2 years. In 2 years I will go and I will not come back again." But prior to this he had said to me I have always given my opinion whether it's wanted or not. Because I have been, I am the oldest, and (name) I came here and did everything that I could do to bring the rest of my family here, and children. Sometimes I tell them "You know I know you guys are adults and you don't care about my opinion but if you need help and I'm not in agreement that's it I'm not going to help, so you may as well listen." So he said to me "Don't think I don't listen to you" He's 58 years old "I have listened to everything you've said." And you said to me, his house is almost as big as my house, and he was trying to sell it, and I say "Do not sell your house, don't sell your house, how will you get the money to build another house like that?" He said "You were right, I'm so glad I didn't sell the house because I'm going home in 2 years."

Therapist: right, it's always good to be able to go back home to Belize and have a place to stay.

Patient: (name) I'm thinking I'm going home in one of these days, pretty soon, maybe next week.

Therapist: Right after we finish?

Patient: (laugh) I have to go home, my father's daughter is sick, my sister is sick, and my nieces called me yesterday, I have go home and see her.

Therapist: Will we be able to reach you if you go back home? In Belize? Your cell phone?

Patient: You guys can reach me.

Therapist: Yeah, good. So does this idea of overcoming limitations, the idea of attitude and using all these other sources of meaning to deal with limitations, does that make some sense to you? Yeah? Could you put it into words? Some simple words?

Patient: Sometimes you have to pick up yourself by the bootstrap, and say you know what, and channel your life in a positive way.

Therapist: yeah

Patient: I am not a negative person and I let things happen, good things happen to me, happen in my life.

Therapist: yeah

Patient: I'm determined and I'm stubborn. Um, sometimes I say that negative or bad things happen in people's lives because they allow them to happen, and that is just the way it's been in my life. And sometimes my husband would say "Oh no, we're not supposed to do this, and he'll say "Oh my wife you're just so stubborn. Sometimes I listen to you and look at what your heading, your heading is, and I have to follow through with you." I say "Because things have to happen in our lives and if you don't work and let it happen it will not happen to you." And that's just the way life is.

Therapist: this was potentially a difficult exercise, cause we talk about things like death and stuff like that. Did you find it difficult?

Patient: No.

Therapist: No, because it sounds like you have been thinking about it a lot. Way before cancer even.

Patient: With life, comes death.

Therapist: yeah, so it's something you've thought about before.

Patient: with life comes death, if you don't have life then you are not going to die. I think both of them are equal.

Therapist: well thanks for your openness and honesty about today's session. I think the next, the next session focuses on creative sources of meaning, that's deriving meaning through creating the life that have, and you know if you haven't noticed already all these sources of meaning we artificially kind of separate them, but its hard to separate them because they are almost always acting. . . .

Patient: Like intermingling

Therapist: Intermingled absolutely. So the next the next session is the creative sources of meaning. You can look at the exercise, is this five?

Patient: This is it here. Creative source of meaning.

Therapist: Let me take it. Yeah, yes, exactly. So you can take a peak at these exercises. It's about basically the responsibility you have to create a life of meaning, identity, direction, connection, transcendence, self-esteem, self-actualization, and so you can go through that exercise, and I know you have been thinking about this legacy project and part of you, rightfully says that your legacy project is you and the life you've lived, but I think you had talked a little bit about last time about music, right?

Patient: I will try to prepare the music

Therapist: So if there's a possibility, maybe the music at some point.

Patient: I'll try it next time.

Therapist: It doesn't . . .

Patient: I'll try to bring . . .

Therapist: it could be next time or the last session.

Patient: Okay

Therapist: so you have plenty of time. So um I don't know if we want to schedule the next meeting today, or we'll have (RSA's name) call you.

Patient: Maybe she should call you

Therapist: Okay, I'll have her call you

Patient: I don't know when I will leave

Therapist: To Belize?

Patient: Mm-hmm

Therapist: it would be great if we could get in these sessions before you go

Patient: I don't know

Therapist: yeah, right

Patient: because my niece called "You know, your sister is not doing well." And I spoke to my sister in the week and she didn't sound like herself, she knew it was me, but she didn't sound like herself.

Therapist: Well you know what we could do is have two sessions in one week if you wanted.

Patient: Oh sure, since I don't have to go over there again

Therapist: Yeah, we can have more than one session in a week, especially if you think you can go to Belize.

Patient: I'm really thinking that I'm going to Belize.

Therapist: Okay, so I'll tell (RSA's name) call you and maybe we can have a few sessions in one week. Maybe even another one before the end of this week or something like that

Patient: Okay, maybe on Friday?
Therapist: yeah
Patient: But I'd like to come early in the morning when the trains aren't . . .
Therapist: Absolutely, absolutely
Patient: So we'll plan that
Therapist: alright
Patient: thank you (name)
Therapist: thank you dear

Session 5: Creative Sources of Meaning—Engaging in Life: Creativity, Courage, and Responsibility

Therapist: So do you have any ideas as to when you're going to Belize?
Patient: I have no idea.
Therapist: not yet, okay
Patient: I was hoping that I would just get a flight and leave.
Therapist: yeah?
Patient: that's how I usually leave, like sometimes on a whim I get a fare and I just go.
Therapist: It's not too expensive, flights aren't too bad?
Patient: Now, it's like 641
Therapist: oh
Patient: and it'll stay like this, its not getting any lower
Therapist: and what's the weather like in Belize now?
Patient: maybe 90 degrees, but that's not . . .
Therapist: is it hurricane season?
Patient: No, hurricane season starts in November.
Therapist: oh
Patient: but it's not humid.
Therapist: It's not humid. So you don't have to worry about hurricanes in July or August.
Patient: Cause my husband got caught in one last year.
Therapist: In a hurricane?
Patient: In the hurricane there
Therapist: I see. Okay, so anything, we just saw each other recently, anything happening medically?
Patient: I just have this abdominal and back pain. I'm even thinking of going there today to ask Dr. (name) if this is how I should feel.
Therapist: No
Patient: because I had severe abdominal pain all day yesterday.
Therapist: okay, I know you're on Oxycodone, which is very mild, do you know what strength? 5? 10?
Patient: 5
Therapist: 5, so you're on a small dose of Oxycodone, which is a mild opioid, you know.
Patient: Mm-hmm
Therapist: and it only lasts the half-life, the duration of the analgesic affect on the pain is only somewhere between 2 and 4 hours. So there are a couple different strategies. He can give you a longer sustained released preparation of the Oxycodone, which is called OxyContin
Patient: OxyContin
Therapist: And he can give you a slightly larger dose, which lasts longer and you can take the Oxycodone if you need it as a rescue. Or they can give you something like a little patch, a fentanyl patch.
Patient: Fentanyl patch
Therapist: Like 25 mg, which is a lose dose, and you use the Oxycodone for breakthrough
Patient: breakthrough
Therapist: But you're on very little, you're on very little pain medicine, so it's reasonable to have the pain better controlled.
Patient: Because its bad now and I had it, I took the pain medication yesterday I got some relief, and then I had this pain all night. I was telling my husband, "I had this abdominal and back pain all night, and in the same token I was still sleeping."
Therapist: yeah, you were tired probably too
Patient: Tired, but I was telling him "I don't know I was just sleeping."
Therapist: Did you get up to?
Patient: Every time I wake up
Therapist: It hurts
Patient: the pain was there.
Therapist: Did you take anything at night?
Patient: Well I took the pain medication at 3 am, and I slept and at 5 am I was awake again.
Therapist: yeah
Patient: But it had taken the edge off
Therapist: definitely, there is, you have such a minimal amount of intervention for the pain; it's such a mild and minimal dose
Patient: My pain. Taking pain medication has been like not me, and maybe something is the tumor is bigger now or
Therapist: You've had bad experiences on pain medication?
Patient: No, I just don't take pain medication.
Therapist: oh, well there are a lot of aches and pains that you kind of tough out
Patient: that was generally my issue as a nurse with sickle cell patients, and I would tell the sickle cell, I would have this discussion with the sickle cell coordinator "Why do you get these patients so hooked on pain medications so early in life. That when they get to be adults they're just stupid."

Therapist: So you're afraid about getting addicted?

Patient: Well, that was not for me, but for everyone.

Therapist: Yeah, you know we're done lots of studies on addiction and pain medications in cancer patients. And less than 1/10th of 1% of cancer patients get addicted

Patient: become addicted

Therapist: yeah, so it's a bit

Patient: Well, I think in cancer you really need the pain medication

Therapist: yeah you really need it, and a lot of it depends on environmental and genetic factors. Um, that lead to the misuse of medicines. But when its used for cancer pain, unless you're someone who had a significant history in your past of abusing drugs, there's less than a .1% chance of becoming addicted, abusing the medicines.

Patient: Because I said (name), my son had brittle bones and I think the bone pain would be so severe. And if needed pain medication I would make sure he got pain medications. And even for his surgeries, and the doctors and the nurses being in there, I would come to the recovery room and they would have given him the pain medication. And as soon as he's awake, he has the pain; he tells them "No, I don't need this pain medication again."

Therapist: Well, let me ask you a slightly difficult question. Do you feel that when people have pain they suffer?

Patient: Yes

Therapist: And I think of two kinds of suffering, there's avoidable suffering, where it's not necessary to suffer and it's only really cruel to make someone suffer.

Patient: It's not necessary.

Therapist: So pain, unnecessary suffering. And then there's unavoidable suffering you know, kind of things you have to face when you have cancer. The losses you anticipate, things like that. Do you think there is something good about suffering? You think for you?

Patient: Oh no

Therapist: No

Patient: Oh no

Therapist: Some meaning for you in some way?

Patient: And if someone needs the pain medication, god I would give it to you.

Therapist: But in other ways, do you feel there's an element, there's something good about suffering?

Patient: No, there is no need. And personally for me and for anyone else that's a no no.

Therapist: the reason I ask is because today's session is about creative sources of meaning right. And I think one of the first things I said to you when we sat down is that in life we have basically one primary responsibility and that's to create a life right? To create a life of meaning, and identity and direction and connection, transcendence you know and to live to our full potential if possible. And so that's a very big job.

Patient: It sure is

Therapist: and you could say that from the beginning it's really quite an impossible job, no one ever succeeds 100%. And so then what happens when you don't quite live up to your full potential or you maybe haven't fulfilled yourself in all those areas of how the life you want to create. Or for some people I know they live very spectacular lives, but not really the life they wanted to live, the life that their mother or father wanted them to live. It wasn't generally theirs, it wasn't authentically theirs. So what people experience is what's called existential guilt, the idea that they didn't quite do enough, and they need to be able to forgive themselves for things that they maybe didn't quite do, because in fact we're human and sometimes it involves just being able to forgive yourself and say "Hey I tried my best" or sometimes in involves saying "Oh I didn't do that right, maybe I can redeem myself and make amends." Or sometimes it's an issue of trying to finish something that's undone in the time that you do have you know. "I never wrote that novel, and I want to write that novel." Or "I never did plant that, I never did finish renovate that part of that house in Belize, and I want to do that." My wife and I have a joke, we in our apartment we have a master bedroom and sorry a bathroom and bathroom that our son uses, and I told my wife, we have a nice apartment but its built in the 60s and the master bathroom hadn't been renovated in quite a while, we have a nice vanity and things like that but you know its white tiles. And I said to my wife "I refuse to die in that bathroom. I want to die in a bathroom that has marble or granite with a walk in shower. If I collapse and die in the bathroom that's not the bathroom I want to die in. And I'm going to renovate that before I die." I know its going to bother me . . .

Patient: If you don't do it

Therapist: If I'm going through cancer treatment or something like that, and I'm lying in that bed and I'm going "I'm going to that bathroom and I might drop dead in that bathroom. I do not want to drop dead in that bathroom." So there are things that you know are unfinished. For me it's finishing certain projects and things like that. Does any of that relate to you?

Patient: My theory has been, um, if it doesn't happen, it doesn't happen, because I tried my best.

Therapist: So forgiving yourself, accepting the life that you tried your best and you accepting who you are is something that you're okay with.

Patient: And this has been my daily life, and at sometimes I won't say I'm sorry. Once I've said all I've had to say that is it, I am not going to apologize. You know and this is how I have lived my life, so for example now at 61 I think I've wrapped up everything that I should have done in life, and that you say some things for some people you know it doesn't happen. The last thing I wrote here was I have no unfinished business except to see my only son married with someone with some children, but it is his life and he should live it as he wishes.

Therapist: So you see the last session that we did was on the limitations of life and we were talking a little bit about what's a meaningful death, and what are you most proud of, what kinds of things do you want to leave, the values you want to leave behind. And it's interesting that with these creative sources of meaning its meaning that you derive through dedicating yourself to something.

Patient: Something

Therapist: something. Something in the world, caring about something and the fact that with creating a life you will inevitably will have some things that are not quite finished.

Patient: finished yes

Therapist: right, not quite finished. The question comes up can something that's unfinished be a masterpiece? So in music there's Brahms's unfinished symphony and people consider that a masterpiece.

Patient: masterpiece

Therapist: but he didn't quite finish it. In Barcelona there's an amazing cathedral.

Patient: Oh my God

Therapist: You've seen it?

Patient: I keep watch it and I keep saying "I should go there."

Therapist: So there is this cathedral

Patient: Sagrada—

Therapist: La Sagrada de Familia, the sacred family, Gaudi's

Patient: Gaudi's yes

Therapist: It is not yet finished, but when you go there it is already a masterpiece.

Patient: yes, watching it on television, it is . . .

Therapist: right so clearly you do not have to finish everything. But the other things about this session, it takes a great deal of commitment and courage to have the audacity you know, to have the will to go out there and make a life in this very

Patient: difficult

Therapist: difficult, vulnerable, dangerous, very often dangerous world where terrible things happen

Patient: happen

Therapist: and beautiful things happen, but terrible things happen. So it takes courage to put yourself out there and do something it takes courage to be who you are

Patient: who you are. Yes

Therapist: and say "I don't say I'm sorry, I am who I am." You get fired for doing that.

Patient: even to my supervisor sometimes she says you know "Well then you have to apologize" I say "I'm not apologizing. My patient has to give me 50, and I have to give him 50, otherwise the patient should not be here. That's not what they're here for."

Therapist: right

Patient: "I'm not apologizing to anyone. Write me up if you have to."

Therapist: Right and this comes from the attitude you take towards your life.

Patient: my life

Therapist: exactly. Which is based on what value? That . . .

Patient: I love me

Therapist: you should be respected

Patient: And I demand it

Therapist: demand respect

Patient: and I give it

Therapist: You deserve respect you demand it and you give it.

Patient: and I give it. I give it. It could be the homeless on the sidewalk, they demand respect, you don't know who that person is.

Therapist: You don't know who that person is. You don't know what that history was.

Patient: What his history was. You know these are the people who have been in the world wars to save this country.

Therapist: You don't even know what would happen if you were to give that person some money, help them out and what they would become and what they would do. The next day they could save your son.

Patient: you never know, you never know, you never know

Therapist: Somebody once asked me when we were doing this therapy "Does everyone in life have meaning? Does everyone's life have meaning? How about that homeless person on the street. Does that person's life have meaning?"

Patient: And sometimes his life has meaning, he went astray at some time for whatever reason

Therapist: yeah

Patient: I knew this guy through the job, oh god I can't remember his name, and I was always so afraid of him, he's burly

Therapist: Mike Tyson

Patient: Something like that

Therapist: the boxer?

Patient: and I was always afraid of him, but he was always respectful. I he speaks so well.

Therapist: okay, this was someone else. Someone in politics or?

Patient: No, he went to Korea; he was in the Korean War. And I had to put in his IV, and the nurses were usually afraid.

Therapist: Oh, one of your patients.

Patient: And then, one of our patients, and I would go to him, I can't remember his name right now, and I would say to him "Mr. so and so, can I put the needle in?" He would say "Well go ahead anyway, because you'll do it anyway." But I was always gentile with him because of my fare, and one day he said "Do you know I wasn't like this growing up. I went into the Korean War and my sergeant would have us drinking and this is why I ended up in this life." But I said he must have been so good, because as many years his wife said she separated from him, she would still come to the hospital to see him. And he spoke fluent Korean and this guy was homeless.

Therapist: homeless, so he wasn't a nobody

Patient: No, he wasn't a nobody. And several of them I would meet. And I said "Oh my goodness, you can't take anyone off the street for granted. You don't know who that person has been." I knew someone, he was at the bowery, he was poor growing up. He is the head of human resources school, its not human resources now they have another name. And he was disabled, he couldn't go to the war, I think one of the world wars, and he designed something for the government and he became a millionaire.

Therapist: There you go

Patient: From the bowery.

Therapist: Right and you know as you're telling me these stories I'm thinking about your son with the bone disease and how people could look at him and discount him and not know what a beautiful person was in there.

Patient: And his personality was such that you could not discount him because he would walk into this room with an aura. Like you said it would take you time to get this together. It wouldn't take him a second. And I would just look. . . .

Therapist: yeah, the audio recorder

Patient: I'd come into the house I say "How did you get this thing together?" He got it together anyway. I couldn't touch anything in his room because I didn't know where to touch. "How did you get these speakers to work?" He has everything in his room connected to something. He just knew how to do things. He was working at the World Trade Center, and when he died he was, they had already offered him a job doing some computer something. Cause he would just sit at the computer and dismantle it. And get it back together. These expensive remote control cars he would just sit there and put them together.

Therapist: He was a remarkable young man

Patient: And I knew, and that's how we ended up with the house. He said to me "Mommy I don't like the winters here. It's too cold. Get the house together."

Therapist: So his legacy is that house in Belize.

Patient: Yes

Therapist: and when you're in Belize you must feel closer to him.

Patient: I feel so close to him. I want to go home, and I want to go home for a whole month. Maybe this is going to be my last trip home, but I feel so close to him. He said "You build a big house and I'm going to get my business going. He had people, he said I'm building a house in Belize, I'm going to have a bed and breakfast." He had all these people lined up to come. He had friends, he had friends that would come to the house, he told this guy, he's a trucker, and "You get me whatever towels you can, I have this business going at home." And the guy came, its 14 years and I haven't seen him, and I said to him "You know what (son's name) got into an accident and died, and I haven't seen (friend's name) since." And another friend of ours he came to the door, he rang the doorbell, because (son's name) would usually come to open the door, and I opened the door and he said "Where is (son's name)?" because he didn't come to open the door. I said to him "Boy (son's name) died. (son's name) died." He turned around and he left, he's also from Belize. And he went to Belize and had an accident and died there too.

Therapist: Oh. Before we move on to the accident, before we move onto the exercise today, any thoughts you have about the last session we did?

Patient: other than um

Therapist: We talked a little bit about death, which sometimes is hard

Patient: And I was talking to my niece about that session you know. Because I was discussing with my niece you know talking about death, and they get so annoyed when I tell them "Listen, I am not talking this medication anymore." They said "Auntie try it. It's not going to be difficult."

Therapist: She couldn't understand why you didn't want to

Patient: No, because, now I'm beginning to feel like myself. I don't know how I'll be with any new treatment, and this is how I want to feel.

Therapist: Right

Patient: My daily life is so important to me, if it's a little, but let it be lucid as it is now.

Therapist: You're willing to give up a little quantity if the quality is better. And your niece was she just so frightened about the idea?

Patient: they want, they don't want to let go you know, they don't want to let go. But I told them realize its my life, and I don't think I'm being selfish, because even my son said "Mommy, you should try." I said "Remember what I told you from the beginning, I'm not afraid. And it will be how I want it to be, its my life."

Therapist: Its living the life you want to live and dying the way you want to die.

Patient: Because that's how I have lived my life

Therapist: that's all we can hope for, that is all we can hope for.

Patient: I have shared my life with everyone that has come into my life, and I know and I think I have shared my life with everyone that has come into my life (name) and I have done, I have accomplished a lot.

Therapist: yeah, when people talk about the creative sources of meaning, most of the time they focus on their work. But there are so many other things that go into creating a life. So for you I think your work is obviously important but it was an expression of the kind of person you made yourself into. A caring person, a sharing person, someone who knew the value of taking care of herself, but that was I think because you saw so much importance in caring for others too, because if you couldn't take care of yourself, you really can't take care of others too well.

Patient: As a little girl, my grandmother's uncle would go fishing and he was an older man, and every time he comes he would call me. I like crabs, and maybe that's why I love crabs, he was a Jehovahs Witness and he wouldn't throw them back into the sea, he would bring them home to me, and every time, that was before I was 5, he would come, I see him and he would come to our landing, and he would call out if I was not there, or he may leave them with my grandmother or with one of my aunts. But half the time I would go myself, because I would look forward to him coming. And as I grew up one day my mother said to me "Grandfather wants you to come to see him," and I said "Alright ma" I didn't know he was dying. And um I went and I said to him "Grandpa, I'm here" and he held my hands and said "I'm going to be leaving, but take care of yourself." I must have been like 12, and I didn't know what that meant.

Therapist: take care of yourself; you didn't know what that meant

Patient: I didn't know what that, I was 12. And as I grew up, I went to high school, college hadn't started in Belize at that time, I was already 20, and I would sew. And I sew real well; I could even make wedding dresses. That was what I did to keep me going to make money. But I said "I'm tired of this" and most of my cousins were leaving Belize, and I said "I'm 20 and I don't want to be relying on anyone anymore. I'm going to make it on my own, the way everyone was doing it." And I was lucky, I came and I made it here. And I knew how important it was for me to fork up a life and help those that I left behind, and which I did, and to this day I'm still doing it. My aunt said to me before I left "Well, what are you going to do for money?" I say "I have money." She said "Well, I have a brand new house, find somebody and sell this house." I say "But this is your brand new house, your first house from your husband." She say "It doesn't matter, I will get another one, and you find market." I told her "I don't feel comfortable doing that." She found market for that house, sold it and gave me that money to make sure that I had enough money to come here. And like I usually tell my husband "Until the day I die, I owe her; I owe her, and her husband." They have been here, a couple of times just like we've had.

Therapist: So now you understand what it means to take care of yourself.

Patient: And (name) I have taken care of myself and everyone else in my family

Therapist: yeah

Patient: I have

Therapist: So caring is very important in your life, it's a big value

Patient: caring is important in my life

Therapist: Does it give your life meaning?

Patient: It gives my life meaning. People have been so good to me, and it's something that I have to return. Even when my son as so sick, the doctors, the nurses would be so good to us, they would be so caring, the um the doctor, I had a father–son team the father died of lung cancer, he would tell me his life story. He says "(name) my uncle could not read or write, but he was my mother's only brother. And from the day I was born he would buy me a book every week and encourage me to read."

Therapist: He knew how important it was to read cause he couldn't.

Patient: "and that is how I became, I went to medical school."

Therapist: In Belize?

Patient: No here.

Therapist: Here

Patient: and these were and he was Jewish and he was just so good to me. He was so good. He would say "Do you have money to take this child to the doctor, Mrs. (name)?" He would send me to John Hopkins, wherever here to these doctors. I said "Yes, Dr. (name)." One day he came to my house and he said to me "Is this your house?" I said "Yes" I said "Why did you ask?" He said "I'm moving to Roslyn, and if you were renting I would just sign over that house to you." I don't think I'm lucky, I think I'm blessed. I really think I'm blessed.

Therapist: I think so too, I think I'm blessed having met you.

Patient: (laugh)

Therapist: So let's do this exercise, you looked at it I guess the other day right?

Patient: Mm-hmm

Therapist: Now I know that we have

Patient: Session 5?

Therapist: Yeah you have different exercises than me (laugh)

Patient: (laugh) creative sources of meaning?

Therapist: right, so we talked a little bit about you know that your responsibility is to create a life right?

Patient: Mm-hmm

Therapist: and so this issue of responsibility is important too, but there are a couple of questions in the exercise, the first is . . .

Patient: Living life

Therapist: Living life

Patient: being creative

Therapist: being creative

Patient: requires courage and commitment. Can you think of a time in your life that you've been courageous taken ownership of your life or made a meaningful commitment to something of value to you?

Therapist: yeah, what did you write for that?

Patient: well, as I love myself and my family I was courageous traveling through Mexico to seek a better life.

Therapist: That's how you got from Belize to here?

Patient: Because its close, its easy to travel to Mexico. And all you had to do in those days try to find a borderline

Therapist: and just cross over

Patient: you can't do that now

Therapist: you can't do it now

Patient: You can't do that now, but back in those days 40 years ago that's how it was done.

Therapist: So you did this to create a better life for you and your . . .

Patient: I did this to create a better life. At that time my uncle's son, he was always the one providing for everyone, cause he had a job, he had a good job. But his children were also growing up; we couldn't leave all this responsibility on him. And I needed something for myself, so I said "This is how I'm going to go" and I came.

Therapist: Was it dangerous in anyway?

Patient: It was.

Therapist: what happened? Anything scary happen?

Patient: Nothing scary happened, other than I don't speak Spanish

Therapist: right

Patient: and they would stop you at the border, no they had check points in those days. And either you tip these Mexicans off, they let you by.

Therapist: and how long were you actually in Mexico?

Patient: that travel was 3 days and 3 nights.

Therapist: 3 days and 3 nights
Patient: because I had a brother who went to medical school in Guadalajara
Therapist: Guadalajara
Patient: Mm-hmm, so I stopped over and continued on.
Therapist: driving?
Patient: on the bus
Therapist: on the bus
Patient: Continued on
Therapist: So on the bus there was you?
Patient: Mm-hmmm and my cousin.
Therapist: and your cousin
Patient: Just the two of us
Therapist: how old were you?
Patient: 21
Therapist: 21. And you were seeking what?
Patient: To earn a better life, the other job that was at home really either you work at an office, and I can't sit still
Therapist: To open up your opportunities, yes?
Patient: Mm-hmm
Therapist: to open up the possibilities of what you could become
Patient: Or um . . .
Therapist: to overcome limitations.
Patient: limitations really because the other thing was to teach and I started teaching and oh the behaviors. And I got turned off right away because I was like into one month and this girl was pregnant in the classroom, I got turned off.
Therapist: Hmm. So remember we talked about attitudinal sources of meaning when you confront limitations how you overcome them and partly it's through your attitude that you take. And your attitude was you had a choice you, you could've said okay I'm staying in Belize
Patient: I'm staying here
Therapist: with limited opportunities to fulfill my unique potential in the world, or I will not be deterred, I will I'm going to do whatever is necessary.
Patient: I'm going to do what I have to. And when my father found out cause my father was here already and my father was here legally. Oh my god, my father was so furious.
Therapist: He was here legally?
Patient: Mm-hmm. So all he had to do was to file the papers for me. So when he filed the papers and I had to go back to Belize and I told them that I came through the back, so they had to penalize me.
Therapist: yeah so it takes courage
Patient: Yes
Therapist: to take that kind of a risk.
Patient: and my father said
Therapist: But you had sense of commitment, you were committed to living a life that you wanted to life.
Patient: My life
Therapist: Your life, my life
Patient: my life, my way
Therapist: My life, my way.
Patient: It sounds selfish, but . . .
Therapist: no, that's the value that you, that's the value that you probably inherited or absorbed from your family, and that's the value that you inculcated in your children right?
Patient: Yes
Therapist: To live your life your way.
Patient: And it's difficult sometimes seeing this in my son now. He says "Mommy, this is how you've brought me up and this is you." Oh God.
Therapist: So when he does some things you don't like
Patient: Cause I can't sway him, and this is me. He says "When you say no, you mean exactly no." So when he says "Mommy, I'm not getting married." There is no way I can convince him.
Therapist: You could always try guilt
Patient: (laugh)
Therapist: (laugh) if there were any Jews at all in Belize, they could've taught you about guilt. You know like "Oh but you know I only have so much time left and I want to see grandchildren."
Patient: Don't you think I've tried that?
Therapist: Oh, you've done that, okay, so it's universal (laugh)
Patient: he said "This is you my mother." That's one thing I did that wasn't right, is what I'll say. He said "It worked for you." He say "This is how you live your life, when you say no you mean no." Then I can't say anything else.
Therapist: there you go. So that did take a lot of courage and commitment if you want to pursue your life and rise above the limitations of where you were born and what kind of environment the opportunity's there, you've got to have some courage and commitment to living the life you want to live you have to take risks.
Patient: You have to take risk, you have to be determined.
Therapist: yeah. I sometimes think about my parents are from Eastern Europe and they were survivors of the concentration camp and I sometimes think if they after they got out of

camp and were in displaced person's camp if they had chosen to go to a different country or to go back to Poland where they, I would've grown up in Poland. And I think to myself "Would I have been able to make the life that I made for myself here? Would I have had the same potential to have the freedom to just live to my full potential? Or would I have had to, I would have been a much more limited place. And would I have had the courage to just leave and get out of there to some place where there was more freedom, more potential?" I'd like to think maybe I would, but you never know until you're tested.

Patient: maybe you would

Therapist: You never know until you're tested.

Patient: it's not easy

Therapist: it's not easy

Patient: When I came to this country, my brother had been here for like 15 years. And then, I would see the attitudes, and I said "What is wrong with these people, they just keep crying they can't do this because they were taken as slaves." We were also from the Caribbean and we came here. I say "Why did these people, some of these people have to die trying to get equality, what did they die for? What was all of this struggle for? Just for you to sit here and cry?"

Therapist: I had a thought in this therapy you know like this is the 5th session, we have two more, and we've been going through the last few sessions the sources of meaning. Lots of times when I tell patients in this therapy "There's this source of meaning, there's this source of meaning, there's legacy, there's attitudes, there's creative source of meaning, there's experiential source of meaning through love, this is something new to them, they hadn't really thought about it." What strikes me about you (name) is that these are the things you have lived natural your whole life.

Patient: These are the things I have lived. . . .

Therapist: And I don't know, has it been interesting for you to actually have them pointed out as sources of meaning?

Patient: Its not, no, because this is how I have lived.

Therapist: this is the way you have lived naturally.

Patient: This is how I have been raised. I know that I was loved

Therapist: hmm

Patient: I know it. When I look into my aunts, my uncles faces I know I was loved. All of us do, all of us. With my grandmother I didn't always feel felt that she loved me, but I think I terrorized her, I think I was just too spoiled. And if my mom wasn't there, my grandma didn't know what to do with me. She didn't know what to do with me, cause if she did my hair I didn't like it I'm going to do it my way, or I wanted it done the way my mom does it. And I would frustrate her.

Therapist: even at a young age you had a clear picture of what you wanted for yourself in your life. Very important. Let's go back. What was the second exercise?

Patient: Do you feel you've expressed what is most meaningful through your life's work, and creative activities? Example job, parenting, hopes, causes, if so how? My meaningful in my life has been my children.

Therapist: your children

Patient: and children, I love children. Oh god, children per se. Um, what did I write here?

Therapist: take your time

Patient: For those that have touched my life I have I have taught to be good to themselves and others. Um, I got into sewing because as I grew up I wanted things done just so.

Therapist: sewing

Patient: and then . . .

Therapist: and the sewing was it right away the wedding dresses or simpler things?

Patient: No, simple things, I would make my dresses. And when people see it "Oh it's so nice, who made it?" "I did" and I got jobs.

Therapist: So you got self-esteem from that

Patient: And I got jobs. Um, but because they were nicely done, and even here people would call "Aren't you sewing anymore?" I say "No it's easier for me to go to the store and buy my clothes instead of sit here sewing." And I got rid, coming here earlier on I would make everything, I got rid of all of the machines.

Therapist: So sewing wasn't quite a hobby, it was a skill you had.

Patient: Mm-hmm

Therapist: it was a way you made some money, but it was also a source of great pride for you was it not?

Patient: Mm-hmm

Therapist: It was a source of great pride, it gave you great self-esteem

Patient: self-esteem

Therapist: And it gave you some independence didn't it. To feel like "Okay now I can become anything I really want." And the sewing was a platform for you to blossom further and the things that you wanted to create in your life was a family, is that right?

Patient: I always wanted children

Therapist: children.

Patient: more than anything else

Therapist: yeah

Patient: I always wanted children

Therapist: and what was that, why do you think?

Patient: I don't know maybe it's because of the way I was brought up. I used to say "My father was here; my mother died, and look at how much these people have given me." What would I do for my children? What wouldn't I do for my children?

Therapist: And I guess, you were so you were so affected by the caring and loving that you received that you realize this is what gave you the spark of life you know, made you feel alive, and it was what you wanted to express with your life. And I guess knowing your family history and all that, I think it was very important to you that there be a continuation of your family.

Patient: Yes. My aunt, my mother's sister, she's the one I call mother, and her husband, oh my goodness, he didn't know what to do for me. And before he died, he said to me "I'm dying. This property is yours." Why would someone who isn't even my father make that effort to leave something for me? But he prepared that, so when he's no longer here, I have something. And I always will have that.

Therapist: So when you dedicate yourself to something or someone, these creative sources of meaning in terms of the life you create, and what we're going to discuss next week in terms of experiential sources of meaning, love, they're so linked, it's sometimes hard to . . .

Patient: differentiate

Therapist: differentiate.

Patient: to separate, yes.

Therapist: to separate them, cause they're almost often, in your case especially, they are very linked, they're very linked. Was nursing important to you in terms of your work? Did that give your life meaning?

Patient: You know initially, I had a friend she said to me from Belize, "(name) why don't you go to nursing school?" I used to sew for her, and she had little ones, she say "You care for these children, why don't you go to nursing school?" I said "No" I wasn't ready. When I came here, my brother said "Why don't you go to nursing school?" He was going to medical school already. I said "Nah I don't want to go to nursing school." He said "No, go to nursing school." "Okay, I'm going to register to go to Kings Country School of Nursing." And I found out I was pregnant; I said "I'm not going to nursing school, I'm pregnant, I'm just going to take care of my baby." And it so happened this child was disabled, with this osteogenesis imperfecta, and I would take care of him, I'd move to the hospital with him. He said to me "You take such good care of me; you seem like you like what you're doing." He said to me "Why don't you go to nursing school?" I say "You too?" And there was free nursing in our neighborhood. There was a free LPN program. He said "Mommy, go to nursing school, so you can learn better how to take care of me." I said "How am I going to do that." He said "I am going to take myself to the doctor." And it was in our neighborhood. I wrote to the board of education about this nursing school and like a year later I heard from them, and I went to nursing school.

Therapist: so interesting so out of a, out of a a . . .

Patient: bad situation

Therapist: Out of a bad situation, something incredible happened. With is the essence of finding meaning through a suffering experience. You took a suffering experience and you came through it and you made it into something rewarding and meaningful. It not only helped you and your son, but so many other people.

Patient: and before I was finished from that LPN program they say you know "You should just go into the RN program" I say "How am I going to do that. I haven't sat for boards." They said "Ms (name) you should just go." I said "I am not going to do that, I'm going to take the boards first and see what happens."

Therapist: So its interesting you know we talked about creating your own, unique life, and people think okay that means I can't take anybody else's advice, I have to only listen to my own internal voice. But here's an example in your life where you got some suggestions and encouragement to move in certain directions that turned out pretty well I guess for you?

Patient: it did

Therapist: it did. And on some level you got to express what was most important to you, caring in your work. You could've actually maybe continued to do that in sewing.

Patient: Maybe, I could have

Therapist: By being like a master wedding dress sewer. And you would've have given, you would've been part of such meaningful experiences for young women getting married and starting families. You could've, you could've . . .

Patient: You could've

Therapist: been very satisfied with that. In fact, do you sometimes think that would've been another alternative?

Patient: I got bored with it.

Therapist: You got bored with it. It was limited.

Patient: And as my son would say sometimes "Mommy, why don't your sewing anymore?" I said to him "No, I don't have time for that."

Therapist: You don't have time. You grew beyond that.

Patient: And I gave away the machines.

Therapist: You don't regret that?

Patient: I don't regret that

Therapist: you moved beyond that

Patient: Because I got into the nursing and thoroughly enjoyed it.

Therapist: yeah

Patient: I said, as I said to him "I didn't know that I would really really enjoy the nursing."

Therapist: See now you're also a somewhat a spiritual person and you I think have a belief in a greater power that guides and influences. And the one way that you might be looking at your life is that you got little messages, little nudges to go in one direction to another that may have been guided by something greater than yourself. Is that true?

Patient: I think so, that's true. And with everyone that I have encountered, if they need a little push, if they need a little nudge I would. My husband would say "(name) you give too much." I say "Yes, but I got a lot."

Therapist: yeah

Patient: and I have to give

Therapist: the secret to life is understanding that you get so much more from giving. That's how you've lived your life?

Patient: That's how my life has been

Therapist: And sometimes when you've been ill, has it interfere with your ability to, I guess when you were on the chemotherapy, it interfered with ability to be who you were? Who you are, right?

Patient: Mm-hmm

Therapist: And that's part of why it is so difficult for you.

Patient: its so difficult for me, its so difficult for me

Therapist: Yeah, you want to still be you

Patient: I ask myself. And even my nieces they say "Auntie, when you were on that chemo you were not yourself." Because they'd be hovering around me. As much as they want me to continue on the chemo, but "You were not yourself." Because they would just see me there just laying there, sleeping, sleeping. They said "This is not you."

Therapist: yeah, lets finish up. I think there's one more or two more.

Patient: Yeah, I think there's two more. What are your responsibilities? Who are you responsible to and for? I didn't, oh; I have been responsible for myself and my family.

Therapist: mainly responsible for yourself. The lesson of self care, its not a selfish thing, its so critical. If you cannot take care of yourself, you cannot fulfill your primary mission.

Patient: I stress self care

Therapist: and it's what dear?

Patient: I stress self care. Sometimes I say "Maybe I'm too indulgent." But its me, it's for me.

Therapist: yeah well you know when you go on the plane to Belize and the stewardess says "Okay I need your attention" and goes through all the things that can happen in case the plane crashes and this and that, the oxygen. And they always say to you if you're traveling with a small child, first put the oxygen mask on yourself

Patient: yourself

Therapist: because if you lose consciousness then you can't help them. And the last one?

Patient: Do you have unfinished business? No.

Therapist: Mm-hmm

Patient: What tasks have you always wanted to do but have yet to undertake? If so, what do you think is holding you back?

Therapist: This is that issue of existential guilt the idea that in life almost impossible to fulfill every potential. And I think you read me that first thing, the first thing what did you say?

Patient: The only unfinished thing is to see my only son married and have some children.

Therapist: Exactly

Patient: But he refuses, but its his life, I have to accept his choice, its his life.

Therapist: yeah, you'd love to see a grandchild

Patient: I would love to see a grandchild.

Therapist: and that's so important to you because you'd like to see continuity of your family continuing. And I think also you know one of the things that was very important to me when my son started to grow up, he's 20 now, it was so important for me to get an idea of whether he had the experience of loving somebody and being love, I wanted him to have that experience. Do you feel like your sons' had that experience?

Patient: Yes Yes

Therapist: That gives me great comfort, I don't know about you.

Patient: More so, they are two different human beings. And I would tell this one "What makes you so different form your brother?" Um, I would hold my children till I can't hold them anymore. He was 12 and 17, and I would tell him "Just come and sit on my lap" that's how much I loved these children. The other one, we would sit until late into the night. He would say "Mommy, come and sleep with me downstairs." He would prepare his bed and he would sleep on the floor and we would have the music going. Oh. We would sit to the table, when the phone rings when I come home from work, my son will say "I cannot be on the phone with you anymore, my mom is here." He would prepare my plate even though he has to eat with me. This one, he's not as close.

Therapist: right, now when you talked about unfinished business, do you think you raised him as a man who is capable of loving someone and who wants to have a marriage and a family?

Patient: I think I have, maybe he's just not ready.

Therapist: So that part of your job is finished, this next part is his job.

Patient: His. That's why I generally say to him "I can't argue. It's your life."

Therapist: Yeah, and the next part is his job. Your job was to raise him to be a man who can love and be loved and have an intimate relationship and see the value of children and loving children.

Patient: and he loves children

Therapist: he loves children. So you did your job actually if you think about it.

Patient: my only fear is (name), that he thinks that he's alone now.

Therapist: He feels alone?

Patient: When we're, he says "Mommy, this is such a burden on me." And why its important for me to generally tell him you know "(son's name) I'm okay with this and these are my decisions. Have no guilt because this is what I want." But he says "It's a tremendous responsibility because I'm alone." I said "It so happens that you're alone but I've done something so that it won't be that difficult for you. Just look at it that way."

Therapist: that's correct. He's not really alone. So, thank you for doing all this, I think the next session is . . .

Patient: Isn't it tomorrow?

Therapist: It's tomorrow right yeah.

Patient: What time am I going to be here tomorrow?

Therapist: I think we said, I'll tell you the time, but the next session tomorrow is experiential sources of meaning. And that's finding meaning through connecting with love, connecting with people, and with love, with beauty, nature, the breezes of Belize, all those kinds of things. I guess there's a little bit of homework you can look at. I think it's the exercise about love, and beauty and humor. Is it over here? Okay, this is the exercise. It's going to be a fun one actually. And we'll see each other, I'll check on the time.

Patient: Mm-hmm, okay

Therapist: I think its something like 9:30, something like that

Session 6: Experiential Sources of Meaning—Connecting with Life Through Love, Beauty, and Humor

Therapist: Good morning (name)

Patient: Good morning (name)

Therapist: So we're up to Session 6, and next week is Session 7, our last session. It went fast

Patient: it sure did.

Therapist: So I just wanted to check in, how are you doing since yesterday?

Patient: Calm

Therapist: Calm. Oh, did you go to the clinic for pain?

Patient: I went there yesterday and they were supposed to call me, but they didn't. And I didn't call back.

Therapist: okay

Patient: Because the doctor was not there. My mistake was not asking her when he was going to be there. But when I came yesterday morning, all I had was that coffee, and for lunch, what did I have?

Therapist: You didn't eat much?

Patient: No, I can't even remember, I had a slice of fruit.

Therapist: you want the doctor to do something about your pain right

Patient: Mm-hmm

Therapist: Is the doctor there today?

Patient: I don't know that was my mistake not asking them.

Therapist: What we can do after we finish I can call (name) to call over to see if they're there, to see if its worth it go over. How is the pain?
Patient: It's not bad
Therapist: Not bad
Patient: It was there, I took some medication last night but I slept all night until this morning
Therapist: oh good
Patient: but yesterday I hardly ate. I drank, and it wasn't as bad.
Therapist: good okay, so you think it had little to do with . . .
Patient: maybe, its not, I don't eat much. And all I would eat is my vegetables and whatever it is that I eat. Which isn't much or I might have a salad and that's it.
Therapist: So uh, so I think today will be an interesting session. We're going to talk about experiential sources of meaning but do you have any thoughts from the last session on the creative sources of meaning, the way we derive meaning through the life we create and the idea of courage and responsibility, and unfinished business really and existential guilt, and the things we're proud of and what we've accomplished.
Patient: It has just reinforced (name) that I have been on the right track with my life.
Therapist: Yes, that's a good feeling.
Patient: and it's a good feeling.
Therapist: Yeah, when you feel, when you look back and you have to do this exercise and it reinforces this idea that you've been on the right track with your life, what emotions does that bring up in you?
Patient: Its um, I've done something right and its calming.
Therapist: like a sense of peace?
Patient: Like a sense of peace. And reflecting yesterday, it's not only my parents, I went to school I went to a Catholic school and those nuns were great.
Therapist: They were great
Patient: Yes
Therapist: because?
Patient: they taught us. They would teach us cooking, they would teach you how to take care of yourself, how to be good to yourself.
Therapist: so they taught some very basic skills in life, how to live.
Patient: Mm-hmm. And as I remember back they would tell you um if you have any problems, don't be afraid to come discuss it with us. And that has helped mold it, in my molding.
Therapist: Did you do that? Did you take advantage of that?
Patient: Mm-hmm. We would go to the convent, we would play music, we would play games. Other than home, we would go there, or at least I would go there, because they were nice to be around.
Therapist: So you know you, when a person looks at your life and hears about your life, like me, what I'm hearing. Its pretty, it's obviously a reflection of who you are and the attitudes and values you have you've created in your life. The person you've created that you at this point in your life can look back and say you know "I did a pretty good job, I feel at peace." Considering that there weren't only just wonderful things that happened in your life, there were difficulties and even tragedies . . .
Patient: there have been difficulties in my life, there have been difficulties
Therapist: And so one can have a sense of feeling that you've done a good job in life and a sense of peace even when . . .
Patient: despite
Therapist: Despite
Patient: the bad things that happened in my life.
Therapist: right, do you see it as a despite the bad things, or that the bad things contributed something uh . . .
Patient: I think that despite
Therapist: is a better word?
Patient: the negativity that has been in my life, it really has pain through separating through death
Therapist: yeah
Patient: and um wonderful things have happened. I have dealt with the pain yes.
Therapist: Yeah
Patient: I have dealt with the pain, but sometimes I tell myself I can't let it consume me
Therapist: does the pain sometimes consume, the death consume you?
Patient: yes
Therapist: your son you're talking about mainly right? Or are you talking about . . .?
Patient: but most of all, my middle brother had died here at 52 years old, and he was the father figure in my life, because my father had been here, and my brother was home and my brother would make sure that I am okay. If he does not see me, he would come to make sure things were right with me. When I came here unknowing to my father, my brother was right there in my corner, "Don't worry about him,

he is going to settle down." But all was well, whatever I did was okay with my brother, the only time my brother would say "(name)" is when he's annoyed with me, otherwise he has a pet name for me. "Shower" and he would say "Shower." But the minute he says "(name)" I know he's angry, but my brother would not be angry with me in front of you or anyone else, it's just when the two of us are together. And I always thought that my sister-in-law had some feelings about that. But that was just the relationship, it was just us. My father was here and he was there with me and he would come from their house to my house to make sure that I'm okay.

Therapist: So when say the death and the losses and death, it's a series from the very beginning of your childhood, your whole life and it has gone through your whole life periodically.

Patient: They have died.

Therapist: yeah

Patient: They have died

Therapist: yeah, people who you have just cherished so much.

Patient: Mm-hmm

Therapist: And in this session today we're going to talk about experiencing the life, the awe of life, the joys of life and that's going to be a loss too for you right?

Patient: Yes

Therapist: if and when you die.

Patient: but

Therapist: and so you're going to lose that too, is that another loss for you?

Patient: I am going to lose that too, but it won't be painful. It's a part of life. Wherever it will take me, I don't know, but it has to be a good place, because that's how my life has been.

Therapist: what has to be a good place?

Patient: no, losing life, my life

Therapist: losing life, yes ma'am

Patient: is going to be good

Therapist: I see

Patient: it's a part of life.

Therapist: Gotcha

Patient: And my life has always been good, and I have only made good out of it, so it can only be good

Therapist: yeah, like you were talking about a few sessions ago about what's a good death, what's a meaningful death. You were talking about being surrounded by your family and things like that; you'll make it into a peaceful

Patient: Yes

Therapist: death, death that only you could . . .

Patient: that's how it should be

Therapist: be yours yeah

Patient: mine

Therapist: you've lived your life

Patient: I've lived it

Therapist: you've created it, and you'll put your mark on it

Patient: oh yes, and I have put my mark

Therapist: already?

Patient: I have put my mark. When our children come now (name), my nephew would come from Detroit, I have another nephew in the Bronx; they would come "Auntie, do you need anything?" I have nieces here they call; you need anything just call, and they make sure that I'm okay. I think I have made my mark.

Therapist: yeah, what role does self-esteem play in all of this?

Patient: a lot

Therapist: A lot

Patient: a lot and I try to impart this throughout

Therapist: right, do you feel you have self-esteem because you played your role so well

Patient: I don't think so, because I've always had it

Therapist: You've always had it? Even before?

Patient: Mm-hmm

Therapist: ah

Patient: but this is the way I have lived.

Therapist: So you had self-esteem before you really sort of started creating your own life.

Patient: I know what I wanted out of life. I'm very; I know what I wanted out of my life.

Therapist: that's interesting

Patient: And I have lived like this. It was like I was brought up trained like this, between my grandma, and my. . . . My grandmother was a reserved woman but proud and with plenty of, lots of self-esteem.

Therapist: So self-esteem and pride are related in your mind.

Patient: I remember the first time I saw my grandma writing her name.

Therapist: Uh-ha

Patient: She was going into Mexico, and those days they needed a permit to go into Mexico. So I go with my grandma everywhere and the police officer said to her "Mrs. (name), can you put your name in the book?" And she says "Okay." And looking at him, I don't think he felt that she knew how to write her name, and my grandma wrote her name. I thought he expected her to put an "X", no but she wrote her name. So leaving the precinct I said to my grandma "Ma I didn't know you knew how to write your name" and my grandma turned around and said "Well, I went to school." I was a little girl I must have been about 7. "I went to school." So that say she said you know "There are these ladies that come here at nights looking for me sometimes, I went to school with them." And then she discussed going to school with me. I come from a proud line of women; I come from a proud family.

Therapist: That's a beautiful story, it brings in like we were talking last week, you know we list these sources of meaning you know from our legacy and overcoming obstacles and suffering, an triumphing over losses and limitations and even tragedies. And then um the creative sources of meaning through the life we have created and all that. We have sort of artificially put them in separated little boxes, but they are all so related aren't they? We were talking about.

Patient: they are

Therapist: and the source of meaning that we're going to talk about today really reflects that being connected to the world through our senses, those experiencing the world through our senses and our emotions, through love, through sight and touch and smell. So the appreciation of the air in the hammock, when you're in the hammock in Belize, the food, listening to the songs, the joys of life in some respect . . .

Patient: the joys of life.

Therapist: holding a baby

Patient: oh yes

Therapist: beautiful art. There was a famous philosopher named, Kierkegaard, who talked about human beings as being perhaps the only animals that have an appreciation for understanding that they are here in the world and they exist, and that because they have this ability to realize that they are here, they also have the ability to perceive the facts of their existence and have emotions related to that. And one of the emotions is part of what we talked about before when we talked about loss and death, in life there is always death, that's a part of life, he called that dread. But the other thing he talked about is because we have these abilities to appreciate our existence we also have the ability to experience the jaw, the joy

Patient: joy

Therapist: of being alive. He called it the awe . . .

Patient: awe

Therapist: the awesome, you know the awesomeness the awe of life. And so actually in this particular exercise when people talk about various experiential sources of meaning, through love and art and beauty and nature and food, whatever, some people travel, some people love to fly. It's usually the joyous things, but sometimes it's very, there are things that are powerfully sad too, but they make you feel something incredibly important.

Patient: And sometimes it's sad, but I think it's what you make of it. When my son died, was the worst pain I've had, and I told my husband "I'm going to Rome." He said "Why do you want to go to Rome?" I said to him "I will see things that have been in my life, from when I was like 15 years old, that I have always wanted to see, and it will help make me forget." My first world history book with a copy of Zeus on the cover

Therapist: a copy of?

Patient: Zeus

Therapist: Zeus.

Patient: on the cover and I never forgot

Therapist: the Greek God, Zeus

Patient: I never forgot, and um . . .

Therapist: why did you not forget that?

Patient: because of the things I read and saw in this book

Therapist: ah

Patient: it was all about Florence, it was all about Rome, it was all about Turkey

Therapist: Turkey

Patient: and

Therapist: Great civilizations

Patient: Yes and the higher Sofia was there, and my grandma had a big bowl and on the bottom was "made in Constantinople" and I've grown up with this bowl.

Therapist: Interesting

Patient: and I don't know how it disappeared.

Therapist: oh, it disappeared.

Patient: there was a hurricane

Therapist: In Belize?

Patient: and we lost everything

Therapist: uh-huh

Patient: and I said it might have gone there, and I never forgot.

Therapist: have you ever been to that part of the world?

Patient: no. and I keep telling my husband, he's afraid of the airplane, so half the time I just leave him here and I'm gone.

Therapist: yeah, you know, I have my friends, patients I talk to, who fly to that area and take these beautiful cruises that take you around the islands there and you really get to see the history of what you read about in that book. The various islands, Greece and Crete, and where a lot of the civilizations. Although, maybe the Garifuna are even more ancient and more greater civilizations, you know what I'm saying.

Patient: who knows? Who knows? Who knows? (Laugh). We went to Rome

Therapist: oh you did go

Patient: we toured Rome, I couldn't go to Venice, because of the weather, and it was raining. And it was just my son and I and we traveled on the train. We went to Venice, and I really really enjoyed that.

Therapist: I love Venice

Patient: We went to the buildings in there, oh my goodness

Therapist: unbelievable

Patient: I said you know "It was worth the trip."

Therapist: We are already starting to talk about the exercise, let's do the exercise. So the exercise has to do with listing a number of things, three ways in which you connected with life and felt most alive through experiential sources of meaning. And we talked about, and they are listed as love, beauty, and we even included humor I guess. And we can even include sorrow I guess at the end. We can even include sorrow. But you were starting to talk about these beautiful trips right, and these beautiful places, Venice and all that, maybe we'll start with beauty.

Patient: Beauty.

Therapist: yeah

Patient: where else did we go? We went to where was that? Vesuvius?

Therapist: Oh, Vesuvius, Naples or something, Pompeii?

Patient: Pompeii and I still want to go to Spain.

Therapist: Spain, yes. So did I categorize it correctly, was it under beauty?

Patient: yes

Therapist: these experiences of traveling were ...

Patient: All these beautiful things.

Therapist: Beautiful things, you saw beautiful things in beautiful places.

Patient: All these beautiful things

Therapist: And beautiful art

Patient: the beautiful art

Therapist: and good food?

Patient: not really, cause I'm wary of what I eat.

Therapist: not really

Patient: Even when I travel through Mexico, there are beautiful places in Mexico, but you know other than going ...

Therapist: You had to fly to these places?

Patient: To Europe

Therapist: To Italy

Patient: but not to Mexico

Therapist: right to Europe you have to fly. Flying, you don't mind flying?

Patient: No

Therapist: You love flying?

Patient: I love flying

Therapist: What do you love about flying?

Patient: I just settle down and I go to sleep until I'm where I'm supposed to be.

Therapist: are you aware of flying when you're flying?

Patient: Nope, I'm sleeping

Therapist: you're sleeping

Patient: Or I tell them you know "I have to be by the window" because I get claustrophobic

Therapist: I see

Patient: but if I'm by the window and I'm looking outside, I'm quite okay

Therapist: So these beautiful places and this beautiful art and the history and all that, what else, what else has been, what else have had of experiences of beauty that has given you a sense of awe about life?

Patient: Little things you know (name), just little daily things.

Therapist: Little daily things

Patient: I don't need much in my life you know. Otherwise I'm at my house.

Therapist: So give me an example of a little daily thing that's just beautiful?

Patient: If I'm in a clean surrounding, I'm happy

Therapist: Good cup of tea?

Patient: A cup of tea. At home they make coffee with rice

Therapist: Coffee with rice how does that work?

Patient: They burn the rice, there's a process that they do with the rice.

Therapist: Oh, instead of using coffee beans they use rice?

Patient: and the best cup of coffee you could have, I'll be angry if you don't give me a cup.

Therapist: I have never heard of this, and I'm going to check it out. Where does one get it?

Patient: Well, it's not bought; it's the natives that do this.

Therapist: you make it?

Patient: I don't make it

Therapist: the natives make it

Patient: yeah, but my sister would make this
Therapist: So you take the rice
Patient: We have these big pans, and then you take rice and they make the fire and they slowly roast the rice until it's burnt.
Therapist: Do they put oil?
Patient: No no no no, it's just the rice
Therapist: Just on the heat and nothing else
Patient: and the heat and then they slowly turn it until it's burnt
Therapist: like roasting coffee
Patient: like roasting coffee, and it smells too wonderful
Therapist: and then they grind it up
Patient: Nope, and the put the water, but I guess they know exactly when the rice has reached that time when they can put the water. That makes the best cup of . . .
Therapist: So for instance you take the rice you burn it, roast it
Patient: Roast it
Therapist: in a certain way. And then what you might do is put it in one of those little decanters
Patient: no they don't
Therapist: you pour water and you just . . .
Patient: they pour the water in there and I guess
Therapist: the coffee is the water that's left
Patient: Yes
Therapist: and you let it steep there I guess for a bit
Patient: And then they let it steep there and they serve it.
Therapist: And it's incredible
Patient: Oh, it's wonderful.
Therapist: any particular kind of rice?
Patient: Nope. Well, I know they just use the white rice
Therapist: yes
Patient: not the brown rice.
Therapist: okay. And that's better than Starbucks?
Patient: Its better. There was this lady I know back in the 70s when coffee was so expensive here, she was my brother's mother-in-law, and she would make this here, and I would just I would go over there just to have a cup of coffee.
Therapist: Would you put sugar or anything in it?
Patient: They put sugar and milk.
Therapist: Oh you put sugar and milk; you treat it like a coffee
Patient: Mm-hmm. You wouldn't know. If you weren't told . . .
Therapist: It looks dark right?
Patient: dark. If you weren't told that that's coffee made of rice you wouldn't know. Wonderful, delicious.
Therapist: you don't have to grind it, that's great.
Patient: Mm-hmm
Therapist: Anything else that comes mind with beauty? I know that you love children.
Patient: I love children. I love children. I love children well taken care of.
Therapist: how about . . .
Patient: I love daybreak
Therapist: you love daybreak
Patient: I love when the sun goes down, I could sit there and watch. My pleasures are simple.
Therapist: You love the sun going down, and you love the sun coming up, both.
Patient: I would sit there and wait for the sun to come up.
Therapist: I remember that you're an early morning person.
Patient: Mm-hmm. And at home the moon is bright and you could see that big moon over the sea and it's the Caribbean Sea and the sea is so calm. And I could sit there and watch that for hours.
Therapist: and you, you know, as opposed to me, I grew up on the streets of Manhattan. I was not I was raised disconnected from nature and the natural world. You grew up in a natural environment so you appreciate the beauty of the natural world. Yeah
Patient: I won't go and bathe at the sea
Therapist: I don't think we can see the sunset, maybe where you live. You would go to the sea you said?
Patient: I won't go and bathe in the sea.
Therapist: Oh, this is back home.
Patient: Yeah I won't go.
Therapist: because they are living things
Patient: because they're . . . and everyone else will go, nope I won't get in there.
Therapist: I'm on your side; there are living creatures in there. I'm not disturbing them.
Patient: That's what I'm thinking of. And on Sundays or when my uncle has time off, he would take us to the beach and we could go crabbing along or um digging up the . . .
Therapist: Clams, mussels
Patient: sea urchins and stuff
Therapist: sea urchins
Patient: I may go, but that's not pleasurable to me.
Therapist: But you like the sea, the horizon and the smell maybe
Patient: Yes, and the smell of the sea. You can just taste the salt air.
Therapist: yeah
Patient: Sometimes when I go home, I could just whiff that air when I get off the plane, because it just smells so clean. It smells different from here, it's totally different, and I find pleasure in that.

Therapist: How about love?
Patient: loving who?
Therapist: I think it's a very broad category
Patient: It is, but I tell you . . .
Therapist: there are so many different kinds of love aren't there?
Patient: I love, yes my family, my children, my husband. My husband is so good to me. He's another one; he's indulgent and even worse now. I know that he's living with his own demons . . .
Therapist: Your husband?
Patient: about me being sick
Therapist: yeah
Patient: when I found out I was sick I told him this is what I want, because I don't know which way this is going to take us. We'll be married this September for 39 years. And he's been good to me. Sometimes I say without him I wouldn't be where I'm at today.
Therapist: you got married at like 16?
Patient: he was, I was 21
Therapist: 21
Patient: and he was 23. And he has worked to provide.
Therapist: he's a good provider
Patient: He's a good provider, he has.
Therapist: Is he the love of your life?
Patient: he's the love of your life
Therapist: how do you? I know as a husband and as a parent, sometimes there's a little bit of a difference in how the love between a husband and a wife and a parent and a child. You experienced that too?
Patient: yes, yes. But my husband also grew up without a father, his father died, and he was raised by his uncle.
Therapist: So you share a lot of that
Patient: And it seems as the middle child, he wanted to provide for his mother. So at home, he's from home, he has always worked also to provide for his mother and his brother and sister, but the brother turned out to be so useless and the sister is mediocre.
Therapist: and you love your sons in a different way?
Patient: I love my sons in a different way
Therapist: Is it more powerful in some way or? It can't compare?
Patient: I can't compare. My love for my oldest son is different, because he was all I had in the beginning.
Therapist: how do you mean?
Patient: I saw this part of me and I was consumed
Therapist: you were consumed. When he was born and he had these problems, that was. . . .
Patient: We didn't know and neither did the doctors know. . . .
Therapist: right away
Patient: until 13 months later
Therapist: yeah
Patient: and he was just a beautiful, beautiful baby. He was so beautiful
Therapist: yeah you forgot to list him under the beauty
Patient: yes, he was so pretty
Therapist: Uh-huh
Patient: he did some modeling. And I told him, you know you should model your fingers, your hands. Because he had big hands with long tapering fingers, beautiful child. That was my gift.
Therapist: your son?
Patient: Yes.
Therapist: with his osteogenesis imperfecta, did it affect his fingers?
Patient: No
Therapist: That was spared
Patient: No, sometimes he would grab me, I would say "Don't grab me; your hands are so big and heavy." But he had, and he kept his, and despite having to roll his wheelchair he would have his gloves on and he kept his fingers. He was taught that he has to take care of himself; he has to be clean and dress well. So that's how he was.
Therapist: So you were saying he was all you had in the beginning. In other words what you mean is . . .
Patient: This was my first child
Therapist: Yeah
Patient: A part of me
Therapist: yes
Patient: and my husband. And from the day I saw this baby I was consumed by him.
Therapist: consumed
Patient: I knew that this child, this is mine, and he has to be but just G-O-O-D 100%
Therapist: D-O?
Patient: G-O-O-D, good
Therapist: Good.
Patient: I told myself that this is what my son is going to be
Therapist: it's not like he was already innately good, by definition, he's my son he's good. It's that you wanted to mold him into a good person. . . .
Patient: the best
Therapist: The best. You succeeded?
Patient: I know I did
Therapist: you did
Patient: I know I did, I know I did. When he looks at me um, that was about the time they stole

Ethan Paitz, and I heard that on the news and I almost went berserk.

Therapist: this was the young boy who was kidnapped in Soho and went missing?

Patient: Yes, uh-huh. And I told him "What is my name?" I asked him "What is my name?"

Therapist: you wanted him to be prepared

Patient: I said you know what "You call me (name), I'm mommy, but I'm (name)." Because I felt that I had to prepare my son also.

Therapist: Yeah, you didn't want anyone or anything taking him away

Patient: No, no no no no no. Despite my son's disability (name), maybe I didn't see it; I didn't treat him like someone was wrong with him.

Therapist: I know

Patient: we went everywhere. I take him to the museums; I take him everywhere there were no restrictions on our life.

Therapist: Given how much you adored him and how you were consumed with him, when this tragic accident happened, how did you keep standing?

Patient: I don't know, I don't know. That's why I don't like a cell phone, I don't want a cell phone with me, I needed just to call to let them know where I'm at, but don't call me, and I turn it off.

Therapist: oh because you got a phone call with the news, and it traumatized you

Patient: And it lives with me. Um, he had called me "I'm coming to get you" I say "Be careful." And when I came downstairs of Mount Sinai and he was not there, I knew something had gone wrong, I knew. And I called home and my mother said "Go to the hospital, something has happened to him." But prior to this, like a month prior to this he said to me "Mommy, if something were to happen to me, what would you do?" I said to him "Like what?" "If I should die, what would you do?"

Therapist: He was worried about whether you would have the will to live

Patient: I said to him "(son's name) I would die."

Therapist: You would die

Patient: He said to me "No you will not."

Therapist: no you would not

Patient: you have to live and take care of my brother

Therapist: you have other reasons to live as well

Patient: and take care of my brother. So he said "If a day comes and I cannot do anything for myself. You make sure that I'm DNR and don't ever put me on a ventilator." And to quiet him down I said to him "You do the same for me also." And this happened, and I didn't know how I got to Elmhurst Hospital and till this day the first thing I saw was the drips.

Therapist: was the?

Patient: The IV drips, and I looked I say "This is it, he's going to die." And to be honest with you, I can't even remember that night, and I called my husband and he came. He said "Well, he's on the ventilator, then let's just go home and then we'll come back." I can't even give you an account of that night, I can't. And my other son was there too, because both of them were in the car.

Therapist: right, he was hurt as well

Patient: but I told myself, and I went to him and I said to him "What happened?" And he said "Mommy somebody hit the car, and that's the last thing I remember." I said to him "Your brother did not look good, he does not look good." I was just trying to prepare him because they were so close. The oldest one I usually tell him "You think you're his father." Because he takes care of his brother, even if I'm reprimanding him, he'll say "No, don't speak to my brother like that." and that's how it was in our house. And he died three days later, but I had made him DNR.

Therapist: you did what dear?

Patient: I had made him DNR. Cause some of you know, that's why I say (name) there is a God. I believe that there is a God, for whatever it is, his name is because I look then and I said you know as painful as it is it could've been worse. The two of them could have died, but he shared them with me, and for that I am grateful.

Therapist: when you look at the beauty of the sunset on the sea, do you also think of God? Yes?

Patient: Who could've made this, who could've made this? It had to have been somebody giving.

Therapist: yeah, and when you think of death as being part of life, you see that as being a design of God?

Patient: Yes

Therapist: so that's why . . .

Patient: and it can't be bad we're left here

Therapist: that's why you think it can't be bad

Patient: Yeah, we're left here baffling and crying and missing, but it could not be bad, it could not be bad. I don't know if people resurrect, I don't know but I usually say, I feel that we go through this life once.

Therapist: and you, you were telling me you are not that religious, but you're spiritual?
Patient: Yes
Therapist: and you were hoping that maybe you would be reconnected with you son
Patient: Yes
Therapist: certainly you haven't lost connection with your son even after he's died. He's a, you remember him every day, you think of . . .
Patient: I think of him every day.
Therapist: yeah
Patient: He has drawings on the wall at my house
Therapist: drawings? He was a great drawer, artist?
Patient: Yes, and little things that he would draw, he would frame them. And my son would buy me beautiful things (name). Since they were little, on Mother's Day I would tell them "Here's money, get me card, and make sure it's pretty."
Therapist: right
Patient: "I have a necklace," he said to me "I want you to have this necklace." It is so pretty; I've worn it once, the day of his funeral.
Therapist: you wore it once, the day of his funeral
Patient: and I haven't worn it since. But everyone says he would get you nice little things that you will definitely like.
Therapist: Yeah, So you wore that on his funeral for a reason. It was something that he gave you. And you didn't wear it again because?
Patient: There is no need for me to
Therapist: There's no need. Because it's so beautiful, and it reminds you are how beautiful he was?
Patient: he was one of the best things that ever happened to me.
Therapist: yeah, and I would venture to say (name) that you were the best thing that happened to him. What do you think?
Patient: Maybe
Therapist: Imagine another mother, could not have done what you did, could not have loved him the way you did.
Patient: Maybe not. Everyone loved him, my whole family.
Therapist: yeah
Patient: Everyone loved him.
Therapist: The big love, its big love
Patient: My sisters they would do anything for him, anything. In fact, I was not the only one who had to take care of him.
Therapist: Other people helped
Patient: my sister's too, my sisters
Therapist: yeah
Patient: If I'm not here, if I want to go home, my sisters will say "Go home." Even if he has to be in the hospital they're there to take care of him.
Therapist: You know I worked here at Sloan–Kettering and I train all these fellows you know
Patient: Mm-hmm
Therapist: young psychiatrists and everyday like last night we were making rounds, we saw 10 or 12 patients and so many of the stories were very tragic. And sometimes there's just so much sadness and so much tragedy you can't allow it to overwhelm you, and one of the ways we handle the profound sadness is we use humor you know we laugh, not at patients, but we to break the. . . . and the last part of the exercise was humor, and is that an important part of your life, is that something that helps you feel alive.
Patient: Yes
Therapist: yeah
Patient: I laugh
Therapist: you're a joker?
Patient: I don't think I'm a joker, I don't think I'm a joker
Therapist: A prankster? No, you just laugh?
Patient: Maybe, maybe
Therapist: yeah
Patient: maybe, maybe, but I'm seldom alone
Therapist: Uh-huh
Patient: I'm seldom alone. I have my moments when I want to be alone
Therapist: yeah
Patient: I love to read, and I had to leave part of that as I had children
Therapist: Uh-huh
Patient: and um, but I find time to be alone. But most of time there is always someone there and we'll be laughing and talking and whatever, and the kids we have I generally say them you know "Steinberg makes so much money, and I don't think he's funny."
Therapist: Seinfeld?
Patient: Seinfeld. He makes so much money, and he would not make me laugh.
Therapist: He doesn't make you laugh?
Patient: He doesn't make me laugh; I don't see what's funny. But come to my house . . .
Therapist: Uh-huh
Patient: . . . when my children are carrying on, and you hear so much nonsense and crap you laugh till you pop.
Therapist: (laugh)
Patient: And my uncle is a comedian

Therapist: Uh-huh

Patient: and he would tell us all these jokes and stories, can't help but laugh. And sometimes are we're sitting together, we would be reminiscing about his jokes, you can't help but laugh.

Therapist: You know sometimes I laugh, and I'm laughing but then there's a certain kind of laugh, that is particularly, it doesn't happen all the time, but it's very cathartic, it's when something strikes me funny and I just laugh in a way that is almost uncontrollable, where I can't, it's not like ha ha ha, it's like prolonged and it's in waves and I can't get over how, and . . .

Patient: then it's funny

Therapist: It's funny, laughing. That's happened to you?

Patient: Yes, oh at my house you would go crazy.

Therapist: Those times are usually when something so true, so true, and so true for me, and it's like, so silly and ridiculous that I you know, it's so true about my nature, and so so silly so unnecessarily serious.

Patient: I don't know where I put my, what I wrote yesterday I don't know what I did with it.

Therapist: Uh-huh

Patient: Because in one of them was beauty

Therapist: yeah

Patient: Was my roosters

Therapist: your rooster, tell me about that

Patient: I think they're majestic

Therapist: roosters

Patient: and chickens.

Therapist: both chickens and roosters?

Patient: and roosters, I think they're just majestic.

Therapist: and you maybe had that growing up, you had them in the . . .

Patient: Uh-huh. But I just love them, so everyone knows if that if they see roosters or chickens, my sons will buy me the chickens, they are all over my window, they're in my living room, they're in my kitchen. Because, "Why do you like these . . ."

Therapist: so pictures or sculpture of chickens?

Patient: Or my kitchen towels or my rugs on my floor of my kitchen. I said "They are just majestic, they are just beautiful creatures, and I just love them."

Therapist: And they also tell you to get up

Patient: They always tell me to wake up. And my son says when he's at home "Mommy, I'm going to kill your roosters. I'm going to . . ."

Therapist: Oh, that's the humor.

Patient: "What did they ever do to you?" "They make so much noise here in the night." I say "No they don't." And I would listen, and say "He's right" because like from 1 am they're crowing and carrying on, I say "Oh my goodness."

Therapist: yeah. Well we've run out of time today, but this is a very interesting session. Um, so next week we're going it'll be our last session. So we'll have a chance to talk about what the whole experience was like for you, um, and maybe we'll talk a little bit about that. I don't know if you had thought a little bit more about the legacy project, I know you you said to me "your life is your legacy." But we can touch base on that, it's not that critically important, but you know don't feel pressured. And then we'll have an exercise about hopes for the future. And then and then I think we'll be done, so you'll be free to maybe go to Belize if you want.

Patient: I'll be free. I'm waiting for my tax bill for my house that is why I'm still delaying here.

Therapist: yeah. And by the way next week at the end of the session I think (RSA's name) is going to want to ask you to try you to fill out the forms. And then we'll be in touch with you, so we'll try to get another set of . . .

Patient: sessions?

Therapist: evaluations

Patient: okay

Session 7: Transitions- Reflections and Hopes for the Future

Therapist: Here we go, so (name) this is our last session; I cannot believe how fast time went.

Patient: It has (name)

Therapist: I can't believe how the time went. Let's talk about that in a second. I just want to check in with you about how you are feeling and how things have been.

Patient: It's just the pain, pain, the pain.

Therapist: You've been having a lot of pain. Where is it? In your back and your belly?

Patient: in my back and in my stomach.

Therapist: And did you manage to go over to the doctor the other day?

Patient: No, because when I left from here the pain was like a three. It was manageable. But the weekend it became so severe, I had to take the medication like twice a day. Last night I had to take it again. I spoke to (name) yesterday. And I'm going over there when . . .

Therapist: when you're finished with me?

Patient: When I'm done here, because they changed my appointments.

Therapist: yeah, like I said you're on a very small dose of a short acting pain medicine, so it would only last 2 to 4 hours at the max.

Patient: 4 hours the max

Therapist: yeah, so you need something that lasts longer. And obviously if you're having pain, you would probably need to take the 4 hour medicine every 4 hours really, if you want to . . .

Patient: And then I sleep (name).

Therapist: You sleep from the medicine?

Patient: I sleep from the medicine.

Therapist: Okay, well after we're done with this if you want I could see you once or twice. And, there are medicines that if you're feeling sleepy on the pain medicine, I could give you something to keep you awake, so that you're not drowsy on it.

Patient: Saturday morning I was in so much pain I took the medication after I ate breakfast, like 9, and I was out like a light.

Therapist: Hmm, yeah, there are medicines that keep you awake that counteract the sedation of pain medicine, so that you can be pain free and awake.

Patient: And I try to distract myself. You know I'm not going to take the medication, maybe I'll walk, no; sometimes the pain gets so severe that I have to take it and I fall asleep.

Therapist: Yeah, that is not too uncommon sometimes a different pain medicine makes you react differently. So you're getting Oxycodone

Patient: Oxycodone

Therapist: So maybe Oxycodone that medicine makes you more sedated, the doctor might give you what's called a Fentanyl patch

Patient: a patch

Therapist: that might make you less sleepy

Patient: I wanted to ask them today to give me at least 25 Fentanyl patch

Therapist: exactly, exactly. If you want I can even prescribe it for you.

Patient: I would appreciate it if you do, and I'll see how I manage with it.

Therapist: Yeah, see how that works. Okay, so before we move on to this session, did you have any thoughts about the last session, the one about experiential sources of meaning, love, beauty and humor? Any residual thoughts?

Patient: (name) it just reinforces that my time here has been worthwhile. My visit here to this planet has been worthwhile, and I have no regrets.

Therapist: Now it's on to other planets.

Patient: Wherever it may take me.

Therapist: Wherever, You're open. You're open to what lies beyond.

Patient: I am.

Therapist: Sometimes I say that you know it takes a great deal of courage to live life, and it because life is finite and you have to give it up at some point right? And it's risky, right, so it takes courage. And it takes courage to love because you can lose people you love. And then ultimately it takes courage to leave this life . . .

Patient: To let go

Therapist: To let go and to move on to what lies beyond. And it's hard for us as human beings because it's either unknown, mysterious, or for some people frightening, uncertain, or certain, they're certain there's nothing. So courage is involved in all of these things. It like we were talking before, before we turned the tape on, in our work when things get very emotional and stressful one has to be able to contain their emotions in order to go through what, and one could say that that's possibly an element of what courage is. You're committed to a job, you act despite fear, and you do what needs to be done despite the fear.

Patient: You do what needs to be done despite the fear. Sometimes I say on the job you have to put the book aside, because it's difficult not to get attached to your patients.

Therapist: Mm-hmm, absolutely

Patient: Sometimes I would come in early, I would promise my patients something, and before I leave I would do it, get them settled. I had a patient that died, she told me, the one that had told me, all she wanted to do was to see her son get married. It was not my place to tell her if I were you I would tell the doctor I would go home. And she died on my shift, and . . .

Therapist: was there a chance for her to see her son get married?

Patient: And her son was getting married that weekend.

Therapist: oh, that weekend

Patient: I've seen children get married while their parents are in the hospital, they would come to the hospital.

Therapist: Yes, I have seen that too, I have helped arrange that.

Patient: And um, she died and it hurt me so cause she told me personally "(name) I don't want to be here." And she relapsed, she had leukemia, and she had to come in for more chemo.

Therapist: Yeah, so the question for me is where does the responsibility for doing what you want to do lie, is it your responsibility because she told you, or is it her responsibility. . . .

Patient: I think it's her responsibility

Therapist: Yeah, now maybe she needed help

Patient: Maybe she needed help, and I thought within my scope of nursing

Therapist: You took it on

Patient: I just let her vent. And I would just talk to her, but I was so hurt.

Therapist: Yeah, I think the one thing about your story and your life that I've hear through all of this is you may have needed help at times in your life, but you never gave up the responsibility for your own life. Even now.

Patient: Even now, and I won't give that responsibility to anyone. It's my life.

Therapist: That's correct. It's your life, and it's your search for meaning.

Patient: I've been searching for meaning. I have known all along that at some point I have to transition, I have to leave this life, and even raising my children, I have lived like this. We have always spoken of death, hoping I would go before them. Even my banking, all of my business, my children are involved. I always told them, if anything would happen to me, you guys are responsible, you should know.

Therapist: Right, so you've taken responsibility for every part of your life including the last part of your life. And you prepared everything . . .

Patient: I think I have.

Therapist: To make it easier for your children when you die. You've taken care of them being involved in the finances, and, so that transition is easy for them.

Patient: easy

Therapist: yeah, my mother did the same thing. My name and my brother's name was ever bank account, everything.

Patient: My children also.

Therapist: She even went with us to the bank to make sure it was okay.

Patient: Yes, yes, yes, cause when my oldest son was 10 years old, I told him you know "Half the time I'm at work, I'll be doing overtime," and my husband is at work also. It's my mom that's at home. I say "You know she could have an emergency and so could you. You know, "here's your bank card. This is not a game; this is not for you to play with."

Therapist: Exactly, and you did this at what point (name), before you got ill?

Patient: Oh, before I got ill

Therapist: way before, you see

Patient: way before, when my oldest son was 10 years old.

Therapist: from the time he was 10?

Patient: yeah, and the youngest one was 5.

Therapist: So you did that even when they were young?

Patient: Even when they were young. Because my oldest was a very bright guy and he knew, I would take him with me to the bank. He's knows every aspect of my life. When he was 13 was when I actually gave him the bank card, he was 13, the other one was 8. And, I say you know "You're only allowed $20 from this account."

Therapist: You didn't do that because you thought "I might die at any time and you may need this."

Patient: For protection

Therapist: For protection

Patient: I didn't want them to have to go out there and feel that they had to need anything from anyone to get into trouble in the first place. I just wanted them protected. But after the older one died, I told the brother "Now it's only you." So "You remain, the bank card remains with you." And he had gone into that account just once, and I had to close it up.

Therapist: So you know we've met 6 other times and what we've tried to do in this treatment is introduce the idea of the importance of meaning. We talked about how cancer has affected meaning. And I think in your case what's was very striking was that the things, the sources of meaning in your life at the core of your life, were essentially the same before and after cancer. Maybe cancer, the only thing that cancer did was make you appreciate them more perhaps.

Patient: Yeah, this cancer, I may have it as a diagnosis but it doesn't have me.

Therapist: it doesn't have you and it didn't change you as a person. You've maintained your identity through cancer. And you've maintained your values; maybe the experience just reinforced how right your values were or how important they were to you.

Patient: Being here and coming here, I told (RSA name) from the beginning, I told my niece too and I told (RSA's name) you know. I'm coming to these sessions, it might help me figure out if there's anything that missed in my life.

Therapist: Yes, exactly

Patient: But (name) coming here reinforced, reinforces that my life has been on an even course. As I've wanted it as it has come, because it's not only me involved in my life, it's my whole family, my husband, my children, you know, um, despite that.

Therapist: Yeah, well that's the feeling I got working with you, when we went through all the various exercises of the sources of meaning through legacy, through history, with the values we inherit, the life that we live, the values and the legacy that we leave behind. Sources of meaning through how we overcome obstacles and limitations and the attitude we have towards life. Experiential sources of meaning through being connected to people and love, and the world and nature and beauty and humor and singing and all these things. And then also through your work as a nurse and through your dedication to your son and all that. My impression of that you are a person who has naturally lived a life of very very intense and full of meaning. You've always been searching for meaning and finding a lot of it and living it.

Patient: my son would say sometimes "You're a bully."

Therapist: a bully? What did he mean?

Patient: I said to him you know what "I'm not a bully. If I feel that I've been wronged, you are going to hear. I'm not going anywhere to cause anyone any distress and I don't expect it from anyone."

Therapist: So in your life, when a person's lived a life of meaning you develop, and who's lived a life where you try to live the life that's guided by the values that are important to you right? And you succeed at that. You have a certain sense of value and self-esteem.

Patient: Self-esteem

Therapist: and you feel, that self-esteem and value and respect for yourself is something that you have and you expect to be respect.

Patient: It's just that

Therapist: yeah

Patient: he went with me to the bank that day, and I asked the bank teller

Therapist: you deserve respect

Patient: something. And she was so rude, she said "Well, then you should know." I can't remember what it was, and I said to her "Well, what do you want me to do. You know the banking rules, I don't, and I'm coming here to ask you." And she was so openly rude. I said to her you know "I don't expect you to answer me. I'm coming here to ask questions and that is not the way you answer." And my son was there just watching the dynamics, and he said "Mommy, you should not have treated her like that." I said "But she was rude, she was rude to me. I came here to ask questions, I expect her to answer."

Therapist: See at his age you had taught him to respect others. He hadn't yet grown up and developed his own sense of self-esteem and respect to understand that he also deserves respect. That hadn't quite happened yet, hopefully it did. I know in your older son that did, I've heard stories of that.

Patient: Oh yes.

Therapist: so in the therapy, we've sort of progressed over the six weeks, introduced the idea and then all these sources of meaning, and when you confront difficult times and you've had some difficult times already and I don't know what lies ahead. You're having some pain we need to deal with that. But I'm hoping these sources of meaning are resources of strength for you. And allow you to, to help you have the courage to do what you need to face, face what you need to face.

Patient: I'm going to (name). I am prepared, I think.

Therapist: You feel prepared

Patient: I think I'm prepared. You know, from the day I tasked out, I remember telling my husband "Hold me." And I woke up in the bed, and I said to him "What happened to me?" That must be how dead is. Because I remember one moment, I remember him holding me and I didn't remember the rest of it, what happened?

Therapist: you think that's what death is like?

Patient: I said "This must be what death is like."

Therapist: to be held

Patient: I was okay one minute, and I remember him holding me, and that was all I remember, that was all I remember.

Therapist: You know they talk about how a person's life, their whole life passes in front of them before they die. I think that's a very interesting sort of a myth or a common belief you know a cultural belief. I don't know, is it true in Belize that people think that? No? It's in the, you see it a lot in movies, and ...

Patient: Mm-hmm, mm-hmm

Therapist: And for me it always represents that really when you approach death the task is to really look back at your life and review your life. And like you said what this all did, this therapy did, is it helped you reaffirm that up until now this life that you lived was pretty meaningful. You did quite a good job.

Patient: And I think about when my brother died, my middle brother and I were so close, he would make sure that I'm well, he would make sure I was okay. And before he died, the day before he died, it was 4th of July, and he said, he called me he said "Come to the party," "You know I'm not coming." And he said like the day after I went over there, he lives around the corner from my house, and he said "Well, I knew you wouldn't come to the party, but I saved us some wine." I said "I want mine with a little orange juice, half and half." And he had, he got some champagne glasses, he said "This is how we're going to drink today." And he said "You know you don't listen to me. You should be driving." I say "Why should I be driving? Who is going to buy me a car, and who is going to pay my insurance. And you drive me wherever I want to go, so why should I drive." He said "Okay, here is money for your lessons, go see about that. And here is money for my nephew for ice-cream." And later on in the evening, he drove me home. I live around the block from my brother, but he will drive me home. And the following morning was when my niece called you know "Come, dad has some problems here." When I got there he was dead. But thinking back, I said "Did he know he was dying?" He was trying to get everything in order.

Therapist: right

Patient: and the money that my brother gave me was the money I paid my ticket with, because he didn't want to be buried here, he wanted to be buried at home.

Therapist: I see

Patient: But often I think that he was trying to get things in order

Therapist: yeah. So I know we had talked a little bit over the course of the previous six sessions about this legacy project, we talked about I think I'm remembering mainly music.

Patient: Mm-hmm, oh, and (niece's name) brought the music.

Therapist: Oh, it's okay. But have you thought about the legacy project, and have you. I know that some people do something very formal and they try to put together a collection of music and this and that. Other people say "You know I've been doing that all my life and it's not necessary." But tell me what you thought about it.

Patient: I have told my sisters that when I die, just get the Garifuna music going and you guys have to play for the good times.

Therapist: This is at the funeral?

Patient: Yes

Therapist: So you sort of planned out the funeral?

Patient: that is all I want

Therapist: An element of the funeral

Patient: that is all I want

Therapist: That's Garifuna music

Patient: and for the good times.

Therapist: and what does that mean for the good time?

Patient: Um, that's a record by one of these guys

Therapist: Oh, that's a song?

Patient: It's a song, right

Therapist: It's a particular song "Just for the Good Times." Oh and how does it go?

Patient: "don't look sad, I know its over, but times go on." And there's more to it.

Therapist: That's beautiful. The words are meaningful I see.

Patient: Mm-hmm. "But life goes on."

Therapist: I got it, the gist of it.

Patient: "don't ever leave me."

Therapist: So that's the song you want played?

Patient: Yes, yes

Therapist: And you said you have a couple drums around right?

Patient: Oh yes, those drums are haunting. I just love the drums.

Therapist: Do you actually have drums?

Patient: There are drums at home, and I keep promising that I would have bought it for my sons, because I love the drums, I love them.

Therapist: And you're going to give the drums to your son? Or someone else?

Patient: The boys

Therapist: the boys

Patient: because they like the music too. We've always played it at home.

Therapist: all the boys in the family.

Patient: Mm-hmm. We've always played it at home. We've had 7 boys and I've always had them while growing up between us 7 boys and I've always had. And I've always played this music at home, they've loved it.

Therapist: okay, so this music is special, it's a legacy project because it's your history; it's your ancestry, its linking you to your past

Patient: past

Therapist: to the Garifuna people. And it's passing on that legacy to your next generation. They know that the Garifuna, they know the tradition, especially the song. I imagine there's some food too that is special.

Patient: Oh yes, but the children don't care.

Therapist: they don't care; they don't care about these foods?

Patient: They do

Therapist: Do they know how to cook it?

Patient: My aunt would cook differently

Therapist: ah, than you

Patient: Than me. I don't like coconut, never had. I do not like the scent of it, but my aunt would make coconut with fish, and she would put eggs. I say "Why are you guys eating all this nonsense?" But the children love it "Oh, no mommy you don't cook the way granny does."

Therapist: So you've been modernizing the traditional cooking but trying to make it healthier.

Patient: It wasn't that, cause even at home I wouldn't eat it cause I don't like the scent of coconut.

Therapist: You don't like the scent of coconut

Patient: But in bread, I make my own bread.

Therapist: you like coconut there

Patient: and then I would put the coconut in it.

Therapist: In bread it feels more, more like in place.

Patient: and it smells different, yes.

Therapist: It's really interesting because in Brazil, I've been in the northeast of Brazil, Bahia, and a lot of the food there is . . .

Patient: made of coconut

Therapist: coconut and fish and all sorts of things, African influence.

Patient: And those people (name) are Garifuna people

Therapist: they are?

Patient: They are. They have lost some of the culture, but this bunch that came to Honduras and to Belize have maintained their language and culture.

Therapist: But the ones that went to northeast Brazil got mixed in with other stuff.

Patient: I was watching CNN one day and they were in Brazil, and there was this person speaking Garifuna, and I was alarmed. I tried to call; I didn't have a computer yet to get the source of where this person was.

Therapist: Well there are two big cities, Bahia, well the region is Bahia, and the big city is Salvador.

Patient: Yes

Therapist: And that's where all that cooking takes place, Salvador Recife, I've eaten there.

Patient: And I watched Andrew Zimmerman one day and there was someone cooking with coconut milk and all this meat and ground food, casafa, and the seaweed all of that they make in Belize, the same way.

Therapist: So next time I go to that part of Brazil

Patient: Think about me

Therapist: I'll ask about it. I haven't been there very often, just once.

Patient: Mm-hmm, yes. And that is how my grandma cooked, with coconut milk, and its good, some people you know.

Therapist: You're just not partial to the coconut.

Patient: Yeah I don't like coconut, never have

Therapist: So I don't know did you actually take a look at the homework that had you look at sort of the questions for the last session. Where we kind of ask, I think that's it where we ask you.

Patient: We have two pages of it, I think.

Therapist: I think there were sort of three questions, one was uh

Patient: Its three questions

Therapist: Yeah, one was, what's it been like for you to go through this experience over the last 7 sessions? Have there been any changes in the way you view your life and cancer experience, ah yeah you did make some comments.

Patient: Not really, I know that death is a part of life. The sessions have reinforced that my life should be lead as I desired and . . .

Therapist: a little bit about what we were talking about before. So these sessions really reinforced that you were doing things right.

Patient: As they should be

Therapist: as they should be. And that gives you a feeling of peace.

Patient: It gives me a feeling of peace. Honestly (name) I don't worry about this or whenever I die or whatever, when it comes it comes. Because I think once you are dead you don't know anything anymore. And as I have been preparing, I've told my son all along you know "When I die, don't open the casket, I never liked people looking at me, and I don't think I will want people looking at me then."

Therapist: Yeah, you don't want an open casket

Patient: No, little things like that. And don't leave me for like two weeks; if no one is here whoever wants to come, my family is so big, just bury me.

Therapist: You don't want a long wake?

Patient: No

Therapist: You want to be buried like a Jew. The next day

Patient: That's what I said to him

Therapist: A Jewish Garifuna

Patient: When my son died I bought three spaces, just put me there, I know that I'm going into that space.

Therapist: You know where you're going

Patient: I know where I'm going. Don't hesitate, don't wait for anyone. And it's just him; I don't want him lingering over things you know, because my husband is dealing with his own demons.

Therapist: Your husband is having a hard time with this?

Patient: But he's not saying

Therapist: He's not saying

Patient: He's not saying, but sometimes I can just see the look in his face. And I tell him you know what, "I'm the one who should be looking like this you know. Just try to be strong." But it's easy for me to say that to him, he hasn't broken down, but I can just see the look in his face. All I have to say is you know and "I want" and he's there.

Therapist: you talked a lot with him about you plan?

Patient: Not really, I have just told him "This is what I want." And he knows me "This is what I want, this is how it's going to be" and that is all I ask.

Therapist: The second question is do you feel like you have a better understanding of the sources of meaning in life and that you are able to use them in your daily life?

Patient: daily life. I live my life daily

Therapist: yeah

Patient: with meaning. I lived everyday as if it were my last.

Therapist: Since when? Since you were that little child who lost her mother?

Patient: Maybe not, but mainly since my son died.

Therapist: Since your son died. That was the event

Patient: yes, yes

Therapist: that made you understand that death is real

Patient: I have not allowed anyone to hold back or to hold me back if there is anything that I desire, not even my husband. This is what I want, this is what I want.

Therapist: So if you were at a party with Denzel Washington, he would not hold you back?

Patient: No, I do exactly as I please.

Therapist: you'd make a bee line to Denzel and you would go.

Patient: I do exactly as I please. That has really, that incident in my life

Therapist: your son?

Patient: has really shown me, has really hurt me

Therapist: yes

Patient: that I will not, to get rid of some of that pain maybe, I will not allow anyone to say "no" to me.

Therapist: So this most profoundly painful moment in your life resulted in a few things that are very dramatic. One is that you will not let anything stop you from doing what you want to do. And you also have, you became fully aware that everyday could be your last, and you live life as if every day is your last. And how do you live life as if every day was your last? What does that exactly translate into?

Patient: If I want to travel anywhere, if I want to go anywhere, if there is anything that I've wanted, it won't be a need, or if I need it

Therapist: you don't put it off

Patient: I'm not going to put it off

Therapist: You don't sacrifice, you don't delay. And I imagine it's not exorbitant, it's not like I want a yacht, I want to go get it.

Patient: No, within reason

Therapist: yeah so

Patient: within reason. And my husband is indulgent

Therapist: Indulgent

Patient: he does. In May, no in June I came out of the hospital from my surgery, September was my birthday; he said "What am I giving you for your birthday?" "I don't know, what am I going to do, I can't even go anywhere." He gave me $1500, he said "This is your birthday gift, do whatever you want with it." I said "Okay" I kept it. I would go and I would buy whatever junk I see out there. He said "Why are you brining all this garbage into this house?" I said "You gave me the money didn't you?"

Therapist: what did you buy?

Patient: Garbage, whatever it is that I want.

Therapist: Garbage

Patient: whatever strikes my fancy

Therapist: shoes huh?

Patient: (laugh) and I can't even wear them. I go home to Belize

Therapist: You go to Belize, that's how you spend the money

Patient: How many times have I been to Belize since I've been sick?

Therapist: So when you have money, you go to Belize?

Patient: Or whatever strikes my fancy. I go to Belize and be quiet.

Therapist: Belize is a place of quiet

Patient: a place of peace

Therapist: peace. Peace and safety maybe. Feels safe there, you feel you feel that you're in the place where you arose or you grew up.

Patient: Yes, you know that's why I have to go

Therapist: Like your childhood where you were surrounded by these loving people

Patient: My sister that's sick, oh my sister would hug me, my sister will kiss me, and when I go home my sister is there with me at my house. She will leave her house every morning to spend the day with me until I come home. She never wanted to come to America. My sister had 10 children, and she never wanted to leave her children. And my father couldn't understand why. Often I'd tell her "You know I'm glad you did not go. These 10 children turned out well, and I have a feeling it's because she stayed with them. It was a struggle for her, but she stayed with her children, and now they are here in the states, she still don't want to come. But that's one of the reasons I generally want to go home, to be with her to spend time with her.

Therapist: how about this last question. What are your hopes for the future?

Patient: You know I didn't answer that question.

Therapist: Okay, do you want to think a little bit about it?

Patient: I just remain hopeful

Therapist: You remain hopeful, yeah about what?

Patient: The lingering thing the most important thing is this diagnosis. I told myself, whatever if I have the chemo, I don't want to be sick as I have been. I don't want to ever feel that way, but I remain hopeful that I will have many more days. It's not for me to say, it's in the stars.

Therapist: It's in the stars. So you're hopefully you'll have many more days?

Patient: how ever many

Therapist: How ever many. And any other hopes about the future?

Patient: I think I have everything wrapped.

Therapist: You have everything wrapped. So there are things that you've hoped for that you've achieved.

Patient: I have

Therapist: what are those things? Achieving a sense of peace about things?

Patient: (name) now I'm at peace with myself. Financially, it may change when I leave from here, I have no problems, um the house that I live in we've paid for and that house was bought because I was having my second baby. I didn't want to raise my children in the projects or, I wanted to be in a house just with them, as we were brought up. And the reason we bought the house and we've struggled and we've paid it off, I've hoped, like I've told my son "Stay on the course you're on. You're an adult now. I won't be with you forever. But I have tried to teach you the right values in life, I've tried to give you a little legacy for example this house." I've taught him how to be frugal with his little monies. And when I die, he has plenty of monies to go around to live by, if he doesn't spend it in one day, because after my father died they said there is monies left from my father. I said "It's not mine. It's not for (son's name), that's for (father's name) he was just my father." And my brother had died and he left three daughters, I said "You guys are responsible; I'm not in that one." And they blew that money, I would say in a couple days, like a hundred thousand dollars.

Therapist: When you think about from now until you die, are things that you hope for? Like having your pain controlled? And things like that?

Patient: My pain controlled

Therapist: Do you hope that you'll die in your own bed?

Patient: I hope that I die at my house

Therapist: At your house in Belize?

Patient: Here

Therapist: here in New York

Patient: Here in New York

Therapist: You don't want to die in Belize?

Patient: No, because my grave is here

Therapist: your grave is here

Patient: And my son's body is here

Therapist: I see

Patient: I carry my death with me wherever.

Therapist: yes

Patient: But my wish is that I die here, at my house here.

Therapist: With your husband, your son?

Patient: My family, and my son. I'm not going to the hospital to die. I'm not going to the hospital.

Therapist: As a nurse you've been there, you've seen a lot of people die in the hospital

Patient: I don't want that

Therapist: I didn't want that for my parents either

Patient: I don't want that. Those are all the things that I ask for. Not much.

Therapist: Not much. Actually it's not much but it turns out to be very important and profound. Not everyone gets to do that, unless they're like you and they get what they want. They have the will, the responsibility to make it happen.

Patient: Yes

Therapist: One of the important things about dying at home is that you have a home DNR. Because what happens is sometimes people panic and they call the police and the EMS shows up and they do resuscitate you even though you didn't want it.

Patient: I have told my husband over and over and even that day that I passed out "Listen, if I pass out and you see that I am not breathing please do not call 911, until . . ."

Therapist: Not even then, don't even call them then, just the funeral home, and the doctor; you call the doctor's office.

Patient: They'll eventually have to call the doctor

Therapist: The doctors are really good here about getting the paperwork done. The funeral home.

Patient: They will eventually have to call the doctor.

Therapist: I had a situation, I thought I took care of everything, nobody would do this, and then there was an aid that worked with my mother and she panicked and she called my wife and my wife wasn't sure, and they called the EMS and I had to run down there, and I didn't have a home DNR. And they wouldn't stop, and I begged them "Please stop, this is not what my mother . . ."

Patient: But you didn't have it written anywhere what her desires were?

Therapist: I didn't have a home DNR, and I couldn't get the DNR from the medical chart. It worked out okay, but it was not I wanted, and it was not what she wanted. So if you have that piece of paper at home even if somebody doesn't know. . . .

Patient: I'll have my home DNR pasted on the wall

Therapist: That's what I was about to say, you have it pasted on the wall.

Patient: I'll have it pasted on the way somewhere, because I told them I want to die at my house. I don't want to die in a hospital.

Therapist: I know we've been talking about how to die, but I think one of the focuses of this therapy, this treatment is even if there is a limited amount of time to live, you're still alive.

Patient: I'm still alive, and I'm doing everything that I want to do.

Therapist: And it's important to live that life fully and with meaning. And we as your doctors need to help you do that as much as possible, by controlling your pain and things like that.

Patient: That's the only thing I was waiting for my bill, I got my bill yesterday and I'm going to take care of it by the weekend.

Therapist: your hospital bill?

Patient: No, my property tax bill

Therapist: ah

Patient: cause I don't want to travel without having to pay it alright, I'm going to take care of that the weekend. (Name) had said "Oh, we changed your appointments." "I'm sorry, other than getting my pain taken care of; I'm going to leave anyway."

Therapist: yeah, Belize

Patient: Yes, I don't care if it's a day or two days. If I run into trouble, I just pay my ticket and I come back. That's it.

Therapist: well, like all good things. Like life, like everything, things come to an end. This has been, I'd appreciate any reflections you have, but I'll just tell you that for me, I've been doing this for 8 years, I mean this therapy, and I've been taking care of patients for almost 30 years here. And you see a lot of patients, but you don't have a unique, powerful and memorable experience with every single one of them, but it has been very very very special for me to get to know you (name) to spend this time with you. You're a remarkable woman in so many ways. You're beautiful, you're beautiful outside and inside. I am never going to forget you, I will always remember you.

Patient: Thank you

Therapist: You've taught me a lot about life and meaning, and how I can help other people too. And so it's been an experience of a lifetime to do this with you, to spend this time with you, and to learn about you.

Patient: That's an honor

Therapist: It's been my honor really

Patient: (name) this has just reinforced that you go through this life once, enjoy every moment, and have no regrets.

Therapist: Thank you for doing this. I know (RSA's name) probably has some papers for you to fill out. While she's doing that I'll get a prescription together for you.

Patient: Okay, and I wanted to get (niece's name) so you could hear some of that music it's on her telephone.

Therapist: Oh ok, thank you. Tell us what we're going to hear.

Patient: which one is this?

Therapist: We're going to hear Garifuna music, yes?

Patient: Garifuna music

Niece: It's hardy

Therapist: what's it called?

Niece: Hardy, um the artist

Patient: Oh, paster hardy

Niece: Paster Hardy

Therapist: Paster Hardy

Niece: Alright

(*Music playing*)

Patient: Oh, you can tap out the music

(*Music playing*)

Therapist: This is an hour long song?

Patient: No no

Therapist: That was it, and that was Garifuna music. In Garifuna language.

Patient: Yes

Therapist: And what's the Paster saying, singing?
Patient: Um, oh lord, I could only tell you as the music is going because they play this as music outside and it's at a church too.
Therapist: At a church too, and in the background is that drums? Or guitars?
Niece: yes, its drums
Patient: Drums and guitars
Therapist: Like tin?
Patient: Nah nah nah nah nah, it's hallowed out from wood and they put a deer skin on the top.
Therapist: So it's not like Jamaican stuff where there's like a little tin drum
(*Music playing*)
Patient: And this guy is just with guitars and I think with drums too
Niece: It's a short cut; I didn't get the whole song.
Patient: Um, that's the maracas
Therapist: The maracas
Patient: He's sick
Therapist: He's sick
Patient: Mm-hmm
Niece: yeah, that's was a short clip
Patient: Ah, that was all you got?
Niece: yeah
Patient: He's singing that when he dies, he wants to be buried with drums and music.
Therapist: He wants to be buried with his drums and music.
Niece: He wants his death to be a celebration and not to let his sister cry for him, at least that's what I remember from this song.
Patient: yes
Therapist: that's a fitting end to this therapy
Patient: It sure is
Therapist: Thank you (name). Thank you for helping bring (name) everyday.

INDEX